INTRAVENTRICULAR CONDUCTION DISTURBANCES

DEVELOPMENTS IN CARDIOVASCULAR MEDICINE

VOLUME 12

Other volumes in this series:

1. Lancée CT, ed: Echocardiology. 1979. ISBN 90-247-2209-8.
2. Baan J, Arntzenius AC, Yellin EL, eds: Cardiac dynamics. 1980. ISBN 90-247-2212-8.
3. Thalen HJT, Meere CC, eds: Fundamentals of cardiac pacing. 1979. ISBN 90-247-2245-4.
4. Kulbertus HE, Wellens HJJ, eds: Sudden death. 1980. ISBN 90-247-2290-X.
5. Dreifus LS, Brest AN, eds: Clinical applications of cardiovascular drugs. 1980. ISBN 90-247-2295-0.
6. Spencer MP, Reid JM, eds: Cerebrovascular evaluation with Doppler ultrasound. 1981. ISBN 90-247-2384-1.
7. Zipes DP, Bailey JC, Elharrar V, eds: The slow inward current and cardiac arrhythmias. 1980. ISBN 90-247-2380-9.
8. Kesteloot H, Joossens JV, eds: Epidemiology of arterial blood pressure. 1980. ISBN 90-247-2386-8.
9. Wackers FJT, ed: Thallium-201 and technetium-99M-pyrophosphate myocardial imaging in the coronary care unit. 1980. ISBN 90-247-2396-5.
10. Maseri A, Marchesi C, Chierchia S, Trivella MG, eds: Coronary care units. 1981. ISBN 90-247-2456-2.
11. Morganroth J, Moore EN, Dreifus LS, Michelson EL, eds: The evaluation of new antiarrhythmic drugs. ISBN 90-247-2474-0.

series ISBN 90-247-2336-1

INTRAVENTRICULAR CONDUCTION DISTURBANCES

by

PAOLO ALBONI, M.D.

Director, Electrophysiology Section
Division of Cardiology
Arcispedale S. Anna
Ferrara, Italy

1981

MARTINUS NIJHOFF PUBLISHERS
THE HAGUE / BOSTON / LONDON

Distributors:

for the United States and Canada

Kluwer Boston, Inc.
190 Old Derby Street
Hingham, MA 02043
USA

for all other countries

Kluwer Academic Publishers Group
Distribution Center
P.O. Box 322
3300 AH Dordrecht
The Netherlands

Library of Congress Cataloging in Publication Data CIP

Alboni, Paolo.
Intraventricular conduction disturbances.

(Developments in cardiovascular medicine; v. 12)
Includes index.
1. Heart block. 2. Heart conduction system — Diseases. I. Title. II. Series.
[DNLM: 1. Heart ventricle — Physiology. 2. Heart ventricle — Physiopathology. 3. Heart block. W1 DE997VME v. 12 / WG 330 A339i]
RC685.B55A42 616.1′2 81-3974
AACR2

ISBN-13: 978-94-009-8289-5 e-ISBN-13: 978-94-009-8287-1
DOI: 10.1007/978-94-009-8287-1

Dedicated to my mother Luisa
and my father Giovanni

CONTENTS

FOREWORD

Rhythm was the first expression of cardiac activity which fell under man's observation, and the heart beat has always represented the very essence of life itself as it accelerates or slows during moments of rest, effort, joy and pain until it comes to a halt at the moment of death. Undoubtedly the heart beat was, for a considerable time, the only semiological element by which man could interpret the dysfunctions of the organism.

Even after thousands of years, research into the alterations of cardiac rhythm still holds a certain fascination, although modern methods and sophisticated devices have changed the approach to such studies. Only about ten years ago, the interpretation of arrhythmias was obtained by a standard electrocardiogram to which experimental findings on animals were still arbitrarily applied. On the other hand, the achievement of diagnostic decisions was of little importance outside the sphere of pure intellectual speculation since valid therapeutical treatments were lacking.

At present, by means of electrophysiological investigations, one can verify and check 'in situ' the different forms and mechanisms through which rhythm and conduction disorders are manifested. Thus, achieving such a methodology which may be defined as a 'functional biopsy', we are àllowed to put forward more accurate therapeutic indications now available using both pharmacological and electrical treatment.

That which until a few years ago was left to the art of reasoning, helped by the cardiologist's intuition and imagination, is now thoroughly analysed, measured and compared. Naturally, the extent of the unknown is still perturbing, but it is gradually being narrowed down.

As always happens, such increasing improvements as regards equipment and instruments require scientific application and specialistic knowledge stretched to their limits since this extension of the possibilities for research work obviously involves higher risks as far as errors are concerned. This is the reason why so few researchers devote themselves to the study of the formation and conduction disturbances of the impulse.

There is a hard point in everyone's life: the circumstances when one chooses one's own way, by which I mean all the wishes, perspectives, expectations and opportunities that push in one or another direction. It is a hard task to determine these choices in young people because some suggestions may interfere heavily with one's life course, so one may direct somebody to a gratifying as well as to disappointing activity.

It is the policy in our Division of Cardiology to allow new assistants to attend to the work that they like best; they are actually free to enter every laboratory: hemodynamics, electrophysiology, ergometry, echocardiography, pacemakers, coronaro-ventriculography, coronary unit, and so on. Before long everyone chooses the most pleasant and interesting for him or herself. At this pont the head of the department must give his suggestions and encouragements.

This happened with Dr. Alboni when he began to be attracted by electrophysiological research. I helped and stimulated him regarding his purpose and sent him for some time to Dr. Narula to learn the most refined techniques in this field. At the same time I directed his interest to peripheral conduction disturbances.

So this was the origin of this book; a unique one in the sense in which an exhaustive review of the literature is completed with new personal ideas.

Dr. Paolo Alboni is 'en route' now; all the best wishes for his journey.

Antonio Masoni
Head of Division of Cardiology
St. Anna Hospital, Ferrara

PREFACE

It gives me great pleasure to write this preface to Dr. Alboni's monograph on intraventricular conduction disturbances. Having read his manuscript, it is difficult for me to describe adequately in a few paragraphs the value of his contribution or the true excellence of the work.

The book represents a complete and completely understandable picture of a complex clinical problem through a lucid synthesis of anatomic, electrocardiographic, vectorcardiographic, electrophysiological and clinical observations. For the first time all of these aspects of intraventricular conduction have been correlated to provide a comprehensive understanding of the subject. It will equip the physician and the cardiologist with an understanding of the fundamentals of intraventricular conduction defects and their variable clinical significance. The material dealing with the diagnosis, clinical course and treatment is complete and convincing. The electrocardiographic illustrations are carefully selected and suitably supplemented with intracardiac electrographic recordings to demonstrate clearly the conduction disturbance under consideration. The style is crisp and clear. The book can be read as well as studied.

The presentation of basic information on anatomy, with emphasis on the complexities of the left bundle branch distribution, and physiology of ventricular excitation are carefully discussed in the first two chapters. An elaborate dissertation of bundle branch blocks as well as peripheral blocks is provided in Chapters 3 to 6. The discussion of peripheral blocks resulting from conduction disturbances distal to the bundle branches and the fascicles is mostly based on the author's personal work. This is an important contribution as little has been discussed on this subject in the English literature.

Chapters 7 to 9 deal with the pathophysiology, ECG, diagnosis and clinical significance of intraventricular conduction disturbances in association with congenital heart defects, cardiac surgery and myocardial infarction. Intermittent intraventricular blocks are presented in Chapter 10. During the past decade electrophysiologic studies have engendered a great deal of interest. Their role in the clinical management of patients, especially the prognostic value of the H-V interval, is reviewed in Chapter 11. The present status and the limitations of non-invasive recordings of the His-Purkinje system is addressed in Chapter 12. The effect of various antiarrhythmic drugs on intraventricular conduction is reported in Chapter

13. The closing chapter deals with therapy of acute and chronic intraventricular conduction defects.

This book clearly is and will remain the definitive description of intraventricular conduction disturbances. This book should be of interest to the internist, cardiologist, cardiac surgeon, electrocardiographer, electrophysiologist, medical student, resident and intensive care nurse.

Onkar S. Narula
Clinical Professor of Medicine
University of Miami, Florida

ACKNOWLEDGMENTS

I should like to give thanks to the many people who have assisted in the preparation of this book. I wish to give special thanks to the following: Prof. Antonio Masoni, who inspired me to write this manuscript and whose guidance and advice have been indispensable; Prof. Onkar Narula, who allowed me to work in his Division of Cardiology, where I could take advantage of his precious teaching on the electrophysiology of the heart; Prof. Lino Rossi, Prof. Bruno Taccardi, Prof. Narasimhan Shantha, Prof. Maria Serratto, Prof. Luigi Tavazzi and Prof. Edoardo Arslan, who kindly reviewed Chapters 1, 2, 3, 7, 10 and 12, respectively; Dr. Carlo Malacarne, Dr. Paolo Pedroni, Dr. Laura Filippi, Dr. Roberto Battaglia and Dr. Elisabeth Jenkins for their help in the compilation of the manuscript; Miss Anna Previati and Miss Lucia Malaguti for their excellent secretarial assistance. Finally, I thank my wife Marina for her encouragement and moral support.

1. ANATOMY OF INTRAVENTRICULAR CONDUCTION SYSTEM

The anatomy of the intraventricular conduction system is a complex and controversial subject. To a large extent the controversy is due to individual variations, and only in a minor degree to differences in the histological techniques employed by the investigators. Among the unsettled anatomical questions concerning the atrio-ventricular (AV) junctional area, there are various opinions as to where the intraventricular conduction system actually begins, i.e. the exact distinction between 'junctional' and 'subjunctional' AV pathway. Hecht et al. [1] consider the bundle branches as part of the intraventricular conduction system, whereas others include the bifurcation or branching portion of the His bundle as belonging to the junctional area [2, 3]. It is difficult histologically to individuate precisely where the AV node ends and the His bundle begins [3, 4]. However, from a clinical and electrophysiological viewpoint, the definition of His boundary is very important, since a block occurring or an arrhythmia originating in either sites may have different therapeutic and prognostic implications [3, 5]. Lately, Jones et al. [6] have emphasized the presence of AV nodal P-cells in the upper AV bundle, further complicating the morphologic question centered upon the anatomo-clinical limits and significance of the diagnostic term of 'His bundle' [7].

The His bundle begins with the AV nodal fibers penetrating the pars membranacea septi. In the majority of human hearts, the anterior portion of the His bundle runs along the left side of the septum and in about 25 % of cases, the His courses along the right side of the septum.

The His bundle in the adult is approximately 6.5 to 20 mm in length and 1.5 to 2 mm in diameter.

The cells of the penetrating as well as those of the branching portion of the His bundle are larger than those in the AV node but smaller than the ventricular fibers. In contrast to the AV node where the cellular arrangement is like a network, the fibers in the His bundle are arranged in organized parallel compartments. These compartments are more or less extensively separated by collagen partitions which are longitudinally oriented extending over the length of many cells. In fact, the loss of interweaving sheets and septa of collagen and the appearance of longitudinally oriented ones are considered useful characteristics in the histological differentiation of the AV node from the His bundle. Transverse intercellular anastomoses are, however, present.

As the common bundle of His reaches the lower membranous septum, the fibers of the left bundle (LBB) are given off over a wide zone in a fan-like arrangement. The His bundle then reaches the bifurcation (or pseudobifurcation) where the right bundle branch (RBB) and the remaining fibers of the LBB are given off.

Some of the cells in the His bundle may look like Purkinje cells and have rectangular or oblong nuclei, a clear perinuclear zone and sparse cellular myofibrils.

The right bundle branch arises as a compact cord, continuous in shape and often in direction with the common bundle. It is a discrete slender fascicle which does not subdivide until its termination at the anterior papillary muscle. The right bundle in the adult is approximately 45 to 50 mm in length and about 1 to 2 mm in diameter. The proximal one third of the RBB is usually intramyocardial and less often subendocardial. This segment is situated near the crest of the right side of the septum and here it is also near the aortic and tricuspid valves. The middle third of RBB is almost always intramyocardial and the distal third of the RBB, as it courses through the moderator band to the right ventricular papillary muscle, is subendocardial. At this point the RBB is supposed to spread out into a wide Purkinje network beneath the ventricle's endocardium. In man, such histologic evidence is very elusive, but it is taken for granted. In rare cases the course of the RBB is entirely intramyocardial [8, 9].

Microscopically, the fibers of the RBB are extensively partitioned by collagen, but are arranged in fairly parallel fashion; they are almost identical to the fibers of the working myocardium.

The *left bundle branch* fans out in a broad sheet as it separates from the His bundle, and courses anteriorly in the left septal endocardium just beneath the aortic noncoronary cusp; a partially intramyocardial variety has been described [10].

Both in optical [11] and electron microscopy [12] the fibers of the LBB often show typical Purkinjean features and a longitudinal arrangement, with incomplete connective sheets; the intercellular connections are Purkinjean. The manner of distribution of the LBB is a controversial subject.

A constant subdivision of the LBB into distinct anterior and posterior fascicles, with consequent 'trifascicularity' of the Tawaran system, has been reported by Rosenbaum et al. [13]. In most studies, however, the manner of distribution of LBB appears more complex [10].

Some authors [14-21] have described a third left fascicle, which they call the septal fascicle. Such a fascicle, which at times is larger than the other two, arises from the main LBB or from the anterior or posterior fascicle and travels to the midseptal surface [21].

A recent study by Massing and James [22] contradicts the fascicular concept; the human left bundle, which was also discovered and described by Tawara in 1906 [23], is highly variable from individual to individual and not composed of distinct fascicles. In fact, the left bundle fibers are arranged like a ribbed fan with the fiber groups arising over a wide zone coursing over the interventricular septum [22, 24-26].

The discrepancy in the results obtained from various studies has not been resolved as yet. However, it cannot be only due to the different techniques employed in the sectioning of the conduction system.

Microscopically, the collagen partitioning from the His bundle continues into the first few millimeters of the LBB.

The blood supply of the conduction system shows marked individual variations. In most cases the proximal portion of the His bundle receives dual blood supply from the AV nodal artery (usually belonging to the right coronary tree) and the first septal branch of the left anterior descending artery. The RBB and the anterior half of the LBB are supplied in almost identical fashion from the first anterior septal branch. The posterior half of the LBB is supplied by the posterior septal perforating branches of the right coronary artery in half of the cases, and in the rest the blood supply is from both the anterior (left) and posterior (right) coronary artery tree.

The His bundle is less richly innervated than the AV node. Contrary to current belief, the bundle branches also seem to have vagal innervation [18, 27].

PERIPHERAL PURKINJE NETWORK

There are very few satisfactory histological demonstrations of the actual ending of the bundle branches and none at all of their alleged trespassing into morphologically distinct Purkinjean networks, which terminate in detectable Purkinje myocardial junctions [10].

The original description of Purkinje in 1845 [28] and the reports that followed [18, 23, 29, 30] illustrate some morphologic features of the Purkinje cells and some aspects of the histoarchitectonic arrangement. These elements are larger than ordinary myocardial fibers and are characterized by peripheral arrangement of the myofibrils with a clear central area and two nuclei.

Great anatomophysiological interest was focused on the statement that the Purkinje cells made up a true syncytium, owing to the absence of intercalated disks and to the continuity of the myofibrils from one element into another [31]. Such an alleged syncytial nature of the Purkinje network was claimed as the strongest histologic support to the physiologic data collected on the high-velocity spreading of the impulse through a pure muscular pathway.

In the fifties, the electron microscopy study of Purkinje cells showed, in addition to the scarcity of myofibrils and mitochondria and the poorly developed endoplasmic reticulum, that they are, indeed, singly cytologic units, separated from each other by intercalated disks, into which the myofibrils end, as in common myocardium [27, 32-35]. Therefore there had to be a new explanation regarding the longitudinal and transverse conduction of impulses which determine the cardiac synchronous contraction.

Rhodin et al. [34], who also gave a schematic representation of the cellular contacts in the conducting system of the steer heart, were inclined to think that the impulse transmission resulted from enzymatically catalyzed chemical processes due to the presence of alkaline phosphatase, succinic dehydrogenase and cholinesterase in the intercalated disks. The conclusion was drawn that the intercalated disks facilitate, instead of initiating, the impulse transmission, which would be mediated by the enzymes present in or near these structures. However there are not at present sufficient data to draw definite conclusions.

REFERENCES

1. Hecht HH, Kossmann CE, Childers RW, Langendorf R, Lev N, Rosen KM, Pruitt RD, Truex RC, Uhley HN, Watt TB: Atrioventricular and intraventricular conduction. Revised nomenclature and concepts. Am J Cardiol 31: 232, 1973
2. Anderson RH, Becker AE, Brechenmacher C, Davies MJ, Rossi L: The human atrioventricular junctional area. A morphological study of the AV node and bundle. Europ J Cardiol 3: 11, 1975
3. Becker AE, Anderson RH: Morphology of the human atrioventricular junctional area. In: The conduction system of the heart. Structure, function and clinical implications, Wellens HJJ, Lie KI, Janse MJ. Stenfert Kroese, 1976, p 263
4. Lev M: The normal anatomy of the conduction system in man and its pathology in atrioventricular block. Ann NY Acad Sci 111: 817, 1964
5. pick A, Langendorf R: Recent advances in the differential diagnosis of AV junctional arrhythmias. Am Heart J 76: 553, 1968
6. James TN, Isobe JH, Urthaler F: Correlative electrophysiological and anatomical study concerning the site of origin of escape rhythm during complete atrioventricular block in the dog. Circ Res 45: 108, 1979
7. Rossi L: His bundle electrocardiographic semantics of A-V block. Anatomoclinical considerations. Pace 3: 275, 1980.
8. Baissus C, Latour H, Grolleau R, Puech P: Branche droite du faisceau de His. De sa morphologie a sa fonction. Arch Mal Coeur 69: 1123, 1976
9. Rossi L, Levy A: Anomalies morphologiques et topographiques de la branche droite du faisceau de His au cours de l'hypertrophie cardiaque. Arch Mal Coeur 53: 154, 1960
10. Rossi L: Histopathology of cardiac arrhythmias, 2nd edn. Milano: Casa Editrice Ambrosiana, 1978
11. Rossi L: Sistema di conduzione e nervi nel cuore dell'uomo. Milano: Casa Editrice Ambrosiana, 1974
12. James TN, Sherf L. Urthaler F: Fine structure of the bundle branches. Br Heart J 36: 1, 1974
13. Rosenbaum MB, Elizari MV, Lazzari JO: The hemiblocks. Oldsmar: Tampe Tracing, 1970
14. Mahaim I: Les maladies organiques du faisceau de His-Tawara. Paris: Masson et Cie, 1931

15. Doer RW: Die Morphologie des Reizleitungsystems, ihre Orthologie und Pathologie. Span K, ed. Stuttgart: Thieme, 1957, p 19
16. Schutz E: Physiologie des Herzens. Berlin: Springer, 1958
17. Uhley HN, Rivkin LM: Peripheral distribution of the canine A-V conduction system. Observation on gross morphology. Am J Cardiol 5: 688, 1960
18. Robb JS: Comparative basic cardiology. New York: Grune & Stratton, 1965
19. Barry A, Pattern BM: The structure of the adult heart. In: Pathology of the heart and blood vessels, 3rd edn Gould SE. Springfield: Thomas, 1968, p 123
20. Uhley HN: Some controversy regarding the peripheral distribution of the conduction system. Am J Cardiol 30: 913, 1972
21. Kulbertus HE, Demoulin JCI: Pathological basis of concept of left hemiblock. In: The conduction system of the heart. Structure, function and clinical implications, Wellens HJJ, Lie KI, Janse MJ. Leiden: Stenfert Kroese, 1976, p 287
22. Massing GK, James TN: Anatomical configuration of the His bundle and bundle branches in the human heart. Circulation 53: 609, 1976
23. Tawara S: Das Reizleitungssystem des Saugetierherzens. Jena: Gustav Fischer, 1906
24. Rossi L: Sistema di conduzione trifascicolare ed emiblochi di branca sinistra. Considerazioni anatomiche ed istopatologiche. G Ital Cardiol 1: 55, 1971
25. Titus JL: Anatomy of the conduction system. Circulation 47: 170, 1973
26. Titus JL: Normal anatomy of the human cardiac conduction system. Mayo Clin Proc 48: 24, 1973
27. Rossi L, Bassi M: Le soubendocarde gauche du septum ventriculaire chez le cobaye. Etude au microscope électronique. Arch Mal Coeur 55: 919, 1962
28. Purkinje JE: Mikroskopisch-neurologische Beobachtungen. Müllers Arch Anat Physiol Med 12: 281, 1845
29. Abramson DL, Margolin MA: A Purkinje conduction network in the myocardium of the mammalian ventricles. J Anat Lond 70: 250, 1936
30. Truex RC: Comparative anatomy and functional considerations of the cardiac conduction system. In: The specialized tissues of the heart. Amsterdam: Elsevier, 1961, p 22
31. Field EJ: The development of the conducting system in the heart of sheep. Br Heart J 13: 129, 1951
32. Caesar R, Edwards GA, Ruska H: Electron microscopy of the impulse conducting system of the sheep heart. Z Zellforsch 48: 698, 1958
33. Kisch B: New investigations on cardiac nerves. II. Protoaxons in contact with heart muscle fibers of men and animals. An electron microscopy study. Exp Med Surg 18: 169, 1960
34. Rhodin JAG, Del Missier P, Reid LC: The structure of the specialized impulse-conducting system of the steer heart. Circulation 24: 349, 1961
35. Bompiani GD: Sugli aspetti ultrastrutturali del sistema specifico di conduzione. XXV Congr Soc Ital Cardiol 2: 159, 1964

2. PHYSIOLOGY OF VENTRICULAR EXCITATION

The physiology of ventricular excitation has been studied by several groups of investigators during the last twenty years. However most of the studies have used canine hearts [1-5]; very few studies describing activation in human hearts are available in literature [6-9].

Various techniques have been utilized to study the sequence of ventricular activation. Durrer et al. [8] described the epicardial and intramural activation sequence in isolated re-perfused human hearts. Other studies [5-7, 9] have utilized recordings from multiple transmural plunge electrodes in isolated cardiac tissue, as well as under direct vision from open chambers of the 'in situ' beating heart during cardiopulmonary by-pass. Although these techniques have provided us with useful information, it is by no means complete. Specifically, the relationship between activation of the specialized conduction system and the functioning myocardial cells still remains to be resolved.

EXCITATION OF THE INTERVENTRICULAR SEPTUM

The activation of the right septal surface depends on the right bundle branch and that of the left septal surface on the left bundle branch. This hypothesis – put forth by Sodi-Pallares et al. [3] – of the existence of a functional barrier between the right and left side of the septum has never been definitely confirmed.

The earliest activity is broadly distributed over the mid and apical portion of the left side of the septum [3, 8, 10, 11]. This is followed almost immediately by activation of the right septal surface. The wave of depolarization moves from left to right and in an apico-basal direction. In some cases, the activation of the right and left side of the septum is simultaneous. However, since the activation of the left septal surface occurs quite rapidly, a major portion of the left surface is excited prior to activation of a comparable area on the right side [11].

The site of earliest activity on the right side of the septum is the inferior portion, near the anterior papillary muscle. The spread of activity over the right septal surface is relatively slow, lasting 35-60 msec, in an upward and somewhat posterior direction. The septal half of the crista supraventricularis is activated late, both by an activation front from the left to right septal surface and a front reaching the crista through the free wall of the right ventricle [12].

EXCITATION OF THE LEFT VENTRICLE

Studies in canine [2] and in human hearts [8], using simultaneous recordings from a great number of sites, have shown that electrical activation of the ventricular walls occurs from the endocardium to the epicardium. Sodi-Pallares et al. [3] have shown that in addition, a portion of the free wall may be activated from outside to inside, owing to penetration by Purkinje fibers. Durrer et al. [8] demonstrated that three areas were activated early: 1) an area high on the anterior paraseptal wall just below the attachment of the mitral valve; 2) a central area on the left surface of the ventricular septum; 3) a posterior paraseptal area at about one third of the distance from apex to base. These three areas were activated simultaneously within 0-5 msec after the start of the left ventricular cavity potential, probably related to excitation of anterior, septal and posterior fascicles. The activation front expands very rapidly, becoming confluent within 15-20 msec, and then moves less rapidly to the epicardial surface overlying these areas of earliest endocardial activation [4]. Wyndham et al. [9] described two breakthrough sites at the left epicardial surface; one anteriorly, adjacent to the midportion of the septum, and the other posterobasally. In some hearts another area of early activation was found near the apex posteriorly. The last site to be activated was the posterobasal left paraseptal region, although in some cases it was more lateral than paraseptal.

EXCITATION OF THE RIGHT VENTRICLE

Endocardial right ventricular activation starts near the base of the anterior papillary muscle, 5-10 msec after the onset of the left ventricular cavity potential, followed by almost simultaneous activation of the adjoining free wall and the septum [5]. Epicardial breakthrough occurs in the area pretrabecularis after 20 msec, and activation front moves tangentially, reaching the pulmonary conus and posterobasal area within 60-70 msec. A recent study by Wyndham et al. [9] described another area of epicardial breakthrough in the inferior right ventricular wall. In some cases it was located near the base adjacent to the septum, in some toward the acute margin posterobasally and in one case toward the right ventricular apex. There is scanty anatomical explanation for this epicardial breakthrough, since the right bundle branch has not been shown to split into major divisions of fascicles. These authors suggested that the relative thinness of the free wall and the inflow region of the right ventricle, compared with the outflow and apical region, may allow early emergence of activation at the basal inferior epicardial surface.

The site of latest activation of the epicardium was always at the atrio-ventricular sulcus, either along the anterobasal right ventricle or posterobasal right or left ventricle [9].

REFERENCES

1. Pruitt RD, Essex HE, Burchell HB: Studies on the spread of excitation through the ventricular myocardium. Circulation 3: 418, 1951
2. Scher AM, Young AC, Malmgren AL, Paton RR: Spread of electrical activity through the wall of the ventricle. Circ Res 1: 539, 1953
3. Sodi-Pallares D, Calder RM: New bases of electrocardiography. St. Louis: Mosby, 1956
4. Myerburg RJ, Nilsson K, Gelband H: Physiology of canine intraventricular conduction and endocardial excitation. Circ Res 30: 217, 1972
5. Myerburg RJ, Nilsson K, Castellanos A, Lazzara R, Befeler B, Gelband H: The intraventricular conduction system and patterns of endocardial excitation. Adv Cardiol 14: 2, 1975
6. Barker PS, MacLeod AG, Alexander J: The excitatory process observed in the exposed human heart. Am Heart J 5: 720, 1930
7. Carouso GJ, Chevalier HA, Latscha BI, Lenegre J: Epicardial electrograms recorded in the course of seven cases of heart surgery. Circulation 5: 48, 1952
8. Durrer O, Van Dam RTh, Freud GE, Janse MJ, Meijler FL, Arzbaecher RC: Total excitation of the isolated human heart. Circulation 41: 893, 1970
9. Wyndham CR, Meeran MK, Smith T, Saxena A, Engelman RM, Levitsky S, Rosen KM: Epicardial activation of the intact human heart without conduction defects. Circulation 59: 161, 1979
10. Venerose RS, Seidenstein M, Stuckey JH: Activation of subendocardial Purkinje fibers and muscle fibers of the left septal surface before and after left bundle branch block. Am Heart J 63: 346, 1962
11. Scher AM: Excitation of the heart: a progress report. In: Advances in electrocardiography, Schlant RC, Hurst JW. New York: Grune & Stratton, 1972, p 61
12. Amer NS, Stuckey JH, Hoffman BF, Cappelletti RR, Domingo RT: Activation of the interventricular septal myocardium studied during cardiopulmonary bypass. Am Heart J 59: 224, 1960

3. BUNDLE BRANCH BLOCKS

The term bundle branch block (BBB) implies a conduction disturbance in one of the two main branches of the His bundle, resulting in delayed activation of either the right ventricle or the left one. The right bundle branch being thinner and longer than the left bundle is more vulnerable to small, focal, fibrotic or inflammatory lesions. Hence, right bundle branch block (RBBB) is more common than left bundle branch block (LBBB) in spite of the fact that diseases involving the right ventricle are less frequent than those affecting the left one.

In clinical electrocardiography BBB is considered to be complete when QRS complex is prolonged to 120 msec or more, and incomplete when the QRS duration is less than 120 msec. However, a mere slowing of the conduction can lead to QRS complex of 120 msec or more [1, 2] (Figure 1). Hence, the term 'complete' does not always signify complete interruption of conduction and it is preferable to omit such a term.

LFT BUNDLE BRANCH BLOCK

In normal hearts, the right and left ventricles are activated almost simultaneously. In LBBB, there is delayed activation of the left septum and left ventricular walls. However the excitation process in this block is controversial and various aspects remain unclear. The greatest contributions to the understanding of the ventricular excitation in LBBB have been made by the Mexican school in studies in the dog [3-5].

The first area to be activated is the low right septal surface, near the base of the anterior papillary muscle. The activation then spreads simultaneously over the endocardial surface of the right ventricle and upward over the right septal surface. As the excitation proceeds transmurally through the apico-lateral free wall of the right ventricle, the inferior and posterobasal portion of the septum undergoes activation in a right to left direction (30-50 msec). The remainder of the septum, i.e. the superior and anterior portions, is activated slowly, after about 70-90 msec.

The first segment of the left ventricular wall to be excited is the apico-posterior after 40-60 msec, followed by the apico-anterior in 50-70 msec. The free wall of the left ventricle is then activated, anterior wall initially (50-70 msec) followed by the

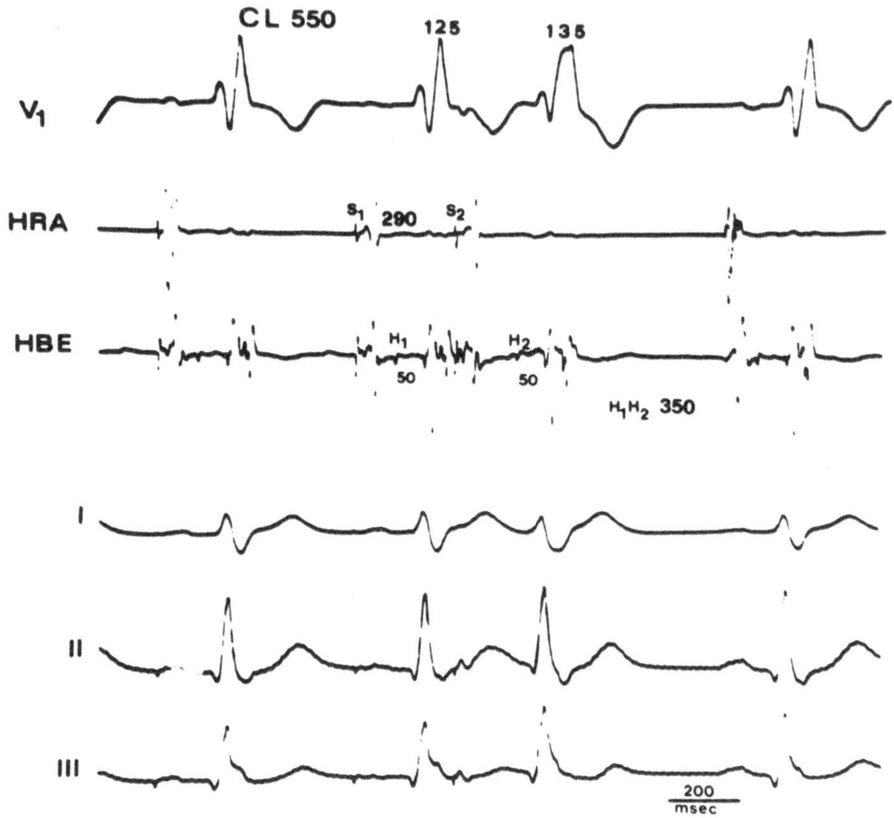

Figure 1. Right bundle branch block pattern. QRS complex measures 125 msec. During programmed premature atrial beats (H_1H_2: 350 msec), QRS duration increases to 135 msec, thus showing that basic RBBB is not complete. HRA: High right atrium. HBE: His bundle electrocardiogram

anterolateral wall (78-80 msec). The posterobasal region of the left ventricle is excited after 45-80 msec and the posterolateral region after 65-105 msec. Other experimental studies [6-9] partly contradict the pattern described above, suggesting that the normal sequence of activation is completely inverted with the posterobasal wall undergoing activation earlier than the anterolateral one.

According to some authors [3-5], the main conduction delay in LBBB is localized to a specific region of the septum, namely, the transition zone between regions of septum, activated by the right bundle branch and those activated by the left bundle branch. Once the activation front crosses this barrier and reaches the ramifications of the left branch, it spreads over the left septal surface and the rest of the left ventricle in a normal fashion. Other authors [6, 7] maintain that the prolongation of ventricular activation time in LBBB is mainly due to differences in rate of conduction, direction and sequence of activation of the free wall of the left ventricle.

In the few studies carried out in man [9, 10] using epicardial mapping during open heart surgery in subjects with LBBB, a slow transeptal epicardial activation from right to left has been observed, whereas there were present widely spaced isochrones over the left ventricular free wall epicardium implying more rapid conduction. It would therefore appear that after completion of septal crossing and upon reaching the left ventricular Purkinje tissue, the impulse accelerates activation of at least part of the left ventricle. Further investigations are, however, necessary in patients with LBBB, since it is possible that the site of the main conduction delay varies from subject to subject.

ELECTROCARDIOGRAPHIC FEATURES

The electrocardiographic changes in typical LBBB are (Figure 2):

- QRS duration of 120 msec or more.
- Absence of q waves in left sided leads I, aVL, V_5 and V_6 in relation to leftward orientation of the first vectors.
- Initial and/or terminal slurring in the left sided leads.
- Broad, notched R waves in leads I, aVL, V_5 and V_6 with middle slurring. According to Rodriguez et al. [3] and Sodi-Pallares et al. [4, 5], this is due to delayed depolarization in the interventricular septum. However, Kennamer et al. [6] and Becker et al. [7] feel that this slurring is due to slow conduction in the free wall of the left ventricle.
- Delayed intrinsecoid deflection time (60 msec or more) in unipolar leads a VL and V_6 in relation to delayed excitation of both latero-superior and latero-inferior walls of the left ventricle. In fact aVL explores the latero-superior wall and V_6 the latero-inferior wall.
- RS or rS pattern in III and aVF.
- rS pattern in V_1 and V_2 with deep and wide S waves. Sometimes a QS pattern is seen due to more posteriorly oriented first vectors.
- R/S ratio increasing progressively from the right to the left precordial leads.
- Depressed ST segment and inverted T wave in the left sided leads due to secondary changes in ventricular repolarization.

VECTORCARDIOGRAPHIC FEATURES

Frontal (F) plane

The QRS loop is generally small and irregular in contour. This is due to a predominant posteriorly directed QRS loop which is thus perpendicular to the frontal plane. The initial deflections are oriented to the left and inferiorly. The efferent

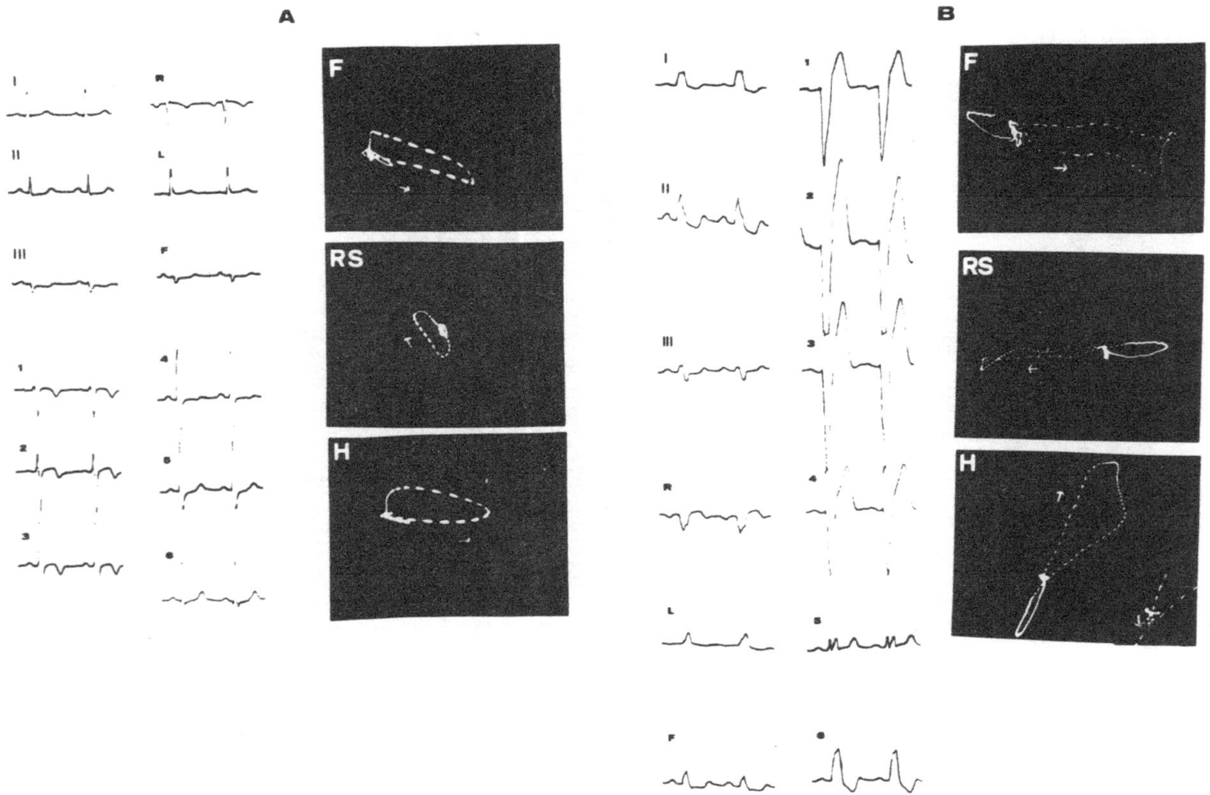

Figure 2. A: Control ECG and VCG tracings. B: Appearance of typical left bundle branch block. ECG: In leads I, aVL, V_5 and V_6 q wave disappears and a middle slurring appears. QRS axis does not significantly change. VCG: Horizontal QRS loops shift posteriorly and rotation becomes clockwise. The first vectors are oriented inferiorly, anteriorly and to the left. A mid-terminal slurring is evident in all three planes.

limb continues in the inferior and leftward course and turns abruptly in a superior direction so that the loop is inscribed counterclockwise or in a figure of eight with the afferent limb being superior to the efferent one. A delay is evident in the mid-terminal and sometimes in the initial part of the QRS complex. The T loop is inscribed in a counterclockwise manner and both the ST vector and T loop are directed to the right and superiorly.

Horizontal (H) plane

The QRS loop, except at times for a small initial segment, is characteristically inscribed in a clockwise fashion. This rotation appears in relation to the earlier activation of the posterior left septal mass compared to that of the anterior one [11]. Sometimes the QRS loop shows a figure of eight configuration, in which case most of the loop is inscribed clockwise. The QRS loop is usually elongated and about 2 mV in magnitude. The initial 10 msec vectors are generally oriented to the left and anteriorly. There is then an abrupt change in direction with the loop moving clockwise to the left and posteriorly. The afferent limb is usually to the left of the efferent one and terminates anteriorly and to the right of the E point. The ST vector and T loop are directed to the right and anteriorly. The T loop is narrow and elongated and its inscription is commonly counterclockwise (Figure 2).

In LBBB the 10 msec vector is a resultant of two main vectors: a right ventricular vector oriented anteriorly and inferiorly due to activation of the low antero-medial wall of the right ventricle and a septal vector directed to the left, posteriorly and inferiorly in relation to activation of the low septal mass [4, 5]. In most cases, this resultant vector is oriented inferiorly, to the left and anteriorly. In a few cases, it may be directed posteriorly. The reason for this change in orientation is probalby due to differences in the activation sequence and the magnitude and direction of the two component vectors [12].

Right sagittal (RS) plane

The QRS loop is elongated and inscribed clockwise; sometimes it shows a figure of eight configuration, in which case most of the loop is inscribed clockwise. The initial forces are commonly directed anteriorly and inferiorly and the remainder of the loop is posterior with mid to terminal delay. The afferent limb is superior to the efferent one. As in the H plane the loop does not close. The ST vector and T loop are oriented anteriorly and superiorly, or inferiorly with a clockwise rotation of the T loop.

Table 1 shows the VCG features of typical LBBB.

Table 1. Vectorcardiographic features of typical left bundle branch block

- Prolonged QRS interval (120 msec or more)
- First vectors directed to the left, anteriorly and inferiorly (rarely posteriorly)
- Mean QRS oriented to the left and posteriorly
- Counterclockwise inscription in frontal plane
- Clockwise or figure-of-eight inscription in horizontal plane
- Mid-terminal and sometimes initial delay of QRS loop
- ST vector and T loop directed to the right and anteriorly

ATYPICAL LEFT BUNDLE BRANCH BLOCK

1) *LBBB with marked QRS axis deviation*

In the majority of cases of LBBB, the electrical axis is between $+30°$ and $-30°$ [1, 13]. This is expected since a delay is present both in the antero-superior and postero-inferior walls of the left ventricle.

A marked axis deviation associated with LBBB poses pathophysiological problems, not yet completely resolved.

LBBB with left axis deviation. A marked left axis deviation (LAD) of $-45°$ or more is not uncommon in LBBB; it has been encountered in 21-28% of cases with LBBB [1, 13]. LAD in the presence of LBBB presumably reflects abnormalities in activation of the septum and distal Purkinje system. This concept was postulated by Rosenbaum et al. [1] based on a study of 98 cases with intermittent LBBB. In 67 of these cases with the occurrence of LBBB, the QRS axis shifted an average of 39.5° (range 2°-160°) toward the left. In 20 cases (20.4%) the complexes with LBBB showed an axis of more than $-45°$. In 6 of these 20 (30%), LAD was present even in the absence of LBBB, and in the remaining 14 cases, the axis shift was caused strictly by the LBBB. These data suggest that in the majority of cases, the LAD is due to LBBB per se.

In the remaining cases the factors responsible for LAD may be the following:

- Incomplete predivisional LBBB associated with anterior fascicular block (AFB) [14, 15]. This possibility has not been confirmed experimentally, but it is believed to be frequent by Lichstein et al. [16]; from an analysis of 24 patients with LBBB and LAD, they observed in a previous ECG without LBBB an AFB pattern in 10 cases.
- AFB associated with incomplete posterior fascicular block (PFB). This possibility is also, at present, only theoretical, since it has not been demonstrated experimentally. The case reported in Figure 3 is, however, highly suggestive; it concerns a patient with atrial fibrillation, LBBB and LAD (ÂQRS: $-70°$). The QRS duration is 150 msec. With RR intervals less than 1200 msec, QRS com-

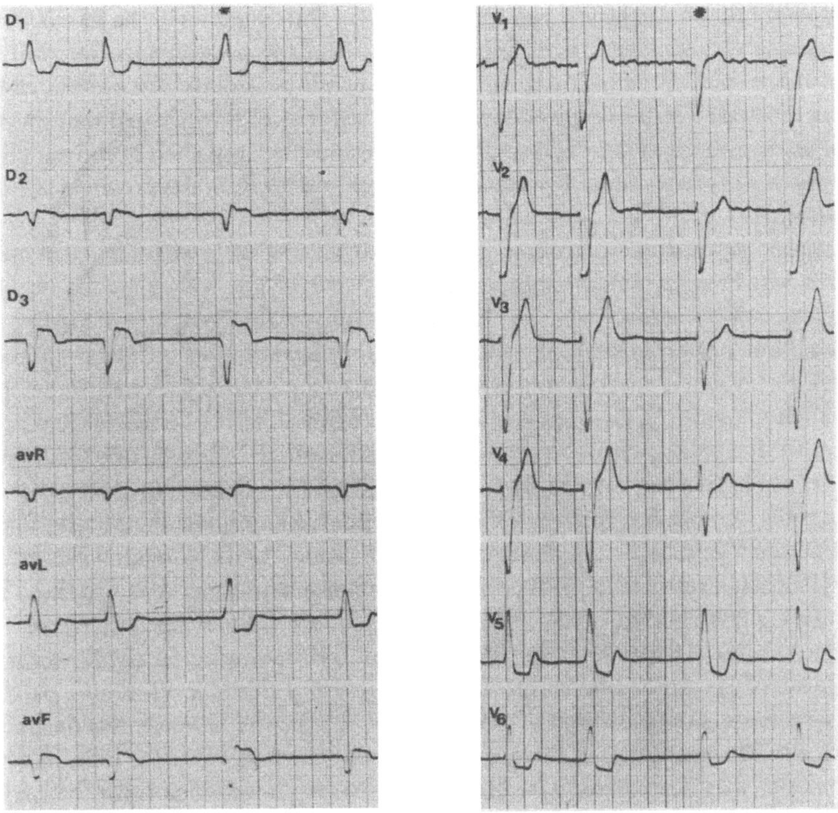

Figure 3. Patient with atrial fibrillation and left bundle branch block with marked left axis deviation. QRS complex measures 150 msec. After RR intervals of 1200 msec or more, QRS duration decreases to 130 msec and further accentuation of left axis deviation is evident (see text for explanation). (From Alboni et al., with permission of G Ital Cardiol [18].) D1: lead I; D2: lead II; D3: lead III

plexes show accentuation of LAD, but they become narrower. The reduction in the duration of the QRS complex means an improvement in conduction. Since such a reduction is associated with accentuation of LAD, it is most likely due to an improvement in conduction, rate dependent, in the posterior fascicle. In this patient, therefore, LBBB appears to be due to involvement of a different degree in both the main fascicles of the left bundle branch.

- Left ventricular enlargement with peripheral block can induce LAD in the presence of LBBB [13, 17]. Hypertrophy and enlargement of the left ventricle have been encountered almost constantly in clinical [17] and post-mortem examinations [13] of patients with LBBB and LAD.
- Right ventricular enlargement, where it occurs in a horizontal heart, may induce LAD [17, 18]. This occurrence, in theory, seems paradoxical. It is, however,

possible that an enlarged right ventricle may shift superiorly the left ventricle.

- Right ventricular peripheral block, localized in the postero-superior wall, can shift the mid-terminal forces superiorly. Such a possibility was experimentally demonstrated in the dog by Marquez-Montes et al. [19], who hold that this type of intraventricular conduction disturbances must be suspected in clinical setting when a slurred terminal R wave is evident in lead aVR, in the presence of LBBB with LAD.
- Inferior myocardial infarction. The association of LBBB with such wall infarction will be discussed in Chapter 9.
- Extracardiac factors such as pulmonary emphysema. The cause of LAD in the disease is not completely understood. The transmission of electrical potentials has been found experimentally to be normal in an inferior to superior direction, but decreased in a superior to inferior direction [20].
- LBBB due to asynchronous conduction within the His bundle (see Chapter 2). Using selective His bundle stimulation, Narula [21, 22] demonstrated that it is possible to localize the site of bundle branch blocks within the His bundle (Figures 4 and 5). In 14 patients with LBBB and LAD, proximal His bundle (HB) pacing resulted in QRS complexes similar in pattern and axis to those seen during sinus rhythm, with a stimulus to R interval equal to the observed HV time. Distal HB pacing resulted in narrow QRS complex in all; however the QRS axis remained unchanged (LAD) in five and normalized in nine patients. These findings suggest that in these 14 patients, the site of lesion responsible for the LBBB was located in the upper half of the His bundle; in the nine, in whom the QRS axis normalized with HB pacing, the lesion responsible for the LAD in all probability was also located in the His bundle.

  If the LBBB or LAD are not intermittent (Figure 6), it is not possible to discriminate the cause of LAD in ECG and VCG tracings.

LBBB with marked right axis deviation. Right axis deviation (RAD) over $+90°$ in LBBB is a very rare occurrence, since it is seen in less than 1% of patients with LBBB [23]. The following factors have been held responsible for the RAD:

- Incomplete predivisional LBBB associated with PFB [14, 15]. This possibility has not been confirmed experimentally.
- PFB associated with incomplete AFB [14, 15]. This occurrence has also not so far been experimentally confirmed.
- Right ventricular overload, secondary to left ventricular failure can shift the QRS axis to the right [24, 26].
- Marked vertical position of the heart [25, 26].
- Increased lung stiffness due to congestive heart failure, as well as emphysema, can alter the conductivity of electrical forces. These circumstances would increase the actual distance between the heart and the right shoulder, with the result that the scalene triangle determined by the vectors of leads I, II, and III

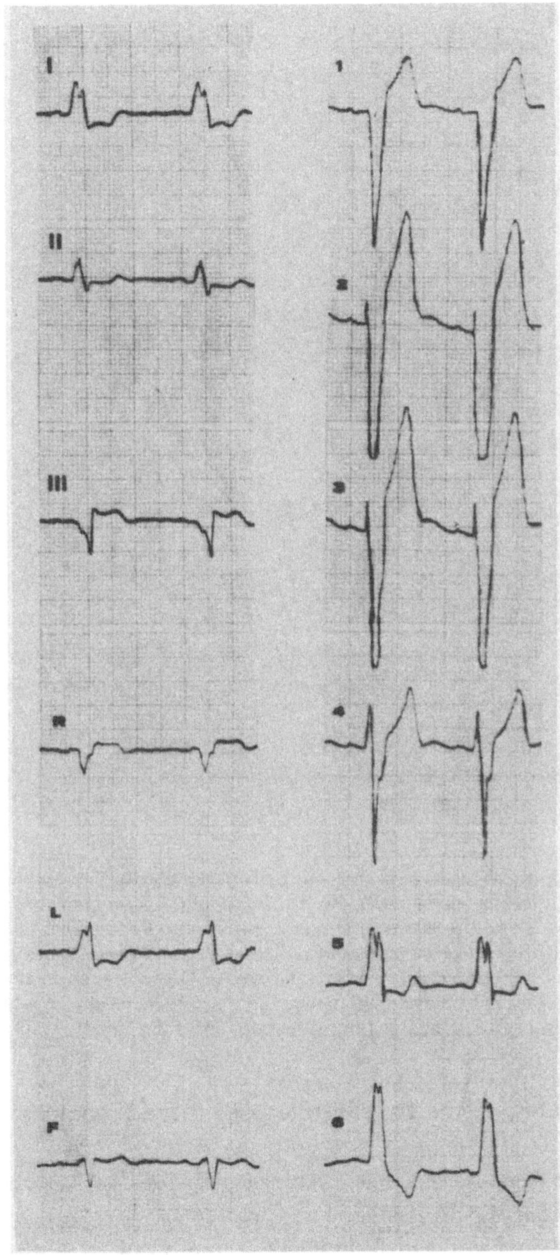

Figure 4. Electrocardiogram shows a typical left bundle branch block. (From Alboni et al., with permission of G Ital Cardiol [145])

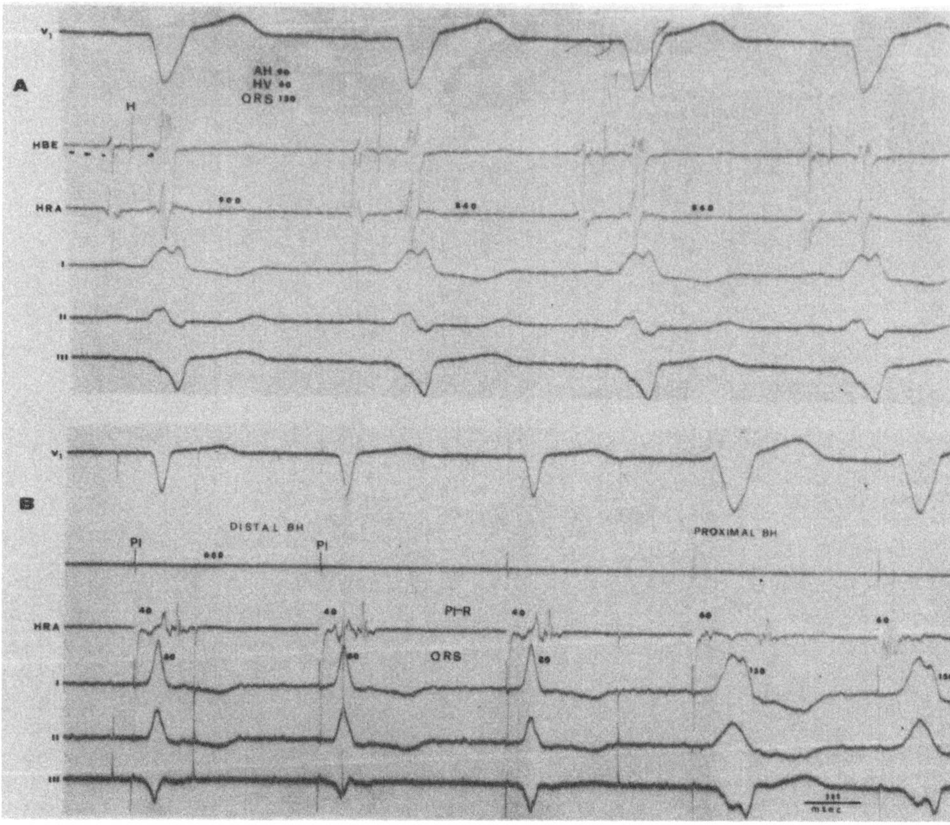

Figure 5. Electrophysiological recording of the same patient as Figure 4. The left bundle branch block is due to a lesion within the His bundle (HB). Normalization of QRS complex with distal HB pacing. A: HV and QRS intervals measure 60 and 150 msec, respectively. B: Proximal HB pacing results in QRS complexes with LBBB identical to the sinus beats and a PI-R interval (60 msec) similar to the HV time (right hand). Distal BH pacing (left hand) normalizes the QRS duration to 80 msec with a PI-R interval (45 msec) shorter by 15 msec than the control HV time. PI-R: Pacing impulse to QRS interval (for details see text). (From Alboni et al., with permission of G Ital Cardiol [145])

would be more oblique and the effective axis of lead I would be shifted to the right [25].

- Infarction of the free wall of the left ventricle [27, 28]. The association of LBBB with this infarction will be discussed in Chapter 9.
- RAD has been noted to occur following evacuation of ascite [29].
- Massive pulmonary embolism can shift the axis to the right in a pre-existing LBBB [30].

The vectorcardiogram of patients with LBBB and RAD shows some interesting features.

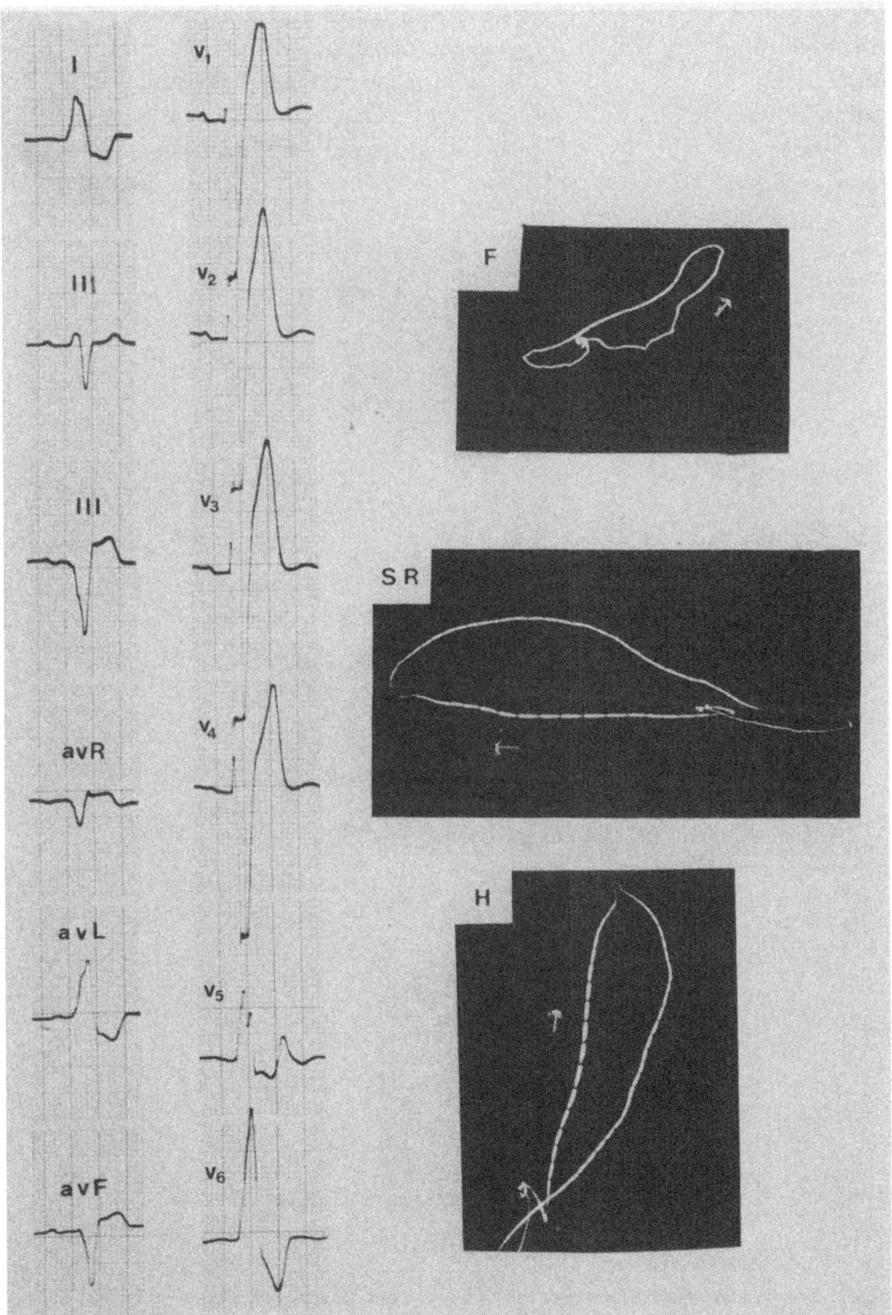

Figure 6. Left bundle branch block with marked left axis deviation. The cause for LAD cannot be evaluated by the ECG and VCG tracings. (From Alboni et al., with permission of G Ital Cardiol [18])

We examined the VCG of 11 patients with LBBB and RAD, without previous myocardial infarction [26]. In F plane the maximum vector was directed to the right between +90° and +150° and in H plane between −90° and −110°. The rotation of the QRS loop was not different in H plane from that seen in LBBB with normal axis, whereas in F plane, in five cases the QRS loop was inscribed clockwise (Figure 7). The same findings can be observed in LBBB coexisting with

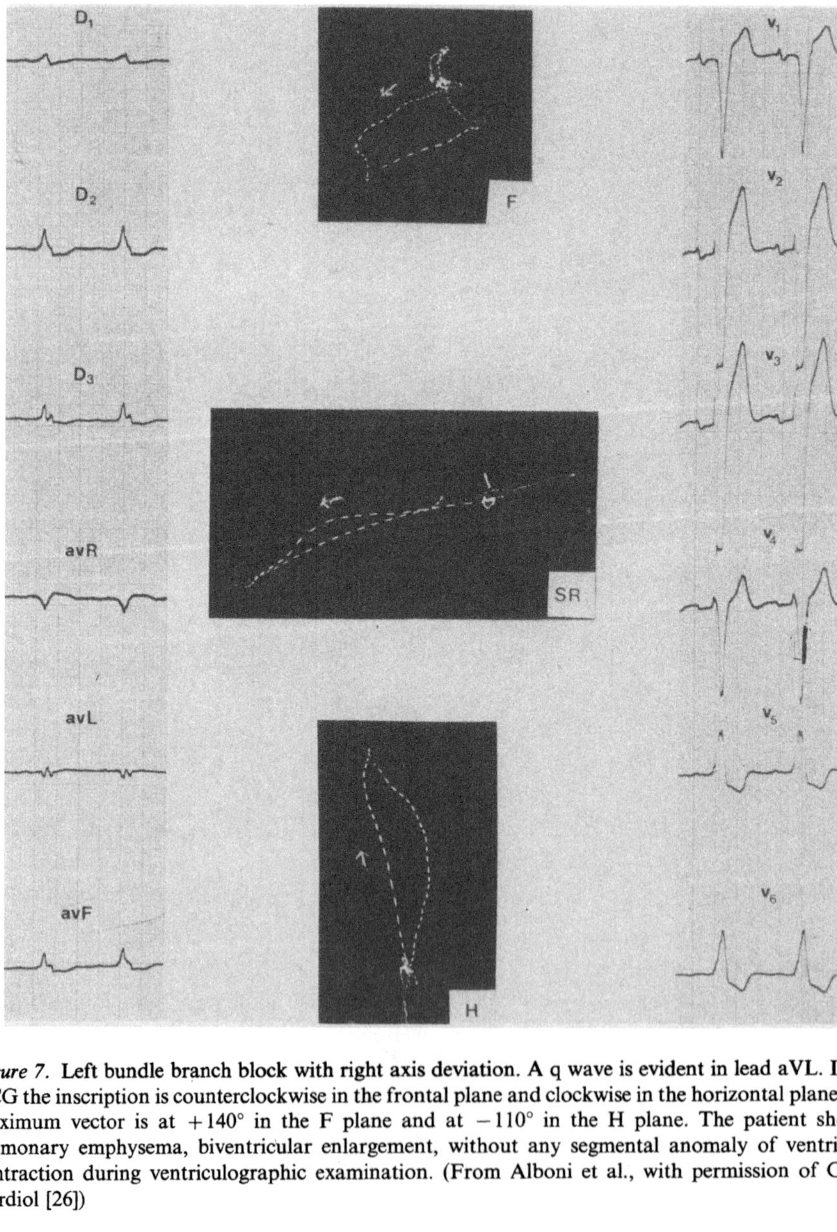

Figure 7. Left bundle branch block with right axis deviation. A q wave is evident in lead aVL. In the VCG the inscription is counterclockwise in the frontal plane and clockwise in the horizontal plane. The maximum vector is at +140° in the F plane and at −110° in the H plane. The patient showed pulmonary emphysema, biventricular enlargement, without any segmental anomaly of ventricular contraction during ventriculographic examination. (From Alboni et al., with permission of G Ital Cardiol [26])

anterolateral myocardial infarction (see Chapter 9). In all 11 patients, evidence of emphysema was present on chest X-ray and in seven, right ventricular enlargement was seen.

If LBBB or RAD are not intermittent, we believe one cannot discriminate the cause of RAD in ECG and VCG tracings.

2) *LBBB with q wave in lead I*

q waves in leads I and/or aVL (Figure 8) coexisting with LBBB are commonly considered an expression of myocardial infarction. However, Laham et al. [17] observed that there is no close correlation between the presence of small q waves in LBBB and myocardial infarction and that it is often seen with LAD. Surprisingly, he noted a higher incidence of right ventricular enlargement when q wave was seen in lead I. The reason for this is not known, but this association could be incidental since in patients with LBBB and LAD, a cardiomegaly is frequently observed (see below).

3) *LBBB with small q wave in lead* V_6

This electrocardiographic finding may be an expression, besides septal necrosis, of LBBB related to a left bifascicular block (AFB + PFB) with normally conducting middle (septal) fascicle (see Chapter 4). Such a type of incomplete LBBB, represents a very rare ECG feature. This interpretation is based on the experimental data of Medrano et al. [31], who recorded ECG and VCG in the dog after cutting the anterior and posterior fascicles without damaging the middle fascicle. The ECG showed an LBBB pattern with small q waves in V_5 and V_6 and the VCG evidenced first vectors of QRS loop directed to the right and anteriorly with counterclockwise rotation. This is consistent with normal septal activation. In the differential diagnosis, myocardial infarction coexisting with LBBB should be considered; however, the q waves are small and narrow and not typical of infarction.

Figure 9 shows the ECG of a 42-year-old man with asymptomatic aortic insufficiency. The PR and QRS intervals measure 170 and 90 msec, respectively. The ECG also shows left ventricular hypertrophy (LVH) with strain pattern. One year later, the patient was still asymptomatic but the ECG showed significant changes (Figure 10): 1) increase in QRS duration to 120 msec; 2) slight downward shift in the QRS axis; 3) small q wave in II, III and aVF; 4) slurring of the initial part of the R wave in III and in the terminal part in II and III; 5) delayed intrinsicoid deflection in aVF as manifested by a middle 'plateau'; 6) mid to terminal slurring of QRS complex in V_4, V_5 and V_6; 7) an increase of the intrinsicoid deflection time to 50 msec in aVL; 8) negative T wave in V_4 and deeper T wave in V_5 and V_6.

The small and narrow q waves seen in the ECG one year ago were still present in leads V_5 and V_6. The PR interval remained unchanged.

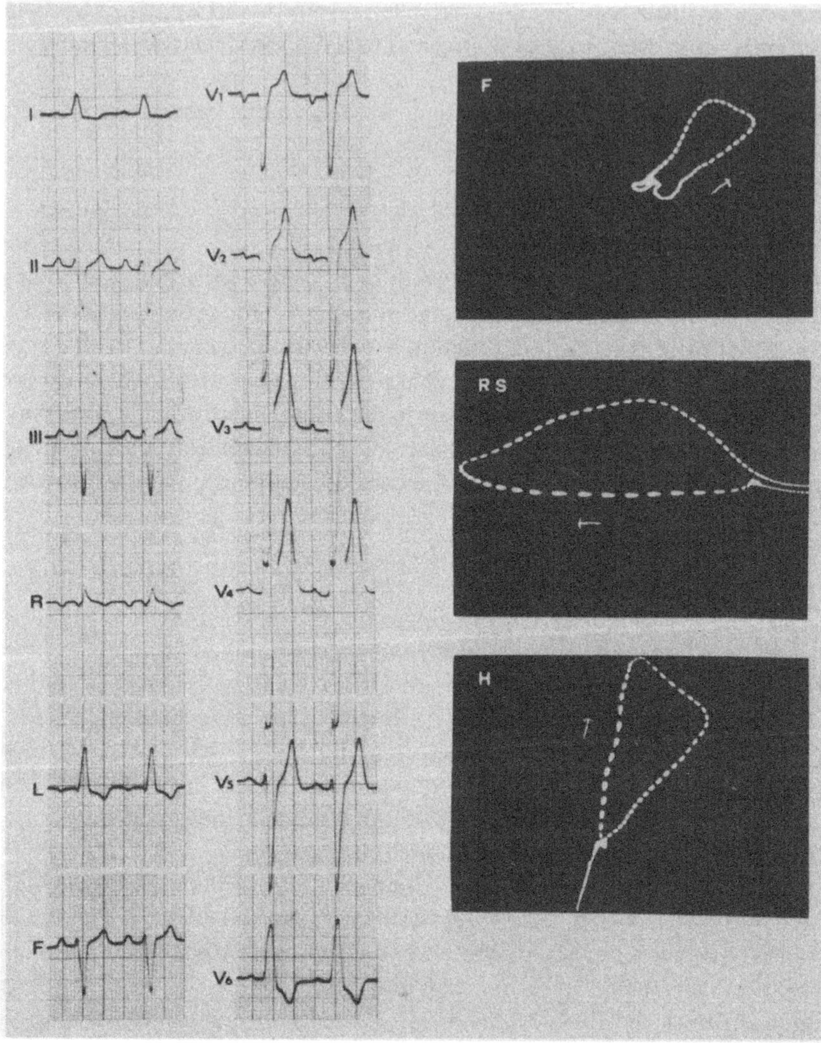

Figure 8. Left bundle branch block with small q wave in lead aVL. QRS complex measures 130 msec. A marked left axis deviation is present. In the frontal plane of the VCG the QRS loop is directed leftward and superiorly with counterclockwise inscription. This tracing suggests predominant involvement of the antero-superior fibers of the left bundle branch

The initial part of the QRS loop, inscribed clockwise the F plane of VCG, showed slight delay, with the first 15 msec vector being oriented to the right and superiorly. The middle part, directed downward, came back upward for a short while and then went downward and leftward. The maximum vector was oriented at $+30°$. In the RS plane the 20 msec vector was directed superiorly; the first half of the loop was clockwise, thus forming a figure of eight. On the H plane the initial

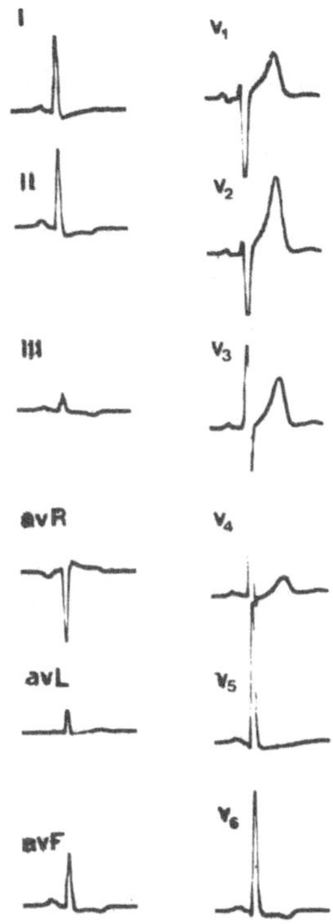

Figure 9. Patient with left ventricular hypertrophy. (From Alboni et al., with permission of J Electrocardiol [32])

vectors were oriented to the right and anteriorly, then to the left and posteriorly with a counterclockwise rotation, while the afferent branch crossed the efferent one at a figure of eight. In all the three planes a mid-terminal delay was clearly seen.

All the above data demonstrate the appearance of incomplete LBBB in a patient with aortic insufficiency and LVH. In addition, evidence for PFB is also present because of the rightward shift in the axis and delay in the intrinsicoid deflection in aVF. The simultaneous presence of a pattern of PFB and incomplete LBBB can be explained on the basis of incomplete main LBBB or by additional incomplete AFB. Predivisional LBBB can be excluded because of the rightward orientation of the first vectors [4, 5]. Associated AFB seems more likely because of the delayed intrinsicoid deflection in aVL. This case, therefore, is suggestive of LBBB due to delayed conduction in both the fascicles, more pronounced in the posterior fascicle [32]. A main or divisional LBBB has always been considered one of the most frequent causes of the leftward orientation of the first vectors. In our case LBBB shows small q waves in V_5 and V_6 and first vectors in the VCG oriented to the right

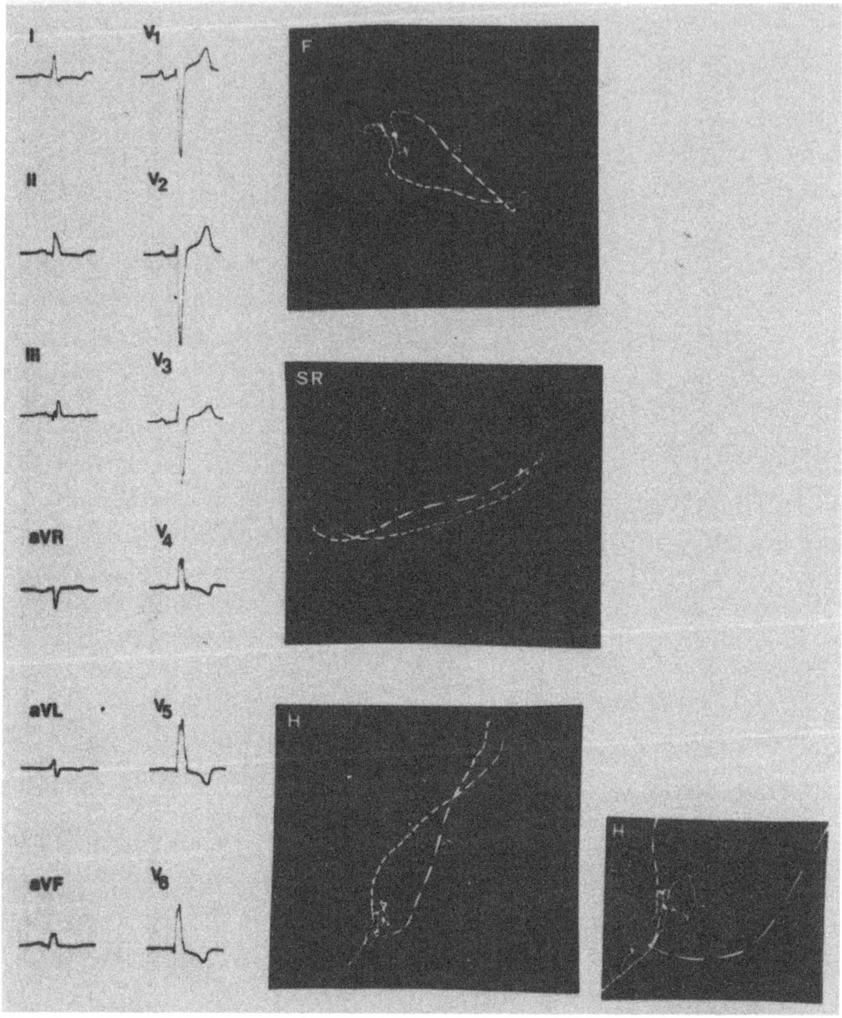

Figure 10. ECG and VCG of the same patient as Figure 9, taken a year later. The tracing is suggestive of left bifascicular block with normally conducting middle (septal) fascicle (see text explanation). (From Alboni et al., with permission of J Electrocardiol [32])

and anteriorly, i.e. a normal septal activation. It seems logical to suppose that the normal septal activation is permitted by a normally middle fascicle activating the inferior two-thirds of the septum. An inferior necrosis cannot be completely excluded since it may be electrically masked by a PFB (see Chapter 9); however the patient did not feel any significant symptoms of myocardial infarction and left ventriculography did not evidence any segmental contraction anomaly.

4) *LBBB with transition zone shifted to the left*

In the majority of cases with LBBB, the transition zone is situated between V_4 and V_5 or V_5 and V_6. In 13% of cases, this zone is shifted to the left with peristence of S wave in V_6 [17]. Laham et al. [17] believe that such a displacement is related to two factors:
- the position of the heart: S wave may in fact appear in left lateral decubitus position;
- right ventricular dilatation in the absence of left ventricular hypertrophy; a displacement of the transition zone to the left has been frequently observed in subjects with LBBB and acute pulmonary embolism.

Moreover S wave in V_6 may express myocardial infarction (see Chapter 9).

5) *Homophasic LBBB*

LBBB is termed homophasic when the T waves are positive in the left sided leads (Figure 11). Most authors feel that homophasic LBBB indicates myocardial ischemia [33-35], others [17, 36] believe that it may be benign. The exact pathophysiology remains to be clarified; however it has been observed that homophasic LBBB often appears when the intraventricular block is intermittent [37-40]. During normal conduction T-wave inversion is present, particularly in leads V_1-V_4, whereas during LBBB upright T waves are evident in the left sided leads.

These T wave changes have been observed in 50-80% of the intermittent LBBB [1, 38-40] and closely resemble the repolarization abnormalities seen after cessation of right ventricular pacing [41-43]. The genesis of such changes is not clear, but they are not related to coronary insufficiency [37-39]. At present, we do not know in how many cases a homophasic LBBB is related to intermittency of the block; however the role of myocardial ischemia in the genesis of this type of block must be reassessed.

DIFFERENTIAL DIAGNOSIS OF LBBB

In most cases, the diagnosis of LBBB is easy. At times, when a marked initial slurring is present, this block may resemble WPW syndrome. Variations in the PR interval associated with change in the QRS morphology would indicate ventricular pre-excitation. In a few cases the diagnosis can be made with certainty only after an electrophysiological study.

Sometimes, in the presence of myocardial infarction, the differential diagnosis between LBBB and peri-infarction block can be difficult. This problem will be discussed in Chapter 6.

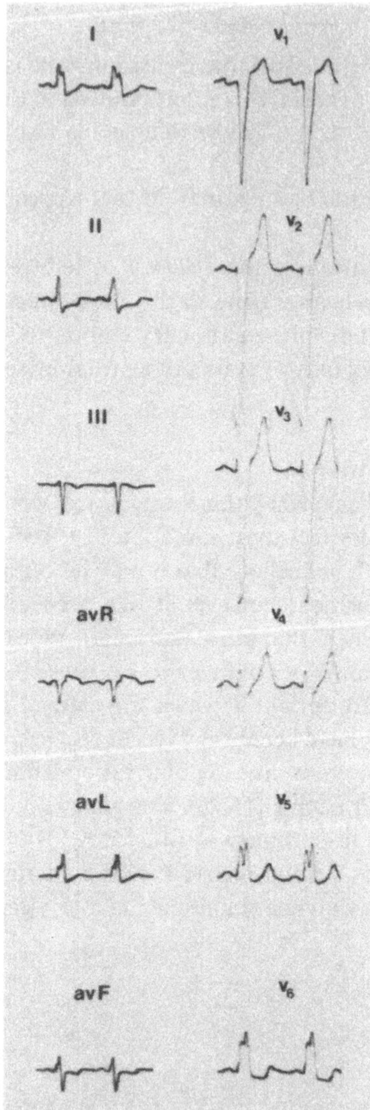

Figure 11. Homophasic left bundle branch block. In leads I, V_5 and V_6 the T waves are positive

LBBB WITH VENTRICULAR HYPERTROPHY

At present there are no definite criteria available for the diagnosis of ventricular hypertrophy in the presence of LBBB; only some suggestive signs are available:

Right ventricular hypertrophy (RVH) may be suspected by the following ECG signs:

- Right axis deviation [17, 25, 26].
- Small q wave in I and/or aVL [17].
- Displacement of the transition zone to the left [17].

In the VCG, the presence of posterior and rightward displacement of the maximum QRS vector in the H plane suggests RVH. Rightward displacement of the QRS vector has also been described in patients with LBBB and infarction of the free wall of the left ventricle [27, 28] but usually only the late forces are involved and the QRS loop in the H plane is often inscribed counterclockwise instead of clockwise as in LBBB with RVH [26].

Left ventricular hypertrophy in the presence of LBBB is difficult to detect. Most authors feel that the voltage criteria for LVH are not applicable in the presence of LBBB and hence unreliable [44-46]. Recently, Cokkinos et al. [47] compared the QRS voltage before and after the appearance of LBBB in 79 cases of intermittent LBBB. They observed that the S wave voltage in V_1 and V_2 increased significantly and the R wave voltage decreased in V_5 and V_6. The Sokolow index did not change significantly. These authors, therefore, suggest that a Sokolow index equal to, or more than, 35 mm indicates LVH even in the presence of LBBB.

INCOMPLETE LEFT BUNDLE BRANCH BLOCK

Incomplete LBBB represents an abnormality as yet undefined and there are some variations in the ECG-VCG criteria listed by different investigators.

The electrocardiographic criteria usually accepted for the diagnosis of incomplete LBBB are those of Barker et al. [48]:

- QRS duration between 100 and 120 msec.
- Absence of Q waves in V_5 and V_6.
- Intrinsecoid deflection time delayed to 50 msec or more in the left precordial leads.
- Slurring in the initial part and sometimes in the descending limb of the R wave in the left sided leads.
- Sometimes inverted T waves in the left precordial leads.

Sodi-Pallares et al. [4, 5], on the basis of their experimental data, subdivided incomplete LBBB into first and second degree. In first degree incomplete LBBB the QRS duration ranges from 70 to 120 msec and only an initial slurring of the R wave in leads V_5 and V_6 is present. In second degree LBBB the QRS duration ranges from 120 to 150 msec and the slurring involves not only the initial portion of the R wave but also the ascending limb and occasionally the descending one (Figure 12).

In first degree LBBB these authors postulated that the functional capacity of the left bundle branch is only slightly affected and that the excitation impulse is conducted down the left branch but more slowly than under normal conditions. The

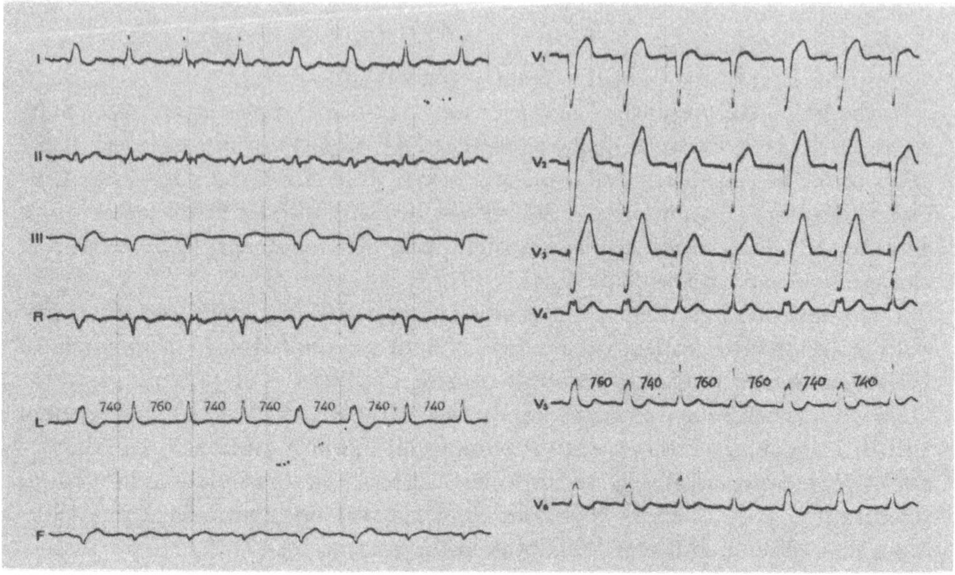

Figure 12. QRS complexes conducted with incomplete left bundle branch block and others with left bundle branch block. The variations of the LBBB do not appear rate-dependent. The QRS complexes conducted with incomplete LBBB measure 100 msec; in leads I, aVF, V_5 and V_6 an initial slurring and a terminal one are present; Q waves are not evident

normal time lag of right septal activation after onset of excitation on the left septal surface therefore tends to be abolished, with the result that the initial forces due to left-to-right septal depolarization are opposed and, in part at least, neutralized. This circumstance is responsible for the disappearance of the Q wave in V_6 lead.

In second degree LBBB the left bundle branch is still functioning but with a very slow rate of conduction. Consequently, while the left branch activates some of the muscle mass of the left septum, the remainder is activated transeptally from the right bundle branch. However, this subdivision of incomplete LBBB does not seem to be of great value in clinical setting.

The vectorcardiogram in incomplete LBBB shows the following features:

In the $\dot{F}$ plane the QRS loop is directed leftward with a maximum QRS loop generally between $+30°$ and $-30°$. The first segment, and at times also the terminal segment of the QRS loop, are delayed. The loop is inscribed counterclockwise, or a major portion of the loop is counterclockwise, if a figure-of-eight inscription is present.

In the H plane the delayed first part of the QRS loop is oriented leftward and anteriorly. Following this there is a change in the loop direction to the left and posteriorly; the maximum vector is generally oriented between $-10°$ and $-50°$.

Most authors describe the rotation of the QRS loop as counterclockwise or as figure-of-eight with first segment of the QRS loop inscribed counterclockwise.

However, on analyzing several cases of intermittent incomplete LBBB, we observed that the QRS loop can also show a figure-of-eight with the first part inscribed clockwise (Figure 13).

In the RS plane the QRS loop is oriented posteriorly and slightly inferiorly or superiorly. The initial deflections are directed anteriorly. Conduction delay is present in the early portion of the loop and often also in the afferent limb.

The ST vector is usually directed rightward, anteriorly, superiorly or inferiorly. The T loop is discordant to the QRS and more or less parallel to the ST vector.

The differential diagnosis of incomplete LBBB must be posed with septal fibrosis [49, 50] and with septal myocardial infarction since such diseases can induce the disappearance of Q wave in V_6.

In septal myocardial infarction the T wave is generally inverted in right precordial leads, an uncommon finding in incomplete LBBB.

The differential diagnosis with septal fibrosis is very difficult, and in most cases impossible, because the latter is often responsible for lesions of the left bundle branch. A normal intrinsecoid deflection time in lead V_6 or a clockwise rotation on the F plane of the VCG are very suggestive of a septal fibrosis (see Chapter 6).

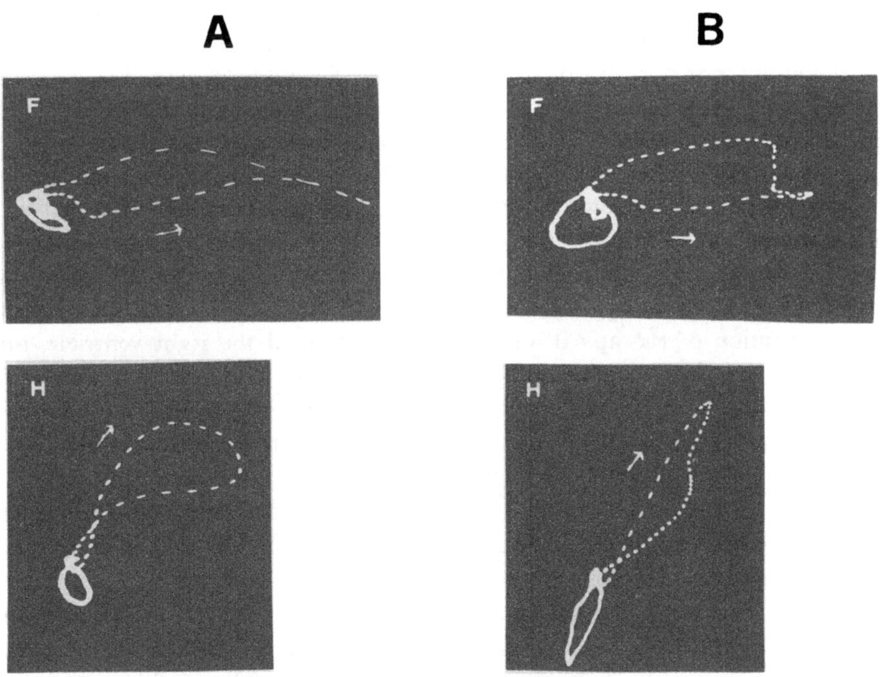

Figure 13. The VCG of the same patient as Figure 12. A: QRS complexes conducted with incomplete LBBB. The first vectors are oriented to the left, anteriorly and inferiorly. The inscription is counterclockwise in frontal plane and clockwise in horizontal plane. A conduction delay is present only in the initial and terminal segments of the QRS loop. B: Typical LBBB.

RIGHT BUNDLE BRANCH BLOCK

Right bundle branch block indicates a delayed activation of the right ventricle as compared to the left ventricle.

According to Sodi-Pallares et al. [4] the impulse spreads normally through the major muscle mass of the septum via the left bundle branch and its ramifications. However, on reaching the transition zone between the portions of the septum activated via the left bundle branch and those activated via the right bundle branch, the excitation impulse is delayed. Once this barrier is jumped by the excitation impulse, the latter activates the right ventricle in a normal fashion. Other authors [51] believe that activation spreads slowly and aberrantly not only in the interventricular septum but also through the right ventricular myocardium in which the Purkinje network is relatively sparse and does not interconnect as in the left ventricle. Thus in RBBB as in LBBB the exact site of the conduction delay is still a controversial subject.

Ventricular activation in RBBB has been schematically divided into four phases [4]. During the first phase (20 msec), since the left branch is intact, the septum is activated normally from left to right. The resultant of initial septal vectors is therefore directed rightward and anteriorly. During the second phase (40 msec) the activation continues in the septum in a left-to-right direction and begins in the apical and anterior portions of the left ventricle. Since the left ventricular potentials are larger thean those produced in the septum, the resultant of the left ventricular and septal vectors is still oriented anteriorly but somewhat leftward. During the third phase (60-80 msec) left-to-right septal activation continues and activation proceeeds through the antero-lateral and basal regions of the left ventricle until it is finally completed in this chamber. For the predominance of the left ventricle the vector is directed leftward, more or less, posteriorly. During the fourth phase (120 msec or more) there is completion of left-to-right septal activation, excitation of the apical and anterior portion of the right ventricle, and finally, activation of the free wall of the remainder of the right ventricle. As activation of the anterior wall occurs after termination of that of the left ventricle, the right terminal vectors are unopposed and oriented, therefore, anteriorly and to the right.

In recent studies carried out in dogs [9] using epicardial mapping, and in man [52], utilizing body surface mapping, this course of ventricular depolarization has been more or less confirmed. The studies show that the onset of right ventricular excitation occurs when the left ventricular activation is for the most part completed. During the first 40 msec, epicardial breakthrough occurs in three areas of the left ventricle, on the anterior and posterior surface. The resulting activation fronts rapidly expand and merge; they result in two wave-fronts invading the right ventricular surface both anteriorly and posteriorly. The wave fronts then advance into the right ventricle and reach the anterior wall and the pulmonary conus. The isochrones are more widely spaced on the posterior side of the right ventricle than anteriorly, indicating a more rapid spread in the posterior wall [9].

ELECTROCARDIOGRAPHIC FEATURES

The following ECG changes are observed in the presence of RBBB:
- QRS interval prolongation to 120 msec or more.
- Electrical axis between 0° and 90°.
- rSR, rsR, R, Rs or Rr morphology, with terminal slurring in right precordial leads.
- Delayed intrinsecoid deflection time in V_1 of 60 msec or more with normal intrinsecoid deflection time in V_5 and V_6.
- Wide and slurred S waves in left-sided leads I, aVL, V_5 and V_6 in as far as the terminal delayed forces are directed rightward.
- Depressed ST segment and interval T wave in right precordial leads due to secondary changes in ventricular repolarization.

VECTORCARDIOGRAPHIC FEATURES

On the F plane the initial vectors are directed rightward and superiorly or inferiorly. The QRS loop is then oriented to the left and inferiorly with clockwise inscription or with figure-of-eight configuration; rarely is the direction of inscription counterclockwise. The maximum QRS vector is directed to the left with a mean value of +25° [53]. The mean voltage is significantly reduced compared to normal, from 1.5 mV to 1 mV [53]. The terminal vectors are slowly inscribed and oriented rightward and inferiorly or superiorly. The ST vector and T loop are generally directed to the left and inferiorly.

On the H plane the initial deflections are normally oriented rightward and anteriorly. It is commonly believed that the RBBB does not alter the instantaneous forces produced during the first 40-50 msec of ventricular depolarization.

Very recently Piccolo et al. [54], recording the VCG of intermittent RBBB and utilizing the extrastimulus method, observed that the 30-40 msec vectors are often shifted anteriorly by RBBB.

In most cases of uncomplicated RBBB the QRS loop is mainly directed to the left, at first anteriorly and later posteriorly with counterclockwise rotation; the afferent limb crosses the midline posterior to E point (Figure 14).

In a few cases the direction of inscription is counterclockwise but the afferent limb is anterior to or through the E point at the midline (Figure 15). The pathophysiology of such development of QRS is not completely clear. Fedor et al. [55] have observed increasing incidences of cardiac failure or severe pulmonary disease

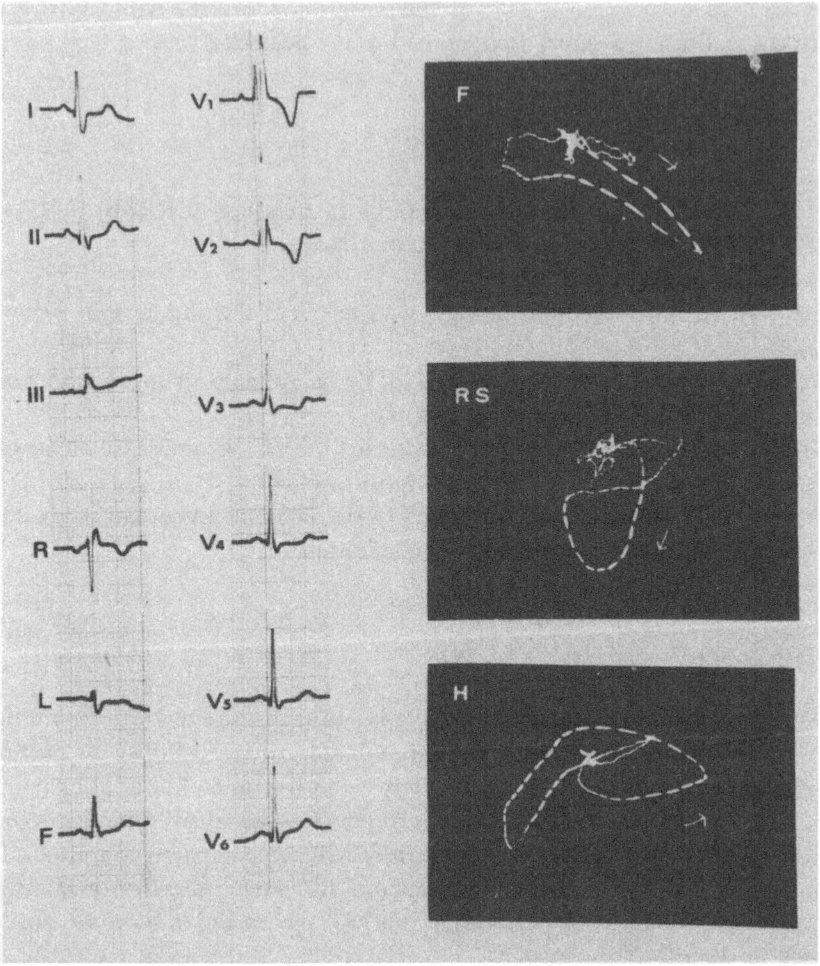

Figure 14. **Typical right bundle branch block. ECG: QRS interval measures 130 msec. In lead V_1, rSR** morphology, delay of intrinsecoid deflection of 90 msec and inverted T wave. Slurred S waves in leads I, aVL, V_5 and V_6. VCG: In horizontal plane the QRS shows counterclockwise rotation. The afferent limb crosses the midline posteriorly to E point. The classical terminal appendage, oriented to the right and anteriorly, is present

in cases of RBBB with anterior-sided afferent limb compared to those with posterior-sided afferent limb.

In some cases the direction of inscription is completely clockwise (Figure 16). Some authors attributed such a rotation to a concomitant RVH [12, 56, 57] or to a posterior myocardial infarction [58, 59]. As a matter of fact, a clockwise rotation in H plane is also observed in patients with RBBB without underlying heart disease. This finding has also been produced in normal hearts by induction of

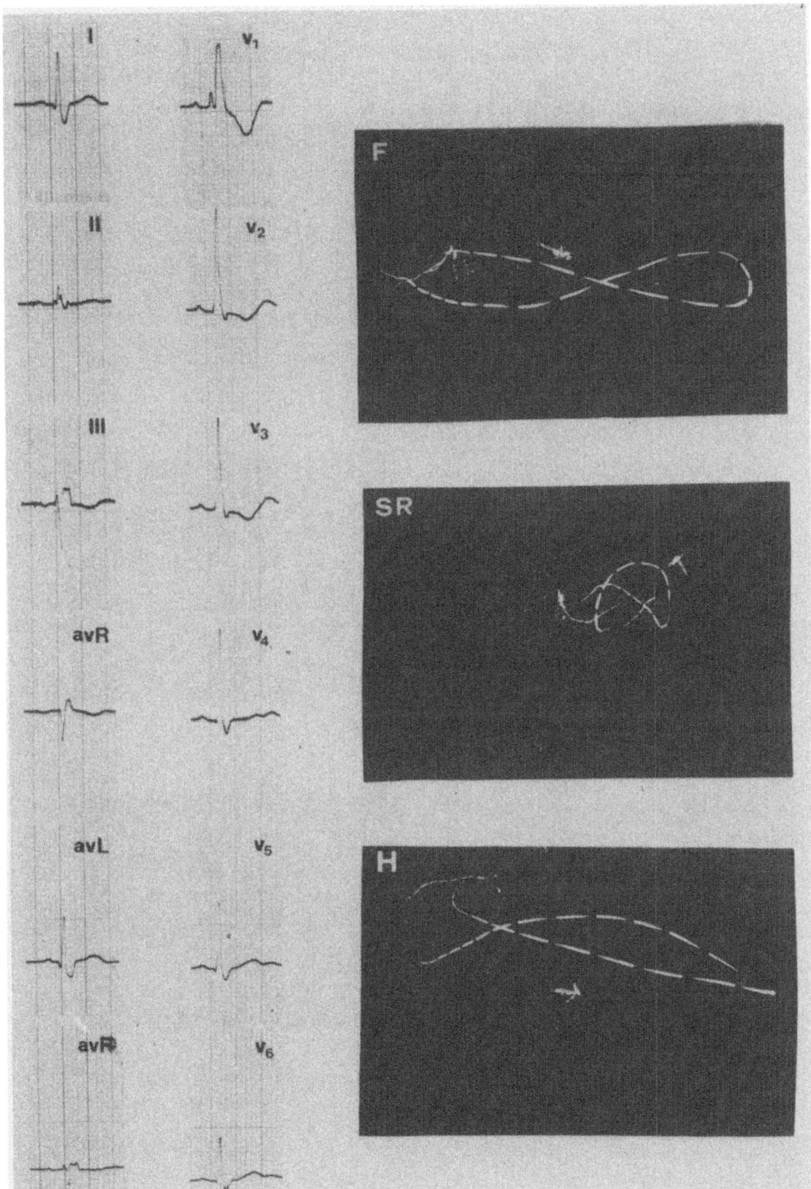

Figure 15. Right bundle branch block pattern. In horizontal plane of the VCG the inscription is counterclockwise, but the afferent limb crosses the midline anteriorly to E point (for details see text)

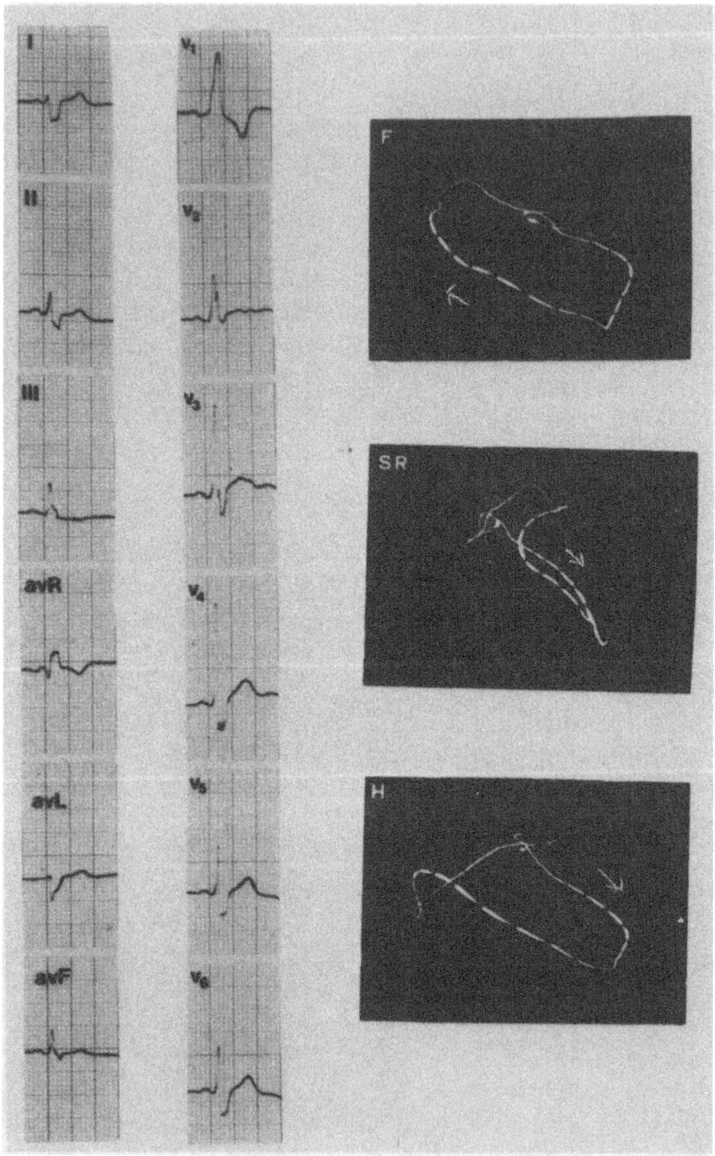

Figure 16. Right bundle branch block pattern. In horizontal plane of the VCG the direction of inscription is clockwise (see text for explanation)

atrial premature beats resulting in aberrant ventricular conduction [60]. Moreover, Kulbertus et al. [61], using the same technique, evidenced in the same patient beats conducted with RBBB with both clockwise and counterclockwise rotation. Therefore, in some cases, the pathophysiology of clockwise inscription in H plane remains unexplained. It is likely that RBBB is associated with a peripheral septal block (see Chapter 6), at times rate-dependent, which determines a delayed excitation of the anterior left septal mass compared to that of the posterior one and consequently a clockwise rotation in H plane.

The direction of the maximal leftward QRS vector has been observed at 0° by Cooksey et al. [62] and at +20° by Chou et al. [53]; the mean voltage is reduced compared to normal from 1.3 mV to 1 mV [53].

The terminal part of the QRS loop is inscribed slowly, with a duration between 40 and 80 msec, and is directed to the right and anteriorly. This characterizes the classical terminal appendage seen in RBBB. The direction of inscription of this appendage can be clockwise, counterclockwise or figure-of-eight. The ST vector and T loop are usually oriented leftward and posteriorly.

On the RS plane most of the QRS loop is directed downward and anteriorly or posteriorly. The inscription can be clockwise, counterclockwise or figure-of-eight. A terminal appendage, oriented anteriorly, superiorly or inferiorly is present, but less evident than in H plane.

DIFFERENTIAL DIAGNOSIS

The diagnosis of RBBB in the majority of cases is easy but this block should be differentiated from conditions inducing anterior shifting of QRS complex.

1) Marked RVH can produce tall R waves in the right precordial leads and an anterior shift of the QRS loop with a clockwise rotation. In this type of RVH, the QRS loop is displaced almost completely to the right with minimal or no terminal delay. The left sided leads show deep but not slurred S wave.
2) Posterior myocardial infarction with a peri-infarction block can show a pattern similar to RBBB in right precordial leads. Again, the terminal delayed appendage is absent in the VCG and slurred S waves are not seen in the leads V_5 and V_6.
3) Peripheral block localized in the anterior wall of the right ventricle can induce delayed terminal forces oriented to the right and anteriorly, and can mimic RBBB [63-65]. There are no definite distinguishing features on ECG and VCG recordings. Within certain limits it is possible to differentiate between the two, introducing an electrode catheter in the right ventricle apex (RVA) and measuring the interval from the beginning of ventricular depolarization to the ventricular electrogram recorded by the catheter in the RVA (V-RVA interval). This interval represents the difference in time between the arrival of impulse at the left septal mass and at the RVA. In the absence of RBBB, V-RVA interval ranges between 15 and 30 msec [66]. Any injury to the main right bundle branch would delay impulse transmission through the right bundle branch to the right ventricular apex and the V-RVA interval would be prolonged. If this interval is

normal in the presence of RBBB pattern, the block has a peripheral localization, most probably in the anterior wall of the right ventricle.

We examined the V-RVA interval in 18 patients with chronic RBBB, unrelated to cardiac surgery (Figure 17). The interval was prolonged in all cases ranging from 40 to 70 msec. These data are similar to those of Castellanos et al. [66] and Kastor et al. [67] and would suggest that in most cases of RBBB, the delay is in the main right bundle branch.

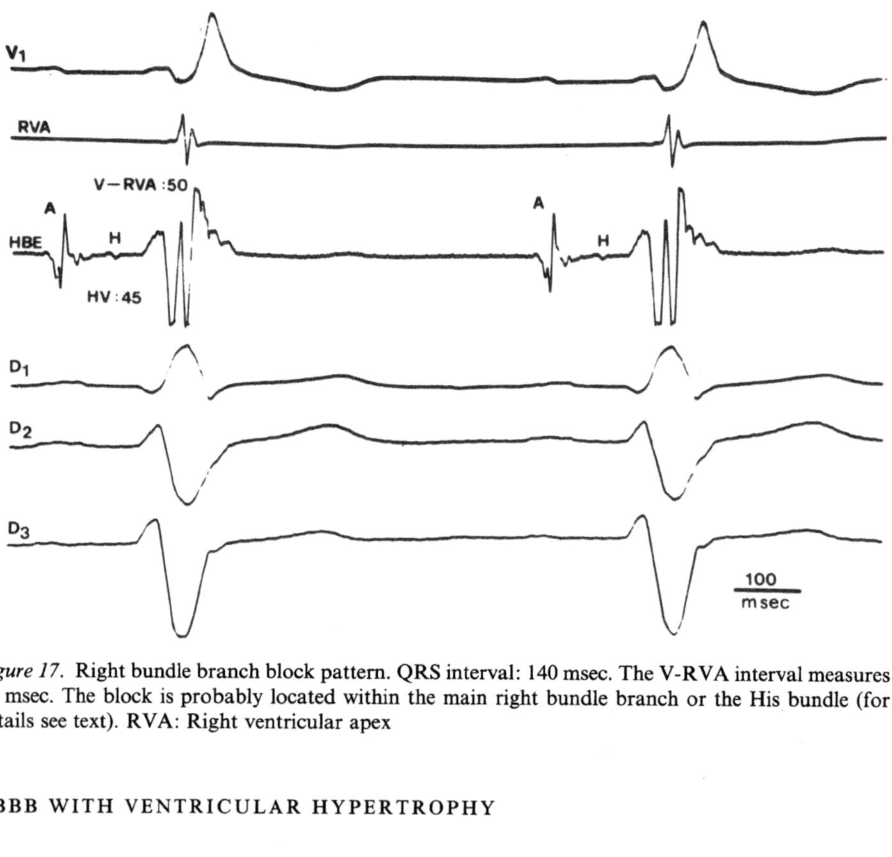

Figure 17. Right bundle branch block pattern. QRS interval: 140 msec. The V-RVA interval measures 50 msec. The block is probably located within the main right bundle branch or the His bundle (for details see text). RVA: Right ventricular apex

RBBB WITH VENTRICULAR HYPERTROPHY

The diagnosis of *left ventricular hypertrophy* in the presence of RBBB is difficult. The commonly used ECG criteria for the diagnosis of LVH [68-70] have limited value in the presence of RBBB with a diagnostic sensitivity of approximately 50 % [71, 72]. The presence of R wave of 20 msec duration or more in V_5 or V_6 is considered to be suggestive of LVH in the presence of RBBB [73], although its validity is yet to be confirmed.

At present there are only a few investigations on the VCG diagnosis of LVH in the presence of RBBB [57, 71-76].

A superior orientation of the QRS loop seems suggestive of LVH [76], as is a posterior displacement of the mid-terminal portions of the QRS loop [57]. However, Murata et al. [77] did not find any correlation between the orientation of the maximum QRS vector and the anatomical findings. In this study, the maximal T angle was found to be a more useful parameter. Although the T loop was directed more posteriorly even in the uncomplicated cases with RBBB than in cases without any conduction abnormalities, the T loop was frequently displaced further posteriorly or sometimes posteriorly and to the right in the presence of LVH.

Recently Holt et al. [72] described a method using 126 ECG leads, referred to as multiple dipole ECG, which increases the diagnostic sensitivity for LVH in the presence of RBBB. The sensitivity index was 93% and the specificity index 96%. However, this method is complicated and cannot be considered at present a routine test.

The diagnosis of *right ventricular hypertrophy* in the presence of RBBB is also difficult. According to Barker et al. [48], RVH can be diagnosed when the R wave in V_1 is greater than 15 mm with such a wave clearly separated by the S wave. Also the R waves recorded in left precordial leads should be relatively small in comparison to the size of the S waves. However, there are many false positive and false negative findings when this criterion is used [71, 78, 79].

In RBBB a qR pattern in lead V_1 is not uncommon; according to Sodi-Pallares et al. [4] such morphology indicates a right atrial enlargement with which in most cases a RVH is associated.

In the vectorcardiogram of uncomplicated RBBB the mid to terminal portion of the loop is slightly posterior to the E point. When RVH and RBBB coexist, the QRS loop is mainly displaced anteriorly and to the right with clockwise rotation [55, 57]. However, as mentioned before, anterior displacement of the QRS loop with clockwise rotation can be present also in uncomplicated RBBB; therefore the question of RBBB can only be posed when the QRS loop is markedly displaced to the right.

Recently, Brohet et al. [79] proposed the following criteria for the diagnosis of RVH associated with RBBB:

- Clockwise rotation of the QRS loop in the H plane.
- r/S ratio in lead X of less than 2.0.
- Mean QRS vector in lead X more negative than $-10°$.
- Maximal vector located between 90° and 270° in the H plane.

This study has certain limitations since it was performed on VCGs taken from a group of young patients with surgically induced RBBB block; it may not therefore be applicable in older patients.

INCOMPLETE RIGHT BUNDLE BRANCH BLOCK

Incomplete RBBB pattern can occur not only in relation to slowing of conduction in the right bundle branch, but also to peripheral conduction disturbance in the presence or absence of RVH. At present reliable ECG and VCG criteria to evaluate the localization of the block (see Chapter 6) do not exist.

Incomplete RBBB is characterized in the ECG by a rSr or rSR morphology in lead V_1 with a QRS duration of 100-120 msec. The left sided leads show slurred S waves.

The vectorcardiographic signs of the incomplete RBBB are (Figure 18):

- Clockwise rotation or figure-of-eight morphology in F plane and counterclockwise rotation in H plane.
- Initial forces normally directed to the right, anteriorly, inferiorly or superiorly.
- Delayed terminal forces, oriented rightward and anteriorly but sometimes posteriorly. At times the classical pattern with terminal appendage is present.
- The ST vector and T loop appear normal or with slight changes.

A recent work by Piccolo et al. [54], using VCG recordings obtained with premature atrial stimuli, demonstrated that an incomplete RBBB can be expressed only by an anterior displacement of the QRS loop without significant shifting to the right of the terminal vectors (Figure 19). Such an anterior displacement, also seen in posterior myocardial infarction, always preceded the appearance of RBBB. It is thus believed by these authors that such findings represent a variant form of incomplete RBBB. In previous studies it was hypothesized that the isolated anterior displacement of the QRS complex was related to an intraventricular conduction disturbance localized in the anterior wall of the left ventricle [80, 81] or in the middle fascicle [82].

ALTERNATING BUNDLE BRANCH BLOCK

Alternating bundle branch block (ABBB) or complete bilateral bundle branch block can be diagnosed when conducted beats with both RBBB and LBBB patterns are seen in the same patient, either in the same or different electrocardiograms (Figures 20 and 21). The ABBB is a rare electrocardiographic pattern. In some cases the alternation in the bundle branch pattern is associated with a change in the PR interval and in other cases the PR interval remains unchanged [22, 83-85]. In three out of seven cases studied by Wu et al. [86], a shift in the bundle branch pattern was accompanied by a variation in the HV interval.

Shift from one bundle branch block pattern to the other can be induced by change in heart rate or by premature atrial beats, which cause a variation in the refractory period of the bundle branches. If the cycle length of spontaneous sinus rhythm is close to the refractory period of the two bundle branches, beats with both left and right bundle branch pattern can be seen [86].

It must be pointed out that in order to observe an ABBB pattern, at least one of the two bundle branch blocks must be incomplete, otherwise a complete atrioventricular block would result.

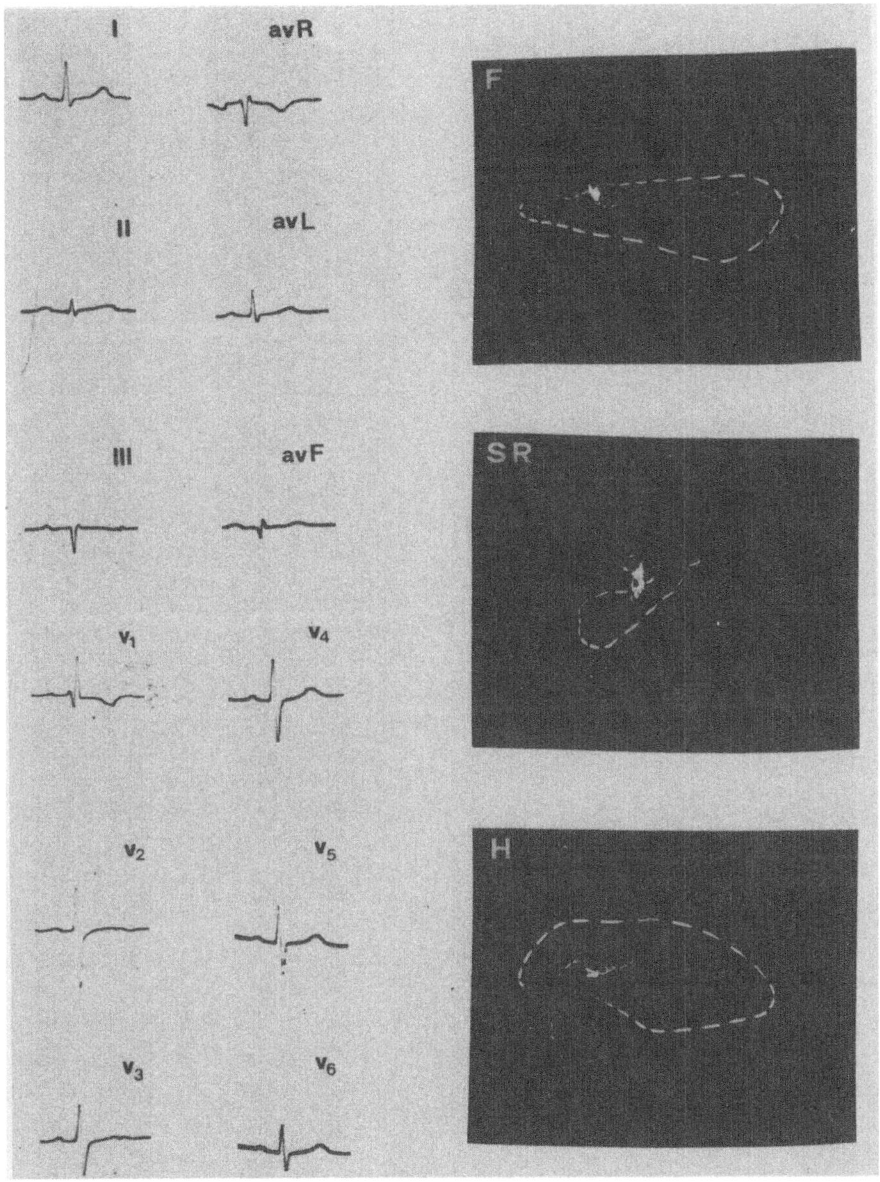

Figure 18. Incomplete right bundle branch block. QRS complex measures 110 msec. rsR morphology in lead V_1. In horizontal plane of the VCG a terminal delay, directed to the right and slightly anteriorly, is present

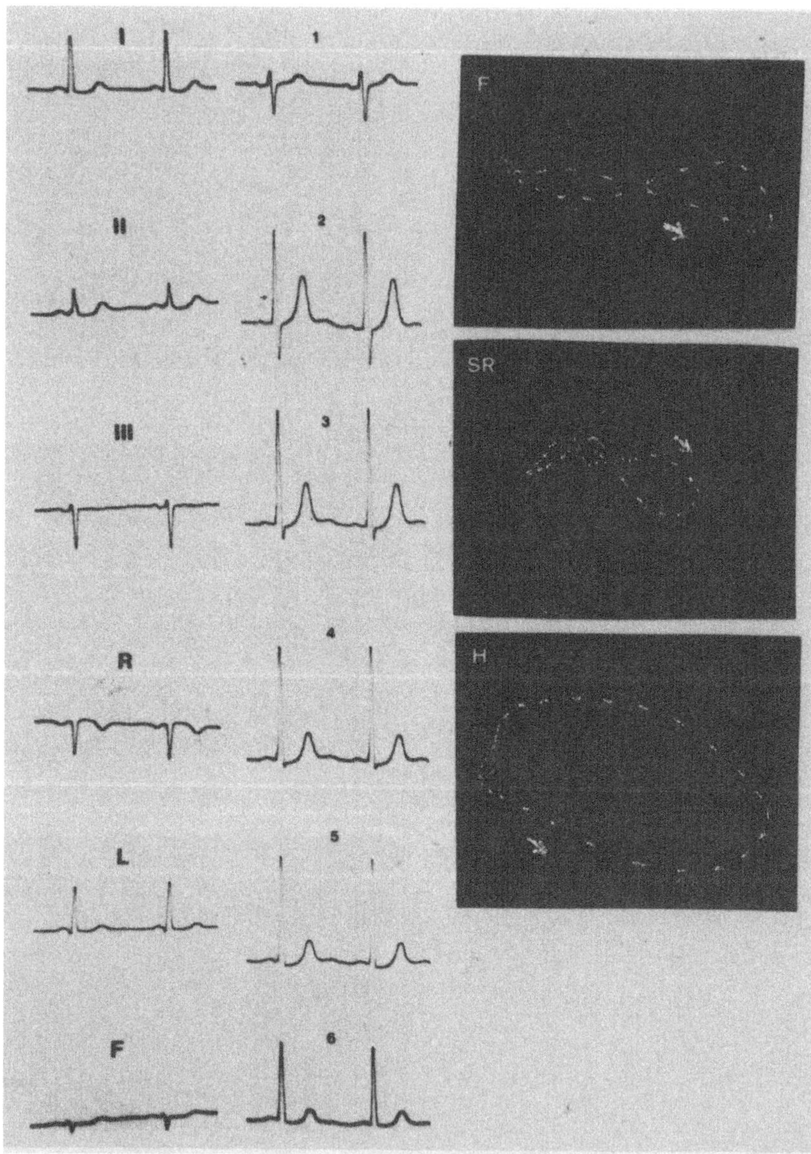

Figure 19. ECG: Tall R waves in leads V_2-V_3. In leads I, aVL, V_5 and V_6 S waves are not present. VCG: In horizontal plane the QRS loop is displaced to the left and mainly anteriorly. This pattern may represent a variant form of incomplete right bundle branch block (for details see text)

Recent studies have suggested that **ABBB** may reflect a lesion involving the distal His bundle and proximal bundle branches [21, 87, 88].

When both ECG and electrophysiological data are available, bilateral bundle branch block can be suspected under the following circumstances:

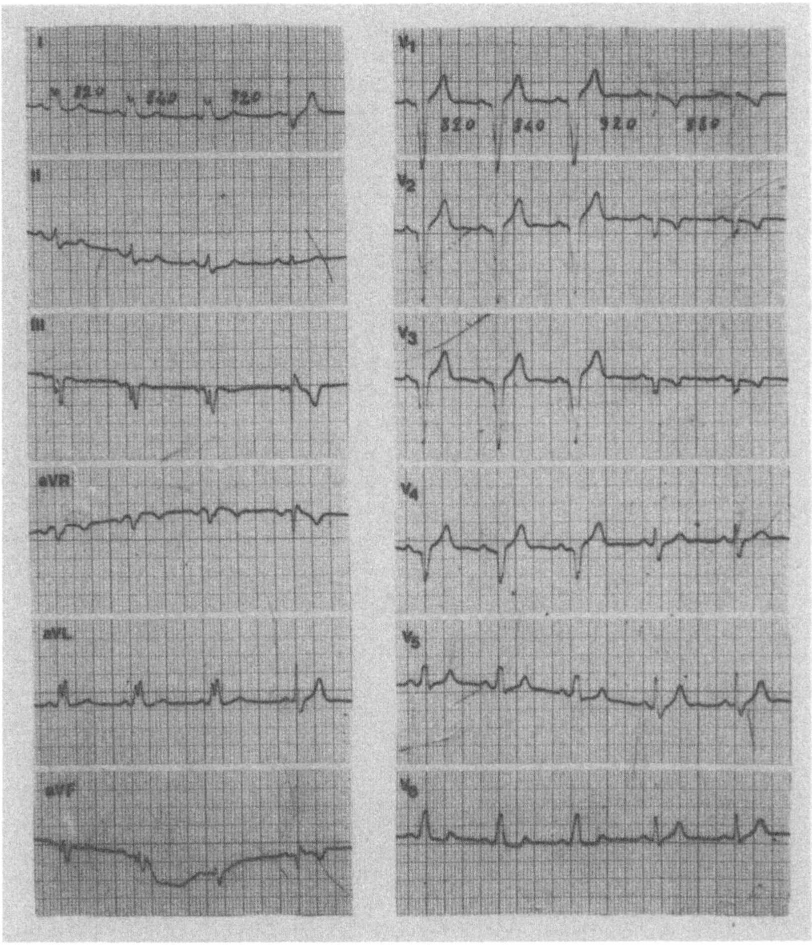

Figure 20. Alternating bundle branch block. Conducted periods of left bundle branch block and incomplete right bundle branch block are present. The PR interval does not change with the alternation of one bundle branch block pattern with another. The incomplete RBBB pattern appears when the sinus cycle length is prolonged more than 900 msec

- Prolonged HV interval with narrow QRS complex (Figure 22). This may indicate either a slow conduction in the His bundle or incomplete block in both the bundle branches.
- Bundle branch block pattern with prolonged HV interval. This may indicate impaired conduction within the controlateral bundle or the His bundle (Figure 23).
- Bundle branch block with second degree atrioventricular block below the AV node. Again, the block can occur in the His bundle or in the controlateral branch (Figure 24).

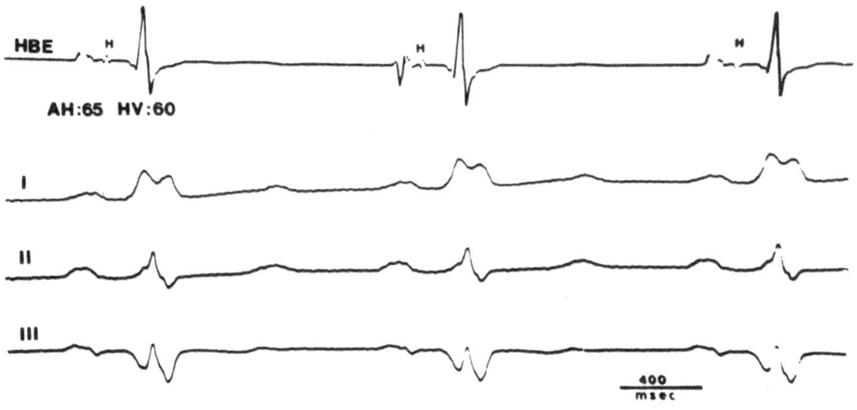

Figure 21. His bundle recording of the same patients as Figure 20. The conducted beats show LBBB pattern. The HV interval measures 60 msec. During the electrophysiological study, beats conducted with incomplete RBBB pattern did not appear

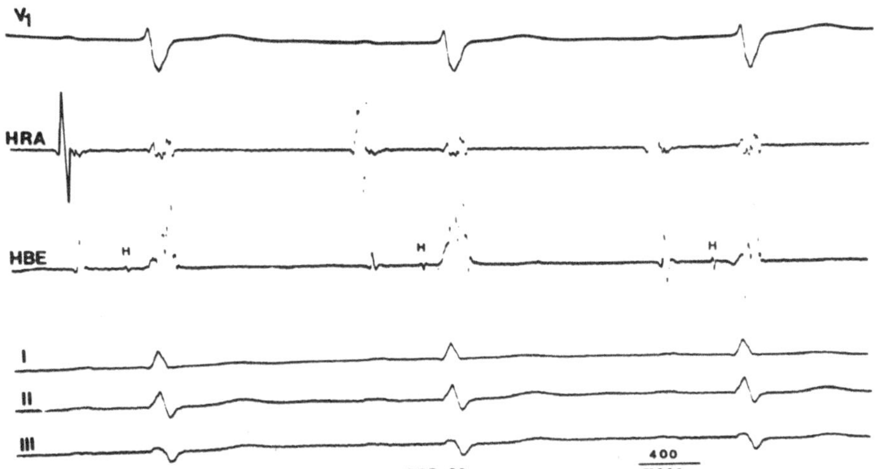

Figure 22. The QRS complex is narrow (90 msec). The HV interval is prolonged (60 msec). Such a pattern may indicate an incomplete block of both bundle branches or a conduction delay within the His bundle

- Complete atrioventricular block with block distal to His, the substitutive rhythm having a wide QRS morphology.

PATHOLOGICAL CORRELATIONS

A good correlation between the electrocardiographic and histological data has

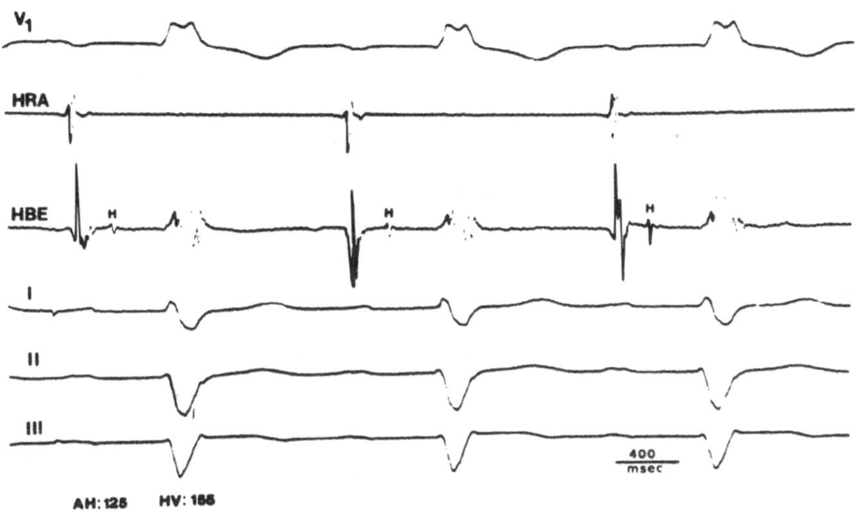

Figure 23. Right bundle branch block pattern. The HV interval is prolonged (155 msec). This pattern may indicate a conduction delay within the left bundle branch or the His bundle

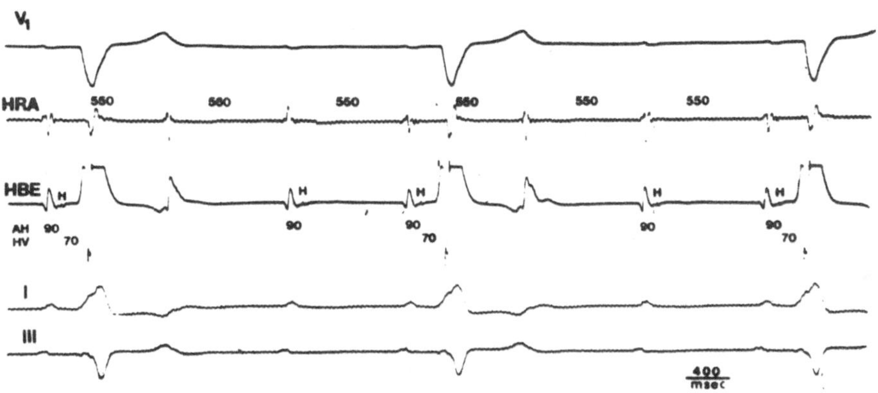

Figure 24. 3:1 atrio-ventricular block distal to His bundle. The conducted beats show LBBB pattern and an HV interval of 70 msec. The 3:1 block can be localized in the right bundle branch or in the His bundle. H wave following the conducted beats is not evident in as far it is superimposed by a ventricular repolarization wave

been found in most patients with LBBB. Visioli et al. [89] investigated four cases, three of which exhibited severe damage to the left bundle branch. Baragan et al. [90] observed significant lesions in the left bundle branch in 44 out of 48 case with LBBB pattern. Sugura et al. [91] found excellent correlation with lesions of left bundle branch in eight cases. Rossi [92], in a postmortem study of five patients with LBBB, observed LVH and marked coronary atherosclerosis in all patients. Significant alterations of the left bundle branch, i.e. sclerosis, inflammation or amyloidosis, were found in four cases, whereas in one case the left branch was fairly well preserved. Lev et al. [93] in a study of eight cases observed a very good correlation between the ECG and histological changes in the left bundle. There was a predilection for the lesions to occur at the origin of the left bundle branch from the His bundle and at the summit of the interventricular septum.

Recently, Bharati et al. [94] performed an anatomo-electrophysiological correlation in four patients with LBBB and prolonged HV interval. In all cases histopathological abnormalities were found in both left bundle branch system and main right bundle branch.

The correlation between the ECG and histological findings in the presence of incomplete LBBB has not been studied extensively. Lenegre [63] found significant lesions of the left bundle branch in 32 out of 37 cases. This author stressed the importance of both the mechanical injury and the pathological involvement of common myocardium of the interventricular septum and left free wall in the etiology of the ECG changes in incomplete LBBB.

Again in the presence of RBBB pattern, good correlation exists between the ECG and histopathological changes. Lev et al. [95] in their study of nine patients with RBBB, observed histopathological alterations in the right bundle branch in all. Lenegre [63] compared the ECG pattern and anatomic changes in 25 cases: in 16 there was total interruption, in eight subtotal disruption and in one partial lesion of the right bundle branch. Rossi [92], in an attempt to localize the lesion in six cases, found that the upper tract was mainly involved in three, the mimetic tract in one and widespread lesions were found in one. Lenegre [63] examined 33 cases of incomplete RBBB and stated that the right bundle branch was significantly altered in eight and normal or subnormal in the remainder. Marked RVH was present in 31 cases and seemed to play an important role in determining the ECG pattern of this type of block. Isokane et al. [96], on the other hand, observed severe lesions in five out of six patients with incomplete RBBB pattern.

In the few histological studies in patients with ABBB, destructive lesions involving the His bundle and both bundle branches were observed [97, 98].

Rossi [92], after analysis of all cases reported in the literature, found that out of 125 cases with both LBBB and RBBB, 67 % showed, in postmortem examination, complete disruption of the bundle branch, 20 % evidenced partial disruption, 4 % slight damage and 9 % showed no significant damage. On the contrary, in the presence of incomplete BBB pattern (left and right), no significant damage to the bundle branch could be demonstrated.

The etiology of the bundle branch block is variable. Lenegre [98] found coronary atherosclerosis in only 25 % of his cases with BBB. He therefore believes that the fibrosis of the conduction system is often 'primary' in nature. According to Lev et al. [95, 98], the lesions of the interventricular conduction system are considered to be due to both direct ischemia and to fibrosis of the summit of the ventricular septum mechanically injuring the bundle branches. Knieriem et al. [99]

were doubtful as to the existence of 'primary' bundle branch blocks, considering coronary atherosclerosis by far the more important etiologic factor. Rossi [92, 100] believes that an altered venous and lymphatic circulation (in the region of the trigonum fibrosum) can offer an alternative explanation to the fibrotic damage to the bundle branches. In fact an impaired venous and/or lymphatic drainage may increase the interstitial pressure and induce eventually atrophy of myocardial fibers and collagenous replacement of the soft tissue.

A complex problem is represented by the discrepancy, evidenced in several cases among the ECG and histological data. The absence of an ECG pattern of a bundle branch block in cases where marked lesions are present in one bundle branch may be explained by the presence of lesions in the controlateral bundle branch [89, 92].

In a few cases, in the presence of an ECG pattern of bundle branch block, no lesions were found in the histological examination. It should be noted that the His bundle was not completely examined in all the studies; in this regard it is now certain that lesions in the His bundle may induce a bundle branch block pattern [21, 87, 88, 101]. One must also consider the possibility of metabolic and biochemical changes such as the etiological factors.

CLINICAL DATA

LBBB

LBBB appears to be extremely rare in young and healthy subjects. Siegman-Igra [102], in a study of Israeli adult males, found an incidence of LBBB of 0.12%. Among aircraft personnel the incidence of LBBB is between 0.02% and 0.05% [103-105]. For some unknown reason, the incidence of such block in the Tecumseh population is high, 0.2% [106]. In elderly and symptomatic patients the frequency of LBBB is higher, 1.0 to 1.2% [1, 107]. LBBB is two to three times more frequent in men than women [63]. The most common causes of LBBB are considered to be hypertensive and coronary heart disease. Graybiel et al. [108] reviewed 395 cases with LBBB; most had coronary or hypertensive heart disease. 118 patients had congestive heart failure, 59 had angina pectoris and 12 had Morgagni-Adam-Stokes attacks. A follow-up of 77% of the total group revealed 223 fatal cases with an average life span of 14 months. Campbell et al. [109] followed 50 patients with LBBB (48 had some form of cardiovascular disease); 39 patients died with a mean survival time of 2 years. Messer et al. [110] in a review of 555 patients with LBBB, reported a mean survival of 3.3 years. It should be noted that these studies were carried out in hospitalized patients. However, when LBBB was discovered on routine ECG, the incidence of both coronary and hypertensive heart disease seems lower [36, 102, 103, 105, 111-115]. Lewis et al. [116] reported on 12 patients with LBBB out of a total study population of 366. Only four of these 12 patients had coronary heart disease. Coronarographic studies were performed by Dizadji et al. [117], on 464 patients, 26 of whom had LBBB; only 11 (42%) out of the 26 had coronary atherosclerosis. Similarly, only one out of nine patients with LBBB, studied by Herbert [118] had coronary artery disease (CAD). It appears that this disease is not a significant etiological factor of the LBBB, a statement supported by some anatomical studies. It was inferred that acquired LBBB is frequently associated with a good prognosis in the asymptomatic patients [102, 103, 105], although a greater incidence of sudden death, compared to asymptomatic patients without such intraventricular block, has been encountered [119-121].

Rare causes of LBBB include heart valve disease, particularly aortic valve disease, myocarditis, idiopathic cardiomyopathy, cor pulmonale, electrolyte abnormalities and myxedema [1, 30, 45, 122, 123]. Myocardial infarction can acutely induce LBBB and this will be discussed in Chapter 8.

The clinical significance of marked LAD in patients with LBBB is controversial. Most authors [13, 17, 36, 124, 125] found a high incidence of myocardial dysfunction. The following clinical variables were more frequent in patients with LBBB and LAD [125]: advanced age, exertional angina, congestive heart failure, cardiomegaly, functional class II-IV and coronary heart disease. The mean HV interval was more prolonged in patients with LBBB and LAD.

A few studies [121, 126, 127] have reported no significant clinical or electrophysiological differences between patients with LBBB and LAD and patients with LBBB and normal axis.

LBBB with RAD seems to imply marked myocardial damage. All the patients reported by Tranchesi et al. [25] and Laham et al. [17] had congestive heart failure. We studied 11 patients with LBBB and RAD without any evidence of myocardial infarction [26]. Four had coronary heart disease, four hypertensive heart disease, one myocarditis, one aortic stenosis, and one idiopathic cardiomyopathy. All of them had pulmonary emphysema and cardiomegaly, thus showing the presence of myocardial damage.

Besides axis deviation, the QRS duration also seems to condition the prognosis of patients with LBBB. Johnson et al. [123], studying LBBB in patients with relatively severe heart disease, observed that survival was inversely proportional to QRS duration, which they believed reflected the severity of the heart disease. On the contrary, for persons without apparent heart disease the QRS duration was not a powerful prognostic factor.

RBBB

The incidence of RBBB was found to be low among healthy individuals, ranging from 0.15% to 0.29% [104, 105, 128, 129].

Among symptomatic subjects, usually in the out-patient population, the frequency of RBBB is about 1.1-3.1% [98, 113].

RBBB is 3-5 times more common in men than in women and is frequently found with the absence of symptoms. In a study by Rotman et al. [105] 97% of 372 patients with RBBB were completely asymptomatic at the time of evaluation; significant CAD was found in only 6% of patients.

However, in hospitalized populations, the clinical meaning is different. Perera et al. [130] studied 104 cases with RBBB. Of 91 cases with adequate follow up, one third had died over a mean follow up period of 4 years. Over 95% of these patients had some form of heart disease. Ischemic etiology may play a less important role in patients with RBBB compared to those with LBBB. In the study by Rotman et al. [105] the incidence of ischemic heart disease was 5% and 16% respectively in RBBB and LBBB.

RBBB is not uncommon in hypertensive heart disease; it is most likely due to subclinical coronary disease or to mechanical stress on the fibrous structures adjacent to the conduction system [1]. RBBB is rarely observed in mitral valve disease or in cor pulmonale [131]. However, it is quite frequently found in aortic valve disease; in fact the lesions of the aortic valve or of the base of the aorta may extend directly into the conduction system and cause RBBB.

A familial incidence of BBB (right or left) has been described. The familial blocks occur in two forms, congenital and adult onset [132]. In the latter form, they often begin as incomplete, then progress to advanced degree BBB. In some cases the mode of inheritance is autosomal dominance [133-135].

The incomplete RBBB is frequently observed in right ventricular enlargement, usually with diastolic overload. Also in experimental studies in animals, ventricular dilatation was demonstrated to cause incomplete RBBB, most probably because of stretching of the right bundle branch [136, 137]. This block can also be seen in acute or chronic cor pulmonale and mitral valve disease, as well as hypertensive and coronary heart disease. Incomplete RBBB is, however, very common in young subjects without any heart disease, probably due to physiological delay in conduction in the postero-basal wall of the right ventricle [63].

Thus the clinical significance of BBB, right or left, complete or incomplete, depends on the underlying heart disease.

The problem of the progression of bundle branch blocks to complete heart block distal to His bundle will be discussed in Chapter 11.

COMMENT

The pathophysiology of bundle branch blocks still presents certain obscure points. In particular it is not clear whether the main conduction delay takes place in the septum or in the left ventricular walls.

At times LBBB pattern is observed with marked initial slurring of the QRS complex, at times only with middle slurring without initial delay. In our opinion, it is likely that in the former the main conduction delay is localized in the septum and in the latter in the ventricular walls. Also, the pathophysiology of some atypical LBBB patterns such as the homophasic one and the LBBB with displacement towards the left of the transition zone, remain in part obscure.

In LBBB the changes of left ventricular activation induce abnormalities of left ventricular contraction, which has been found to be delayed [126, 138]. Some authors [7, 118, 139] have also observed an asynchronous contraction, mainly related to an apical emptying delay.

In patients with intermittent LBBB the appearance of intraventricular block induces a reduction in systolic pressure, cardiac output and left ventricular contractility [138, 140]. Ventricular wall motion has also been investigated with contrast ventriculography in patients with LBBB without underlying heart disease and the results appear contradictory. Williams et al. [141] observed in about half of their cases segmental wall motion abnormalities which were not confirmed by Wong et al. [142]. The reasons for such discrepancy do not appear clear. However echocardiographic studies demonstrated asynergy of the interventricular septum in patients with LBBB without signs of heart disease [143, 144]; this finding also seems to stress the possibility of contraction abnormalities in patients with LBBB without manifestation of cardiac disease.

It is commonly thought that RBBB alters only the terminal phases of ventricular depolarization. Instead it was recently demonstrated [54] that the first 30-40 msec vectors can also be anteriorly shifted. At present the reason for this shifting is not clear.

Also inexplicable to a great extent is the presence of clockwise rotation of horizontal QRS loop in subjects with RBBB without underlying heart disease. This is possibly the coexistence of a peripheral septal block, sometimes rate-dependent, which induces a delayed excitation of the anterior part of the left septum, and consequently a clockwise rotation of the H loop.

The ECG and VCG recordings do not allow an evaluation of the anatomical localization of a bundle branch block pattern (right or left), which can take place within the His bundle, the bundle branches or the peripheral subdivisions. In some cases of LBBB, by means of selective His bundle stimulation, it is possible to localize the site of the block within the His bundle (Figure 5). The utility of this technique in order to localize the lesion of a RBBB appears uncertain at present, in that a right septum pacing could normalize a LBBB pattern, even if His bundle is not selectively stimulated [22, 145].

In the presence of an RBBB pattern by the evaluation of the V-RVA interval it is possible to exclude a peripheral localization of the block, but not to state whether the lesion is situated within the His bundle or the right bundle branch.

The problem of the localization of a bundle branch block is not purely speculative, as it is extremely likely that the more proximal the seat of the block, the more the latter is likely to progress to complete heart block distal to His bundle.

In this connection, the evaluation of conduction of the remaining His-Purkinje system (HV interval) appears particularly useful (see Chapter 11). In patients with LBBB, HV interval has been found prolonged in 50-80% of cases [22, 146-150], whereas in patients with RBBB and normal axis, only in 30% [22]. These data suggest that LBBB expresses a more widespread involvement of intraventricular conduction system and/or a more frequent involvement of His bundle.

The clinical significance of bundle branch blocks is still uncertain since such blocks can coexist in normal hearts and in greatly compromised hearts. However, it should be noted that the incomplete LBBB and the LBBB with marked axis deviation are very rarely observed in patients with a normal heart.

We therefore believe that patients with BBB without underlying heart disease must also be periodically checked, not only because these blocks may represent the first sign of sublinical heart disease, but also because they may progress to complete AV block distal to His bundle.

REFERENCES

1. Rosenbaum MB, Elizari MU, Lazzari JO: Los hemibloques. Buenos Aires: Ed. Paidos, 1968
2. Cannom DS, Goldreyer BN, Damato AN: Atrioventricular conduction system in left bundle branch block with normal QRS axis. Circulation 46: 129, 1972
3. Rodriguez MI, Sodi-Pallares D: The mechanism of complete and incomplete bundle branch block. Am Heart J 44: 715, 1952
4. Sodi-Pallares D, Calder RM: New bases of electrocardiography. St. Louis: CW Mosby, 1956
5. Sodi-Pallares D, Bisteni A, Testelli MR, Medrano GA: Ventricular activation and the vectorcardiogram in bundle branch blocks: clinical and experimental studies with a critical appraisal of the vectorcardiographic methods of Frank and Grishman. Circ Res 9: 1098, 1961
6. Kennamer R, Prinzmetal M: Depolarization of the ventricle with bundle branch block: X. Studies on the mechanism of ventricular activity. Am Heart J 47: 769, 1954
7. Becker RA, Scher AM, Erickson RD: Ventricular excitation in experimental left bundle branch block. Am Heart J 55: 547, 1958
8. Walston A, Boineau JP, Spach MS, Ayers CR, Estes EH Jr: Relationship between ventricular depolarization and QRS in right and left bundle branch block. J Electrocardiol 1: 155, 1968
9. Van Dam RTh: Ventricular activation in human and canine bundle branch block. In: The conduction system of the heart. Structure, function and clinical implications, Wellens HJJ, Lie KI, Janse MJ. Leiden: Stenfert Kroese, 1976, p 377
10. Wyndham CRC, Smith T, Meeran MK, Mammana R, Levitsky S, Rosen KM: Epicardial activation in patients with left bundle branch block. Circulation 61: 696, 1980
11. De Micheli A, Medrano GA: Electrocardiograma y vectocardiograma. Mexico: La Prensa Medica Mexicana, 1971
12. Kennedy RJ, Varriale P, Alfenito JC: Textbook of vectorcardiography. New York: Harper & Row, 1970

13. Blondeau M: Le bloc complet de la branche gauche avec forte déviation axiale gauche de QRS. I. Etude clinique. Arch Mal Coeur 67: 621, 1974
14. Pryor B, Blount SG Jr: The clinical significance of true left axis deviation. Left intraventricular blocks. Am Heart J 72: 391, 1966
15. Warembourg H, Lekieffre J, Thery CL: Blocs pariétaux et blocs peri-infarctus. Leur responsabilité dans l'apparition des blocs auriculo-ventriculaires. Coeur et Med Intern 9: 35, 1970
16. Lichstein E, Mahapatra R, Gupta PK, Chadda KD: Significance of complete left bundle branch block with left axis deviation. Am J Cardiol 44: 239, 1979
17. Laham J, Gerbaux A: Les blocs de branche gauche atypiques. Ann Cardiol Angiol 23: 1, 1974
18. Alboni P, Malacarne C: Problemi di asincronismo fascicolare nel blocco di branca sinistro avanzato con marcata deviazione assiale sinistra. G Ital Cardiol 6: 255, 1976
19. Marquez-Montes J, Juffe A, Artaza M, Castillo-Olivares LJ: Bloqueo de rama izquierda troncular asociato a bloqueo periférico de rama derecha. Estudio experimental en perros. Rev Esp Cardiol 28: 399, 1975
20. Warembourg H, Thery CL, Pauchant M, Lekieffre J, Ketelers JY: Les hyperdéviations de ÂQRS d'origine extracardiaque (Etude expérimentale. Considérations sur l'emphysème). Arch Mal Coeur 64: 1295, 1971
21. Narula OS: Longitudinal dissociation in the His bundle. Bundle branch block due to asynchronous conduction within the His bundle in man. Circulation 56: 996, 1977
22. Narula OS: Intraventricular conduction defects: current concepts and clinical significance. In: Cardiac arrhythmias. Electrophysiology, diagnosis and management, Narula OS. Baltimore: Williams & Wilkins, 1979, p 114
23. Lepeschkin E: Modern electrocardiography, Vol 1. The P-Q-R-S-T-U complex. Baltimore: Williams & Wilkins, 1951
24. Chou TC, Helm RA: The diagnosis of right ventricular hypertrophy in the presence of left bundle branch block. In: Vectorcardiography 2, Hoffman I, Hamby RI, Glassman E. Amsterdam: North-Holland, 1971, p 289
25. Tranchesi J, Moffa P, Ebaid M: Right axis deviation in left bundle branch block. An electro-vectorcardiographic study. In: Vectorcardiography 2, Hoffman I, Hamby RI, Glassman E. Amsterdam: North-Holland, 1971, p 283
26. Alboni P, Longhini C, Malacarne C, Giovannini G: Il blocco di branca sinistro con asse elettrico deviato a destra. Studio clinico ed elettro-vettocardiografico. G Ital Cardiol 5: 543, 1975
27. Neuman J, Blackaller J, Tobin JR, Szanto PB, Gunnar RM: The spatial vectorcardiogram in left bundle branch block. Am J Cardiol 16: 352, 1965
28. Doucet P, Walsh TJ, Massie E: A vectorcardiographic and electrocardiographic study of left bundle branch block with myocardial infarction. Am J Cardiol 17: 171, 1966
29. Cordeiro A: Contribucao para o estudo da syndrome de Wolff-Parkinson-White. Dissertation, Lisbon, 1947
30. Zuckermann R, Estandia A, Zamora J, Barbato E: Cor pulmonale agudo. Arch Inst Cardiol Mex 18: 582, 1948
31. Medrano GA, Brenes PC, De Micheli A, Sodi-Pallares D: El bloqueo simultaneo de los subdivisiones arterior y posterior de la rama izquierda del haz de His (bloqueo bifascicular) y su asociacion con bloqueo de la rama derecha (bloqueo trifascicular). Arch Inst Cardiol Mex 40: 752, 1970
32. Alboni P, Malacarne C, Baggioni GF, Masoni A: Left bifascicular block with normally conducting middle fascicle. J Electrocardiol 10: 401, 1977
33. Taccola A, Fulle F, Straneo G: Contributo alla conoscenza del blocco di branca

omofasico. Min Cardioangiol 11: 395, 1963
34. Giorgetti C, Pistelli G: I blocchi di branca. La Medicina Internazionale 73: 1, 1965
35. Blondeau M: Les blocs de branche intermittents. Ann Cardiol Angiol 24: 499, 1975
36. Beach TB, Grace JG, Peter RH: Benign left bundle branch block. Ann Intern Med 70: 269, 1969
37. Tavazzi L, Salerno JA, Bobba P: Meccanismo e implicazioni cliniche degli emiblocchi e dei blocchi di branca intermittenti. Boll Soc Ital Cardiol XXXV Italian Meeting of Cardiology, 1974, p 235
38. Denes P, Pick A, Miller RH, Pietras RJ, Rosen KM: A characteristic precordial repolarization abnormality in patients with intermittent left bundle branch block. Ann Intern Med 89: 55, 1978
39. Engle TR, Shah R, De Podesta LA, Frankl WS, Krause RL: T-wave abnormalities of intermittent left bundle branch block. Ann Intern Med 89: 204, 1978
40. Abben R, Rosen KM, Denes P: Intermittent left bundle branch block: anatomic as reflected in the electrocardiogram during normal conduction. Circulation 59: 1040, 1979
41. Chatterjee K, Harris AM, Davies JG, Leatham A: Electrocardiographic changes subsequent to artificial ventricular depolarization. Br Heart J 31: 770, 1969
42. Gola E, Arosio G, Riva S, Rusconi C: Alterazioni delle ripolarizzazioni correlate con l'elettrostimolazione endocavitaria destra. G Ital Cardiol 2: 257, 1972
43. Antonioli GE, Alboni P, Baggioni GF, Fischer D: Sulle alterazioni della ripolarizzazione nell'elettrocardiogramma spontaneo susseguente a stimolazione endocavitaria permanente. Cardiol Prat 25: 275, 1974
44. Goldman MJ: Principles of clinical electrocardiography, 5th edn. Oxford: Blackwell, 1964
45. Friedberg CK: Diseases of the heart, 3rd edn. Philadelphia: WB Saunders, 1966
46. Lipman BS, Massie E, Kleiger RE: Clinical scalar electrocardiography, 6th edn. Chicago: Year Book Medical Publishers, 1972
47. Cokkinos DV, Demopoulos JN, Hemonas ET, Mallios C, Papazoglou N, Vorides EM: Electrocardiographic criteria of left ventricular hypertrophy in left bundle branch block. Br Heart J 40: 320, 1978
48. Barker JM: The unipolar electrocardiogram: a clinical interpretation. New York: Appleton-Century-Crofts, 1952
49. Burch GE: An electrocardiographic syndrome characterized by absence of Q in leads I, V_5 and V_6. Am Heart J 51: 487, 1956
50. Alboni P, Malacarne C, Masoni A: Physiopathological and diagnostic hypotheses in peripheral block. J Electrocardiol 10: 87, 1977
51. Dodge HT, Grant RP: Mechanisms of QRS complex prolongation in man: right ventricular conduction defects. Am J Med 21: 534, 1956
52. Sugenoya J, Sugiyama S, Wada M, Niimi N, Oguri H, Toyama J, Yamada K: Body surface potential distribution following the production of right bundle branch block in dogs: effects of breakthrough and right ventricular excitation on the body surface potentials. Circulation 55: 49, 1977
53. Chou TC, Helm RA, Kaplan S: Clinical vectorcardiography, 2nd edn. New York: Grune & Stratton, 1974
54. Piccolo E, Delise P, Raviele A, D'Este D, Totaro G, De Piccoli B, Artusi L, Cazzin R: The anterior displacement of the QRS loop as an incomplete RBBB. Electrophysiologic and vectorcardiographic study in man. 13: 267, 1980
55. Fedor JM, Walston A, Wagner GS, Starr J: The vectorcardiogram in right bundle branch block: correlation with cardiac failure and pulmonary disease. Circulation 53: 926, 1976

56. Milnor WR: Electrocardiogram and vectorcardiogram in right ventricular hypertrophy and right bundle branch block. Circulation 16: 348, 1957
57. Baydar ID, Walsh TJ, Massie E: A vectorcardiographic study of right bundle branch block with the Frank system. Clinical correlation in ventricular hypertrophy and chronic pulmonary disease. Am J Cardiol 15: 185, 1965
58. Saltzmann P, Linn M, Pick A: Right bundle branch block with left axis deviation. Br Heart J 28: 703, 1966
59. Rothfeld EL, Zucker IR, Tiu R, Parsonnet V: The electrocardiographic syndrome of superior axis and right bundle branch block. Dis Chest 55: 306, 1969
60. Cohen SI, Lau SH, Stein E, Young MY, Damato AN: Variations of aberrant ventricular conduction in man: evidence of isolated and combined block within the specialized conduction system. An electrocardiographic and vectorcardiographic study. Circulation 38: 899, 1968
61. Kulbertus HE, Collignon PG, Humblet L: Right bundle branch block with left axis deviation. A vectorcardiographic study of 40 cases. In: Vectorcardiography 2, Hoffman I, Hamby RI, Glassman E. Amsterdam: North-Holland, 1971, p 272
62. Cooksey JD, Dunn M, Massie E: Clinical vectorcardiography and electrocardiography. Chicago: Year Book Medical Publishers, 1977
63. Lenegre J: Contribution à l'étude des blocs de branche comportant notamment les confrontations électriques et histologiques. Arch Mal Coeur 50: 1, 1957
64. Noseda V, Santi A, Aguggini G, Filotto V, Bergamaschi M: Experimental focal block in the sheep and the dog. An electrocardiographic and hystological study. Cardiologia 42: 243, 1963
65. Boineau JP, Spach MS, Ayers CS: Genesis of the electrocardiogram in atrial septal defect. Am Heart J 68: 637, 1964
66. Castellanos A Jr, Agha AS, Befeler B, Castillo CA, Berkovits BV: A study of arrival of excitation at selected ventricular sites during human bundle branch block using close bipolar catheter electrodes. Chest 63: 208, 1973
67. Kastor JA, Goldreyer BN, Moore EN, Shelburne JC, Manchester JH: Intraventricular conduction in man studied with an endocardial electrode catheter mapping technique. Patients with normal QRS and right bundle branch block. Circulation 51: 786, 1975
68. Sokolow M, Lyon TP: Ventricular complex in left ventricular hypertrophy as obtained by unipolar precordial and limb leads. Am Heart J 37: 161, 1949
69. Scott RC, Seiwert VJ, Simon DL, McGuire J: Left ventricular hypertrophy. Circulation 11: 89, 1955
70. Grant RP: The septal vector approach. New York: McGraw-Hill, 1957
71. Booth RW, Chou T, Scott RC: Electrocardiographic diagnosis of ventricular hypertrophy in the presence of right bundle branch block. Circulation 18: 169, 1958
72. Holt JH Jr, Barnard ACL, Kramer JO: A study of the human heart as a multiple dipole source. IV. Left ventricular hypertrophy in the presence of right bundle branch block. Circulation 56: 391, 1977
73. Scott RC: Left bundle branch block. A clinical assesment. Am Heart J 70: 535, 1965
74. Abildskow JA, Jackson CE, Burch GE, Cronvich JA: The spatial vectorcardiogram in right bundle branch block. Circulation 31: 600, 1951
75. Grishman A, Scherlis L: Spatial vectorcardiography. Philadelphia: WB Saunders, 1952
76. Massie A, Walsh TJ: Clinical vectorcardiography. Chicago: Year Book Medical Publishers, 1960
77. Murata K, Matsushita S, Kuramochi M, Terasawa F: Vectorcardiographic diagnosis

of coexisting left ventricular hypertrophy in right bundle branch block. Jap Circ J 35: 209, 1971
78. Scherlis L, Yu-Chen L: Right bundle branch block following open heart surgery. Electrocardiographic and vectorcardiographic study. Am J Cardiol 8: 780, 1961
79. Brohet CR, Styns M, Arnaud P, Brasseur LA: Vectorcardiographic diagnosis of right ventricular hypertrophy in the presence of right bundle branch block in young subjects. Am J Cardiol 42: 602, 1978
80. Hoffman I, Jawahar M, Hilsenrat J, Hambi RI: Anterior conduction delay: a possible cause for pseudo-dorsal infarction. In: Vectorcardiography 3, Hoffman I, Hamby RI. North-Holland, 1976, p 129
81. Kulbertus HE, De Leval R, Rutten F, Casters P: Vectorcardiographic study of aberrant conduction. Anterior displacement of QRS: another form of intraventricular block. Br Heart J 38: 549, 1976
82. De Padua F, Lopes MG, Dosreis DD, Pereirinha A, Lopes V, Nunes R: Anterior displacement of the QRS forces. Ethiologic assessment by echocardiography. XX. Electrocardiological Symposium (Abstr) Yalta, 1979, p 174
83. Rosenbaum MB, Lepeschkin E: Bilateral bundle branch block. Am Heart J 50: 38, 1955
84. Schloff LD, Adler L, Donoso E, Friedberg CK: Bilateral bundle branch block. Circulation 35: 790, 1967
85. Brusca A, Rosettani E: Criteri diagnostici del blocco di branca bilaterale (BBB), apporto delle indagini elettrofisiologiche. XXXV Congresso Soc. Ital Cardiol. Montesilvano, 1974, p 220
86. Wu D, Denes P, Dhingra R, Amat-y-Leon F, Wyndham CR, Chuquimia R, Rosen KM: Electrophysiological and clinical observations in patients with alternating bundle branch block. Circulation 53: 456, 1976
87. Fabregas R, Tse W, Han J: Conduction disturbances of the bundle branches produced by lesions in the non-branching portion of His bundle. Am Heart J 92: 356, 1976
88. El-Sherif N, Amat-y-Leon F, Schonfield C, Scherlag B, Rosen K, Lazzara R, Wyndham C: Normalization of bundle branch block patterns by distal His bundle pacing. Clinical and experimental dissociation in the pathologic His bundle. Circulation 57: 473, 1978
89. Visioli O, Piccoli P: Correlazioni anatomo-cliniche nei disturbi della conduzione cardiaca. G Clin Med 40: 1, 1959
90. Baragan J, Maurice P, Lenegre J: Bloc complet de branche gauche et infarctus du myocarde (étude anatomo-électrique de 48 observations). Arch Mal Coeur 56: 445, 1963
91. Sugura M, Okada R, Ohkawa S, Shimada H: Pathohistological studies on the conduction system in 8 cases of complete left bundle branch block. Jap Heart J 11: 5, 1970
92. Rossi L: Histopathology of cardiac arrhythmias. Milan: Casa Editrice Ambrosiana, 1978
93. Lev M, Unger PN, Rosen KM, Bharati S: The anatomic substrate of complete left bundle branch block. Circulation 50: 473, 1974
94. Bharati S, Lev M: Histological and electrophysiological correlations in atrioventricular block and bundle branch block. In: Cardiac arrhythmias. Electrophysiology, diagnosis and management, Narula OS. Baltimore: Williams & Wilkins, 1979, p 164
95. Lev M, Unger PN, Lesser ME, Pick A: Pathology of the conduction system in acquired heart disease. Complete right bundle branch block. Am Heart J 61: 593, 1961
96. Isokane N, Fernandez F, Iris L, Gerbaux A: Les lésions de la branche droite du

faisceau de His. Etude clinique, électrocardiographique et histologique de 33 cas. Arch Mal Coeur 70: 9, 1977
97. Unger PN, Lesser ME, Kugel VH, Lev M: The concept of masquerading bundle branch block. Circulation 17: 397, 1958
98. Lenegre J: Etiology and pathology of bilateral bundle branch block in relation to complete heart block. Prog Cardiovasc Dis 6: 409, 1964
99. Knieriem HJ, Finke E: Morphologie und Aetiologie des totalen AV Blocks. Munich: Urban & Schwarzenberg, 1974
100. Rossi L: Case of cardiac lymphangitis with atrioventricular block. Br Med J 2: 32, 1965
101. Sciacca A, Sangiorgi M: Trouble de la conduction intraventriculaire droite due à la lésion du tronc commun du faisceau de His. Acta Cardiol 12: 486, 1957
102. Siegman-Igra Y, Yahini JH, Goldbourt U, Neufeld HN: Intraventricular conduction disturbances: a review of prevalence, etiology, and progression for ten years within a stable population of Israeli adult males. Am Heart J 96: 669, 1978
103. Lamb LE, Kable KD, Averill KH: Electrocardiographic findings in 67, 375 asymptomatic subjects. V. Left bundle branch block. Am J Cardiol 6: 130, 1960
104. Hiss RG, Lamb LE: Electrocardiographic findings in 122, 043 individuals. Circulation 25: 947, 1962
105. Rotman M, Triebwasser JH: A clinical and follow up study of right and left bundle branch block. Circulation 51: 477, 1975
106. Ostrander LD: Bundle branch block. An epidemiologic study. Circulation 30: 872, 1964
107. Edmands RE: An epidemiological assessment of bundle branch block. Circulation 34: 1081, 1966
108. Graybiel A, Sprague HB: Bundle branch block: an analysis of 395 cases. Am J Med Sci 185: 395, 1933
109. Campbell M: The outlook with bundle branch block. Br Heart J 31: 575, 1969
110. Messer AL, Birmingham A, Johnson RP, Schreenivas A, White PD: Prognosis in bundle branch block. III. A comparison of right and left bundle branch block with a note on the relative incidence of each. Am Heart J 41: 239, 1951
111. Rodstein M, Gubner R, Mills JP, Lovell JF, Ungerleider HE: A mortality study in bundle branch block. Arch Intern Med 87: 663, 1951
112. Vazifdar JP, Levine SA: Benign bundle branch block. Arch Intern Med 89: 568, 1952
113. Reusch CS, Vivas JR: Clinical analysis of right bundle branch block. Am Heart J 58: 543, 1959
114. Blackburn H, Taylor HS, Keys A: The electrocardiogram in prediction of five year coronary heart incidence among men aged forty through fifty-nine. Circulation (Suppl I) 41-42: 154, 1970
115. Tunstall Pedoe HD: Effect of previous manifestations of coronary heart disease. Br Heart J 40: 630, 1978
116. Lewis CM, Dagenais GR, Friesinger GC, Ross RS: Coronary arteriographic appearances in patients with left bundle branch block. Circulation 46: 299, 1970
117. Dizadi H, Tahmooressi P, Cernock WF: Etiology of LBBB Haemodynamic and angiographic studies. J Electrocardiol 7: 221, 1974
118. Herbert WH: Left bundle branch block and coronary artery disease. J Electrocardiol 8: 317, 1975
119. Schneider JF, Thomas HE, Kreger B, McNamara P: Left bundle branch block in Framingham. Circulation (Abstr) 53-54 (Suppl II): 128, 1976
120. Rose G, Baxter PJ, Reid DD, McCartney P: Prevalence and prognosis of electrocar-

diographic findings in middle aged men. Br Heart J 40: 636, 1978
121. Rabkin SW, Mathewson AL, Tate RB: Natural history of left bundle branch block. Br Heart J 43: 164, 1980
122. Merril JP, Levine HD, Somerville W: Clinical recognition and treatment of acute potassium intoxication. Ann Intern Med 33: 797, 1950
123. Johnson RP, Messer L, Shreemivas A, White PD: Prognosis in bundle branch block. II. Factors influencing the survival period in left bundle branch block. Am Heart J 41: 225, 1951
124. Spurrel RAJ, Krickler DM, Sowton E: Study of intraventricular conduction times in patients with left bundle branch block and normal QRS axis using His bundle electrograms. Br Heart J 31: 1244, 1972
125. Dhingra RC, Amat-y-Leon F, Wyndham C, Sridhar S, Wu D, Denes P, Rosen KM: Significance of left axis deviation in patients with chronic left bundle branch block. Am J Cardiol 42: 551, 1978
126. Haft JI, Herman MV, Gorlin R: Left bundle branch block: etiologic, hemodynamic and ventriculographic considerations. Circulation 43: 279, 1971
127. Wiberg TA, Richman HG, Gobel FL: The significance and prognosis of chronic bifascicular block. Chest 71: 329, 1977
128. Packard JM, Graettinger JS, Graybiel A: Analysis of electrocardiograms obtained from 1000 young healthy aviators. Circulation 10: 384, 1954
129. Johnson RL, Averill KH, Lamb LE: Electrocardiographic findings in 67, 375 asymptomatic subjects. VI. Right bundle branch block. Am J Cardiol 6: 143, 1960
130. Perera GA, Levine SA, Erlanger H: Prognosis of right bundle branch block. A study of 104 cases. Br Heart J 4: 35, 1942
131. Lenegre J, Soulie P: Maladies de l'appareil cardiovasculaire. Paris: Flammarion, 1968
132. Sarachek NS, Leonard JJ: Familial heart block and natural history. Am J Cardiol 29: 451, 1972
133. Antonioli G, Zanardi F, D'Agostino F, Masoni A: Degenerazione familiare del sistema di conduzione. G Ital Cardiol 3: 519, 1973
134. Vallianos G, Sideris DA: Familial conduction defects. Cardiology 59: 190, 1974
135. Stephan E: Hereditary bundle branch system defect. A new genetic entity? Am Heart J 97: 708, 1979
136. Rasmussen H: Experimental production of bundle branch block. ECGs by acute dilatation of the right and left heart. Acta Med Scand 110: 32, 1942
137. Moore EN, Hoffman BF, Patterson DF, Stuckey JH: Electrocardiographic changes due to delayed activation of the wall of the right ventricle. Am Heart J 68: 347, 1964
138. Takeshita A, Basta LL, Kioschos JM: Effect of intermittent left bundle branch block on left ventricular performance. Am J Med 56: 251, 1974
139. Braunwald E, Morrow AG: Sequence of ventricular contraction in human bundle-branch block: a study based on simultaneous catheterization of both ventricles. Am J Med 23: 205, 1957
140. Bourassa MG, Boiteau GM, Allenstein BJ: Hemodynamic studies during intermittent left bundle branch block. Am J Cardiol 10: 792, 1962
141. Williams RS, Behar VS, Peter RH: Left bundle branch block: angiographic segmental wall motion abnormalities. Am J. Cardiol 44: 1046, 1979
142. Wong B, Rinkenberger R, Dunn M, Goodyer A: Effect of intermittent left bundle branch block on left ventricular performance in the normal heart. Am J Cardiol 39: 459, 1977
143. Abbasi AS, Eber LM, MacAlpin RN, Kattus AA: Paradoxical motion of the interventricular septum in left bundle branch block. Circulation 49: 423, 1974

144. McDonald IG: Echocardiographic demonstration of abnormal motion of the interventricular septum in left bundle branch block. Circulation 48: 272, 1978
145. Alboni P, Pedroni P, Malacarne C: Problematica dei blocchi di branca a localizzazione nel fascio di His. G Ital Cardiol 10: 1583, 1980
146. Berkowitz WD, Lau SH, Patton RD, Rosen KM, Damato AN: The use of His bundle recordings in the analysis of unilateral and bilateral bundle branch block. Am Heart J 81: 340, 1971
147. Javier RP, Narula OS: Analysis of left bundle branch block by His bundle recordings. Circulation (Abstr) 44: 183, 1971
148. Ranganatham N, Dhurandhar R, Phillips JH, Wigle ED: His bundle electrocardiogram in bundle branch block. Circulation 45: 282, 1972
149. Rosen KM, Ehsani A, Rahimtoola SH: HV interval in left bundle branch block: clinical and electrocardiographic correlations. Circulation 46: 717, 1972
150. Puech P, Grolleau R, Guimond C: Incidence of different types of A-V block and their localization by His bundle recordings. In: The conduction system of the heart, Wellens HJJ, Lie KI, Janse MI. Leiden: Stenfert Kroese, 1976, p 467

4. FASCICULAR BLOCKS

The term fascicular block implies a conduction disturbance involving the main divisions of the left bundle branch (LBB). The concept of fascicular block is limited to the LBB system, since the right bundle branch (RBB) does not subdivide into fascicles but ends directly into the Purkinje network (see Chapter 1).

As early as 1917, Rothberger et al. [1] in experimental studies observed that the electrical axis shifted superiorly when the anterior division of LBB was sectioned. In 1934, Wilson et al. [2] similarly hypothesized a block in the anterior division of the LBB as an explanation for the superiorly directed axis. Grant [3], in 1956, observed that marked left axis deviation (LAD) occurred frequently in anterolateral myocardial infarction and designated this finding peri-infarction block, suggesting the presence of an infarction even in the absence of Q waves. Since then many studies have confirmed the correlation between marked axis deviation and fascicular block, but have excluded a constant coexistence of myocardial infarction.

Rosenbaum et al. [4, 5] first introduced the concept of 'hemiblock' in clinical setting. According to these investigators, the intraventricular conduction system consists of three main fascicles: one fascicle is destined to the right ventricle (right bundle branch) and two fascicles of the LBB, i.e. anterior and posterior, without any anatomical and functional interconnections, supply the left ventricle. Block in any one of the latter two fascicles has been labelled hemiblock.

However, as pointed out in Chapter 1, the distribution of the left intraventricular conduction system is more complex. Several histological studies have demonstrated the presence of an additional middle (septal) fascicle which activates the inferior two thirds of the septum [6-10]. However, others [11-13] have contradicted the fascicular concept and have described the distribution of the left bundle branch fibers as fan-shaped.

From a functional standpoint, Durrer et al. [14], in isolated perfused human hearts, have shown that the earliest activation of the left ventricle occurs simultaneously at three sites in the septum, i.e. anterior, middle and posterior. These three septal sides correspond to the areas activated by the three divisions (or fascicles) of LBB as described by Uhley et al. [7, 8]. Subsequently, others have confirmed this pattern of activation [15-17]. Recently, some electrophysiological characteristics peculiar to the fibers of the middle fascicle have been documented;

they show an action potential duration shorter than that of the fibers of the anterior and posterior fascicles [18].

The concept of 'trifascicular' intraventricular conduction system is still widely accepted in most of the international literature. However it appears over-simplified and the nomenclature of 'Hemiblock' as proposed by Rosenbaum et al. [4] does not seem appropriate. The term 'fascicular block', despite some limitations due to the inconsistency in the subdivision into fascicles of the LBB, is preferable from a functional point of view. In 1973, a group of electrophysiologists [19] evaluated the nomenclature of cardiac conduction disturbances and suggested that the term 'hemiblock' was inappropriate and preferred that of 'fascicular block' [19].

ANTERIOR FASCICULAR BLOCK

The anterior fascicle of LBB courses superiorly and anteriorly and the posterior fascicle inferiorly and posteriorly. At the base of the anterior and posterior papillary muscles, each fascicle divides into the Purkinje network, which extensively anastomoses with each other. Under normal conditions, the anterior and posterior fascicles of the LBB practically activate the antero-superior and postero-inferior walls of the left ventricle simultaneously.

In the anterior fascicular block (AFB) the activation of the antero-superior wall of the left ventricle is delayed as the depolarizing impulse reaches this wall via the intact posterior fascicle. In this connection Watt et al. [20] experimentally showed that left anterior divisional block in dogs and primates resulted in delay in antero-superior left ventricular epicardial activation by 30 to 40 msec and in a superior shift in mean QRS electrical axis. More recently, Gallagher et al. [21], utilizing intramural endocardial and epicardial recordings, showed that damage of the anterior LBB fibers in dogs uniformly produced delays of 6 to 60 msec in the blocked Purkinje fibers, 3 to 25 msec delays in the associated endocardial areas, and 4 to 25 msec delays in the epicardial surface confined to the anterolateral surface of the left ventricle. When lesions were placed in the septal fascicle of the LBB, in addition to the anterior fascicle damage, epicardial surface delays of greater magnitude (7 to 35 msec) as well as marked LAD were encountered.

Similar changes of ventricular depolarization have been observed during epicardial [22, 23] and body surface mapping [24] in man. Four patients with marked LAD were studied with epicardial mapping during coronary by-pass surgery [23]. All patients had normal right ventricular and inferior left ventricular epicardial breakthrough sites and activation sequence. The latest site of left ventricular activation was the basal segment of the anterolateral wall, a site never found to be the latest activated in previously studied patients without conduction defects [25].

ELECTROCARDIOGRAPHIC FEATURES

The most commonly accepted criteria for the diagnosis of AFB are [4, 5]:
1) Left axis deviation greater than $-45°$, and
2) Q_1 S_3 pattern with an rS morphology in leads II, III and aVF.

Since the Q_1S_3 pattern is highly nonspecific, the diagnosis is only suggested by the LAD.

It must be pointed out that a leftward shift of QRS axis may be due to other causes [3, 26-28] such as left ventricular hypertrophy (LVH), horizontal position of the heart, left ventricular peripheral block located in the postero-superior wall, pulmonary emphysema, inferior myocardial infarction, or Wolff-Parkinson-White syndrome (Table 1). In the literature it is popularly stated that these alterations by themselves rarely induce LAD of $-45°$ or more. This statement, though mostly true in an experimental setting, is not applicable clinically as the various

Table 1. Causes of left axial deviation, besides anterior fascicular block

- Left ventricular hypertrophy
- Horizontal position of the heart (due to counterclockwise rotation on the longitudinal axis, to elevation of diaphragm, to anomaly of the chest)
- Left ventricular peripheral block
- Right peripheral ventricular block located in the postero-superior wall
- Pulmonary emphysema
- Inferior myocardial infarction
- W.P.W. syndrome

above-mentioned conditions are often associated in a clinical setting and can produce a marked LAD due to a summation effect. This possibility has also been confirmed experimentally [27]. Therefore, the deviation of the QRS axis is not a specific diagnostic feature for AFB. In our opinion, for the diagnosis of AFB, the presence of LAD is necessary although, in itself, not sufficiently reliable unless other findings indicative of asynchrony in left ventricular activation are also present.

On the basis of their experimental studies, Medrano et al. [29-31] defined the following ECG criteria for the identification of asynchronous left ventricular activation:
1) Intrinsicoid deflection time (IDT) in lead aVL delayed by 50 msec or more as it explores the antero-superior wall of the left ventricle
2) Intrinsicoid deflection time delayed for a comparatively longer time (15 msec or more) in lead aVL than in lead V_6 as the latter explores the latero-inferior wall of the left ventricle, normally activated by the posterior fascicle (Figures 1 and 2). From an analysis of intermittent or transient AFB, we have found these criteria to be valid (Figures 3 and 4).

Although no precise limits exist between the normal and pahtological pattern,

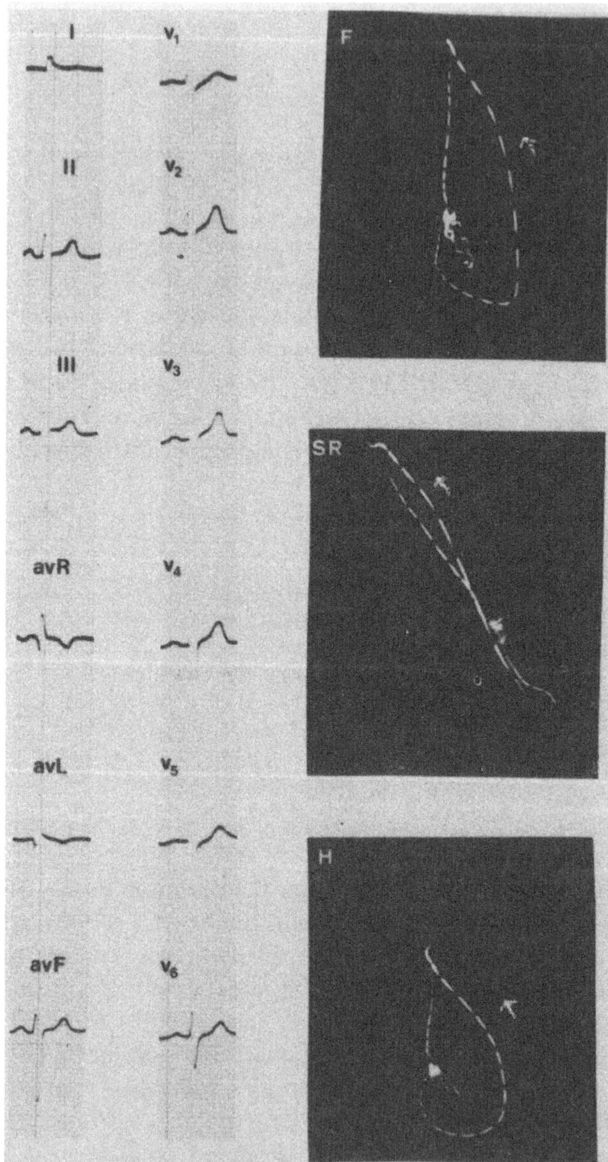

Figure 1. Anterior fascicular block. ECG: Marked left axis deviation (−75°). The intrinsecoid deflection time is 50 msec in aVL and 25 msec in V_6. Terminal R wave in aVR and S wave in V_6. Lead aVL shows a negative T wave. VCG: The first vectors are oriented inferiorly, anteriorly and to the right. In the frontal plane the mid-terminal forces are oriented upward and to the left with counterclockwise rotation. In the horizontal plane a good development of the QRS loop antero-posteriorly and a slight one to the left is evident. Terminal delay, lasting 20 msec (for details see text)

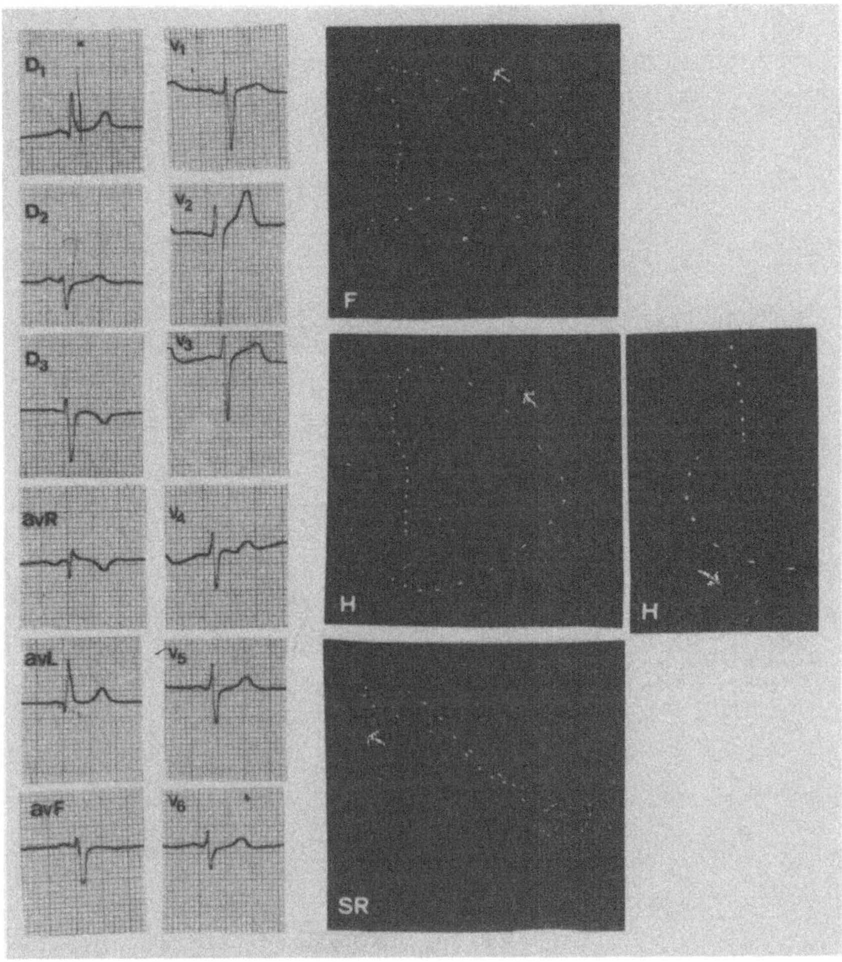

Figure 2. Anterior fascicular block. EGC: Left axis deviation ($-55°$) A q wave is evident in leads I and aVL. The intrinsecoid deflection time is 50 msec in aVL and 30 msec in V_6. Terminal slurring is evident in aVL. VCG: The QRS loop is mainly oriented superiorly and antero-posteriorly (for details see text). D_1: lead I, D_2: lead II, D_3: lead III

we believe that the ECG features of asynchronous left ventricular activation when associated with LAD are of special diagnostic value.

Medrano recommends the diagnosis of AFB simply on the basis of ECG signs of asynchronous left ventricular activation, considering the presence of LAD to be superfluous for the diagnosis of AFB. His conclusions may be valid in experimental animal models, especially the canine heart, as: 1) It occupies a different position in the chest. The right septal surface and the entire right ventricle is oriented more superiorly; 2) The right ventricle is anatomically and electrically

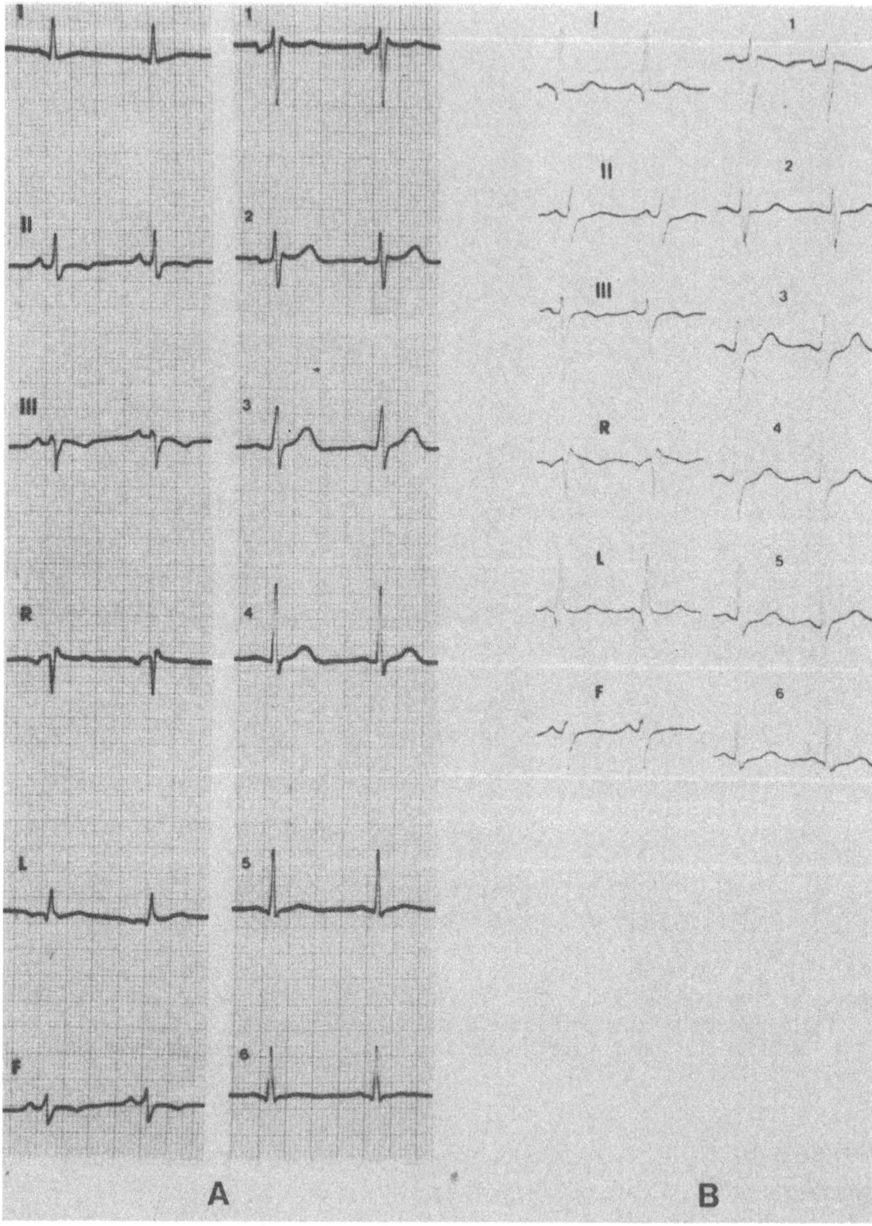

Figure 3. Transient anterior fascicular block. A: Control tracing. B: ECG, 2 months later, shows the appearance of AFB. Besides the left axis deviation at $-30°$, there is an increase in the depth of q wave in I and a VL. Intrinsecoid deflection time increases from 40 msec to 50 msec in lead aVL

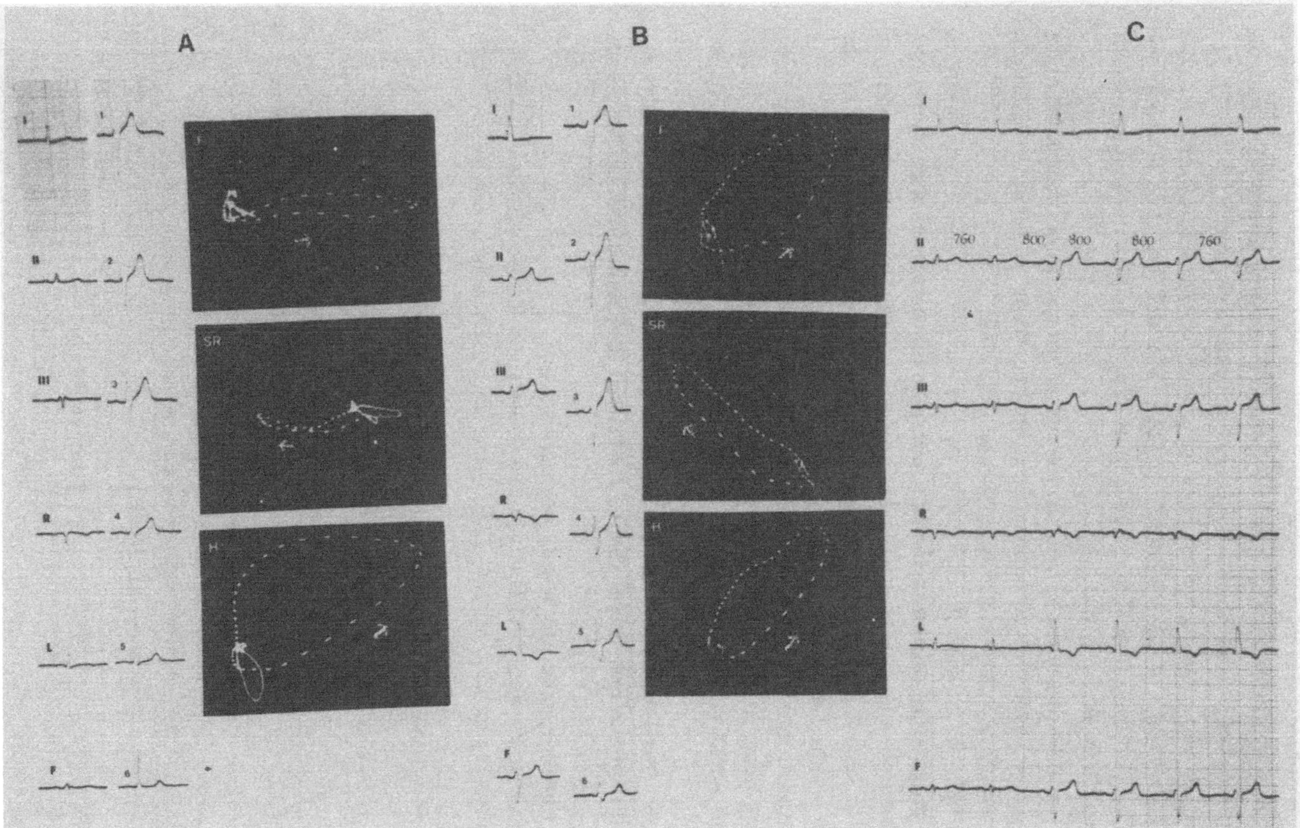

Figure 4. Intermittent anterior fascicular block. A: Control ECG and VCG tracings. B: ECG showing all typical features of AFB. The electrical axis is shifted superiorly (−45). In a VL the intrinsecoid deflection time increases from 40 to 50 msec and a negative T wave appears. In the VCG the frontal QRS loop is directed more superiorly than in control tracing. In the horizontal plane the posterior development of the QRS loop increases while the leftward forces decrease. C: The intermittent nature of AFB is evident.

more predominant than in the human heart; and 3) A control tracing preceding the induction of block is always available for a comparison. However, on the basis of the currently available clinical data, we believe it is dangerous to diagnose an AFB in humans only on the basis of the IDT in leads aVL and V_6.

Summarizing, the most important ECG features of AFB are LAD of more than −30° along with signs of asynchronous left ventricular activation. In addition, the following ECG findings are often observed and may be helpful in the diagnosis of AFB (Figures 1 to 4):

a) Q waves in leads I and aVL, due to the rightward and inferior orientation of the first vectors. These may sometimes be deep, according to the modification in septal activation, and they are sometimes absent [32-34].

b) Terminal r or R wave in aVR and s or S wave in V_6, due to an abnormal inferior to superior activation of the left ventricle. RS pattern in lead V_6 results, therefore, from the fact that the electrodes are located (in relation to the spread of activation) in such a fashion that the terminal QRS forces move away from the electrode in a superior direction.

c) Terminal or mid to terminal slurring in aVL and rarely in I. This results from a conduction delay in the antero-superior wall of the left ventricle.

d) Flat or negative T wave in aVL, due to secondary alterations in repolarization.

e) Narrow, small and not slurred q wave in V_2-V_3 leads. This results from a posterior shift of the first vector due to AFB itself and septal fibrosis (discussed later).

d) QRS duration generally within normal limits.

In fact, in studies where AFB developed acutely, as during cardiac catheterization or following cardiac surgery [35], the QRS duration has been observed to increase only by 10-20 msec.

Table 2 shows the ECG features and pathophysiology of AFB.

Table 2. Pathophysiology and ECG changes in anterior fascicular block

ECG FEATURES	PATHOPHYSIOLOGY
q wave in I and aVL	Downward and rightward orientation of the first vectors
Delay of intrinsecoid deflection more prolonged in aVL than in V_6 (15 msec or more)	Asynchronous left ventricular activation
Delay of intrinsecoid deflection in aVL of 50 msec or more Left axial deviation of −30° or more Terminal r or R wave in aVR. S or s wave in V_6	Abnormal inferior to superior activation of the left ventricle
Terminal or mid-terminal slurring in aVL	Conduction delay in the anterosuperior wall of the left ventricle
Flat or negative T wave in aVL	Secondary alterations of repolarization

VECTORCARDIOGRAPHIC FEATURES

In the frontal (F) plane, the first vectors are directed to the right and inferiorly. The QRS loop is then inscribed to the left and superiorly in a counterclockwise fashion. In horizontal hearts, the terminal vectors are oriented slightly to the right. In most cases a terminal delay of about 15-20 msec is present. The appearance of the maximum vector is delayed to 50 msec or more.

In the horizontal (H) plane, the first vectors are directed to the right, anteriorly or slightly posteriorly. The QRS loop is then inscribed to the left and posteriorly in a counterclockwise fashion or less often in a figure of eight. The terminal vectors, often delayed, are oriented either to the left or slightly to the right.

According to many authors, the QRS morphology in the H plane is nonspecific and, therefore, believed to be useless in the diagnosis of AFB. However, from an analysis of the VCG of experimental AFB [29-31, 36, 37] and of intermittent AFB [38, 39] it appears that the horizontal QRS loop indeed shows a definite pattern in the H plane: this consists of alterations of the middle phases, i.e. a good development of the loop antero-posteriorly and a slight one to the left (the relation between the X axis and the Z axis is in favor of the latter, see Figures 1, 2 and 4).

In our opinion, this change, even if not pathognomonic, provides important evidence for asynchronous left ventricular activation and is due to the fact that the electrical forces of the antero-superior and the postero-inferior walls of the left ventricle manifest themselves at different times; therefore there is not the full manifestation of the resulting vectors directed to the left.

In the right sagittal (RS) plane, the initial vectors are oriented inferiorly and anteriorly or slightly posteriorly. The QRS loop is then inscribed in a clockwise fashion or figure-of-eight configuration and is directed superiorly.

Controversies exist regarding some ECG and VCG manifestations of AFB. These deserve special mention because of their particular implication.

q waves in V_2-V_3 leads

In AFB, small, narrow and not slurred 'q' waves, not characteristic of infarction, are often seen in the right precordial and/or transitional leads, particularly V_2-V_3 (Figure 5).

The incidence of such q waves in our analysis of 1008 cases of AFB was 13.7%. Since the clinical significance of these q waves was not known in the available literature, we analyzed the clinical data of these patients [40]. They were divided into two groups: group 1 AFB included patients without q waves in leads V_2-V_3, and group 2 AFB consisted of 139 patients (13.7%) with the characteristic q waves. The clinical diagnosis of these patients is reported in Table 3. There was a slightly higher incidence of arteriosclerotic heart disease in group 2 patients, 64.8% as compared to 51.8% in group 1 patients. On the other hand, myocardial

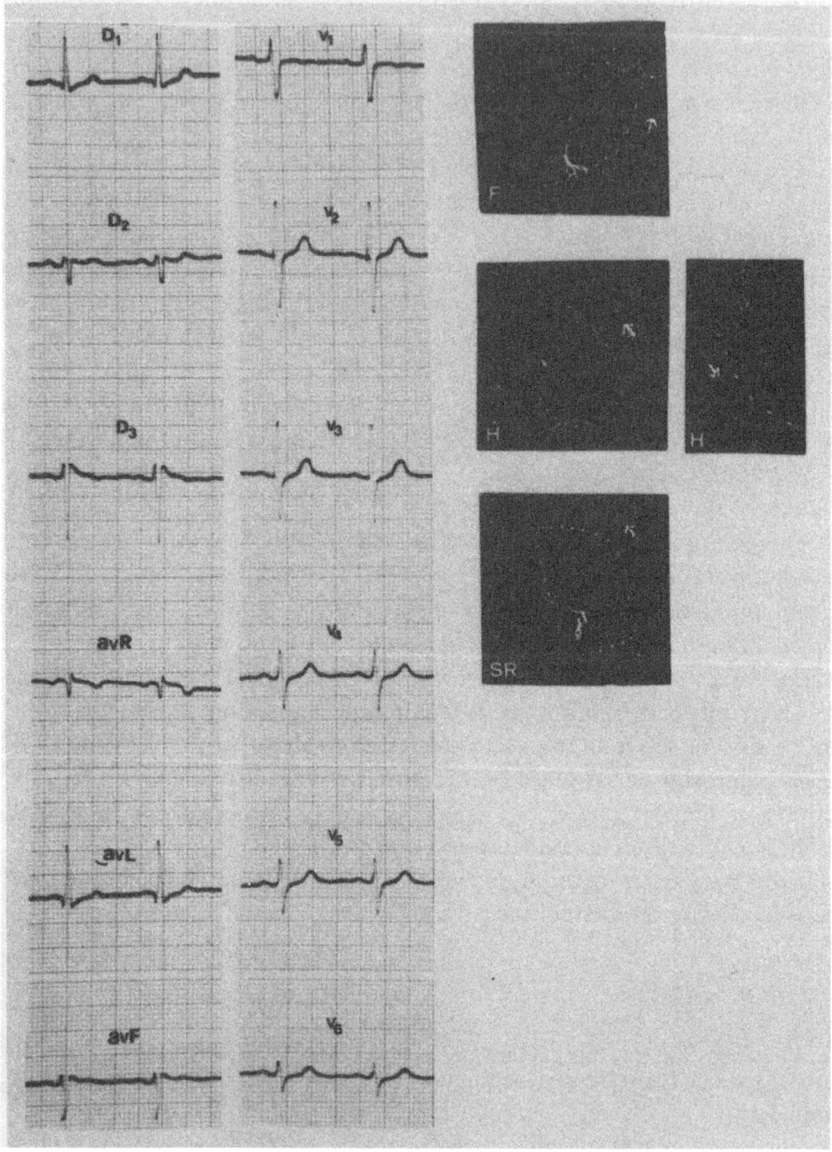

Figure 5. Anterior fascicular block. In the ECG, lead V_2 shows a small, narrow and not-slurred q wave. In the horizontal plane of VCG the first vectors or QRS loop are directed to the right and slightly posteriorly with counterclockwise rotation

Table 3. Clinical diagnosis of patients showing anterior fascicular block with and without q waves in V_2–V_3. (From Alboni et al., with permission of J Electrocardiol [40])

Clinical diagnosis	AFB without small q waves Total cases: 869 Diagnosis made: 814	AFB with small q waves Total cases: 139 Diagnosis made: 128
No cardiopathy	39 (4.77%)	
Congenital heart disease	10 (1.22%)	
Rheumatic heart disease	20 (2.4%)	2 (1.56%)
Hypertension	170 (20.88%)	29 (22.65%)
Coronary artery disease	423 (51.88%)	84 (64.83%)
Myocardial infarction	100 (12.28%)	3 (2.3%)
Chronic cor pulmonale	37 (4.54%)	7 (5.46%)
Rare cardiopathies	15 (1.84%)	3 (2.34%)

infarction was more common in group I. The reason for this higher incidence is obvious since antero-septal infarction causing AFB would produce wide and slurred Q waves and thus would be excluded from group 2. The incidence of other diseases was nearly equal in the two groups. It must be emphasized that patients who showed no clinical and radiological manifestations of cardiac disease, who were most likely to be affected by idiopathic degeneration of intraventricular conduction system, i.e. Lenegre disease [41], and patients with congenital heart disease showed no q waves.

Incidence based on the age of the patient was compared (Table 4). Patients in group 2 were all over 60, and patients in group 1 were distributed over all age groups.

Vectorcardiograms of 35 control patients with normal electrocardiogram, 32 patients with AFB without q waves, and 30 patients with AFB and q waves were analyzed and compared. Figure 6 summarizes the range and mean orientation of the 10 and 20 msec vectors in the three groups of patients. When compared to the

Table 4. Distribution of the various decades of life of patients showing anterior fascicular block with and without q waves in V_2-V_3. (From Alboni et al., with permission of J Electrocardiol [40])

Age	AFB without small q waves Total cases: 869	AFB with small q waves Total cases: 139
1-9	10 (1.14%)	
10-19	12 (1.38%)	
20-29	12 (1.38%)	
30-39	25 (2.8%)	2 (1.43%)
40-49	60 (6.90%)	3 (2.15%)
50-59	111 (12.77%)	19 (13.66%)
60-69	262 (32.45%)	55 (39.56%)
70-79	247 (28.45%)	43 (30.93%)
80-89	94 (19.81%)	16 (11.51%)
90-99	9 (1.03%)	1 (0.71%)

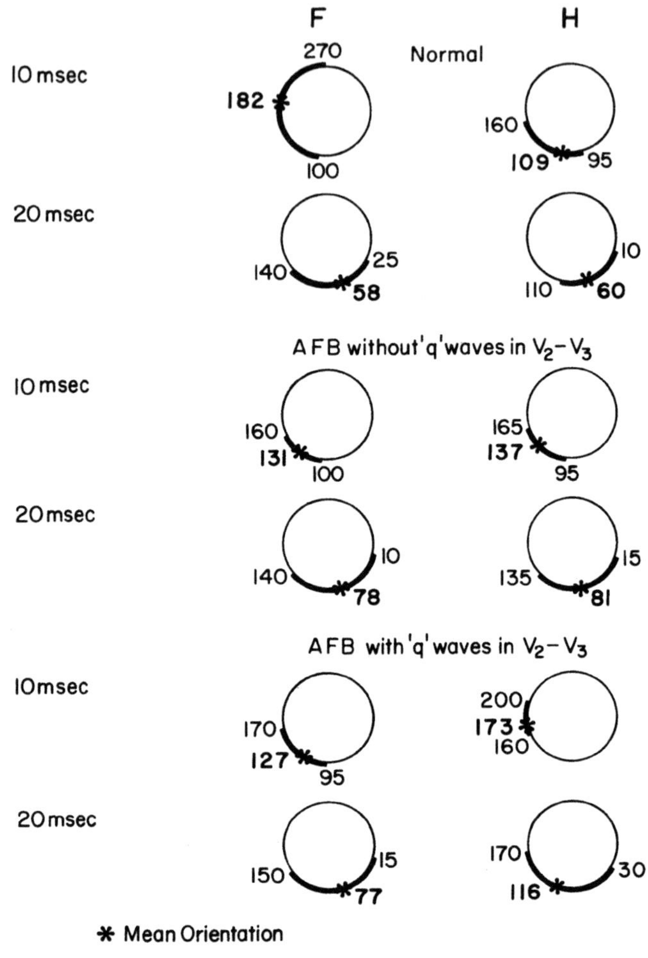

Figure 6. Mean orientation with limit values of the 10 and 20 msec vectors in the frontal and horizontal planes, in the control patients and in the patients showing anterior fascicular block with and without q waves. (From Alboni et al., with permission of J Electrocardiol [40])

control group, the patients with AFB showed a significant difference with a more posterior and inferior orientation of 10 and 20 msec vectors. Between the two groups of patients showing AFB with and without q waves, no difference was noted in the orientation of these vectors in the F plane ($P > 0.4$). However, in the H plane these vectors were directed more posteriorly in the group of AFB patients with q waves compared to those without q waves ($P < 0.001$).

The q wave in AFB has been attributed by some authors to modification in septal activation, i.e. due to AFB per se [4, 42-44], and to septal fibrosis by others [45]. Our data support both hypotheses. The higher incidence of coronary artery disease (CAD) in the group showing q waves (Table 3) and the fact that q waves were not present in the younger patients and in those without underlying heart disease (Tables 3 and 4) suggest that septal fibrosis is the reason for the q waves. Moreover such q waves were not seen in experimental AFB [4, 6, 20, 29-31, 46-48].

The data in favor of AFB per se as a cause of these q waves are:

- High incidence (13.78 %) of the q waves in V_2-V_3 in patients with AFB and the extreme rarity of these q waves in the other intraventricular conduction disturbances.
- In AFB with and without q waves the 10 msec vector is directed more posteriorly than in the control group ($P < 0.001$); in fact a posterior shift of the first vectors, due to any cause, favors the appearance of q waves in right precordial and/or transitional leads.

The analysis of our data shows that AFB, because of the posterior shift of the first vectors as a result of modification of septal activation, represents a factor facilitating but not sufficient for the appearance of q waves in V_2-V_3 leads. It seems logical, therefore, that such q waves are either due to concomitant septal fibrosis or to peripheral septal block involving the Purkinje and/or muscular fibres [49-51]. Such alterations, therefore, induce right precordial q waves by shifting posteriorly the first vectors.

Some authors [4] postulate that the q waves are related to AFB per se because of a more inferior rather than more posteriorly directed first vectors. In support of this postulation they report that such waves are not evident or less evident if the precordial electrodes are placed in a lower intercostal space. In our experience, when the electrodes are placed in a lower intercostal space, there is an increase in the amplitude of normal r waves and a decrease of the infarctional Q waves in the right precordial leads. This finding has also been observed in the ECG tracings published by other authors [52]. To our knowledge, the reason for this change in amplitude has not been explained. Hence, we believe this is not specific for q waves seen in association with AFB. In addition, our data show that the 10 and 20 msec vectors in the F plane have the same direction whether or not q waves are present in AFB (Figure 6).

Theoretically such q waves can also be observed in patients without heart disease when there is a backward rotation of the septum or when a variation of distribution of conduction system is present. However, AFB q waves were not seen in patients without underlying heart disease and we believe that this would be a rare exception rather than a rule.

DIFFERENTIAL DIAGNOSIS

AFB should be differentiated from conditions inducing left axis deviation:

1) Left ventricular hypertrophy. Both a marked LAD and delayed intrinsicoid deflection time in aVL can occur in LVH [53]. However, the IDT is also delayed in

lead V_6 and the ECG signs of asynchrony in left ventricular activation are not present [54]. The VCG shows a marked leftward displacement of the QRS loop [55, 56] not present in isolated AFB. Figure 7 shows the ECG and VCG of a patient with LAD of $-45°$ and delayed IDT in aVL (150 msec). Since no signs of

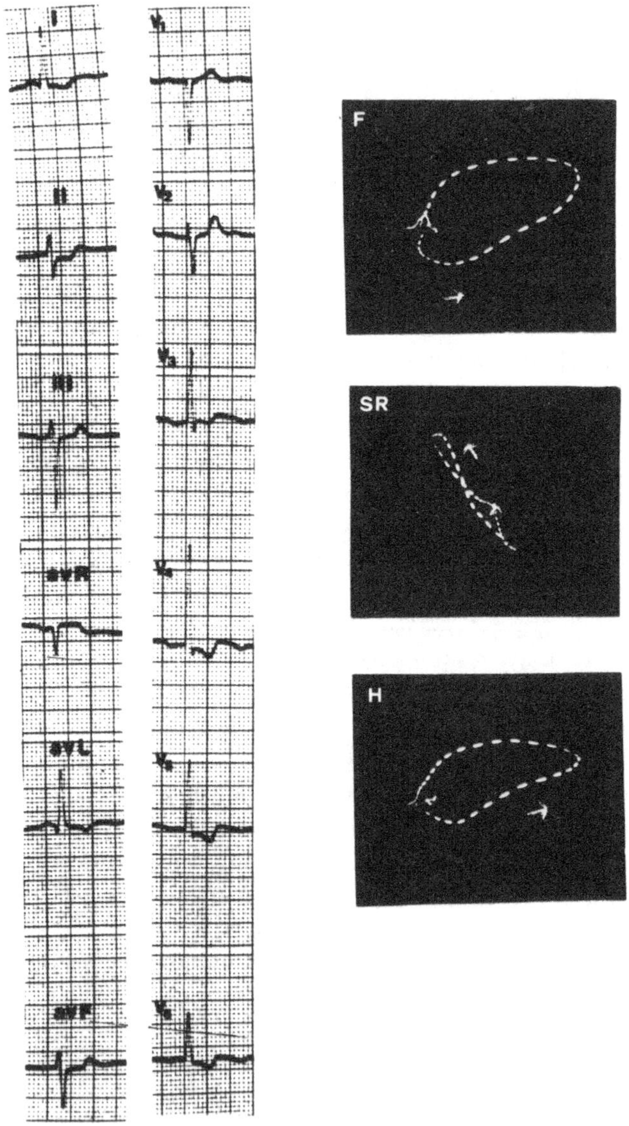

Figure 7. The ECG shows left axis deviation of $-45°$. The intrinsecoid deflection time is prolonged in aVL (50 msec) and in V_6 (40 msec) with a difference of only 10 msec. The QRS loop shows a marked leftward orientation. In the absence of the ECG and VCG signs of asynchronous left ventricular activation the left axis deviation can be mainly attributed to left ventricular hypertrophy

asynchronous left ventricular activation are present, the LAD is ascribed to LVH. However, a slight lesion of the antero-superior fibers of the LBB cannot be ruled out.

It is difficult to diagnose LVH in the presence of AFB, since such a block would enhance the ECG criteria for LVH in the extremity leads and decrease the sensitivity in the precordial leads [57]. Thus, the usual indices of Lewis [58] and Sokolow [59, 60] are not valid in the presence of AFB.

The following criteria have been suggested for the diagnosis of LVH in the presence of AFB:

a) V_6 showing an IDT delayed by 40 msec or more, in the presence of asynchronous left ventricular activation [30].
b) S wave amplitude in lead III of more than 1.5 mV [4].
c) Maximum vector voltage of 2 mV in the H plane [61].
d) QRS loop with a figure-of-eight configuration in the H plane [61].

None of these criteria, however, let us diagnose with certainty an LVH in the presence of AFB.

2) Inferior wall infarction frequently induces LAD. However, the ECG shows pathological Q waves in the diaphragmatic leads. The initial portion of the QRS loop shows a clockwise rotation in the F plane. When the two conditions coexist, it is sometimes difficult to make the diagnosis (see Chapter 10).

3) Left peripheral block localized in the antero-superior wall, can produce LAD in a few cases [26] (see Chapter 6). Experimental [26, 62, 63] and clinical studies [26, 50, 51, 64, 65] have shown that this block produces a terminal and sometimes a mid to terminal delay of QRS complex, lasting 30 msec or more.

It is still not clear whether a left ventricular peripheral block can induce the ECG signs of asynchronous left ventricular activation, even if they have not been observed in clinical studies [64-66].

At present it is not possible to define whether an AFB pattern expresses lesions localized in the septum or in the antero-superior wall of the left ventricle. According to some authors [70], the absence of q waves in leads I and aVL is indicative of a peripheral localization of the block. In our opinion, the presence of such q waves do not represent a discriminating criterion in that they can be missing due to coexisting septal sclerosis, which shifts the first vectors to the left, or due to the fact that the AFB is incomplete. In Figure 8 an AFB pattern without q wave in lead I is present. During slowing of sinus rate the AFB is accentuated and q wave appears in lead I.

The presence of a marked terminal slurring ($>$ 30 msec) of QRS complex indicates, in our opinion, a peripheral block since if in isolated AFB a terminal slurring is present, it is generally of short duration (10-20 msec). In Figure 9 the ECG tracing shows LAD of $-45°$ and a QRS duration of 125 msec. Slurred S waves are present in leads I and aVL. The IDT in aVL and V_6 is 60 and 70 msec, respectively. VCG shows leftward orientation of the QRS loop with a terminal

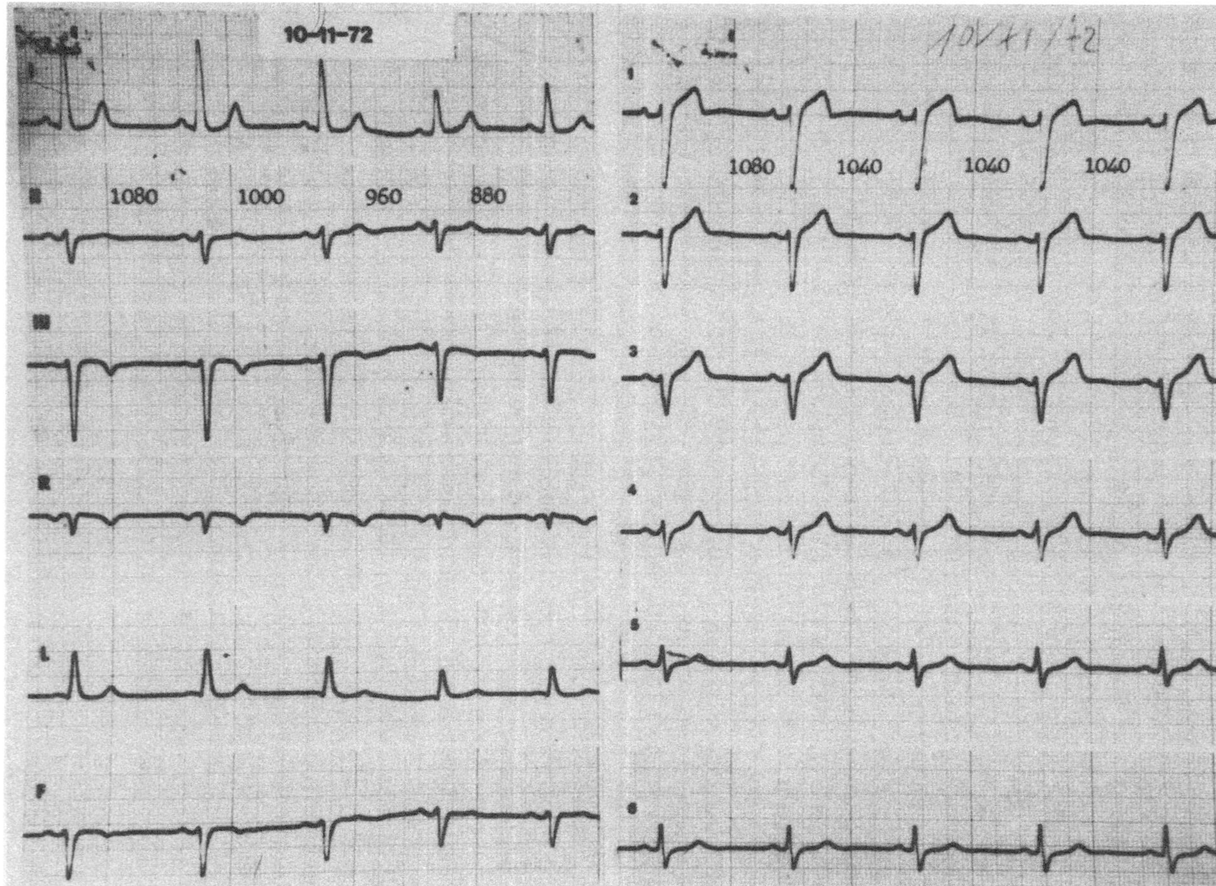

Figure 8. Anterior fascicular block pattern without q wave in lead I. When the sinus cycle length is prolonged to 1000 msec or more, the AFB accentuates and a q wave in lead I appears (for details see text)

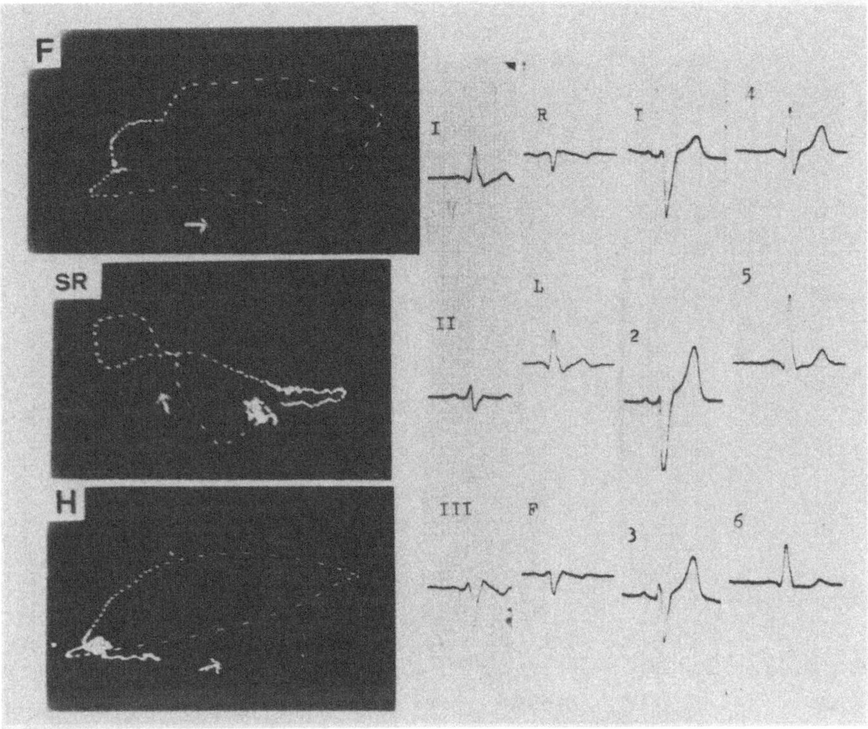

Figures 9. ECG shows left axis deviation of $-45°$. The QRS complex measures 125 msec. Intrinsecoid deflection time is 70 msec in aVL and 60 msec in V_6. Slurred s waves are present in I and aVL. In the VCG, the QRS loop is oriented markedly to left and there is a terminal delay, lasting 50 msec. This tracing is very suggestive of a peripheral block, located in the antero-superior wall of the left ventricle which, together with left ventricular hypertrophy, induces left axis deviation (for details see test)

delay of 50 msec. Since there are no signs of asynchronous left ventricular activation, the LAD is probably due to left ventricular peripheral block.

It must, however, be pointed out that a true AFB and a peripheral block may coexist in the same patient and therefore the presence of a marked terminal slurring does not represent a discriminating diagnostic criterion. In Figure 10 the ECG tracing shows a peripheral block evidenced by a terminal slurring in leads II, III, aVF and V_5. When the sinus rate increases, a 2:1 AFB with marked terminal slurring appears. This case clearly shows that an AFB with terminal slurring can express two or more intraventricular blocks, coexisting in the same patient at various levels.

4) A right peripheral block located in the postero-superior wall (see Chapter 6) can induce pseudo LAD if the mid-terminal forces are directed superiorly as
6) Horizontal position of the heart, elevation of the diaphragm and severe chest

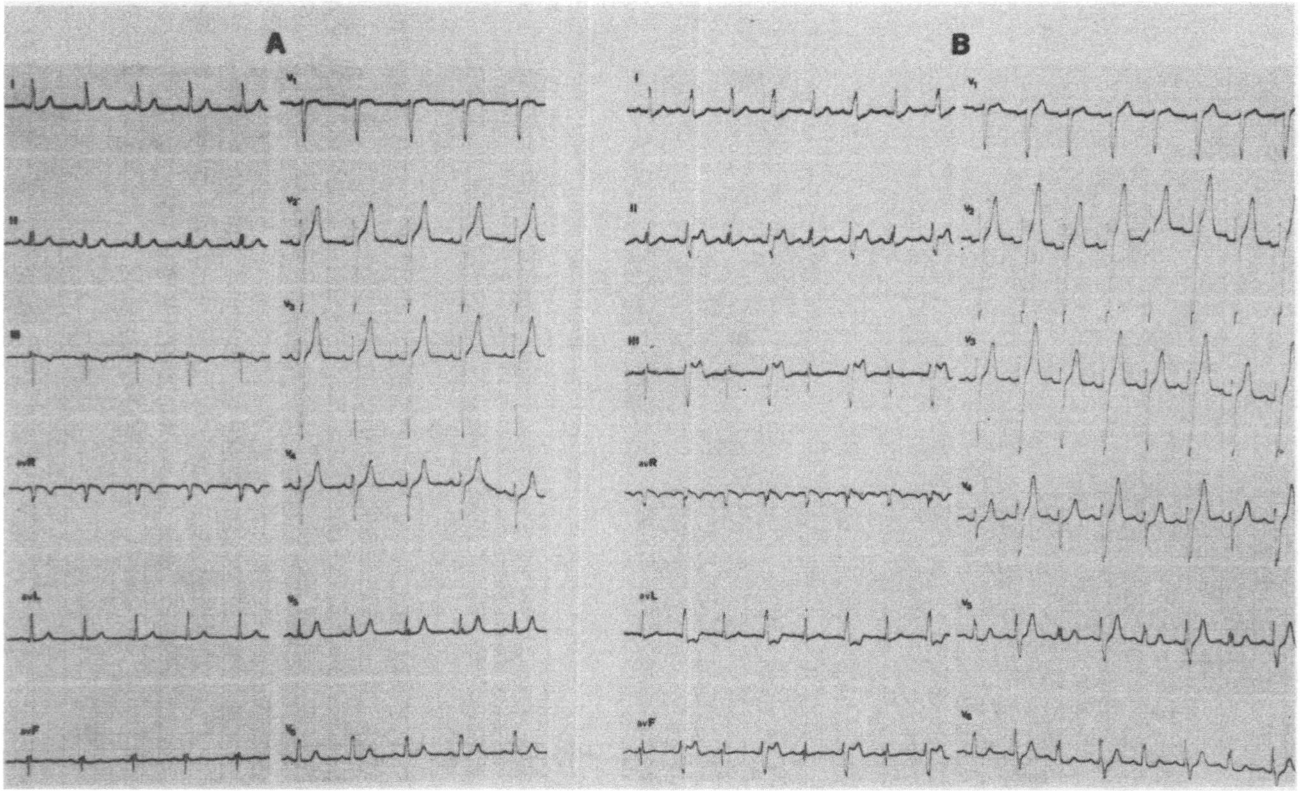

Figure 10. A: Sinus rhythm at a rate of 90/min. QRS complex measures 90 msec. Small q wave, related to normal septal activation, is present in leads I, aVL and V_6. A terminal slurring in II, III, aVF and V_5 suggestive of ventricular peripheral block. B: With an increase in sinus rate up to 110/m′, intermittent 2:1 anterior fascicular block appears. The QRS complexes conducted with AFB have a duration of 110 msec and there is a slurred s wave in leads I and a VL, denoting a ventricular peripheral block associated with AFB (for details see text)

indicative of a right peripheral block, is present. VCG recording is useful; if frontal QRS loop shows clockwise rotation, it excludes an AFB (Figure 11); if, on the other hand, it shows counterclockwise rotation, the maximum QRS vector is generally oriented under 0° [28]; this pattern is contrary to the presence of AFB.

5) Pulmonary emphysema is sometimes associated with LAD. The cause of such QRS deviation is not completely clear; however in experimental emphysema it was observed that the transmission of electrical potential remained normal in an in-

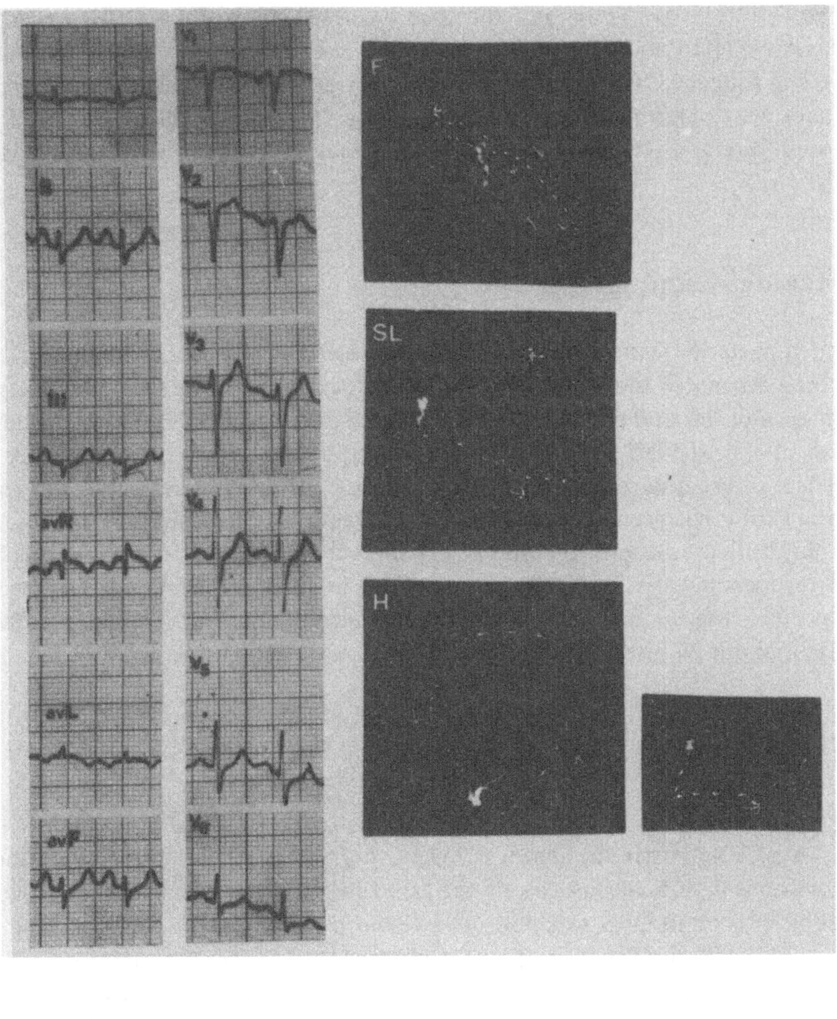

Figure 11. Right ventricular peripheral block located in the postero-superior wall simulating an anterior fascicular block. Pseudo left axis deviation. The presence of an s wave in lead I and, above all, of a clockwise rotation in the frontal plane of VCG excludes an anterior fascicular block

ferior to superior direction but it decreased in a superior to inferior direction [27]. The ECG shows S wave in lead I – absent in isolated AFB – and normal IDT in aVL. The presence of P pulmonale and low voltage of the QRS complex are additional helpful signs in making the diagnosis.

6) Horizontal position of the heart, elevation of the diaphragm and severe chest deformities rarely produce a LAD of more than $-30°$. However, unlike the AFB, the ECG generally shows an $S_1S_2S_3$ pattern.

7) Wolff-Parkinson-White syndrome can be associated with LAD. However, the ECG shows the typical diagnostic features; short PR interval, initial slow delta wave and widened QRS complex. The difficulty arises when Mahaim fibers are the cause of pre-excitation as they are associated with a normal PR interval; in these cases additional electrophysiological studies may be required to make the diagnosis.

POSTERIOR FASCICULAR BLOCK

Isolated posterior fascicular block (PFB) represents a very rare ECG feature; this has been attributed to the fact that this fascicle is short, with a dual blood supply from the anterior and posterior arteries, as well as its location in the less turbulent inflow tract of the left ventricle. When conduction in this fascicle is impaired, the electrical forces due to the functioning anterior fascicle predominate. In experimental PFB it has been observed that the activation of the posterior portions, and in a third of cases also of the middle portions of the septum is delayed [68]. The antero-superior wall is normally activated by the functioning anterior fascicle and the postero-inferior wall is abnormally activated by the Purkinje fibers, after a delay of about 20 msec, in a superior to inferior direction [68, 69].

ELECTROCARDIOGRAPHIC FEATURES

PFB is commonly diagnosed by right axis deviation (RAD) of more than $+100°$ with an S_1Q_3 pattern in the absence of right ventricular hypertrophy (RVH) and of an anatomical vertical position of the heart [4, 70, 71]. Other authors attribute diagnostic value to QRS axis deviation between $+60°$ and $90°$ [72, 73].

As with AFB, the criterion of axis deviation does not appear sufficient to diagnose PFB, since many conditions such as RVH, anatomic vertical heart, pulmonary emphysema, right ventricular conduction disturbance, lateral infarction, pulmonary embolism [74], and paracentesis [75], could cause RAD.

From the analysis of experimental data [29, 31, 54] and of intermittent PFB [76-

79], we believe that, in order to diagnose PFB, the evidence for asynchronous left ventricular activation due to delayed excitation of the inferior wall must be present in addition to RAD.

In PFB asynchrony is manifested as: 1) delayed IDT (50 msec or more) in lead V_6 (or aVF), as it explores the latero-inferior wall of the left ventricle, and 2) IDT in lead V_6 delayed for a comparatively longer time (15 msec or more) than that in lead aVL, which normally explores the antero superior wall [29, 31, 54] (Figure 12).

In addition, the following ECG changes may be helpful in the diagnosis of PFB:

a) Q waves in leads II, III and aVF, due to superior orientation of the first vector. These may sometimes be deep according to modification in septal activation.

b) Absence of terminal r wave in aVR and of s wave in V_6 since the left ventricle is abnormally activated in a superior to inferior direction.

c) Terminal or mid to terminal slurring in leads II, III, aVF and V_6. This results from a conduction delay in the inferior wall of the left ventricle.

d) Flat or negative T wave in diaphragmatic leads due to secondary alterations in repolarization.

e) QRS duration generally within normal limits. Table 5 shows the ECG features and pathophysiology of PFB.

VECTORCARDIOGRAPHIC FEATURES

In the F plane, the QRS loop shows clockwise rotation. The first vectors, sometimes delayed, are directed superiorly and to the right or sometimes to the left. The middle vectors are oriented inferiorly and to the left with a maximum vector generally between $+60°$ and $+80°$. The terminal vectors are directed inferiorly and to the left or sometimes slightly to the right. A terminal delay of about 20-25 msec is sometimes seen, but it is more evident in ECG leads II, III and aVF [40].

In the H plane, the QRS loop is inscribed in a counterclockwise fashion. The initial vectors are directed anteriorly and to the right or sometimes to the left. The maximum vector is oriented posteriorly and to the left.

In the RS plane, the QRS loop is inscribed in a clockwise fashion. The initial vectors are directed superiorly and anteriorly, the middle vectors posteriorly and the terminal vectors inferiorly and posteriorly.

DIFFERENTIAL DIAGNOSIS

PFB should be differentiated from conditions causing right axis deviation:

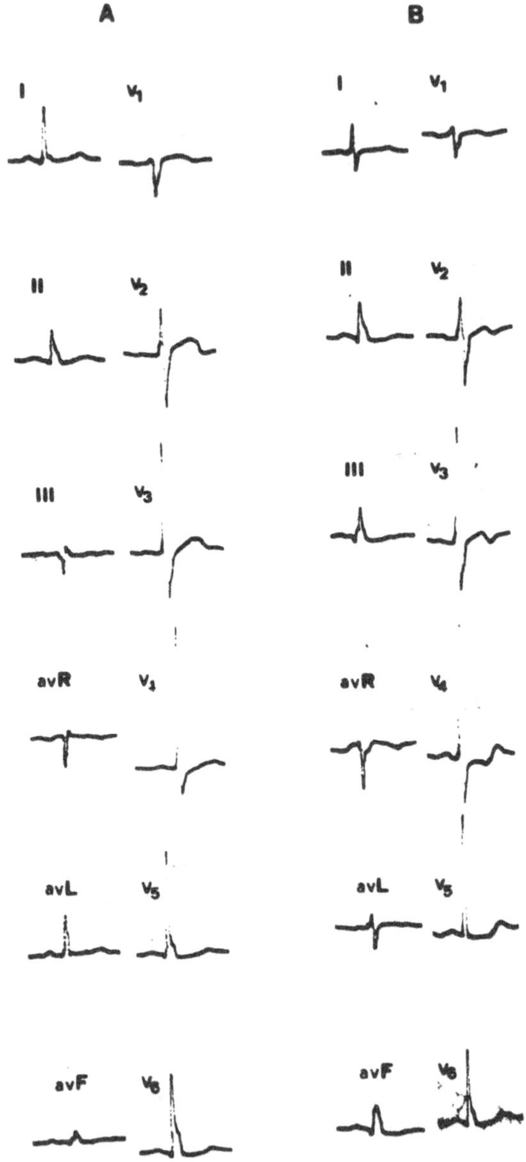

Figure 12. Transient posterior fascicular block. A: ECG tracing with intermediate electrical axis. The QRS complex measures 90 msec. The intrinsecoid deflection time is 55 msec in aVF and 40 msec in aVL. There is an initial slurring in aVF and a terminal one in II, III, V_5 and V_6. B: ECG recorded during angina; the appearance of posterior fascicular block can be observed. The electrical axis shifts to the right (+90°). The QRS complex duration increases to 100 msec. The terminal r wave in aVR disappears, whereas the terminal slurring remains. In A, in spite of the intermediate electrical axis, an incomplete PFB is most likely to be present because of the prolonged intrinsecoid deflection time in aVF and of terminal slurring in the diaphragmatic leads

Table 5. Pathophysiology and ECG changes in posterior fascicular block

ECG FEATURES	PATHOPHYSIOLOGY
q wave in II, III, aVF	Upward orientation of the first vectors
Delay of intrinsecoid deflection more prolonged in V_6(or aVF) than in aVL (15 msec or more)	Asynchronous left ventricular activation
Delay of intrinsecoid deflection in V_6 (or aVF) of 50 msec or more Right axial deviation of more than $+90°$ Absence of terminal r wave in aVR Absence of S wave in V_6	Abnormal superior to inferior activation of the left ventricle
Terminal or mid-terminal slurring in II, III, aVF	Conduction delay in the inferior wall of the left ventricle
Flat or negative T wave in II, III, aVF	Secondary alterations of repolarization

1) According to most authors [4, 70, 71] right ventricular hypertrophy, in the absence of clinical and radiological data, is impossible to differentiate from PFB. In fact they evaluate PFB as a diagnosis of exclusion only possible in the absence of RVH. This can be true if one considers only the axis criterion for diagnosing PFB. In ou opinion the differential diagnosis is possible in some cases. In fact, in PFB, a terminal r wave in aVR and a S wave in V_6 are not present (Figure 12). These features are incompatible with RVH. However, it must be pointed out that when RVH is present, it is difficult, if not impossible, to make the diagnosis of PFB.

2) Vertical position of the heart. In this position, the ventricular activation is directed mainly inferiorly with a clockwise rotation of the QRS loop, thus giving a finding very similar to that of PFB. Moreover, the activation appears earlier in aVL than in V_6, producing left asynchronous activation as in PFB [80]. According to Medrano [30] (Figure 13)a delayed IDT of 50 msec or more in V_6 (or aVF) excludes vertical position of the heart as the cause of RAD. However, this criterion needs further validation. The terminal slurring in the diaphragmatic leads, frequent in PFB, is often observed in the absence of such fascicular block; hence it cannot be used as a differentiating feature for PFB [80]. The electrical axis of P wave can be of particular help in the ECG diagnosis; if this is shifted downward (flat or negative P waves in lead I), it very likely expresses a vertical position of the heart (Figures 14 and 15). However, in all cases in which the presence of PFB is suspected, a chest X-ray is useful to evaluate the position of the heart since reliable EGG and VCG criteria to differentiate a PFB from a vertical heart do not exist.

3) Inferior wall myocardial infarction. PFB can produce deep Q waves in diaphragmatic leads – due to superior orientation of the first vectors – which can simulate an inferior wall infarction. However, these Q waves are not wide and a vertical axis is quite rare in inferior infarction [81, 82]. The coexistence of the two

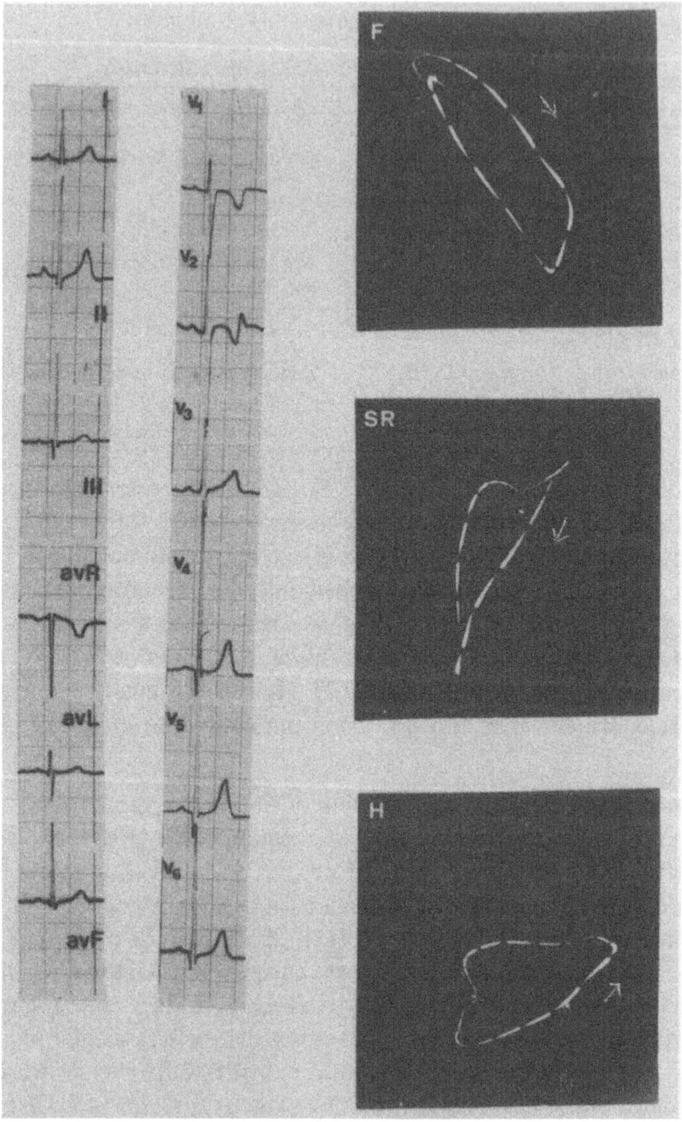

Figure 13. A patient, whose chest X-ray shows a vertical position of the heart. In the ECG the electrical axis is vertical and a posterior fascicular block must be considered. Absence of prolonged intrinsecoid deflection time in aVF (40 msec) tends to exclude the fascicular block

affections can produce both infarctional Q waves and vertical axis (see Chapter 10).

3) Lateral wall infarction can sometimes induce marked RAD. However, infarctional Q waves are observed in lead I and aVL and the VCG shows a QRS loop

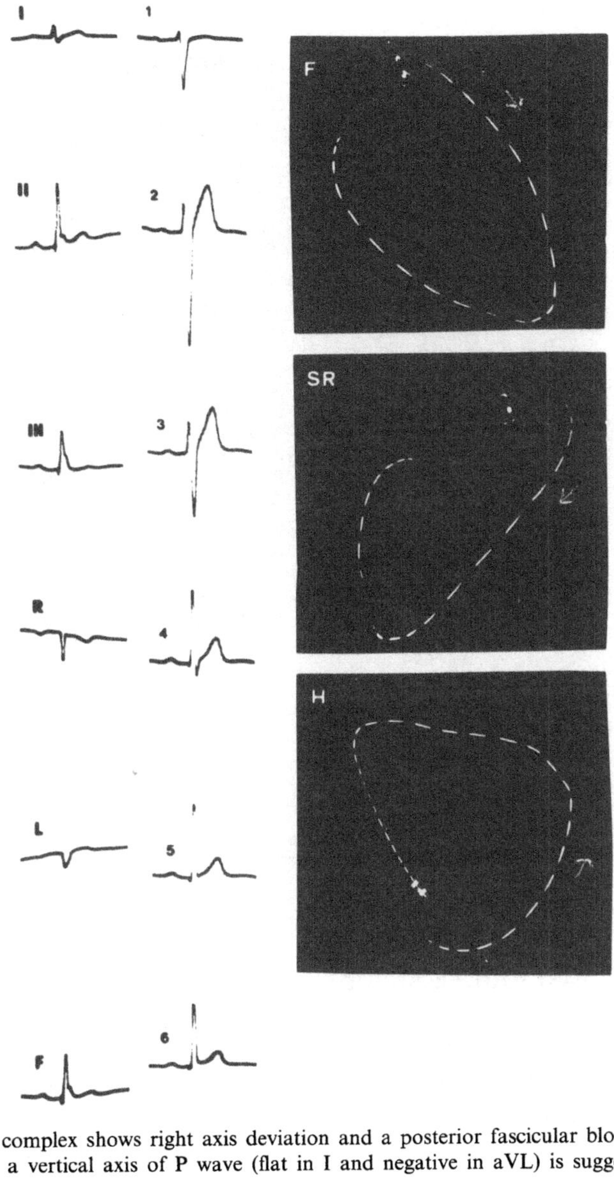

Figure 14. QRS complex shows right axis deviation and a posterior fascicular block must be considered. Instead, a vertical axis of P wave (flat in I and negative in aVL) is suggestive of vertical anatomic position of the heart

oriented to the right with clockwise rotation or figure of eight in the H plane.

5) Wolff-Parkinson-White is at times associated with RAD. However, as mentioned previously, the ECG shows typical features and only in a few rare cases is an electrophysiological investigation necessary to make the diagnosis.

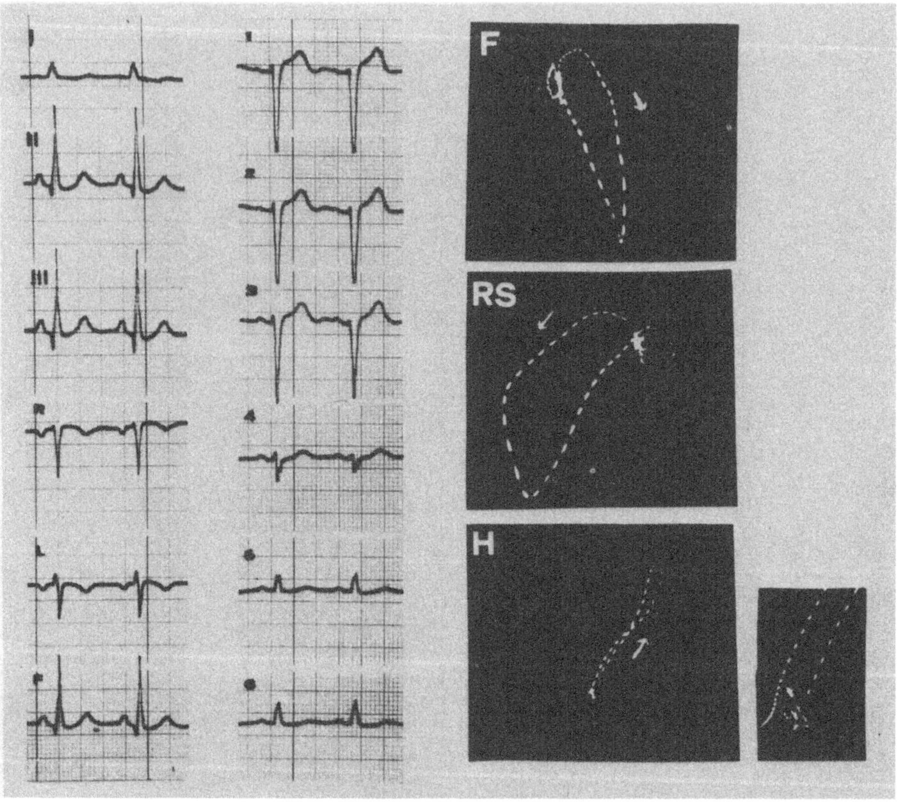

Figure 14. Right axis deviation and terminal slurring in leads III and aVF. A posterior fascicular block must be considered. Instead, a vertical axis of P wave (flat in I and negative in aVL) is suggestive of vertical anatomic position of the heart

LEFT SEPTAL FASCICULAR BLOCK

The few experimental studies in which the septal (middle) fascicle has been damaged produced different results, all difficult to interpret since the functional characteristics of such a fascicle are not well defined.

Uhley et al. [6, 8], following sectioning of the septal fascicle, found a prolongation of the QRS complex by 10 msec with disappearance of q wave in leads V_5 and V_6. Other authors [21] observed a leftward deviation of the electrical axis. By cutting into the left side of the interventricular septum of a dog, Dabrowka et al. [10] produced a pattern of incomplete LBBB with a slight prolongation of the QRS complex. This finding could be related to sectioning blindly in the area of the left bundle branch.

Since the available experimental data are controversial and the subdivision of

LBBB is variable, it is difficult, if not impossible, to diagnose a left septal fascicular block in ECG and VCG tracings.

In some rare cases, it appears possible to evaluate the integrity of the middle fascicle when the anterior and posterior fascicles are blocked [6] (see Chapter 3).

PATHOLOGICAL CORRELATIONS

Very few studies correlating the histopathological lesions and the ECG changes in fascicular blocks have been published and their results are contradictory. Some authors feel that AFB is clearly related to damage to the anterior division of the LBB [4, 83, 84] but this correlation is less evident in other studies. Demoulin et al. [9] found that patients with AFB when compared to those without ECG signs of intraventricular blocks, had a consistent and significantly greater density of fibrosis throughout the left intraventricular conduction system. In eight patients with AFB, the fibrosis appeared to be evenly distributed throughout the conduction system, in four cases it was located predominantly in the anterior, and midseptal fibers in one patient. In the remaining three patients, there was an increasing density of fibrosis from the posterior to midseptal and anterior fibres. These authors concluded that the AFB is a reliable sign of LBB disease, but that the underlying lesions are more widely distributed than would be expected from the ECG findings. Rossi [85] studied serial sections of the conduction system in eight cases with AFB and found pathological changes in the LBB in all of them but a significant involvement of the anterior division occured in only two cases. Similarly, Blondeau et al. [86] and Entman et al. [87] found in their cases a poor correlation between the ECG and anatomical lesions in the anterior fascicle.

With PFB, gross anatomy of the hearts in most patients revealed diffuse involvement. Inferior wall myocardial infarction was often present, although not always evident in the ECG [88].

Recently, Demoulin et al. [89] studied 13 patients with PFB. In nine of the patients the conduction disorders were observed during an episode of acute myocardial infarction. Of these nine patients, four showed interruptive lesions at the level of the posterior radiation of the left bundle or of the posterior portion of the main LBB. Two were found to have severe alterations scattered throughout the LBB system. All four patients with chronic PFB had major alterations of the left-sided conduction system that were consistently maximal at the level of the posterior fibers or posterior portion of the main LBB. In two of these patients scattered lesions were found throughout the LBB fibers. In general, the alterations underlying PFB were less widely spread than in AFB; however, they were more severe and more proximally located.

From the limited available data it is possible to conclude that AFB and PFB do not always have a clear cut histopathological basis. This discrepancy in the anatomical and functional correlation should provide an incentive to improve the diagnostic criteria. In most studies the diagnosis of AFB and PFB was based only on the axis criterion, which is not very specific and can result in false positives.

In addition, the design of the histological studies should be modified as in most of the cases His bundle was not examined. Recent studies have shown that a discrete lesion in the His bundle may manifest AFB pattern [90-92]. The role of metabolic and biomedical changes which may alter the action potential of the conducting fibers without an associated histological change should be kept in mind. Sophisticated electronic microscopes could clarify some of these discrepancies.

CLINICAL DATA

Our analysis of 61900 out-patient ECGs, showed AFB in 1008 cases, which were diagnosed utilizing the criteria mentioned previously. The overall incidence of AFB was 1.6% and was similar to that described in other studies utilizing an axis of −45° as a diagnostic criterion for AFB [93-95]. However, other investigators have reported a higher incidence with a range of 2.4%-11% [4, 96-99]. In similar reports, the incidence of AFB was higher (78.8%) in the male population and increased with age, being highest in the 7th and 8th decades of life (Table 4). There was no clinical evidence of heart disease in only 3.7% of our cases.

As reported by others [4, 53, 96, 100], CAD was the most common (53.8%) etiological factor. This association is understandable as arteriosclerosis induces degenerative changes not only in the working myocardial fibers, but also in the fibers of the conduction system despite their greater resistance to ischemia.

Hypertension was noted in 21.1% of patients: subclinical CAD, hypertrophy and dilatation of the left ventricle, which causes elongation and stretching of the anterior fascicle and an acceleration of the process of sclerosis of the cardiac skeleton, may all be contributing factors in the production of AFB in hypertensive heart disease.

In our series, rheumatic heart disease was a rare cause (2.3%) of AFB and the aortic valve was most commonly involved.

Congenital heart disease was present in 1% of the cases and the most common lesion was endocardial cushion defect. However, in this situation, the fascicular block pattern is not due to a true conduction disturbance, but is caused by anomalous distribution of the intraventricular conduction system (see Chapter 7). Chronic pulmonary disease was present in 4.6% and rare causes like alcoholic cardiomyopathy and collagen diseases were present in 1.9% of cases.

A small group (3.7%) of patients had no clinical evidence of heart disease and AFB may be attributed to the following etiological factors: a) sclerodegenerative disease, as described by Lenegre [41], involving only the intraventricular conduction system; b) anomalous distribution of the LBB system as seen in endocardial cushion defect; c) sclerosis of the cardiac skeleton primarily involving the anterior fascicle; d) old subclinical myocarditis [101]; e) subclinical CAD.

The incidence of various heart diseases in our group of patients is similar to those in other series [53, 96, 100, 102]. Rosenbaum et al. [4] described a higher incidence of myocarditis in South America which is probably related to a higher incidence of Chagas disease.

The incidence of AFB in the absence of heart disease is higher in other series. Ostrander [97] described an incidence of 59% and Yano et al. [94] one of 60% of cases. The reasons for the discrepancies are possibly related to the fact that: a) Ostrander considers an axis of more than $-30°$ as diagnostic of AFB. Hence, his series probably includes patients in whom the LAD was due to causes other than AFB; and b) Yano's study was carried out in an outpatient population of a Hawaiian Island, where the society is still partly primitive. It is well known that industrialization increases both the incidence and severity of CAD. It is also possible that many patients considered normal did have subclinical heart disease.

AFB has rarely been reported to have been induced by hyperkalemia [103, 104], diphtheria [105], chest trauma [106], neuromyopathies [107, 108] or mitral and aortic valve prosthesis [109]. Aravindakshan et al. [110] reported some patients in whom AFB occurred following tricuspid valve surgery. It is unclear as to how the anterior fascicle, which is a left ventricular structure, could be damaged during an operation involving only the right ventricular chamber. It hs been proposed by these authors that the damage is located within the His bundle. The appearance of AFB following corrective procedures for congenital heart disease is well recognized, particularly after repair of tetralogy of Fallot (see Chapter 7).

A familial incidence of fascicular block has been described. In these cases, the block was not limited to a single fascicle, but it progressively involved the entire conduction system [59, 111-115]. In some cases the genetic transmission was of the autosomal dominant type [112, 115].

From the available data, it is difficult to define the clinical implication of AFB. Data are confused since various types of intraventricular blocks are often included and some studies involved hospitalized patients whereas others analyzed outpatient population. To the best of our knowledge, ours is the only clinical study in which diagnosis of AFB is based on the criteria of left ventricular asynchrony in addition to the LAD. The incidence of AFB in our study (1.6%) may be higher than expected as we analyzed outpatients. However, like many other authors [4, 53, 96, 100], we believe that AFB in most cases underlies some cardiac pathology. Even if an underlying heart disease is not detected, these patients should be followed as AFB may represent sublinical heart disease.

Few data are available on the long-term follow-up of persons with AFB [94, 97, 116-118] and hardly any of these studies report the development of other intraventricular conduction disturbances. Schneider et al. [116] analyzed the Framingham data and found that AFB was an uncommon precursor of LBBB; only 6% of the subjects had prior LAD. Also in the study by Rabkin et al. [118], few cases of LAD progressed to LBBB (0.8%). The likelihood of developing RBBB increased in males with marked LAD. The risk of this conduction disturbance, which was only 2.4% (6 out of 247) for men of all ages during the 12 years follow-up period, might be considered too low to be clinically significant. Although the number of such cases of LAD progressing to RBBB is small, the proportion is larger than for the rest of the population without LAD. In the absence of the intercurrent development of CAD, complete AV block did not develop in any subject [118].

Siegman-Igra et al. [119], in a study performed in a stable Israeli population, followed 74 patients with AFB for 10 years. In seven patients (9.5%) progression was observed; in five to bifascicular block, in one to bifascicular block and complete heart block and in one to complete AV block without bifascicular block. Progression was closely connected with presence or subsequent appearance of CAD.

From these few data obtained from the general population it may be deduced that in patients with AFB the development of complete AV block represents a very rare complication and almost always appears in relation to the presence of CAD.

Because of the rarity of PFB, it is difficult to draw conclusions on the epidemiology and the clinical significance of PFB. De Padua et al. [120] reported an incidence of 0.5% of PFB. This datum may not be very accurate as only an axis of more than +90° was used for the diagnosis of PFB. It has been pointed out that PFB is not uncommon in aortic insufficiency due to the trauma induced by the regurgitant stream on the diaphragmatic wall [121].

COMMENT

According to most authors, the ECG diagnosis of anterior and posterior fascicular blocks is based on the presence of marked QRS axis deviation. Since many conditions can produce the shift in the axis (Table 1), this criterion can lead to false positives. Based on experimental and clinical works, the demonstration of asynchrony in left ventricular activation appears to be a very important diagnostic feature of fascicular blocks. However, there are certain limitations to the ECG criteria of asynchronous left ventricular activation as with the heart in a vertical position the lead aVL may explore the anterior paraseptal region or the left atrium [122] instead of the antero-superior wall. Consequently, in patients with vertical heart, the delay of IDT, in aVL and V_6 can be worthless.

According to most authors, in the absence of clinical and radiological data it is impossible to differentiate in ECG recording a PFB from an RVH or a vertical heart. We believe that the differentiation between isolated PFB and RVH can be made since in PFB a terminal R wave in aVR and often an S wave in V_6 are lacking; this finding is incompatible with RVH.

Various investigators have placed little importance on the VCG features for the diagnosis of AFB. We have shown that in this block the horizontal QRS loop evidences a definite pattern, most probably related to asynchronous left ventricular activation; this consists of a good development of the loop antero-posteriorly and in a slight one to the left. This finding is not specific since it is also seen in pulmonary emphysema, anterior myocardial infarction, and vertical heart.

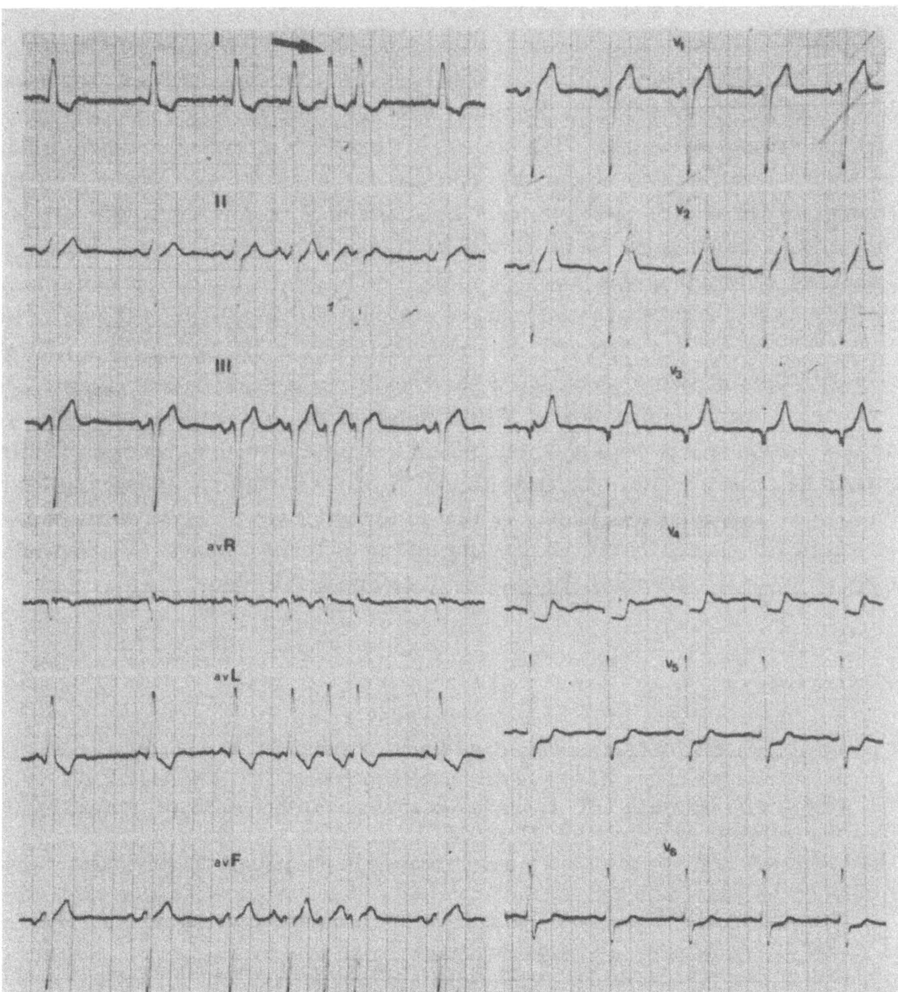

Figure 16. Anterior fascicular block with marked left axis deviation (−75°). During premature atrial beats one can observe further leftward shift of the QRS complex, thus showing that the fascicular block is not complete, in spite of marked left axis deviation

Moreover, it has also been noted in children without heart disease, probably because of anatomical and electrical preponderance of the outflow tract over the inflow tract of the right ventricle. Nevertheless, if not pathognomic, this behavior of the horizontal QRS loop is highly characteristic of AFB.

As for bundle branch blocks, it is not possible to evaluate in ECG and VCG tracings whether a fascicular block pattern expresses a complete interruption of conduction or only a mere slowing of conduction. In Figure 16 an AFB with marked LAD ($-75°$) is reported; during premature atrial beats one can observe further leftward shift of the QRS complex, thus showing that the fascicular block was not complete, in spite of marked LAD.

A difficult problem is to define the anatomo-functional location of the lesion causing the AFB pattern. In fact, the fibers destined to the fascicles are grouped at the level of the His bundle and the main LBB. Therefore the lesion responsible for AFB pattern can be located in His bundle, in main LBB, in anterior fascicle and in the antero-superior wall of the left ventricle. By means of selective His bundle stimulation the site of fascicular block pattern may be located within the His bundle [92] (see Chapter 3). ECG and VCG recordings do not allow a reliable evaluation of whether the lesion is within the anterior fascicle or the antero-superior wall. The presence of a marked terminal slurring suggests the latter location (Figure 9), but does not, however, represent a discriminating criterion, because lesions at two or more levels can coexist in the same patient (Figure 10).

On the clinical significance of AFB, literature offers contradictory data. In various studies it has been encountered almost always in the presence of heart disease, in others a high incidence (50-60%) of AFB without underlying heart disease has been reported. It may be that in the latter cases, AFB expresses subclinical heart disease. However it is important to point out that this fascicular block, if isolated, very rarely progresses to complete AV block.

REFERENCES

1. Rothberger CY, Winterberg H: Experimentelle Beiträge zur Kenntnis der Reizleitungsstörungen in den Kammern des Saugetierherzens. Z Ges Exp Med 5: 264, 1917
2. Wilson FN, Herrman GR: Electrocardiograms of an unusual type in right bundle branch block. Am Heart J 9: 472, 1934
3. Grant RP: Left axis deviation. An electrocardiographicpathologic correlation. Circulation 14: 233, 1956
4. Rosenbaum MB, Elizari MV, Lazzari JO: Los hemibloqueos. Buenos Aires: Paidos, 1968
5. Rosenbaum MB, Elizari MV, Lazzari JO: The hemiblocks. Oldsmar: Tampa Tracing, 1970
6. Uhley HN, Rivkin LM: Electrocardiographic patterns following interruption of the main and peripheral branches of the canine left bundle of His. Am J Cardiol 13: 41, 1964

7. Uhley HN: Some controversy regarding the peripheral distribution of the conduction system. Am J Cardiol 30: 913, 1972
8. Uhley HN: The quadrifascicular nature of the peripheral conduction system. In: Cardiac arrhythmias, Areifus LS, Likoff W:. New York: Grune & Stratton, 1973
9. Demoulin JC, Simar LJ, Kulbertus HE: Quantitative study of left bundle branch fibrosis in left anterior hemiblock: a stereologic approach. Am J Cardiol 36: 751, 1975
10. Dabrowka B, Ruka M, Walczak E: The electrocardiographic diagnosis of left septal fascicular block. Europ J Cardiol 6: 347, 1978
11. Rossi L: Sistema di conduzione trifascicolare ed emiblocchi di branca sinistra. Considerazioni anatomiche ed istopatologiche. G Ital Cardiol 1: 55, 1971
12. Titus JL: Anatomy of the conduction system. Circulation 47: 170, 1973
13. Massing GK, James TN: Anatomical configuration of the His bundle and bundle branches in the human heart. Circulation 53: 609, 1976
14. Durrer D, Van Dam RTh, Freud GE, Janse MJ, Meijler FL, Arzbaecher RC: Total excitation of the isolated human heart. Circulation 41: 899, 1970
15. Myerburg RJ, Nilson K, Gelband H: Physiology of canine intraventricular conduction and endocardial excitation. Circ Res 30: 217, 1972
16. Brusca A, Rosettani E: Activation of the human fetal heart. Am Heart J 86: 79, 1973
17. Lazzara R, Yeh BK, Samet P: Functional anatomy of the cardiac left bundle branch. Am J Cardiol 33: 623, 1974
18. Lazzara R, El-Sherif N, Befeler B, Scherlag BJ: Regional refractoriness within the ventricular conduction system. Circ Res 39: 254, 1976
19. Hecht HN, Kossmann CE, Childers RW, Langendorf R, Lev M, Rosen KM, Pruitt RD, Truex RC, Uhley HN, Watt TB: Atrioventricular and intraventricular conduction. Revised nomenclature and concepts. Am J Cardiol 31: 232, 1973
20. Watt TB, Freud GE, Durrer D, Pruitt RD: Left anterior arborization block combined with right bundle branch block in canine and primate hearts. Circ Res 22: 57, 1968
21. Gallagher JJ, Ticzon AR, Wallace AG, Kasell J: Activation studies following experimental hemiblock in the dog. Circ Res 35: 572, 1974
22. Meeran MK, Wyndham CR, Levitsky S, Engelman RM, Rosen KM: Comparison of epicardial activation in patients with normal conduction and left anterior fascicular block. Circulation 56 (Suppl III): 107, 1977
23. Wyndham CRS, Meeran MK, Smith T, Engelman RM, Levitsky S, Rosen KM: Epicardial activation in human left anterior fascicular block. Am J Cardiol 44: 638, 1979
24. Sohi GS, Flowers NC: Effects of left anterior fascicular block on the depolarization process as depicted by total body surface mapping. J Electrocardiol 13: 143, 1980
25. Wyndham CR, Meeran MK, Smith T, Saxena A, Engelman RM, Levitsky S, Rosen KM: Epicardial activation of the intact human heart without conduction defects. Circulation 59: 161, 1979
26. Ribeiro CS: Estudo da activação ventricular nos bloqueios intraventriculares esquerdos (Contribuição experimental para o seu diagnostico clinico). Arquivo de Patologia 41: 151, 1969
27. Warembourg H, Thery CL, Pauchant M, Lekieffre J, Ketelers JY: Les hyperdéviations de ÂQRS d'origine extracardiaque (Etude expérimental. Considérations sur l'emphysème). Arch Mal Coeur 64: 1295, 1971
28. Nava A, Rusconi L, Silvani S, Schivazappa L, Buja GF: I blocchi di branca destra con ansa dorsalizzata. G Ital Cardiol 6: 265, 1976
29. Medrano GA, Brenes CP, De Micheli A, Sodi-Pallares D: El bloqueo simultaneo de la subdivision anterior y posterior de la rama izquierda del haz de His (bloqueo

bifascicular) y su asociaction con bloqueo de la rama derecha (bloqueo trifascicular). Estudio electrocardiografico experimental y clinico. Arch Inst Cardiol Mex 40: 752, 1970
30. Medrano GA, De Micheli A: El electrocardiograma y el vectorcardiograma en los bloqueos mono- y polifasciculares. Arch Inst Cardiol Mex 44: 421, 1974
31. Medrano GA, De Micheli A, Brenes PC, Sodi-Pallares D: Experimental bases for diagnosis of left bifascicular and trifascicular block. G Ital Cardiol 5: 8, 1975
32. Rosenbaum MB, Shabetai R, Peterson KL, O'Rourke RA: Nature of conduction disturbances in selective coronary arteriography and left heart catheterization. Am J Cardiol 30: 334, 1972
33. Jacobson LB, Lafollette L, Cohn K: An appraisal of initial QRS forces in left anterior fascicular block. Am Heart J 94: 407, 1977
34. Burchell HB, Tuna N: The interpretation of gross left axis deviation in the electrocardiogram. Europ J Cardiol 10: 259, 1979
35. Samson WE, Bruce RA: Left ventricular parietal block produced by transventricular aortic commissurotomy. Am Heart J 63: 41, 1962
36. Medrano GA, Cisneros F, De Micheli A, Sodi-Pallares D: The anterior subdivision block of the left bundle branch of His. 2. Experimental vectorcardiographic observations. J Electrocardiol 3: 13, 1970
37. Medrano GA, De Micheli A, Brenes PC, Alatriste VM, Sodi-Pallares D: Necrosis posterior complicada con bloqueo bifascicular y trifascicular. Arch Inst Cardiol Mex 42: 375, 1972
38. Alboni P, Fantini F, Nava A, Masoni A: Criteri elettrocardiografici attuali per la diagnosi dei blocchi fascicolari. G Ital Cardiol 6: 118, 1976
39. Alboni P: Revisione del concetto di emiblocco. Atti IX Congresso Nazionale ANMCO. Rome: Pozzi, 1978, p 205
40. Alboni P, Malacarne C, De Lorenzi E, Pirani R, Baldassarri F, Masoni Q: Right precordial q waves due to anterior fascicular block. Clinical and vectorcardiographic study. J Electrocardiol 12: 41, 1979
41. Lenegre J: Etiology and pathology of bilateral bundle branch block in relation to complete heart block. Cardiovasc Dis 6: 409, 1964
42. Cerqueira-Gomez M, Abreu-Lima C, Ramalhao C: Acerca da importancia da orientaçao des forcas iniciais no diagnostico dos hemibloqueios. Boll Soc Port Cardio 8: 227, 1970
43. Lemberg L, Castellanos A Jr, Arcebal AG: Revaluation of septal activation in the human heart with special reference to the spatial orientations of the initial QRS vectors in intermittent left hemiblocks. In: Vectorcardiography II: Proceedings of the XI International Symposium on Vectorcardiography, Hoffman I. Amsterdam: North Holland, 1971, p 257
44. McHenry PL, Philips JF, Fisch C, Corya BR: Right precordial qrS pattern due to left anterior hemiblock. Ann Heart J 81: 498, 1971
45. Medrano GA, De Micheli A, Alatriste VM, Sodi-Pallares D: Necrosis septal complicada con bloqueo bifascicular y trifascicular. Arch Inst Cardiol Mex 43: 715, 1973
46. Pruitt RD, Watt RB, Murao S: Left axis deviation: its relation to experimentally induced lesions of the anterior left bundle branch system in canine and primate heart. Ann NY Acad Sci 127: 204, 1965
47. Okuma K: ECG and VCG changes in experimental hemiblock and bifascicular block. Am Heart J 92: 473, 1976
48. Watt TB: Features of fascicular block unposed upon existing right bundle branch block in the dog and baboon. Am J Cardiol 39: 1000, 1977

49. Burch GE: An electrocardiographic syndrome characterized by absence of Q in leads I, V_5 and V_6. Am Heart J 51: 487, 1956
50. Masoni A, Alboni P: Ipotesi fisiopatogenetiche nel blocco periferico. G Ital Cardiol 6: 812, 1976
51. Alboni P, Malacarne C, Masoni A: Physiopothological and diagnostic hypotheses in peripheral block. J Electrocardiol 10: 87, 1977
52. Smith MGB, Lamb LE: Electrocardiographic findings in 67, 375 asymptomatic subjects. IX. Myocardial infarction. Am J Cardiol 6: 190, 1960
53. Pryor R, Blount SGJr: The clinical significance of true left axis deviation. Left intraventricular blocks. Am Heart J 72: 391, 1966
54. Medrano GA, De Micheli A, Cisneros F, Sodi-Pallares D: The anterior subdivision block of the left bundle branch of His. 1. The ventricular activation process. J Electrocardiol 3: 7, 1970
55. Chou TC, Helm RA: Clinical vectorcardiography. New York: Grune & Stratton, 1967
56. Benchimol A: Vectorcardiography. Baltimore: Williams & Wilkins, 1973
57. Kulbertus HE, Collignon P, Humblet L: Vectorcardiographic study of the QRS loop in patients with left anterior focal block. Am Heart J 79: 293, 1970
58. Lewis T: Observations upon ventricular hypertrophy with special reference to preponderance of one or other chamber. Heart 5: 367, 1914
59. Tsagaris TJ, Bustamante RA; Priesendorff RA: Familial heart disease. Dis Chest 52: 153, 1967
60. Bozzi G, Figini A: Influenza dell'emiblocco anteriore sinistro sui caratteri elettrocardiografici di diagnosi di ipertrofia ventricolare sinistra. G Ital Cardiol 6: 658, 1976
61. Llamas Lombardia A, Isokane N, Montoyo J, Gausi C: Criterios vectorcardiograficos de hypertrofia ventricular izquierda en presencia de hemibloqueo anterior. Rev Esp Cardiol 30: 249, 1977
62. Frau G: La pathogenie des troubles de la conduction ventriculaire. Contribution experimentale. Cardiologia 19: 2, 1951
63. Noseda V, Santi A, Aguggini G, Filotto U, Dergamaschi M: Experimental focal block in the sheep and the dog. An electrocardiographic and histological study, Cardiologia 42: 243, 1963
64. Alboni P: Diagnostic problems pertaining to the left parietal block. In: Electrocardiology: I. Proceedings of World Congress on Electrocardiology, Gandhi MJ, Mehta AB, Pahlajani DB. Bombay: Tata, 1975, p 118
65. Alboni P, Malacarne C, Masoni A: Diagnosis of left ventricular parietal block (Abstr II). 7th European Congress of Cardiology. Amsterdam: Excerpta Medica, 1976, p 352
66. Alboni P, Malacarne C, Masoni A: Left ventricular parietal block: diagnostic and clinical study. J Electrocardiol 9: 139, 1976
67. Fernandez F, Scebat L., Lenegre J: Electrocardiographic study of left intraventricular hemiblock in man during selective coronary arteriography. Am J Cardiol 26: 1, 1970
68. Medrano GA, Brenes PC, De Micheli A, Sodi-Pallares D: Block of the posterior subdivision of the left bundle branch of His. Experimental study. J Electrocardiol 3: 309, 1970
69. Medrano GA, Brenes PC, De Micheli A: Alteraciones de la activacion ventricular producidas por el bloqueo de la subdivision posterior de la rama izquierda del haz de His. Estudio experimental y clinico. Gac Med Mex 101: 53, 1971
70. Benchimol A, Desser KB, Massey BJ: The Franck vectorcardiogram in left posterior hemiblock. J Electro-cardiol 4: 129, 1971
71. Castellanos A Jr, Chaprunoff E, Lemberg L, Porvillo B: The vectorcardiogram in left

posterior hemiblock. In: Vectorcardiography 2; Proceedings of the XI International Symposium on Vectorcardiography, Hoffman I. Amsterdam: North Holland, 1971, p 264
72. Schweizer P, Mellen NS, Rubenfire M: Left posterior hemiblock. I. Electrocardiol 4: 204, 1971
73. Polu JM, Gilgenkrantz JM, Faivre G: Le diagnostic des hémiblocs de branche gauche isolés et associés à un bloc de branche droit ou à un infarctus du myocarde. Arch Mal Coeur 65: 1041, 1972
74. Zucherman R, Estandia A, Zamora J, Barbato E: Cor pulmonale agudo. Arch Inst Cardiol Mex 18: 582, 1948
75. Alboni P, Longhini C, Malacarne C, Giovannini G: Il blocco di branca sinistro con asse elettrico deviato a destra. Studio clinico ed elettro-vectorcardiografico. G Ital Cardiol 5: 543, 1975
76. Bobba P, Salerno JA, Casari A: Transient left posterior hemiblock: report of four cases induced by exercise test. Circulation 46: 931, 1972
77. Gorfinkel HJ, Inglesby TV, Lansing AM: ST-segment elevation, transient left posterior hemiblock and recurrent ventricular arrhythmias unassociated with pain. A variant of Prinzmetal's anginal syndrome. Ann Int Med 79: 795, 1973
78. Colonna L, Bacca F, Cristallo E: Hémibloc postérieur gauche transitoire dans la cardiopathie ischémique aiguë. Arch Mal Coeur 68: 853, 1975
79. Jaillon P, Rosensztajn L, Wargon H, Catinat J: Hémibloc postérieur gauch paroxistique en cours d'une crise angineuse. A propos de 2 observations d'ondes Q transitoires. Coeur et Med Int 14: 169, 1975
80. Nava A, Alboni P, Rusconi L, Malacarne C: Difficoltà diagnostiche nel blocco fascicolare posteriore sinistro isolato. G Ital Cardiol 5: 42, 1975
81. Horan LG, Flowers NC, Johnson JC: Significance of the diagnostic Q waves of myocardial infarction. Circulation 43: 428, 1971
82. Alboni P, Malacarne C, Pradella A, De Lorenzi E: Evoluzione della depolarizzazione ventricolare nella fase acuta dell'infarto inferiore e postero-inferiore. G Ital Cardiol 7: 132, 1077
83. Hawley RL, Pryor R: Quantitative and electrocardiographic correlation of the conduction system of the heart (abstr). Am J Cardiol 15: 132, 1965
84. Sugiura M, Okada R, Hiraoka K: Histological studies of the conduction system in 14 cases of right bundle branch block associated with left axis deviation. Jap Heart J 10: 121, 1969
85. Rossi L: Histopathology of conducting system in left anterior hemiblock. Br Heart J 38: 1304, 1976
86. Blondeau M, Lenegre J: Bloc atypique de la branche droite. Paris: Masson, 1970
87. Entman ML, Estes EH, Hackel DB: The pathologic basis of the electrocardiographic pattern for parietal block. Am Heart J 74: 202, 1974
88. Strickland AW, Horan LG, Flowers NC: Gross anatomy associated with pattern called left posterior hemiblock. Circulation 46: 276, 1972
89. Demoulin JC, Kulbertus HE: Histopathologic correlates of left posterior fascicular block. Am J Cardiol 44: 1083, 1979
90. Sciacca A, Sangiorgi M: Trouble de la conduction intraventriculaire droite dû à lésion du tronc commun du faisceau de His. Acta Cardiol 12: 488, 1957
91. Sciacca A, Di Giacomo V, Neri A, Carmenini G: Turbe di conduzione di tipo bi- e trifascicolare e loro interpretazione anatomo-funzionale. Progr Med 31: 694, 1975
92. Narula OS: Longitudinal dissociation in the His bundle. Bundle branch block due to asynchronous conduction within the His bundle in man. Circulation 56: 42, 1977

93. Testoni F, Coppotelli L, Tommaselli A: Frequenza, eziopatogenesi e significato clinico-prognostico del blocco focale sinistro della conduzione intraventricolare. G Ital Cardiol 1: 204, 1971
94. Yano K, Peskoe SM, Rhoas GG, Moore JO, Kagan A: Left axis deviation and left anterior hemiblock among 8000 Japanese-American men. Am J Cardiol 35: 809, 1975
95. Fadayomi MO, Stephens MR: Left anterior hemiblock in adult Africans. Europ J Cardiol 7: 35, 1978
96. Curd GW, Hicks WM Jr, Gyorkey F: Marked left axis deviation. Indication of cardiac abnormality. Am Heart J 62: 462, 1961
97. Ostrander LDJ: Left axis deviation. Prevalence, associated conductions and prognosis. Ann Intern Med 75: 23, 1971
98. Das G: Left axis deviation. A spectrum of intraventricular conduction block. Circulation 53: 917, 1976
99. Corne RA, Beamish RE, Rollwagen RL: Significance of left anterior fascicular block. Br Heart J 40: 552, 1978
100. Bahl OP, Walsh TJ, Massie E: Left axis deviation. An electrocardiographic study with post-mortem correlation. Br Heart J 31: 451, 1969
101. Lev M: Anatomic basis for atrioventricular block. Am J Med 37: 742, 1964
102. Corne RA, Parkim, TW, Brandenburg RP: Significance of marked left axis deviation. Electrocardiographic-pathologic correlative study. Am J Cardiol 13: 605, 1965
103. Ewy GA, Kalirner J, Bedynek JL: Electrocardiographic QRS axis shift as a manifestation of hyperkalemia. JAMA 215: 429, 1971
104. Punja MM, Schneebaum R, Cohen J: Bifascicular block induced by hyperkalemia. J Electrocardiol 6: 71, 1973
105. Christofani M: Emiblocco sinistro anteriore con blocco di branca destro in corso di difterite. Riporto di 4 casi. Cardiol Prat 25: 39, 1974
106. Harris LK: Transient right branch block following blunt chest trauma. Am J Cardiol 23: 884, 1969
107. Perloff JK: Myocardial disease of heredofamilial neuromyopathies. In: Myocardial disease. New York: Grune & Stratton, 1973, p 319
108. Perloff JL, Roberts NK, Cabeen WR: Left axis deviation. A reassessment. Circulation 60: 12, 1979
109. Gannon PG, Sellers RD, Kanjnh VI, Edwards JE, Lillehei VW: Complete heart block following replacement of the aortic valve. Circulation (suppl I) 33: 152, 1966
110. Aravindakshan V, Elizari MU, Rosenbaum MB: Right bundle branch block and left anterior block (left anterior hemiblock) following tricuspid valve replacement. Circulation 42: 895, 1970
111. Steemkamp WF: Familial trifascicular block. Am Heart J 84: 758, 1972
112. Antonioli GE, Zanardi F, D'Agostino F, Masoni A: Degenerazione familiare del sistema di conduzione. G Ital Cardiol 3: 519, 1973
113. Husson GS, Blackman MS, Rogers MC, Bharati S, Lev M: Familial congenital bundle branch system disease. Am J Cardiol 32: 365, 1973
114. Sangiorgi M, Cannata D, Pierangeli L: Emiblocco anteriore sinistro familiare. Boll Soc Ital Cardiol 19: 29, 1974
115. Vallianos G., Sideris DA: Familial conduction defects. Cardiology 59: 190, 1974
116. Schneider JF, Thomas HE, Kreger B, McNamara P: Left bundle branch block in Framingham (abstr). Circulation (Suppl II) 54, II: 128, 1976
117. Blackburn H, Taylor HS, Keys A: The electrocardiogram in prediction of five-year coronary heart disease incidence among men aged forty through fifty-nine. Circulation (Suppl I) 51, 52: 154, 1970

118. Rabkin SR, Mathewson FAL, Tate RB: Natural story of marked left axis deviation (left anterior hemiblock). Am J Cardiol 43: 605, 1979
119. Siegman-Igra Y, Yahini JH, Goldbourt U: Intraventricular conduction disturbances: a review of prevalence, etiology, and progression for ten years within a stable population of Israeli adult males. Am Heart J 96: 669, 1978
120. De Padua F, Lopes VM, Pereira MJ: Left posterior hemiblock. Good prognosis? Adv Cardiol 14: 157, 1975
121. Warembourg H, Pauchant T Cl, Lekieffre J, Ducloux, G, Gosselin B: Bloc intraventriculaire postérieur au cours de l'insuffisance aortique. Arch Mal Coeur 63: 408, 1970
122. De Micheli A, Medrano GA: Electrocardiograma y vectocardiagrama en el infarto del miocardio. Mexico: La Prensa Medica Mexicana, 1971

5. BIFASCICULAR AND TRIFASCICULAR BLOCKS

The term bifascicular block refers to a combination of right bundle branch block (RBBB) with either anterior fascicular block (AFB) or posterior fascicular block (PFB).

Such a term is not, however, completely suitable due to inconsistency in the subdivision into fascicles of the left bundle branch (see Chapters 1 and 4). For this reason some authors [1, 2] prefer the term RBBB with left axis deviation (LAD) or with right axis deviation (RAD).

In this chapter only the features resulting from interference between RBBB and AFB will be discussed. The characteristics of each block are refered to in their respective chapters.

RIGHT BUNDLE BRANCH BLOCK AND ANTERIOR FASCICULAR BLOCK

Right bundle branch block with anterior fascicular block is the most common type of bifascicular block. Due to the scarcity of experimental data we know very little about ventricular activation in this type of block. The postero-inferior wall of the left ventricle is normally activated, whereas both the right ventricle and the antero-superior wall of the left ventricle show delayed excitation [3-6].

Watt [6], who studied ventricular activation both in the dog and in the baboon during experimentally induced RBBB and AFB, observed that RBBB caused greater delay in right ventricular excitation in the dog than in the baboon (46 versus 42 msec). Conversely the antero-superior wall of the left ventricle was activated later in the baboon (25 msec versus 18 msec).

At present, epicardial mapping during open heart surgery has not been performed in man as it has been for isolated AFB [7] and LBBB [8].

Electrocardiographic features

In this bifascicular block the ECG features of both isolated RBBB and isolated AFB are observed as well as some ECG signs related to the combination of the two blocks. The most commonly accepted criteria for the diagnosis of RBBB with AFB are those proposed by Rosenbaum et al. [9]: *RBBB pattern with QRS axis more negative than* $-45°$ *and with a small q wave in lead I.*

However, an LAD can be related to other causes such as left ventricular hypertrophy, pulmonary emphysema, inferior myocardial infarction, horizontal position of the heart, and left ventricular peripheral block. These conditions are often associated in a clinical setting and can produce a marked LAD due to a summation effect. Therefore LAD is not a specific diagnostic feature for AFB associated with RBBB.

On the basis of experimental data [3-6] RBBB with AFB can be diagnosed if, besides LAD, the ECG signs of asynchronous left ventricular activation are also present (see Chapter 4).

The following ECG characteristics are helpful in the diagnosis of RBBB associated with AFB (Figures 1 and 2):

- QRS interval of 120 msec or more.
- Right bundle branch block morphology in right precordial leads.
- Left axis deviation greater than $-45°$, due to an abnormal inferior to superior activation of the left ventricle. In RBBB with AFB, LAD is more marked than in isolated AFB [9].
- q wave in I and aVL, due to downward and rightward orientation of the first vectors.
- Delay of intrinsecoid deflection in aVL of 50 msec or more, because of a delayed activation of the antero-superior wall of the left ventricle.
- Delay of intrinsecoid deflection more prolonged in aVL than in V_6 for asynchronous left ventricular activation (see Chapter 4). Such a feature is, however, of more importance for the diagnosis of isolated AFB; in fact isolated RBBB can also change the intrinsecoid deflection time in the left-sided leads.
- Deep S wave in V_5 and V_6, in so far as such a wave is accentuated both by RBBB and AFB.
- Sometimes small q waves in V_2-V_3 leads due to a more posterior orientation of the first vectors in relation to AFB and septal fibrosis (see Chapter 4).
- Small or absent s wave in I and aVL; this finding contrasts with the presence of RBBB.

The latter electric feature was defined by Rosenbaum et al. [9] as 'masquerading bundle branch block'. In fact, when the QRS complex is prolonged and the S wave in leads I and aVL is very small or absent, the extremity leads may simulate a left bundle branch block (LBBB) although the precordial leads show RBBB. For this reason some authors considered these cases as LBBB [10], or called then 'LBBB masquerading as RBBB' [11, 12]. The late leftward and superiorly oriented forces related to AFB tend to cancel out the late rightward forces related to RBBB; consequently the S waves in I and aVL decrease or disappear (Figures 1 and 2). In effect, the higher the degree of AFB, the smaller the S_1.

Such an ECG pattern is very useful for the diagnosis of bifascicular block in cases where the presence of AFB associated with RBBB is doubtful.

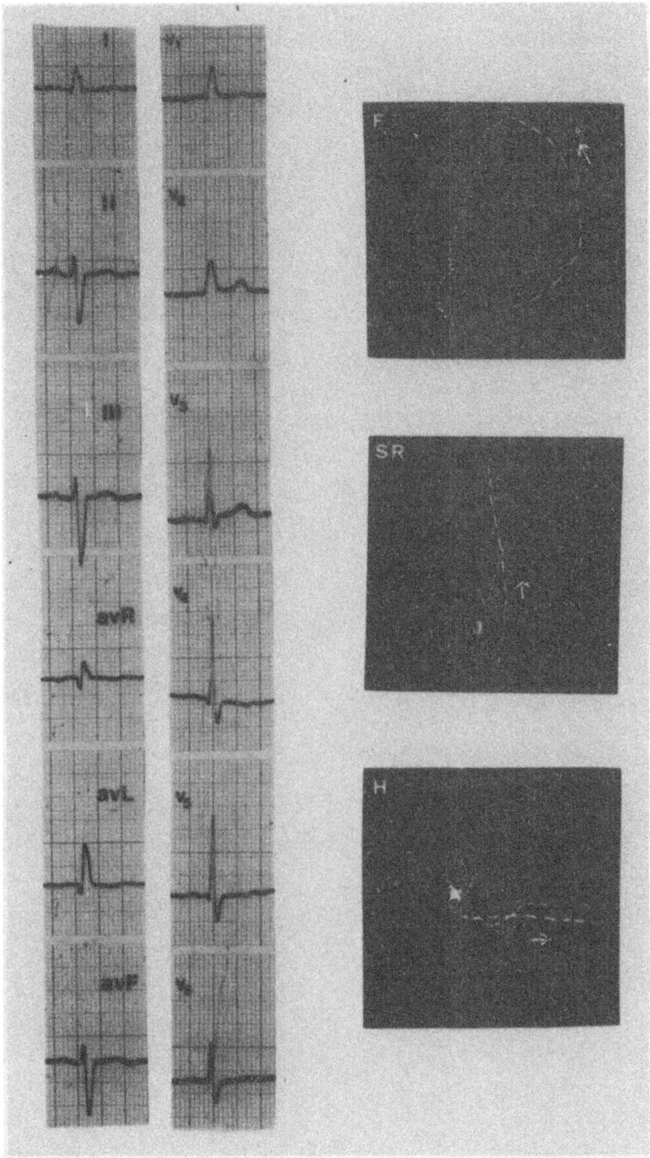

Figure 1. Right bundle branch block (RBBB) with anterior fascicular block (AFB). ECG: RBBB clearly evident in right precordial leads. Marked left axis deviation. The delay of intrinsecoid deflection is 60 msec in aVL and 30 msec in V_6. *In I and aVL leads the S wave is absent.* VCG: The frontal plane shows counterclockwise rotation of the QRS loop woth marked superior orientation of the mid-terminal forces. Even in the horizontal plane the rotation is counterclockwise. In both planes the rightward displacement of the terminal forces is very slight; this pattern represents the vectorcardiographic espression of a 'masquerading bundle branch block pattern'

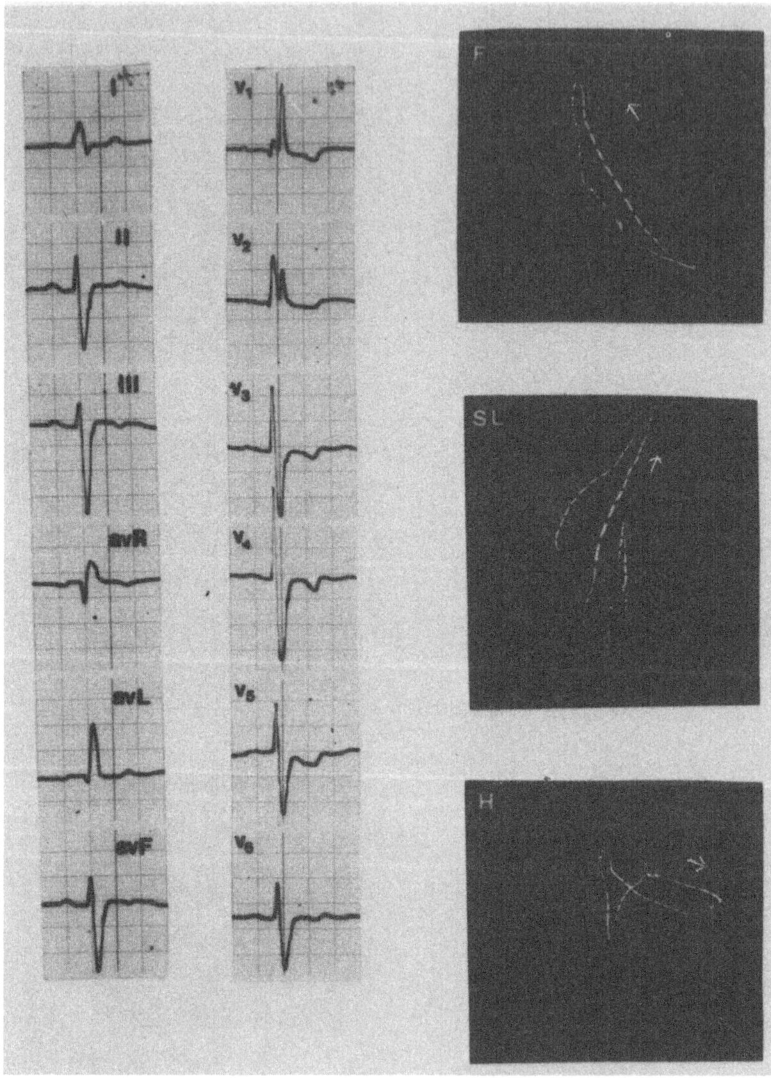

Figure 2. Right bundle branch block with anterior fascicular block. The ECG shows RBBB in right precordial leads; in addition there is marked left axis deviation. The delay of intrinsecoid deflection is 80 msec in aVL and 40 msec in V_6. *S wave is absent in aVL and small in I.* In the VCG the inscription of the QRS loop is counterclockwise in the F plane, whereas in the H plane the initial and middle forces show clockwise rotation. The delayed terminal forces are displaced to the right, superiorly and anteriorly

Rosenbaum et al. [13] described three cases in which AFB obscured the diagnosis of RBBB also in right precordial leads. The RBBB was incomplete in one case and of advanced degree in the other two. The AFB abolished not only the S waves in I and aVL, but also the terminal R^1 wave in V_1. The late posteriorly oriented forces related to AFB cancel out the rightward and anteriorly oriented forces related to RBBB (Figure 3).

The possibility that RBBB can be totally missed in the presence of AFB may imply a limitation in clinical setting, because some of the well known diagnostic and prognostic connotations of this association of conduction disturbances may then be overlooked. However, if the QRS interval is excessively wide or more than expected for isolated AFB, a concealed RBBB may be suspected.

Rosenbaum et al. [13] suggest the recording of additional right precordial leads, one interspace above the conventional level, to uncover the RBBB. In our experience, however, the appearance of a terminal R wave in such leads is quite frequent, as in normal subjects, and appears therefore not to be specific for a concealed RBBB.

Table 1 shows the ECG features of RBBB associated with AFB.

Vectorcardiographic features

In the frontal (F) plane the first 10-20 msec vectors are directed to the right and inferiorly. The QRS loop is then oriented superiorly and only slightly to the left in a counterclockwise fashion. The delayed terminal forces are directed to the right and superiorly. The rightward displacement of the terminal vectors is however less marked than in isolated RBBB. Such a pattern represents the vectorcardiographic expression of the masquerading bundle branch block.

In the horizontal (H) plane the first vectors are directed to the right, anteriorly or slightly posteriorly. The QRS loop may rotate in a counterclockwise or clockwise fashion. The loop shows slight development of the QRS to the left. The terminal segment of the QRS loop is inscribed slowly and oriented to the right and anteriorly.

In the right sagittal (RS) plane the efferent limb shows a markedly superior orientation and may be more or less anteriorly directed, depending on whether the horizontal QRS loop is clockwise or counterclockwise, respectively. The afferent limb inscription is delayed and shows an antero-superior orientation (Figures 1 and 2).

Differential diagnosis

The diagnosis of RBBB is generally easy for the typical morphology of the QRS complex in right precordial leads. Recognition of AFB associated with RBBB is more complicated. As for the isolated AFB, the differential diagnosis must be

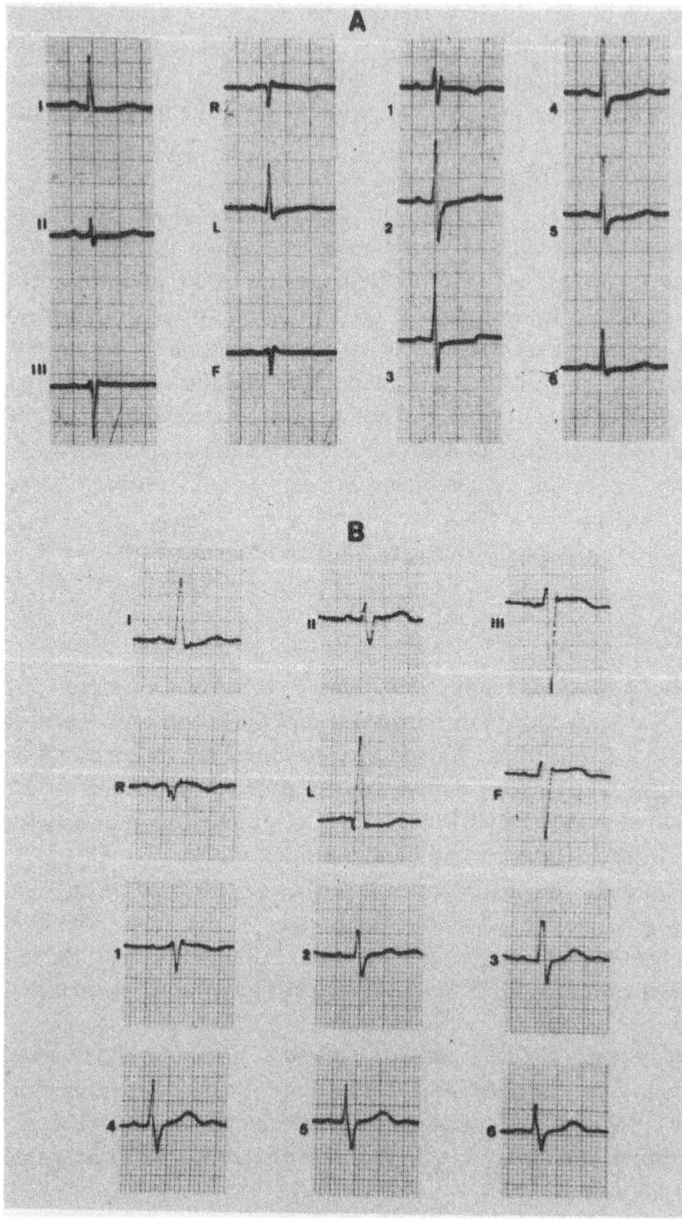

Figure 3. A: Incomplete right bundle branch block pattern. AQRS: +10°. B: ECG registered after 4 days. Appearance of anterior fascicular block is evident. The incomplete RBBB pattern is lead V_1 is partly obscured (see text for explanation)

Table 1. Electrocardiographic features in right bundle branch block with anterior fascicular block

- QRS interval of 120 msec or more
- Right bundle branch block pattern in right precordial leads
- Left axis deviation greater than $-45°$
- Q waves in lead I and aVL
- Delay of intrinsecoid deflection time in aVL of 50 msec or more
- Delay of intrinsecoid deflection time more prolonged in aVL than in V_6
- Deep S wave in leads V_5 and V_6
- At times small q wave in V_2-V_3 leads

made with the other conditions causing LAD, such as left ventricular hypertrophy, inferior myocardial infarction, pulmonary emphysema and horizontal position of the heart.

The ECG signs of asynchronous left ventricular activation are important diagnostic criteria (see Chapter 4).

It must, however, be stressed that such criteria are of less value in the bifascicular block since the RBBB often also changes the QRS complex morphology in the left-sided leads.

For the diagnosis of RBBB and AFB the electrical pattern of the 'masquerading bundle branch block' is very useful: if in leads I and aVL, deep and slurred S waves are evident, the presence of AFB associated with RBBB, is in our opinion often doubtful (Figure 4).

RIGHT BUNDLE BRANCH BLOCK AND POSTERIOR FASCICULAR BLOCK

Right bundle branch block associated with posterior fascicular block is relatively uncommon. The ventricular activation in this block has not been greatly investigated. Watt [6], who studied ventricular activation both in the dog and in the baboon during experimentally induced RBBB and PFB, observed that the antero-superior wall of the left ventricle is normally activated; the excitation of the right ventricle and of the postero-inferior wall of the left ventricle is instead delayed: 42 and 22 msec in the baboon and 46 and 20 msec in the dog, respectively.

At present, epicardial mapping in man has not been performed in patients with this bifascicular block.

Electrocardiographic features

The ECG diagnosis of RBBB with PFB is often puzzling and more difficult than that of AFB associated with RBBB, since isolated RBBB can, at times, also induce a marked RAD.

Also in this bifascicular block one can observe ECG features of both isolated

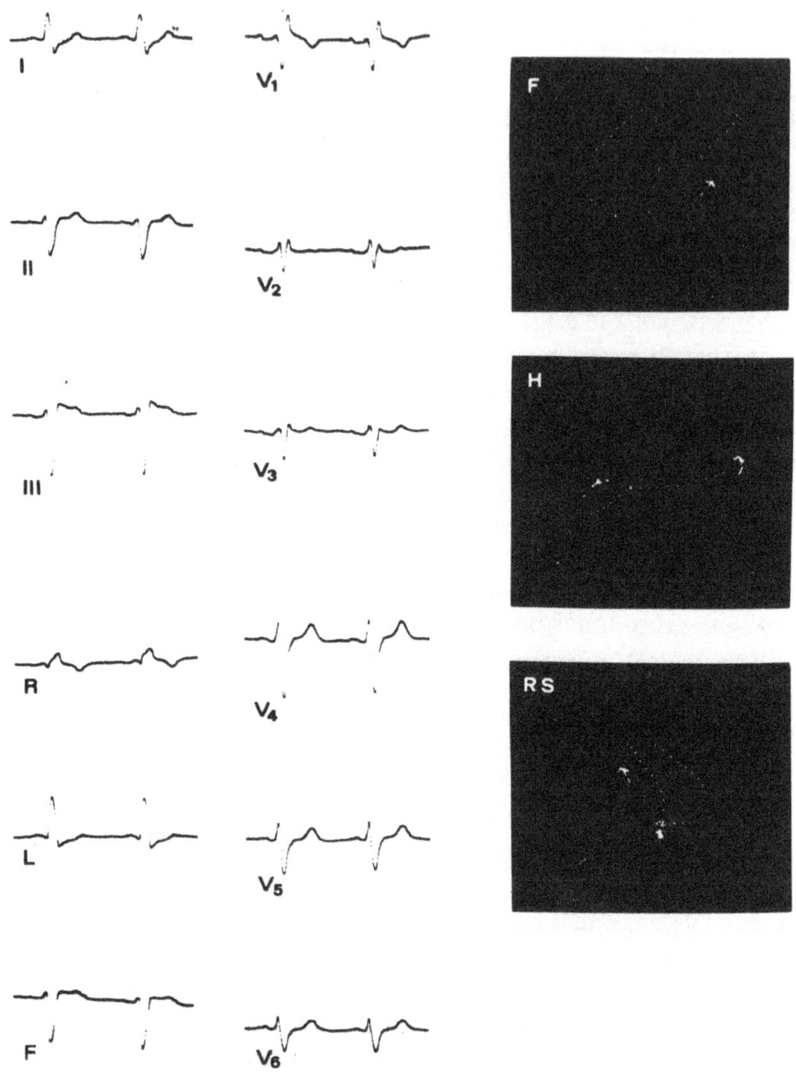

Figure 4. Although RBBB is incomplete (the R′ in V_1-V_2 is small), in I and aVL leads deep and slurred S waves are evident. The presence of AFB associated with RBBB is dubious in spite of the left axis deviation and the counterclockwise rotation of QRS loop in the H plane of VCG (see text for explanation)

RBBB and isolated PFB, as well as some ECG signs related to the combination of the two blocks.

The most commonly accepted criteria for the diagnosis of RBBB with PFB are those proposed by Rosenbaum et al. [9]:

RBBB pattern with right axis deviation greater than 120° and with q waves in diaphragmatic leads. An RAD can be related to other causes such as right ventricular hypertrophy, anatomic vertical heart, pulmonary emphysema, lateral myocardial infarction and pulmonary embolism, besides RBBB per se. Therefore, RAD is not a specific diagnostic feature for PFB associated with RBBB. On the basis of experimental data [3-6] PFB associated with RBBB can be diagnosed if, besides RAD, the ECG signs of asynchronous left ventricular activation, due to delayed excitation of the postero-inferior wall, are present (see Chapter 4).

The following electrocardiographic features are helpful in the diagnosis of RBBB with PFB (Figures 5, 6 and 7):

- QRS interval of 120 msec or more.
- Right bundle branch block morphology in right precordial leads.
- Right axis deviation greater than $+90°$ due to an abnormal superior to inferior activation of the left ventricle.
- Q wave in II, III and aVF leads, due to a superior orienyation of the first vectors.
- Delay of intrinsecoid deflection in V_6 (or aVF) of 50 msec or more, due to the delayed activation of the inferior wall of the left ventricle.
- More prolonged intrinsecoid deflection time in V_6 (or aVF) than in aVL for asynchronous left ventricular activation (see Chapter 4). Such a feature, however, is of greater importance in the diagnosis of isolated PFB; in fact, the isolated RBBB can also change the intrinsecoid deflection time in the left-sided leads.
- Deep and slurred S wave in lead I and aVL since such a wave is accentuated by both RBBB and PFB.
- Terminal r wave in aVR and s wave in V_6 small or absent; this finding contrasts with the presence of RBBB (Figures 5, 6 and 7). In fact the late inferiorly and leftward oriented forces related to PFB tend to cancel out the late rightward forces related to RBBB; consequently the terminal R wave in aVR and the S wave in V_6 decrease or disappear [14-16]. In effect, the higher the degree of PFB the smaller the terminal r wave in aVR. This feature represents a scarcely known type of 'masquerading bundle branch block', resulting from interference between RBBB and PFB. In our opinion it is the most important ECG sign for the diagnosis of this bifascicular block.

Table 2 shows the ECG features of RBBB associated with PFB.

Vectorcardiographic features

In the F plane the QRS loop shows a clockwise rotation. The initial deflections are directed superiorly and to the right or more rarely to the left. The efferent limb is then directed inferiorly and to the left. The delayed terminal forces are oriented to the right and inferiorly.

In the H plane the QRS loop is very similar to that seen in isolated RBBB, but

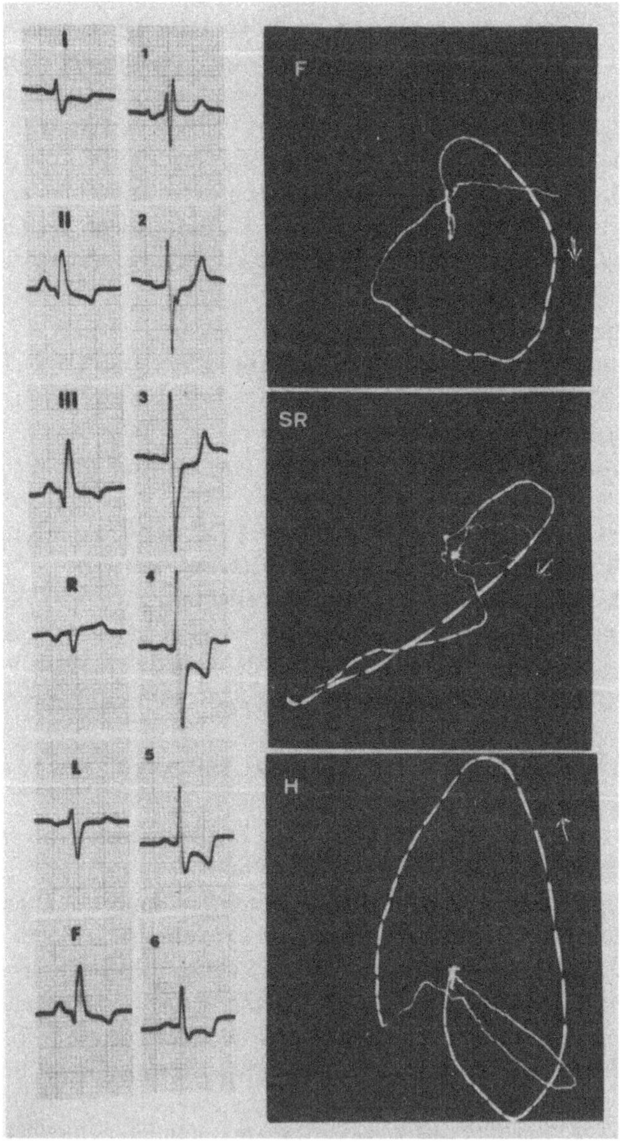

Figures 5. Right bundle branch block with posterior fascicular block. ECG: RBBB clearly evident in the right precordial leads. Marked right axis deviation. The delay of intrinsecoid deflection is 60 msec in aVF and 30 msec in aVL. *In aVR a terminal R wave is absent and in V_6 the S wave is small:* such a characteristic expresses the masquerading bundle branch block. VCG: The first vectors are oriented superiorly. Frontal and right sagittal planes show clockwise rotation of QRS loop with markedly inferior orientation of the mid-terminal forces. In the horizontal plane the rotation is counterclockwise

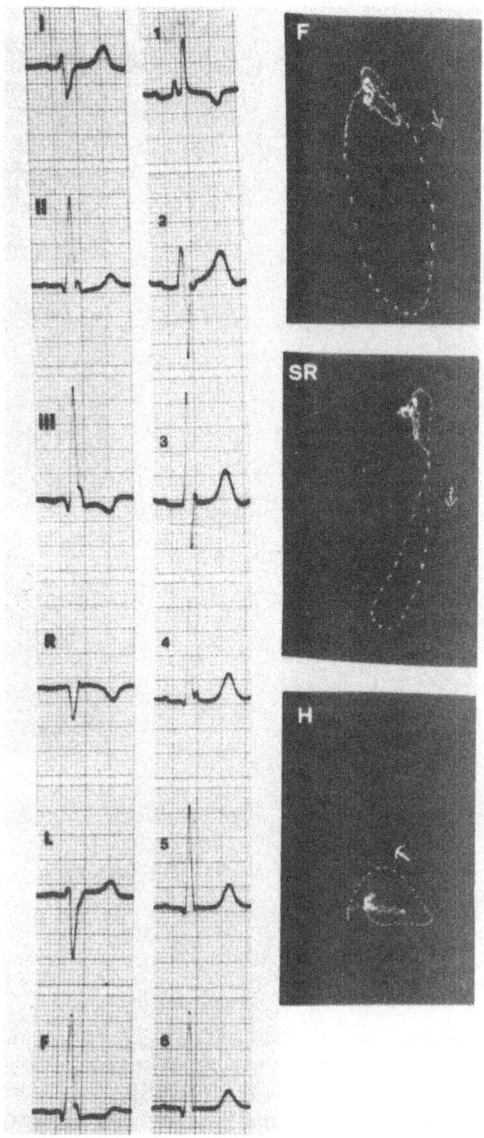

Figure 6. Right bundle branch block with posterior fascicular block. ECG shows RBBB in the right precordial leads; in addition there is marked right axis deviation. The delay of intrinsecoid deflection is 70 msec in aVF and 40 msec in aVL. *Terminal R wave in aVR and S wave in* V_6 *are very small.* In VCG the inscription of the QRS loop is clockwise in frontal and right sagittal plane and counterclockwise in horizontal plane. The mid-terminal forces are oriented inferiorly

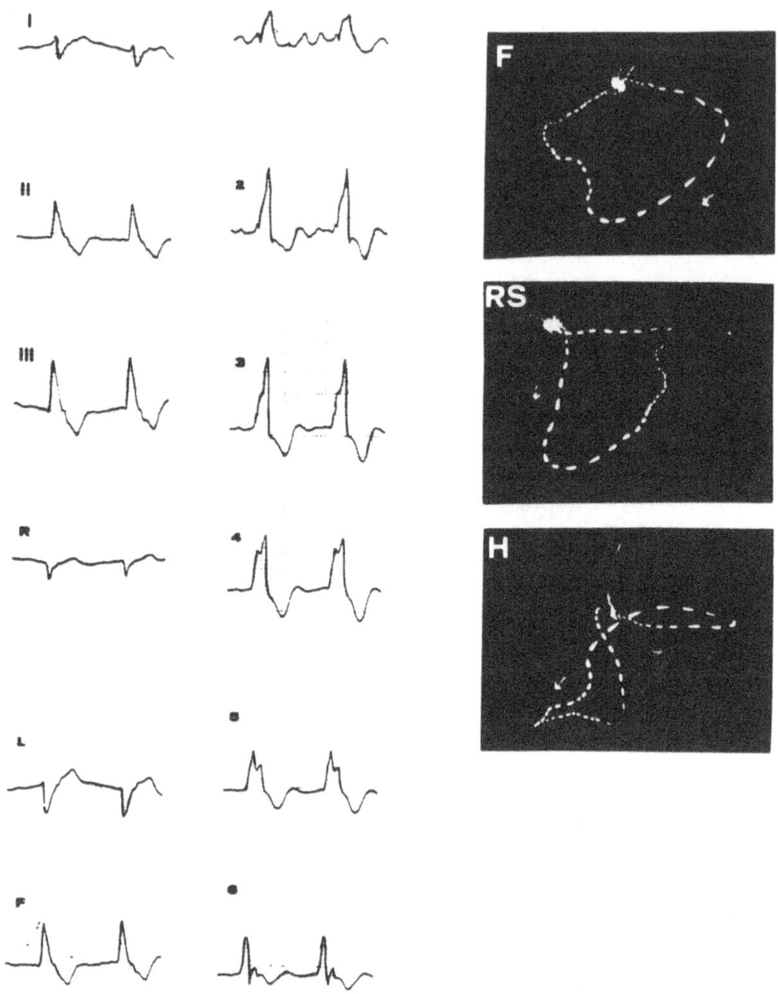

Figure 7. Right bundle branch block and posterior fascicular block. Patient with atrial fibrillation. RBBB pattern is evident in right precordial leads. Marked right axis deviation. *In aVR a terminal R wave is absent and V_6 shows a Rsr morphology.* In F and RS planes of VCG the rotation is clockwise and the middle forces are markedly oriented inferiorly. The terminal vectors are characteristically directed inferiorly

generally shows less leftward development. The initial vectors are directed anteriorly and to the right or more rarely to the left. The efferent limb of the QRS loop is inscribed either clockwise or counterclockwise, to the left and anteriorly or posteriorly. The delayed terminal vectors are oriented anteriorly and to the right.

In the RS plane the QRS loop is inscribed in a clockwise fashion or shows a figure-of-eight morphology. The initial vectors are directed superiorly and ante-

Table 2. Electrocardiographic features in right bundle branch block with posterior fascicular block

- Small or absent s wave in leads I and aVL
- QRS interval of 120 msec or more
- Right bundle branch block pattern in right precordial leads
- Right axis deviation greater than +90°
- Q wave in II, III and aVF leads
- Delay of intrinsecoid deflection time in V_6 (or aVF) of 50 msec or more
- Deep and slurred S wave in leads I and aVL
- Terminal r wave in aVR and s wave in V_6 small or absent

riorly. The mid terminal forces show a morphology very similar to that of isolated RBBB (Figures 5, 6 and 7).

Differential diagnosis

In this bifascicular block the diagnosis of RBBB is easy whereas recognition of PFB is difficult and differential diagnosis must be made with the other conditions causing RAD.

Right ventricular hypertrophy associated with RBBB can induce marked RAD, but in such an association deep S wave in V_6 and high terminal R wave in aVR are present; on the other hand, such waves are small or absent if RAD is in relation to PFB.

In patients with RBBB and anatomic vertical position of the heart, a marked RAD can be present as well as ECG signs of asynchronous left ventricular activation (see Chapter 4), but a delay of intrinsecoid delfection in aVF more than 50 msec tends to exclude such a position of the heart [4] (Figure 8). However, this criterion needs further validation. Therefore, in all cases with RBBB and marked RAD, a chest X-ray is useful in order to evaluate the position of the heart.

Occasionally, a lateral myocardial infarction associated with RBBB may elicit a marked RAD; however, in this case, infarctional Q waves are evident in I and aVL and the QRS voltage in the extremity leads is characteristically small.

Sometimes the Wolff-Parkinson-White syndrome can induce an RBBB pattern with RAD. However, the ECG shows the diagnostic features of a short PR interval and an initial delta wave. The difficulty arises when Mahaim fibers are the cause of pre-excitation as they are associated with a normal PR interval; in this case an electrophysiological study may be required for the differential diagnosis.

The ECG pattern of 'masquerading bundle branch block' is particularly useful to recognize PFB associated with RBBB. In our opinion, if this is lacking the diagnosis of this bifascicular block can only be made with any degree of certainty if PFB is intermittent.

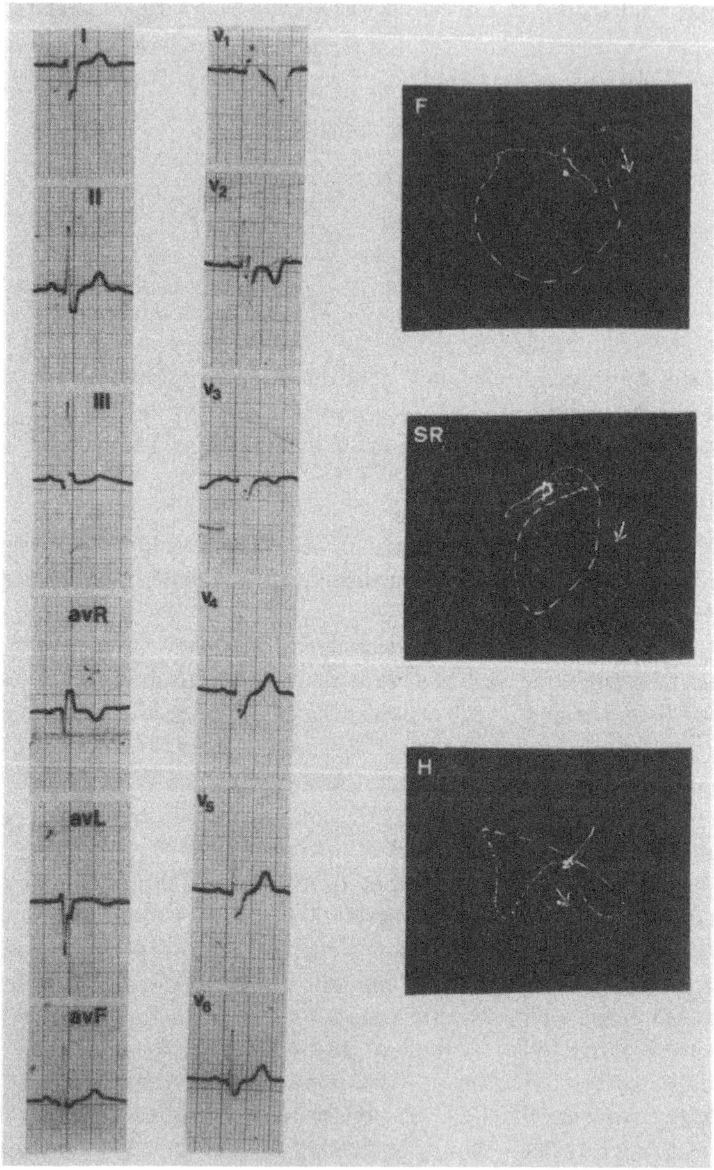

Figure 8. A patient, whose chest X-ray shows a vertical anatomic position of the heart. RBBB pattern in right precordial leads. In the ECG a marked right axis deviation is present and a posterior fascicular block associated with RBBB must be considered. A normal intrinsecoid deflection time in aVF (35 msec) and V_6 (40 msec) tends to exclude a PFB

TRIFASCICULAR BLOCK

The term trifascicular block should be employed to indicate cases in which RBBB with AFB and PFB are observed in the same or different electrocardiograms of a patient (Figure 9). It would not be correct to define as trifascicular block a bifascicular one with a first degree atrioventricular (AV) block since the conduction delay can originate, not only in the remaining fascicle of the left bundle branch, but also in the AV node or in the His bundle.

Rosenbaum et al. [9] described eight morphological types of trifascicular block: 1) RBBB with AFB and PFB, or trifascicular complete heart block; 2) permanent RBBB and PFB with intermittent AFB; 3) permanent RBBB and an AFB with intermittent PFB; 4) permanent AFB and PFB, with intermittent RBBB; 5) permanent RBBB with intermittent AFB and PFB; 6) permanent PFB, with intermittent AFB and RBBB; 7) permanent AFB, with intermittent PFB and RBBB; 8) RBBB, AFB and PFB, all intermittent.

In most cases, however, the block is permanent in the right bundle branch and in the anterior fascicle and intermittent in the posterior one. The block is rarely intermittent in the right bundle branch or in all three fascicles; in the latter, QRS complexes conducted with LBBB pattern, when anterior and posterior fascicles are concomitantly blocked, can be observed.

In an electrophysiologically studied case the alternation of one fascicular block with another was associated with changes in HV time [17].

When both ECG and electrophysiological recordings are available, a trifascicular block can only be suspected under the following circumstances:

- Bifascicular block with prolonged HV interval. Such a pattern can indicate a slowing of conduction in the remaining fascicle of the left bundle branch or in the His bundle (Figure 10).
- Bifascicular block with post-His second degree AV block (Figures 11, 12 and 13). Under such circumstances the 2° AV block can reflect a lesion in the remaining left fascicle or in the His bundle.
- Complete AV block distal to H deflection with wide QRS complexes can indicate a block in the right bundle branch and in the two main fascicles of the left bundle branch, as well as a complete block within the His bundle or both the two main bundle branches.

PATHOLOGICAL CORRELATIONS

Very few data correlating the ECG changes and the histopathological lesions in bifascicular block have been reported and their results are dissimilar.

Sugiura et al. [18] examined the conduction system of 16 patients with RBBB and RAD. Right bundle branch was interrupted with fibrosis in all cases; complete

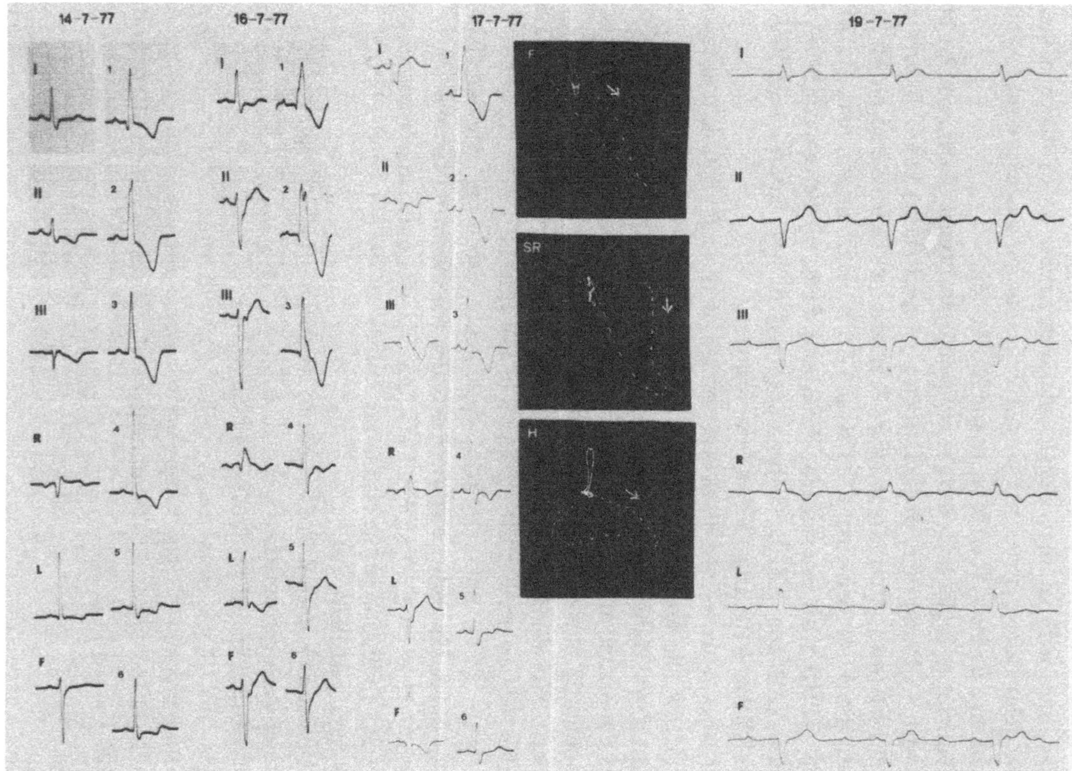

Figure 9. Child aged 7 with acute viral myocarditis. A trifascicular block is present. ECG of 14-7-77 shows right bundle branch block. Two days later an anterior fascicular block appeared. In the ECG of 17-7-77 one can observe the appearance of marked right axis deviation, as an expression of posterior fascicular block associated with RBBB. Two days later a complete atrio-ventricular block was present

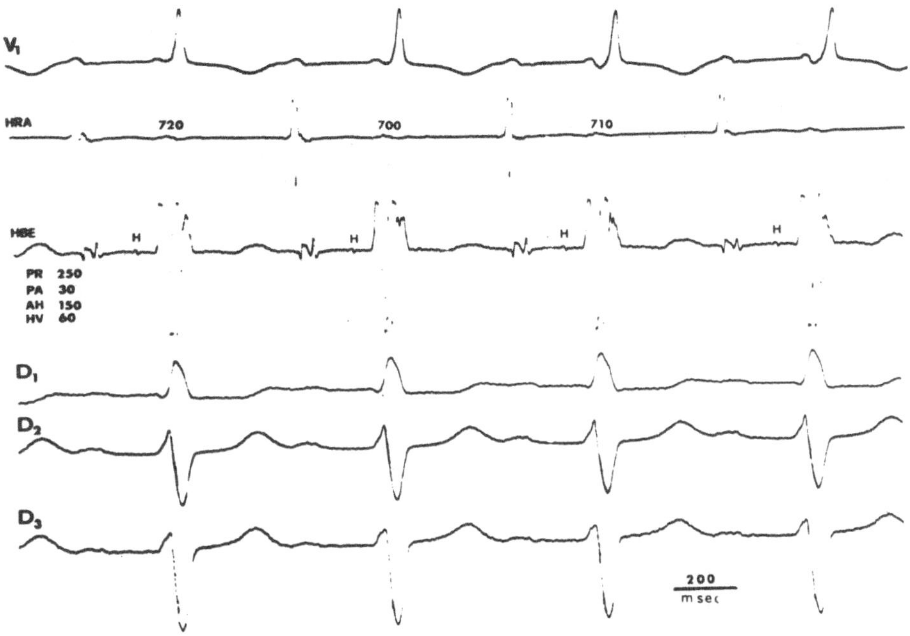

Figure 10. Right bundle branch block with anterior fascicular block; PR and HV intervals are prolonged, 250 and 60 msec, respectively. Such a pattern may indicate a conduction delay in the left posterior fascicle or in the His bundle. HRA: High right atrium. HBE: His bundle electrocardiogram. D_1: lead I, D_2: lead II, D_3: lead III

interruption was found in 87% of the left posterior fascicles and in 28% of the left anterior fascicles. These authors concluded that the electrocardiographic pattern of RBBB with RAD is extremely suggestive of interruption of right bundle branch and left posterior fascicle. Andrade et al. [19] found an excellent correlation between ECG and histopathologic abnormalities in 17 patients with bifascicular block secondary to chronic Chagasic myocarditis.

In other studies such a correlation is poor. In 10 cases of bifascicular block, five of RBBB and AFB and five of RBBB and PFB, Rossi [20] found that only the RBBB pattern correlated with histopathological lesions, whereas the precise topographic-segmentary implication of the diagnosis of anterior and posterior fascicular block respectively, did not rely on sound morphologic grounds at all. The lesions were seen to be commonly scattered all over the left bundle branch and no significant difference was found in type and severity of the left bundle branch injury between AFB and PFB.

Blondeau and Lenegre [21] in the cases of RBBB and AFB found that the involvement of the left bundle branch was not necessarily anterior but in some cases was medial and posterior. Such observations were confirmed in a later study by Fernandez and Lenegre [22].

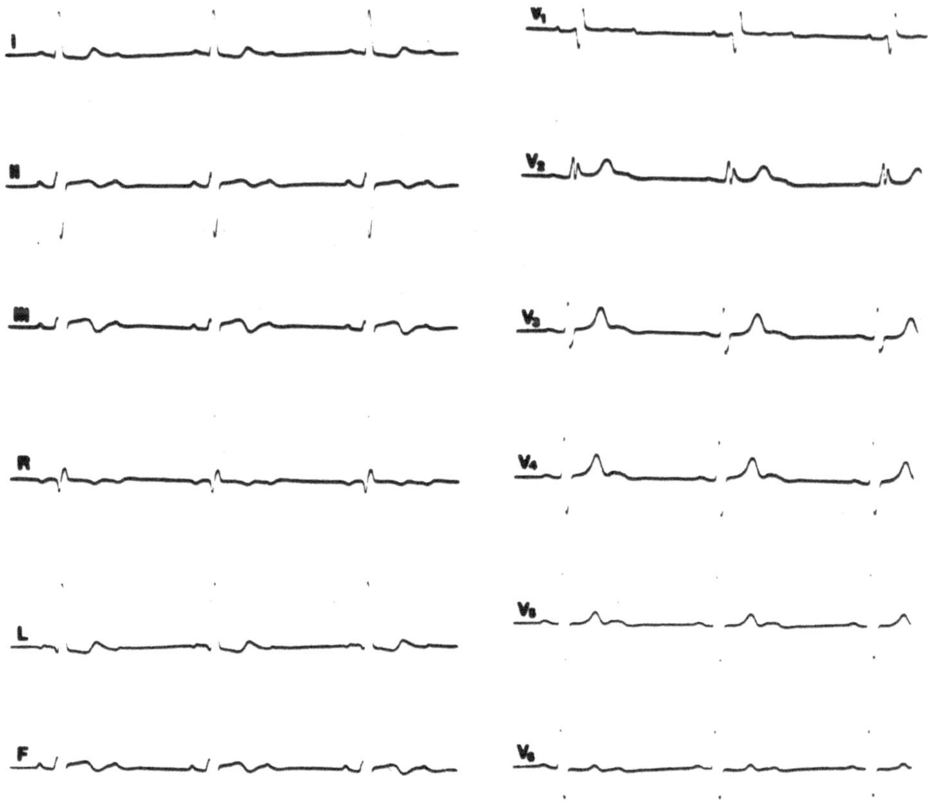

Figure 11. Right bundle branch block with anterior fascicular block and 2:1 AV block

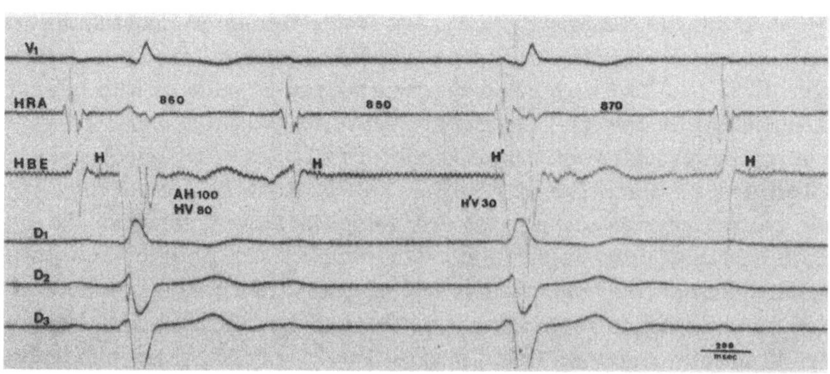

Figure 12. Electrophysiological study of the same patient as Figure 11. The blocked P waves are followed by His bundle deflection. Junctional premature beats, preceded by a His bundle deflection (H′) at interval of 30 msec are present. The 2:1 block can be localized in the left posterior fascicle or in the distal part of the His bundle

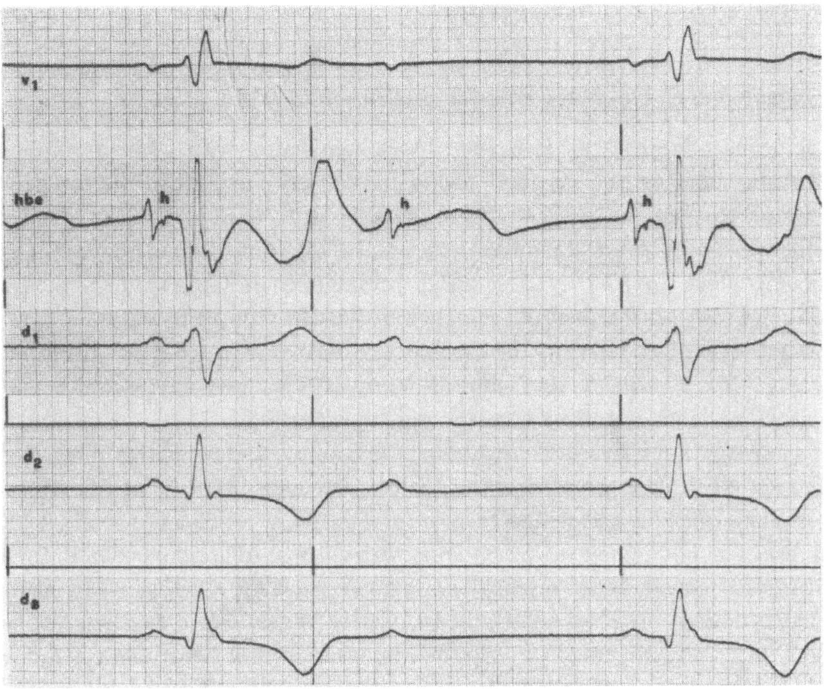

Figure 13. Right bundle branch block with posterior fascicular block and 2:1 post-His AV block (the blocked P waves are followed by His bundle deflection). The AH and HV intervals measure 60 and 65 msec, respectively. The 2:1 block can be localized in the left anterior fascicle or in the His bundle

Bharati et al. [23] performed an anatomo-electrophysiological correlation in three patients with RBBB, LAD and prolonged HV interval; in all cases histopathological abnormalities in right bundle branch and in left bundle branch system were found. However, the LAD did not necessarily correspond with greater involvement of the anterior than the posterior left fascicular fibers.

From the limited studies available, it is possible to conclude that bifascicular blocks do not always have a clear-cut histopathological basis. The correlation between ECG changes and histopathological lesions is generally good in RBBB, whereas in fascicular blocks discrepancies appear.

The causes of such discrepancies appear the same as those reported for the isolated fascicular blocks (see Chapter 4).

Right bundle branch block and anterior fascicular block

The incidence of right bundle branch block associated with anterior fascicular block is uncertain since very few studies have been carried out on the general population. Rotman et al. [24] found RBBB with AFB in 0.08% of aircraft personnel and applicants. Siegman-Igra et al. [25] found an incidence of such bifascicular block in 0.17% of a stable population of Israeli adult males. In Kulbertus's study [2] the overall incidence of RBBB with AFB was 0.35%.

Among hospitalized patients the incidence of RBBB with AFB was found to be about 1% [26, 27] and a very similar figure (0.9%) was encountered among ambulatory patients attending a cardiological center [9].

Little information is available regarding the etiology and clinical implications of RBBB with AFB. The most common factors are considered to be hypertension and coronary artery disease (CAD).

Dhingra et al. [28] reviewed 452 patients with chronic bifascicular block. In 40% of cases hypertensive heart disease was present, in 38% CAD, in 9% primary myocardial disease, in 7% valvular heart disease and in 6% miscellaneous heart disease. Eighty-six patients (19%) had no apparent organic heart disease and were categorized as a primary conduction disease group. Cardiovascular mortality (including sudden death) was higher in patients with underlying heart disease compared to those with primary conduction disease, 29% and 12%, respectively. Scanlon et al. [29] studied 129 patients with RBBB and AFB. The most common etiology was CAD. In 15% of cases clinical and electrocardiographic signs of underlying heart disease were not present. Mortality was higher in patients with Lenegre's disease: 17% and 7%, respectively. However, there was no information as to whether the deaths were due to cardiovascular causes, sudden or not. In 83 patients with chronic RBBB and AFB, De Pasquale et al. [30] found hypertension or CAD in 82% of cases. In only five patients were there no signs of cardiovascular disease. In 140 cases of RBBB and AFB, reported by Rosenbaum et al. [9], hypertension or CAD was present in 52%, Chagasic myocarditis in 27%, and aortic stenosis in 4%. In only 10% of patients was there no evidence of underlying heart disease. Of the 83 patients with RBBB and LAD analyzed by Narula et al. [31], 33 had clinical or ECG evidence of CAD, with or without hypertension; another 14 had hypertension alone. There were three patients with rheumatic heart disease. Thirty (34%) of the 83 patients had no apparent underlying cardiovascular abnormality.

It should be noted that these studies were carried out on hospitalized or ambulatory patients. A few papers have dealt with RBBB and AFB in patients in whom such a block was discovered during routine electrocardiograms [2, 24, 25]. In 16 out of 18 patients with RBBB and LAD, reported by Rotman et al. [24] no sign of cardiovascular disease was encountered. Of the nine patients reported by Siegman-Igra et al. [25] only four showed organic heart disease. The incidence of patients without underlying heart disease was not clearly reported, but hypertension was present in 57% of cases, angina in 24%, cardiomegaly in 22%, marked dilatation of the aortic root in 15% and chronic pulmonary disease in 2%.

The clinical data also appear contradictory in the studies obtained from the general population. In effect LAD, which constituted the only diagnostic criterion for AFB, is not pathognomic of a conduction defect in the anterior divisions of the left bundle branch. Therefore, patients with a RBBB and LAD pattern may not represent a homogeneous group since partial bilateral bundle branch block may not be present in all cases.

As for isolated AFB, it is difficult to understand the clinical implication of such a bifascicular block. Like many other authors [9, 29, 30], we believe that in most cases RBBB with AFB underlies some cardiac pathology. Even if an underlying heart disease is not detected, these patients should be followed closely since RBBB associated with AFB may represent subclinical heart disease or primary degeneration of the conduction system, which in some cases progresses to complete AV block distal to His bundle (see Chapter 11).

Right bundle branch block and posterior fascicular block

The available clinical data on RBBB associated with PFB are at present very scarce.

As for RBBB with AFB, in all the studies such a bifascicular block appears more frequently in men than in women.

Rotman et al. [24] found only 17 cases (0.007%) of RBBB with RAD greater than +120° out of 237,000 individuals. In one case hypertensive heart disease was present and in the rest there were no signs of underlying heart disease. To our knowledge, this is the only study obtained from the general population in which such a bifascicular block has been investigated.

Rosenbaum et al. [9] examined 29 out-patients with RBBB and PFB; CAD was present in eight cases (27%). In six of them the disease was severe, with protracted angina, there was evidence of an inferior myocardial infarction in three, and both anterior and inferior infarction in three. In the remaining cases, angina was also severe, but ECG evidence of myocardial infarction was lacking. In 10 cases (34%) the clinical diagnosis was chronic Chagasic myocarditis and in nine (31%) clinical examination did not reveal any clear-cut etiology. Varriale et al. [32] reported 12 cases with RBBB and PFB. Five patients had CAD diagnosed on the basis of clinical and ECG evidence of myocardial infarction. In all but one, a bifascicular block developed years after the acute infarction. Two patients had aortic valve disease; a definite etiology was not established in five patients who were thought to have Lenegre's disease. Out of 24 patients reported by Scanlon et al. [29], 10 had

CAD, two of whom also had hypertension. Another four patients had hypertension alone. Three patients had rheumatic disease of the aortic valve. Two patients were obese, one of whom had diabetes. One patient was felt to have myocarditis. The remaining five had no apparent cardiovascular abnormality. Out of 21 cases examined by Dhingra et al. [33], 10 (48 %) had hypertensive heart disease, three (14 %) CAD, one (5 %) primary myocardial disease and seven (33 %) primary conduction disease.

From the few studies reported in literature it appears that a frequent cause of RBBB associated with PFB is myocardial infarction, especially if located in both anterior and inferior walls.

The only paper which has dealt with RBBB and PFB in patients in whom such a bifascicular block was discovered during routine electrocardiograms is the one reported by Rotman [24]. In 16 out of 17 patients no signs of underlying abnormalities were observed. However, the low number of cases and the lack of autopsy data preclude any clinical conclusion.

The progression of bifascicular blocks towards complete AV block will be discussed in Chapter 11.

Trifascicular block

The syndrome of RBBB with intermittent AFB and PFB (trifascicular block) implies a marked involvement of the intraventricular conduction system. Therefore, generalized myocardial damage or at least generalized involvement of the conduction system should be anticipated. In the six patients studied by Rosenbaum et al. [9] the clinical diagnoses were CAD in two, chronic Chagasic myocarditis in one and Lenegre's disease in three. The cases are nevertheless too few to draw definite conclusion.

A patient aged 31 has been described [34] with trifascicular block which satisfies Lenegre's criteria: absence of underlying heart disease and infrahision conduction defects. However, cardiac catheterization showed abnormalities suggestive of an early-stage non-obstructive cardiomyopathy although there were no radiological signs of cardiomegaly or clinical signs of heart failure. These subclinical changes of myocardial function could be interpreted as the first signs of idiopathic cardiomyopathy. This case suggests that further clinical and hemodynamic investigations are necessary in patients who are presumably affected by Lenegre's disease.

However, from a clinical point of view and disregarding the causal disease, the most characteristic feature of the RBBB with intermittent AFB and PFB is its tendency to progress to complete AV block [9].

COMMENT

The criterion commonly accepted for the diagnosis of PFB associated with RBBB is the presence of marked QRS axis deviation. This criterion is not, however, specific since other conditions, in particular RBBB alone, can produce a shift in the electrical axis.

The ECG signs of asynchronous left ventricular activation are useful in diagnosing a fascicular block coexisting with RBBB, but play a lesser role than in

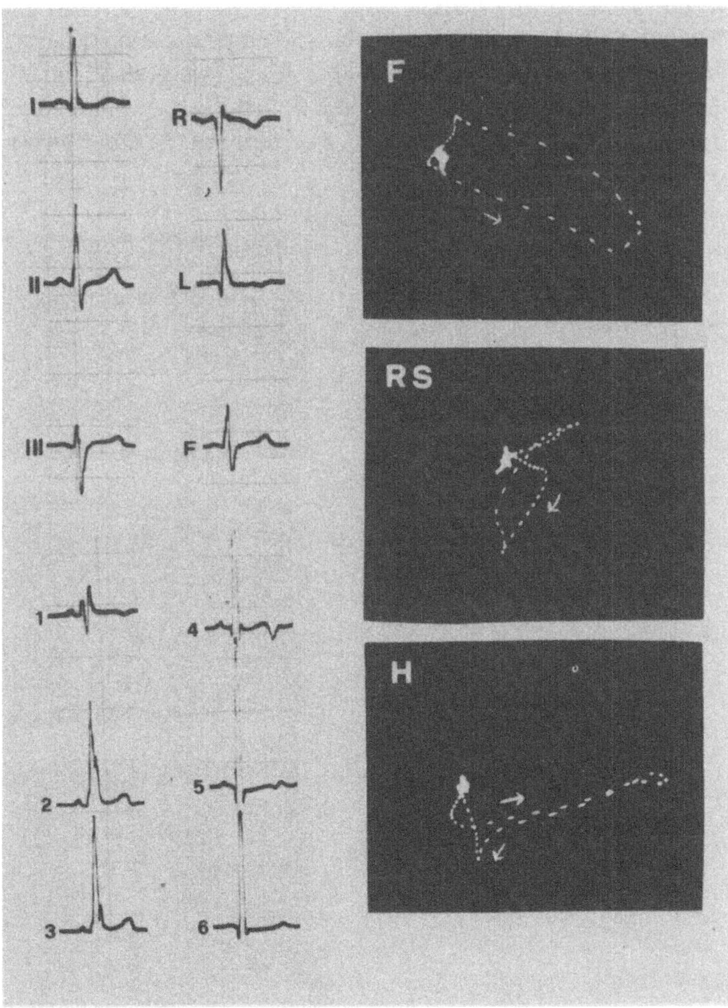

Figure 14. **ECG tracing shows incomplete right bundle branch block (rsR morphology in V_1) and left** ventricular hypertrophy (LVH). S wave is absent in I and very small in V_6. Horizontal plane of VCG shows terminal vectors oriented anteriorly, but to the left. Probably, the LVH shifts to the left the delayed rightward terminal forces related to incomplete RBBB (see text for explanation)

the diagnosis of isolated fascicular blocks since RBBB often changes the intrinsecoid deflection time in the unipolar left-sided leads. Consequently, the ECG evaluation of asynchrony of left ventricular activation is less reliable. The 'masquerading bundle branch block' pattern represents the most important ECG sign for the diagnosis of both bifascicular blocks. This feature in RBBB associated with AFB is manifested by small or absent s waves in leads I and aVL, which contrast with the presence of RBBB (Figures 1 and 2); this is due to late leftward and superiorly oriented forces related to AFB, which tend to cancel out late rightward forces related to RBBB.

In RBBB with PFB the 'masquerading bundle branch block' pattern is revealed by very small (or absent) terminal r wave in aVR and s wave in V_6, which contrast with the presence of RBBB (Figures 5, 6 and 7). This is due to late inferiorly and leftward forces related to PFB which tend to cancel out the late rightward forces related to RBBB.

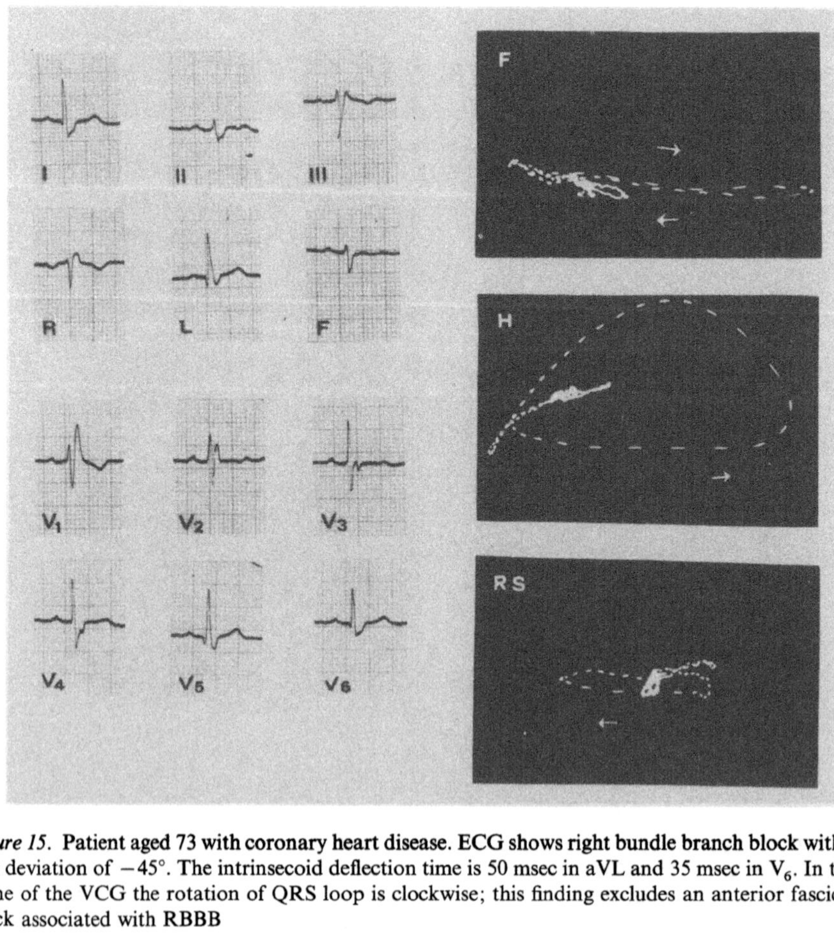

Figure 15. Patient aged 73 with coronary heart disease. ECG shows right bundle branch block with left axis deviation of −45°. The intrinsecoid deflection time is 50 msec in aVL and 35 msec in V_6. In the F plane of the VCG the rotation of QRS loop is clockwise; this finding excludes an anterior fascicular block associated with RBBB

When these features, resulting from interference between RBBB and fascicular block, are lacking, the diagnosis of bifascicular block, in our opinion, is always dubious. However, at present, it is not clear if a left ventricular hypertrophy or a left ventricular peripheral block associated with RBBB can also induce a 'masquerading buncle branch block' pattern (Figure 14).

Vectorcardiographic recording is more useful in diagnosing isolated fascicular blocks than the bifascicular ones. In cases in which the ECG does not definitely evidence a bifascicular block pattern, the VCG rarely clarifies it. At times VCG recording can exclude electrocardiographically suspect AFB associated with RBBB, if the rotation of the frontal QRS loop is clockwise (Figure 15). In fact, on the basis of clinical and experimental data [3-6] in RBBB associated with AFB, the QRS rotation is definitely counterclockwise in frontal plane.

An electrophysiological study appears of particular use in defining the conduction in the remaining His-Purkinje system (HV interval), which in most studies appeared involved in a high percentage of cases. In Narula's patients with RBBB and LAD, the incidence of HV interval prolongation (> 45 msec) was 62% and 88% with a normal PR interval and 1° AV block, respectively. In patients with RBBB and RAD the HV time was abnormal in 80% with a normal PR interval and in 100% with a prolonged one [35]. In other studies in which 55 msec was used as the upper limit of normal HV time, a variable incidence of HV abnormalities ranging from 28 to 64% in RBBB with LAD (36-39) and from 50 to 87% in RBBB with RAD [33, 37, 39, 40], has been reported.

The clinical significance of the fascicular blocks is at present uncertain since the results obtained in studies on the general population are contradictory. Until diagnostic criteria are more reliable, it will not be possible to clarify the clinical significance of bifascicular blocks. We therefore believe that patients with bifascicular block, even without evident manifestation of heart disease, must be checked periodically not only because such a block may represent the first sign of subclinical heart disease, but also because it may develop towards a complete AV block (see Chapter 11).

REFERENCES

1. Narula OS, Samet P: Right bundle branch block with normal, left or right axis deviation: analysis by His bundle recordings. Am J Med 51: 432, 1971
2. Kulbertus HE: Reevaluation of the prognosis of patients with LAD-RBBB. Am Heart J 92: 665, 1976
3. Medrano GA, Brenes CP, De Micheli A, Sodi-Pallares D: El bloqueo simultaneo de la subdivision anterior y posterior de la rama izquierda del haz de His (bloqueo bifascicular) y su asociacion con bloqueo de la rama derecha (bloqueo trifascicular). Estudio electrocardiografico experimental y clinico. Arch Inst Cardiol Mex 40: 752, 1970

4. Medrano GA, De Micheli A: El electrocardiograma y el vectorcardiograma en los bloqueos mono- y polifasciculares. Arch Inst Cardiol Mex 44: 421, 1974
5. Medrano GA, De Micheli A, Brenes PC, Sodi-Pallares D: Experimental bases for diagnosis of left bifascicular and trifascicular block. G Ital Cardiol 5: 8, 1975
6. Watt TB: Features of fascicular block imposed upon existing right bundle branch block in the dog and baboon. Am J Cardiol 39: 1000, 1977
7. Windham CRS, Meeran MK, Smith T, Engelman RM, Levitsky S, Rosen KM: Epicardial activation in human left anterior fascicular block. Am J Cardiol 44: 638, 1979
8. Wyndham CRC, Smith T, Meeran MK, Mammana R, Levitsky S, Rosen KM: Epicardial activation in patients with left bundle branch block. Circulation 61: 696, 1980
9. Rosenbaum MB, Elizari MV, Lazzari JO: The hemiblocks. Oldsmar: Tampa Tracing 1970
10. Grant RP: Spatial vector electrocardiography. A method for calculating the spatial electrical vectors of the heart from conventional leads. Circulation 2: 676, 1950
11. Richman JL, Wolff L: Left bundle branch block masquerading as right bundle branch block. Am Heart J 47: 383, 1954
12. Unger PN, Lesser ME, Kugel VH, Lev M: The concept of masquerading bundle branch block. An electrocardiographic-pathologic correlation. Circulation 17: 397, 1958
13. Rosenbaum MB, Yesuron J, Lazzari JO, Elizari MV: Left anterior hemiblock obscuring the diagnosis of right bundle branch block. Circulation 48: 298, 1973
14. Palmieri M, Ruggeri G, Zappala' A, Nava A: Studio dell'emiblocco posteriore sinistro associato a blocco della branca destra. Contributo clinico, elettro e vettocardiografico. G Ital Cardiol 4: 463, 1974
15. Alboni P, Fantini F, Nava A, Masoni A: Criteri elettrocardiografici attuali per la diagnosi dei blocchi fascicolari. G Ital Cardiol 6: 118, 1976
16. Alboni P: Revisione del concetto di emiblocco. Atti IX Congresso Nazionale ANMCO. Rome: Pozzi, 1978, p 205
17. Bloch Thomsen PE, Steendorff B, Gotzsche H: Intraventricular trifascicular block verified by His bundle electrocardiography. Am Heart J 92: 497, 1976
18. Sugiura M, Hiradka K, Ohkawa S: A histological study on the conduction system in 16 cases of right bundle branch block associated with right axis deviation. Jap Heart J 15: 113, 1974
19. Andrade ZA, Andrade SG, Oliveira GBI, Alonso DL: Histopathology of the conducting tissue of the heart in Chagas' myocarditis. Am Heart J 95: 316, 1978
20. Rossi L: Histopathology of cardiac arrhythmias, 2nd edn Milan: Casa Editrice Ambrosiana, 1978
21. Blondeau M, Lenegre J: Blocs atypiques de la branche droite. Paris: Masson & Cie, 1970
22. Fernandez F, Gay J, Lenegre J: Bloc de la branche bilatéral; étude des aspects électrocardiographiques et des corrélations anatomo-électriques dans 100 cas avec des lésions histologiques majeures des deux branches du faisceau de His. II. Etude des corrélations anatomo-cliniques. Arch Mal Coeur 67: 655, 1974
23. Bharati S, Lev M: Histological and electrophysiological correlations in atrioventricular block and bundle branch block. In: Cardiac arrhythmias. Electrophysiology, diagnosis and management, Narula OS. Baltimore: Williams & Wilkins, 1979, p 164
24. Rotman M, Triebwasser JH: A clinical and follow-up study of right and left bundle

branch block. Circulation 51: 477, 1975
25. Siegman-Igra Y, Yahini JH, Goldbourt U, Neufeld HN: Intraventricular conduction disturbances: a review of prevalence, etiology and progression for ten years within a stable population of Israeli adult males. Am Heart J 96: 669, 1978
26. Lasser RP, Haft JI, Friedberg CK: Relationship of right bundle branch block and marked left axis deviation (with left parietal or peri-infarctional block) to complete heart block and syncope. Circulation 37: 429, 1968
27. Watt TB Jr, Pruitt RD: Character, cause and consequence of combined left axis deviation and right bundle branch block in human electrocardiogram. Am Heart J 77: 460, 1969
28. Dhingra RC, Wyndham C, Bauernfeind R, Denes P, Wu D, Swiryn S, Rosen KM: Significance of chronic bifascicular block without apparent organic heart disease. Circulation 60: 33, 1979
29. Scanlon P, Pryor R, Blount G: Right bundle-branch block associated with left superior or inferior intraventricular block. Clinical setting, prognosis and relation to complete heart block. Circulation 42: 1123, 1970
30. De Pasquale NP, Bruno MS: Natural history of combined right bundle branch block and left anterior hemiblock (bilateral bundle branch block). Am J Med 54: 297, 1973
31. Narula OS, Gann D, Samet P: Prognostic value of HV interval. In: His bundle electrocardiography and clinical electrophysiology. Nacula OS. Philadelphia: FA Davis, 1975, p 437
32. Varriale P, Kennedy RJ: Right bundle branch block and lef posterior fascicular block. Vectorcardiographic and clinical features. Am J Cardiol 29: 459, 1972
33. Dhingra RC, Denes P, Wu D, Chuquimia R, Amat-y-Leon F, Wyndham C, Rosen KM: Chronic right bundle branch block and left posterior hemiblock. Clinical, electrophysiologic and prognostic observations. Am J Cardiol 36: 867, 1975
34. Meilhac B, Noblet-Meilhac D, Le Pailleur CL: Bloc trifasciculaire chez le sujet jeune avec atteinte infraclinique de la contractilité myocardique. Arch Mal Coeur 72: 793, 1979
35. Narula OS: Intraventricular conduction defects: current concepts and clinical significance. In: Cardiac arrhytmias. Electrophysiology, diagnosis and management, Narula OS. Baltimore: Williams & Wilkins, 1979, p 114
36. Berkowitz WD, Lau SH, Patton RD, Rosen KM, Damato AN: The use of His bundle recordings in the analysis of unilateral and bilateral bundle branch block. Am Heart J 81: 340, 1971
37. Haft JI, Weinstock M, De-Quia PK, Gupta F, Fano A: Assessment of atrioventricular conduction in left and right bundle branch block using His bundle electrocardiogram and atrial pacing. Am J Cardiol 27: 424, 1971
38. Denes P, Dhindra RC, WU D, Chuquimia R, Amat-y-Leon F, Wyndham C, Rosen KM: HV interval in patients with bifascicular block (right bundle branch block and left anterior hemiblock). Clinical, electrocardiographic and electrophysiologic correlations. Am J Cardiol 35: 23, 1975
39. Puech P, Grolleau R, Guimond C: Incidence of different types of AV block and their localization by His bundle recordings. In: The conduction system of the heart. Structure, function and clinical implications, Wellens HSJ, Lie KI, Janse MS. Leiden: Stenfert Kroese, 1976, p 467
40. Levites R, Haft JI: Significance of first degree heart block in bifascicular block. Am J Cardiol 34: 259, 1974

6. PERIPHERAL BLOCKS

We define peripheral block as a conduction disturbance localized below the main intraventricular pathways (bundle branches and fascicles), i.e. in the Purkinje and muscular fibers. As long ago as 1916, Oppeheimer et al. [1] hypothesized conduction defects located in the periphery of the intraventricular conduction system. Since then, however, few experimental [2-7] and clinical studies [8-19] have been performed and our knowledge on this topic is very limited. Peripheral blocks have been defined in various ways: block of the arborization [1], focal block [8] and parietal block [9]. In previous papers on peripheral blocks, most likely located in the left ventricular walls, we defined them as parietal blocks [14-16]. However, if we consider that these blocks can be present in any part of the heart, including the interventricular septum, the term 'parietal' is not adequate for all localizations, and the definition 'peripheral block' would, therefore, seem more appropriate.

DIAGNOSIS AND LOCALIZATION

The problems relative to localization of peripheral blocks not related to myocardial infarction are:

- Localization of the ventricle and of the ventricular wall.
- Intraparietal localization: subendocardial or subepicardial.
- Level of the block: Purkinje fibers, synapses or muscular fibers.

The most important problem appears to be the localization of the involved ventricle, left or right.

LEFT PERIPHERAL BLOCKS

A left peripheral block can be localized in the left ventricular walls (left ventricular peripheral block) or in the left part of the septum (left septal peripheral block).

Left ventricular peripheral block

We posed the problem of diagnosing in clinical setting a left ventricular peripheral block, not related to myocardial infarction, and we extrapolated diagnostic criteria (ECG and VCG) on the basis of clinical data and the few available experimental data.

After an injection of 1-2 cm^3 of cocaine or bichlorhydrate of quinine into the ventricular walls of a dog or sheep, the following changes in epicardial QRS complexes were observed [2, 5-7]: a) increase in QRS duration; b) notching or thickening of the terminal segment of QRS complexes; c) appearance of Rsr′ of Rsr′ s′ morphology; d) prolongation of intrinsecoid deflection time; e) slight deviation of QRS axis; f) at times, decrease in amplitude of QRS complexes. Such changes, clearly evident in the epicardial leads, did not always appear in the extremity leads.

Ribeiro [7] also registered the vectorcardiogram after cocaine injection into the left ventricular walls. In this recording no variations in the initial vectors were observed; the middle vectors generally shifted posteriorly, slightly superiorly or inferiorly. The most important alterations were evident in the terminal part of QRS loop, which appeared delayed, at times irregular and more or less shifted to the left.

These data, therefore, suggest that a left ventricular peripheral block induces a terminal delay of the QRS loop, oriented to the left and posteriorly, without significant changes in initial and middle phases of ventricular depolarization.

On the basis of these results we have selected VCG recordings with QRS duration of 100 msec or more and with a terminal delay evident in all three planes, lasting at least 30 msec and oriented to the left and posteriorly. Not included were cases with alterations in initial and middle phases, i.e. bundle branch blocks, fascicular blocks and myocardial infarctions.

We encountered 55 cases with these VCG characteristics and we presume that, in such cases, the conduction disturbance takes place in the left ventricular walls.

The duration of the QRS loop ranged from 100 to 140 msec and that of terminal delay 30-50 msec. In 22 cases irregularities of the delayed segment were present. The orientation of the 20 msec vector, of the maximum vector and of the vector corresponding to the beginning of the terminal delay are reported in Figure 1.

The 20 msec vector in the frontal (F) and horizontal (H) planes had a greater concentration between $+80°$ and $+10°$; the maximum vector in the F plane between $+30°$ and $-10°$ and in the H plane between $0°$ and $-60°$; the terminal slurring vector in the F plane between $0°$ and $-60°$ and in the H plane between $0°$ and $-80°$.

The rotation in the three planes is reported in Table 1. In frontal plane it was clockwise, counterclockwise or figure of eight; in right sagittal plane, clockwise or figure of eight; in horizontal plane, always counterclockwise or figure of eight with counterclockwise beginning.

In 30 cases a left ventricular hypertrophy pattern was evident.

In the electrocardiogram a terminal slurring in at least three leads was present in

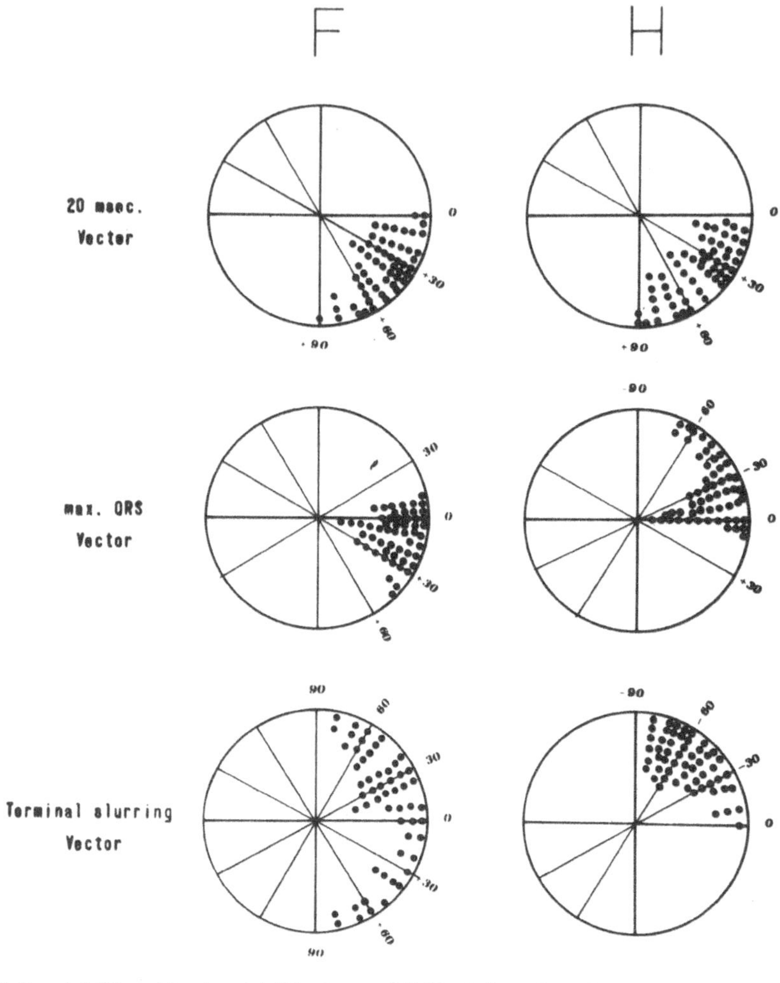

Figure 1. Frontal (F) and horizontal (H) planes of VCG. Orientation of the 20 msec vectors, of the maximum vectors and of the terminal vectors of QRS loop. (From Alboni et al., with permission of J Electrocardiol [16])

all cases, at times on R wave, at others on S wave. The most affected leads were I, II, III, aVL, aVR, aVF and V_5-V_6 (Figure 2).

In most cases, in the left sided leads (I, aVL, V_6) the terminal slurring appeared on R wave, but quite often on S wave (Figure 2): comparing ECG (Figure 2) and VCG data (Figure 1) there appeared to be a discrepancy. In fact, assuming that an ECG lead should have a terminal positive deflection if the terminal QRS forces are placed in the positive half of the axis of this lead, an excess of S waves in left sided leads appears, compared to what one would expect from VCG data.

In ECG recording a scattering of the morphology of the delayed terminal forces

Table 1. Rotation of QRS loop in the three planes of VCG

	F	RS	H
CW	10	43	—
CCW	36	—	51
∞	9	12	4

F = frontal
SR = right sagittal plane
H = horizontal plane
CW = clockwise rotation
CCW = counterclockwise rotation
∞ = figure of eight

is therefore evident. For this reason, in our opinion, only in some cases can an ECG diagnosis of left ventricular peripheral block be made, i.e. when the terminal slurring is positive (on R wave) in left sided leads. In fact, in such cases it may be deduced that the delayed terminal vectors are directed to the left and posteriorly. If the terminal slurring is on S wave in one or more of the left sided leads it is not possible to detect whether the delayed forces are directed to the left or to the right.

The ECG and VCG discrepancies are probably due to the greater sensitivity of the ECG leads in intercepting local forces; consequently the ECG gives a less exact picture of the development of ventricular depolarization.

On the basis of the above-mentioned experimental data and our clinical observations, we propose the following *electrocardiographic criteria* to diagnose a left ventricular peripheral block (Figures 3, 4 and 5):

- QRS duration of 100 msec or more.
- Normality of initial and middle phases of ventricular depolarization or else alterations due to concomitant left ventricular hypertrophy.
- Terminal slurring, evident in at least three leads and positive (on R wave) in the left sided leads I, aVL and V_6. If the terminal slurring is on S wave in one or more of these leads, the localization of the involved ventricle is doubtful.

And the following vectorcardiographic criteria (Figure 3):

- QRS duration of 100 msec or more.
- Normality of initial and middle phases of ventricular depolarization or else alterations due to concomitant left ventricular hypertrophy.
- Terminal delay, lasting 30 msec or more, sometimes with irregularities, directed to the left and posteriorly, at times superiorly, and others inferiorly.

These depolarization alterations express an intraventricular disorder. The normality of initial and middle phases of ventricular depolarization leads us to exclude that terminal delay is related to bundle branch block, incomplete or of advanced degree, or to fascicular blocks (see Chapter 4). We believe, therefore, the

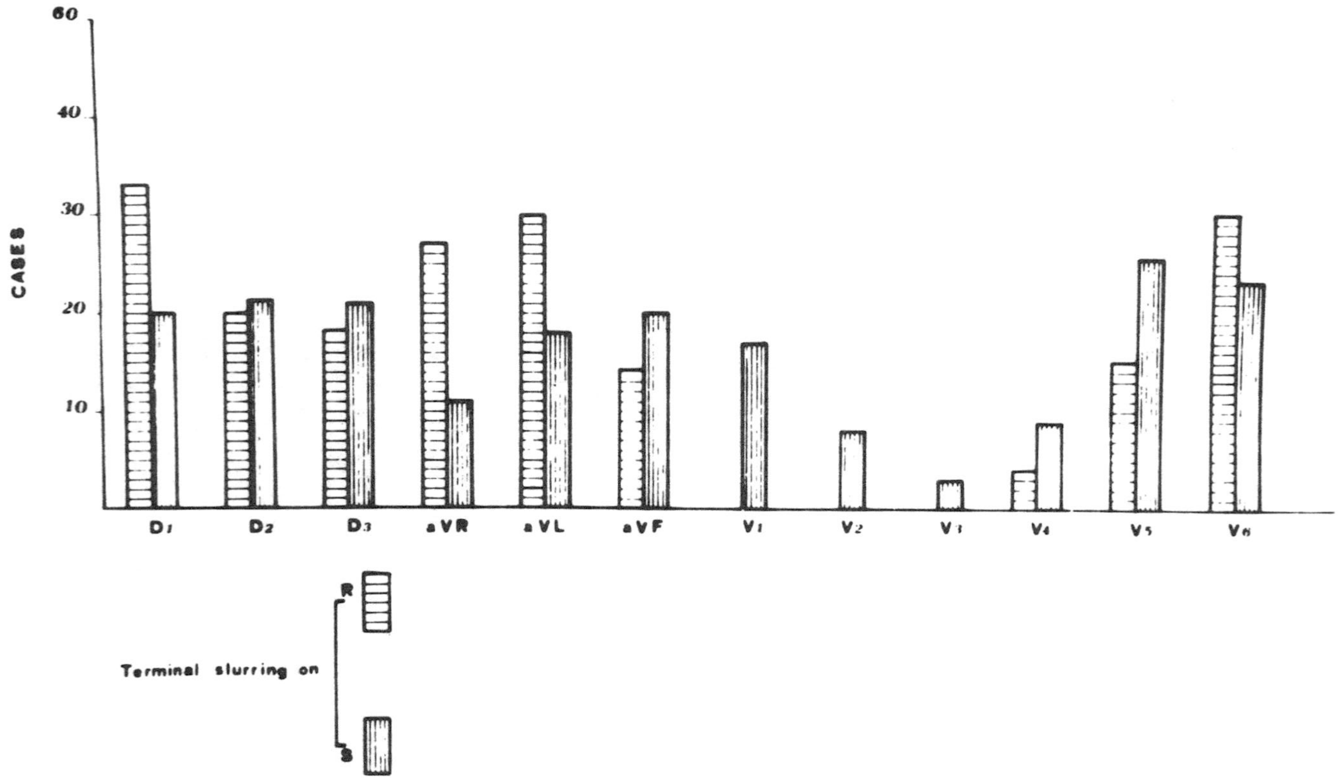

Figure 2. Terminal slurring on R and S waves in the ECG leads: D_1: lead I, D_2: lead II, D_3: lead III. (From Alboni et al., with permission of J Electrocardiol [16])

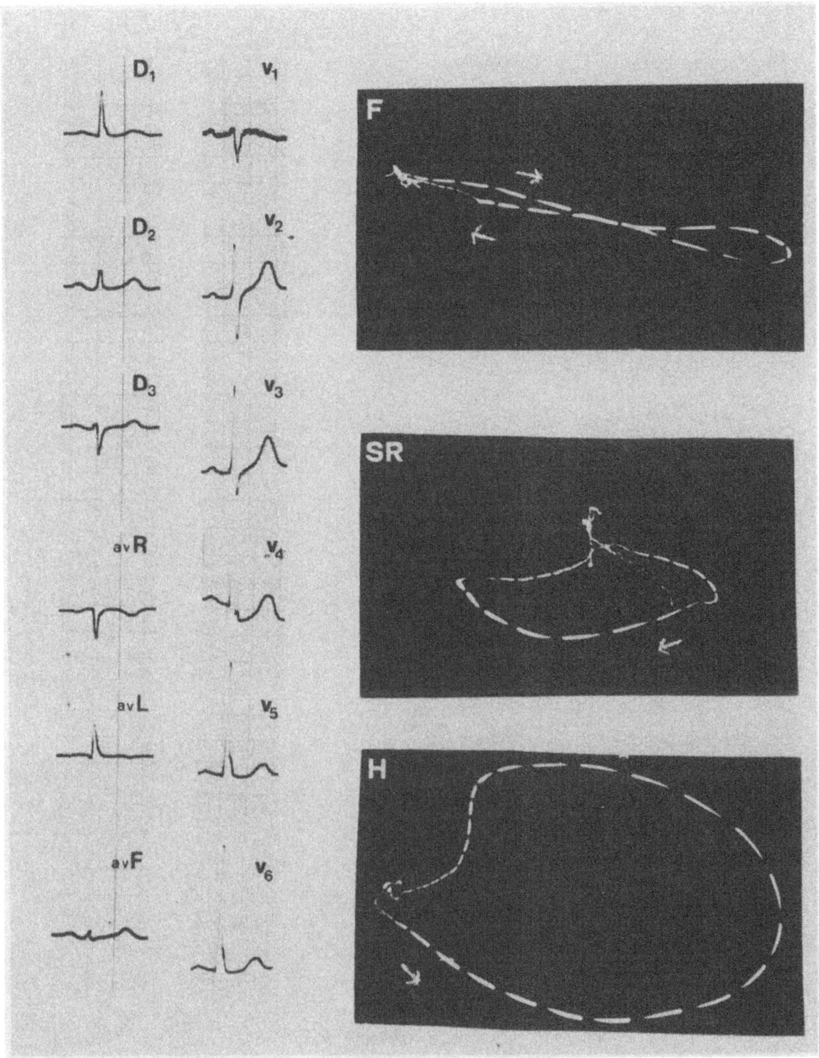

Figure 3. Left ventricular peripheral block. ECG: QRS = 100 msec. Terminal slurring on R wave in I, aVL, V_5 and V_6. Terminal slurring on S wave in aVR, aVF, and V_1. VCG: Terminal delay lasting 30 msec, with irregularities, oriented to the left posteriorly and inferiorly. (From Alboni et al., with permission of J Electrocardiol [16])

most likely cause is a peripheral conduction disturbance. The orientation of the terminal delay to the left and posteriorly, in accordance with Ribeiro's experimental data [7], allows location of these peripheral blocks within the left ventricular walls.

These diagnostic criteria are, however, of limited value when a left ventricular

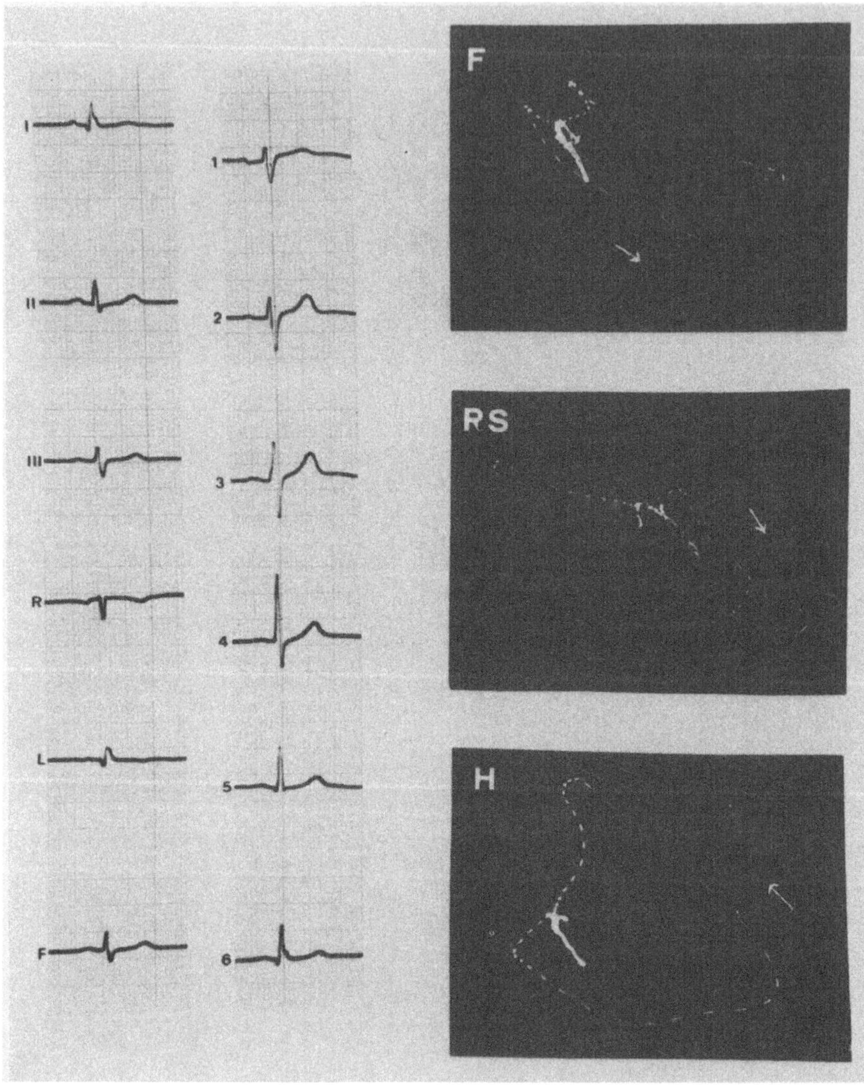

Figure 4. Left ventricular peripheral block. ECG: QRS = 100 msec. Terminal slurring on R wave in I, aVL and V_6. Terminal slurring on S wave in III, aVF and V_1. VCG: Terminal delay lasting 35 msec, with irregularities, directed to the left, posteriorly and superiorly

hypertrophy is present. As a result of the electric preponderance of the left ventricle it is possible that delayed terminal vectors shift to the left, even if peripheral slowing of conduction is located in the right ventricle.

At present we hold that it is possible, within certain limits, to localize only the ventricle affected by the peripheral block, but not the involved ventricular walls.

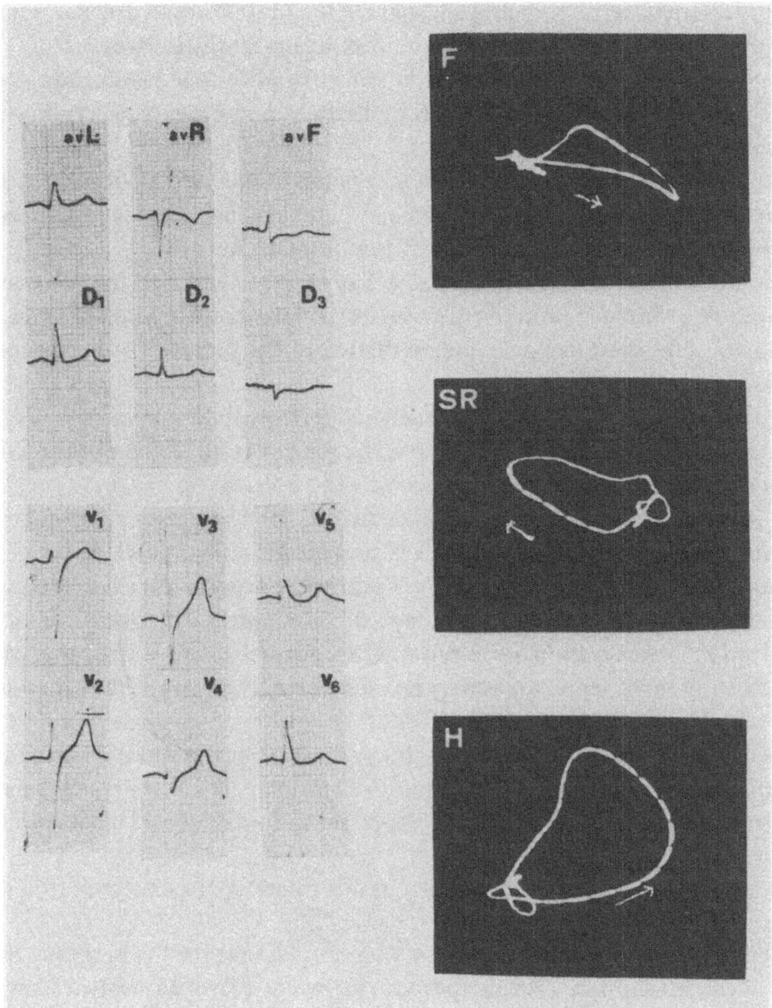

Figure 5. Left ventricular peripheral block. ECG: QRS = 120 msec. Terminal slurring on R wave in aVL, II, V_5 and V_6. Slurred S wave in III, aVF, V_1 and V_4. VCG: Terminal delay, lasting 35 msec, oriented to the left, posteriorly and superiorly. (From Alboni et al., with permission of J Electrocardiol [16])

Left septal peripheral block

Up to now the interventricular septum, regarding intraventricular conduction, has always been considered as a starting point and the ventricular walls as a periphery (Purkinje network and muscular fibers). In effect, a periphery exists also in the septum and can manifest its own pathology. At present, the latter only represents a theoretical possibility since there are no experimental studies in which the septal

Purkinje fibers have been damaged, sparing the main intraventricular conduction pathways. This shortcoming is due to great technical difficulties.

However, in our opinion, there do emerge from literature some data suggestive of this type of peripheral block; from these, some diagnostic criteria may be deduced:

- Burch [20] observed in post-mortem examination a septal fibrosis in patients whose ECG showed small r wave in V_1V_2 and absence of q wave in leads V_5-V_6, without other ventricular depolarization alterations.
- In some studies [21, 22] a discrepancy has emerged between the presence of QS morphology in V_1-V_3 and the discovery of anteroseptal myocardial infarction at autopsy. This discrepancy could be related to the presence of peripheral septal block.
- In order to explain a rate-dependent widening of Q waves in V_2-V_3 in two patients with antero-septal infarction, Gambetta et al. [23] hypothesized a focal block in the left septum associated with the necrosis.
- Conde et al. [24] and Zeft et al. [25] described the reappearance of anterior QRS forces after coronary arterial bypass surgery in patients with previous antero-septal infarction pattern (Figure 6). These authors point out that, although these patients represent a small percentage of those with a preoperative pattern of infarction, regeneration of anterior QRS forces demonstrates that the prior electrically silent septal areas may be only partially damaged and are not always synonymous with myocardial cell death.
- The results of one of our studies [26] suggests that the small q waves in V_2-V_3 leads, at times associated with anterior fascicular block (AFB) are related to a loss of septal forces, probably an expression of a left septal block (see Chapter 4).

  The above-mentioned data suggest, in our opinion, the existence of a left peripheral septal block.

A septal necrosis or other types of lesion can damage the Purkinje and muscular fibers of the left septum, sparing the main intraventricular pathways. These lesions can induce a conduction delay, which should be manifested — in contrast to left ventricular peripheral block — by an *initial slurring* of the QRS complex, in that the left septum is the first ventricular area to be activated. It may be that ECG recordings, interpreted as Wolff-Parkinson-White syndrome, actually express a left peripheral septal block.

This block, particularly if related to septal fibrosis, can also induce a loss of electrical forces. If the block is localized in the lowest part of the septum, one can observe a healed inferior infarction pattern, whereas if it is localized in the third middle of the septum, there should be a shifting to the left of the first vectors with reduction in amplitude of the r wave in V_1-V_2 and disappearance of the q waves in V_5-V_6 (Figures 7 and 8).

The latter ECG pattern may be present also in the anatomic vertical heart [27],

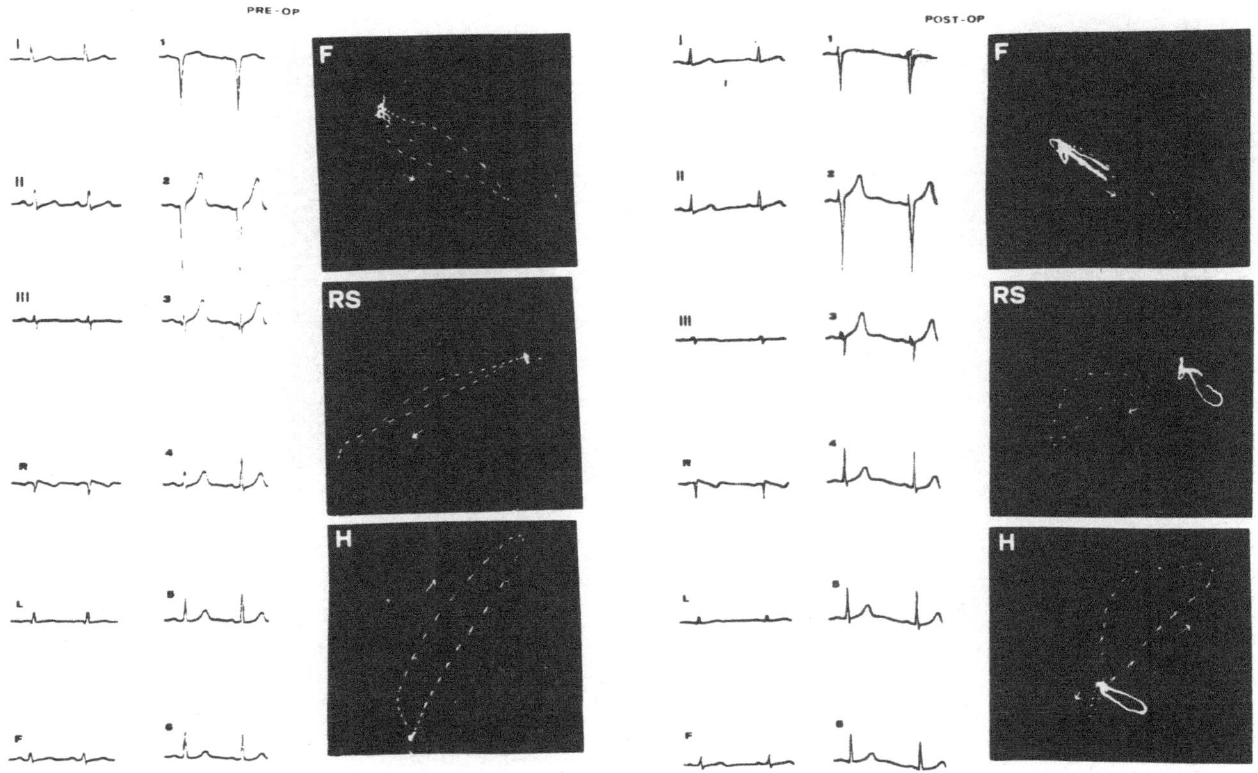

Figure 6. Patient with unstable angina with no history of acute myocardial infarction. Preoperative ECG and VCG recordings (left) show anteroseptal myocardial infarction pattern. ECG and VCG registered after coronary bypass surgery (right) evidence regeneration of anterior QRS forces (see text for explanation)

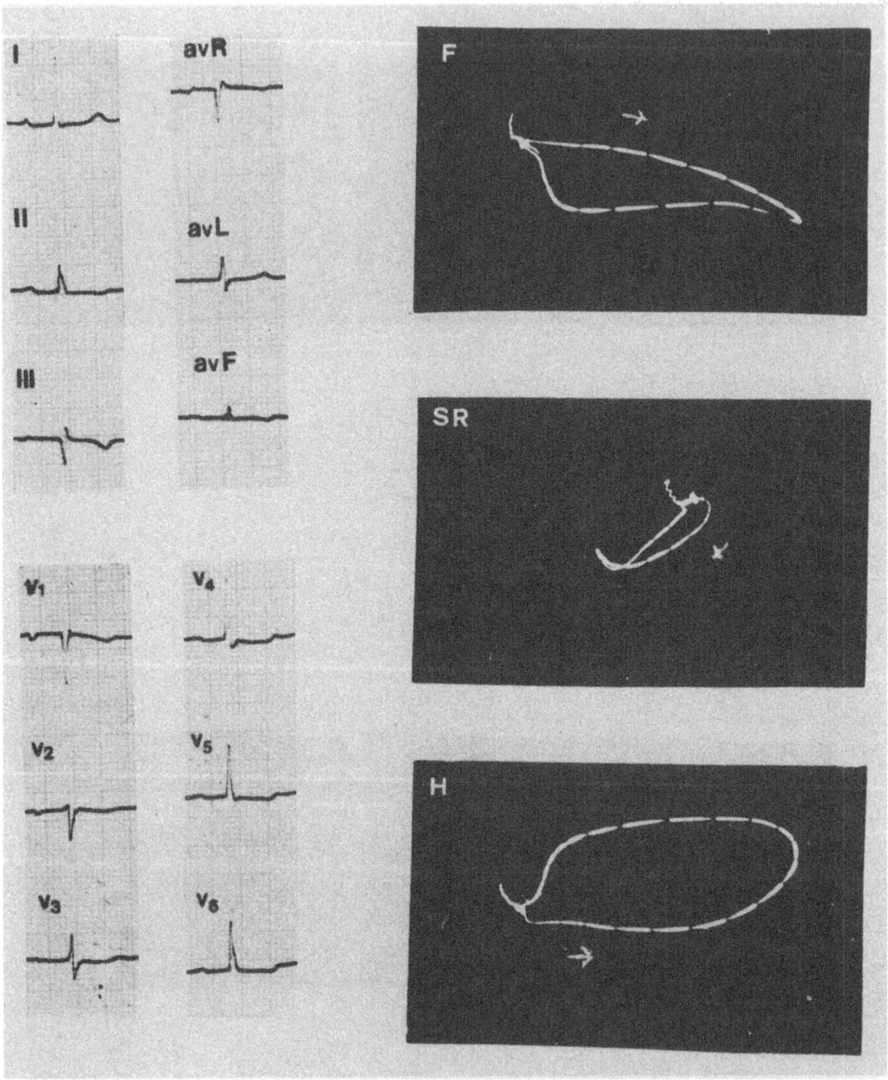

Figure 7. ECG: QRS = 80 msec. QS morphology in V_1 and small r wave in V_2. In V_5-V_6 q wave is absent and the delay of intrinsecoid deflection is only 20 msec. Such a pattern is highly suggestive of a left peripheral septal block

pulmonary emphysema [28], right ventricular hypertrophy [29]. However, all these conditions are fairly easy to individualize.

Of greater difficulty appears to be a differential diagnosis with incomplete left bundle branch block (LBBB). The latter induces, besides the above-mentioned ECG changes, a delayed activation of the left ventricular walls with subsequent

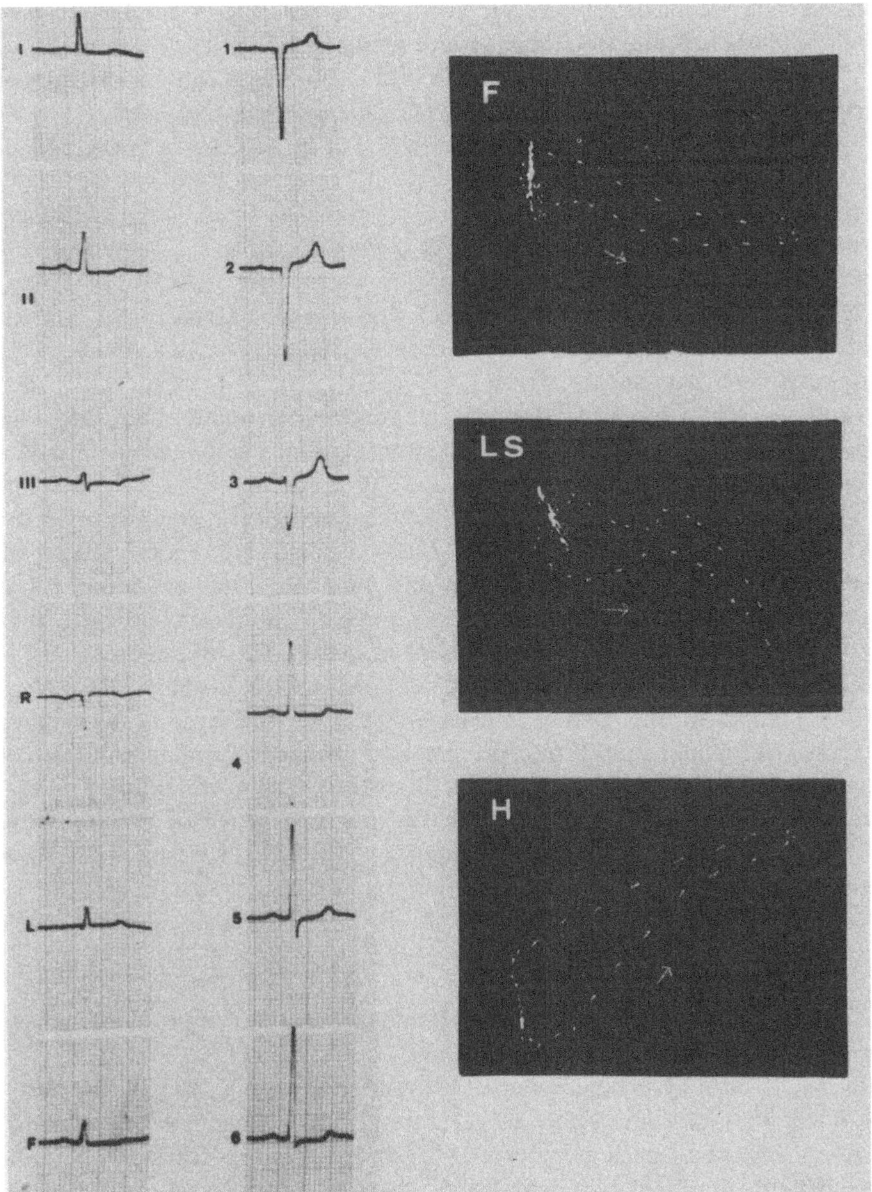

Figure 8. ECG: QRS = 80 msec. QS morphology in V_1-V_2 and small r wave in V_3. In V_5-V_6 q wave is absent and the delay of intrinsecoid deflection measures 30 msec. In the VCG the first vectors are directed to the left and anteriorly. Such a pattern suggests left septal peripheral block

delayed intrinsecoid deflection time in V_6 (Sodi-Pallares). A conduction defect localized in the septum should not induce such a delay.

Thus we propose the following ECG criteria for the diagnosis of left septal peripheral block, until reliable experimental confirmation is available:

- *Slurring of the initial part of QRS complex, in the absence of ventricular pre-excitation.*
- *Absence or reduction in amplitude of the r wave in V_1-V_2 and disappearance of q wave in V_5-V_6, with normal intrinsecoid deflection time in V_6 and without other ventricular depolarization alterations.*

If the left septal block manifests itself with a healed myocardinal infarction pattern, anteroseptal or inferior, the differential diagnosis with a true healed infarction is practically impossible.

In Figure 9-14 a case of intraventricular conduction trouble is reported whose morphological characteristics would seem to confirm the diagnostic criteria we proposed.

The patient was a 45-year-old man without cardiological symptoms, apart from palpitations during exercise. Chest X-ray showed slight cardiomegaly. Electrocardiogram (Figure 9) revealed normal sinus rhythm with a rate of 75/min, PR and QRS intervals of 160 and 120 msec, respectively. A QS morphology in II, II and aVF suggested a healed inferior myocardial infarction. This infarction pattern was evident also in the vectorcardiogram. In V_2-V_3 leads and in the H and RS planes of VCG an initial slurring, lasting 25 msec, was present. In Figure 10 the sinus rate increased to 100/min and PR interval remained unchanged. An anterior fascicular rior myocardial infarction pattern (see Chapter 8). The initial slurring in V_2-V_3 remained. During exercise (Figure 11) the sinus rate increased to 130/min and PR interval to 180 msec. The disappearance of the initial slurring in V_2-V_3 was evident. Owing to this behavior ECG tracings were suggestive of W.P.W. syndrome.

Coronary arteriograms and ventricular angiograms did not evidence any segmental anomaly of ventricular contraction.

During electrophysiological study, the initial slurring in V_2 was evident and the HV interval was prolonged (55 msec) (Figure 12); the QRS complex measured 110 msec. During atrial pacing (cycle length 380 msec) initial slurring in V_2 disappeared, QRS duration decreased to 90 msec and HV interval did not change (Figure 13).

In Figure 14 driving cycle length was 530 msec. For an H_1H_1 interval of 510 msec, H_2V_2 and QRS intervals measured 55 and 105 msec, respectively; the initial slurring in V_2 was present. For an H_1H_2 of 405 msec, initial slurring disappeared, QRS duration decreased to 90 msec, whereas HV interval did not change (55 msec).

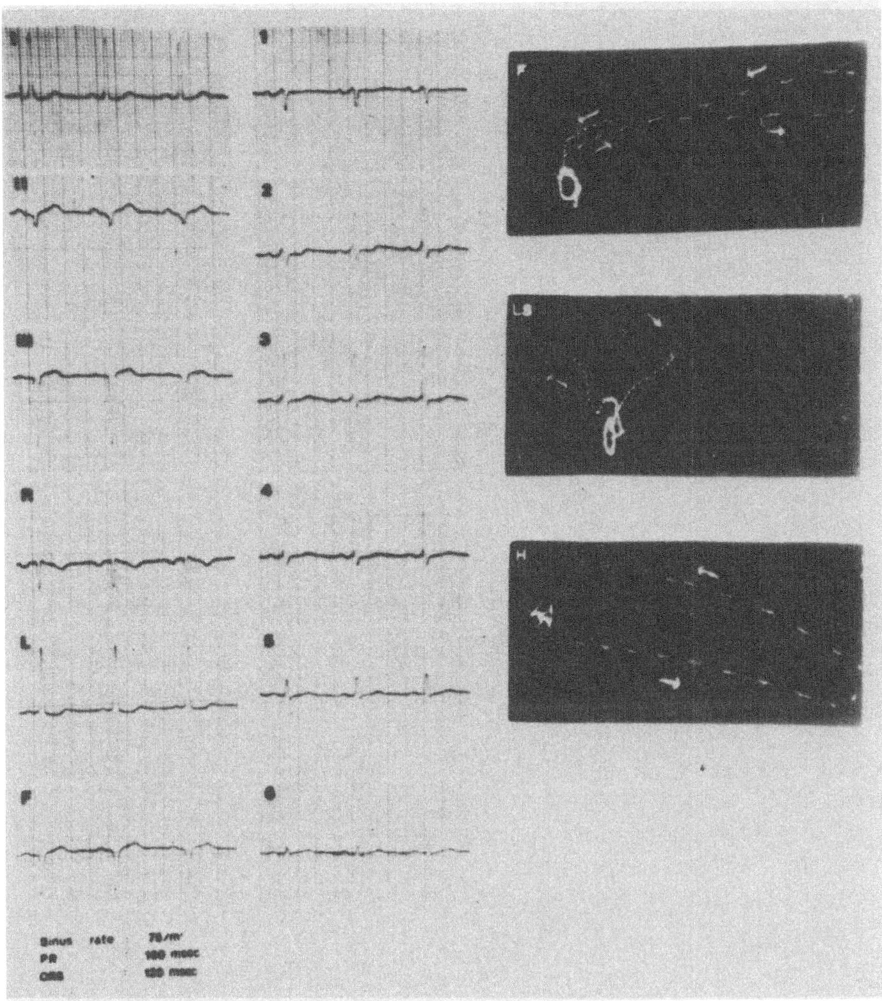

Figure 9. In ECG and VCG recordings an inferior myocardial pattern is present (QS morphology in II, III, aVF). In V_2-V_3 an initial slurring is evident. Such a slurring, in the three planes of VCG, lasts 25 msec. (From Alboni, with permission of G Ital Cardiol [19])

The constancy of such an interval, in the presence and in the absence of the initial slurring, excludes a WPW syndrome. This case may be interpreted as a rate-dependent left peripheral septal block, localized in the inferior part of the left septum, which manifests itself with both an initial slurring of QRS complex and a loss of electric forces.

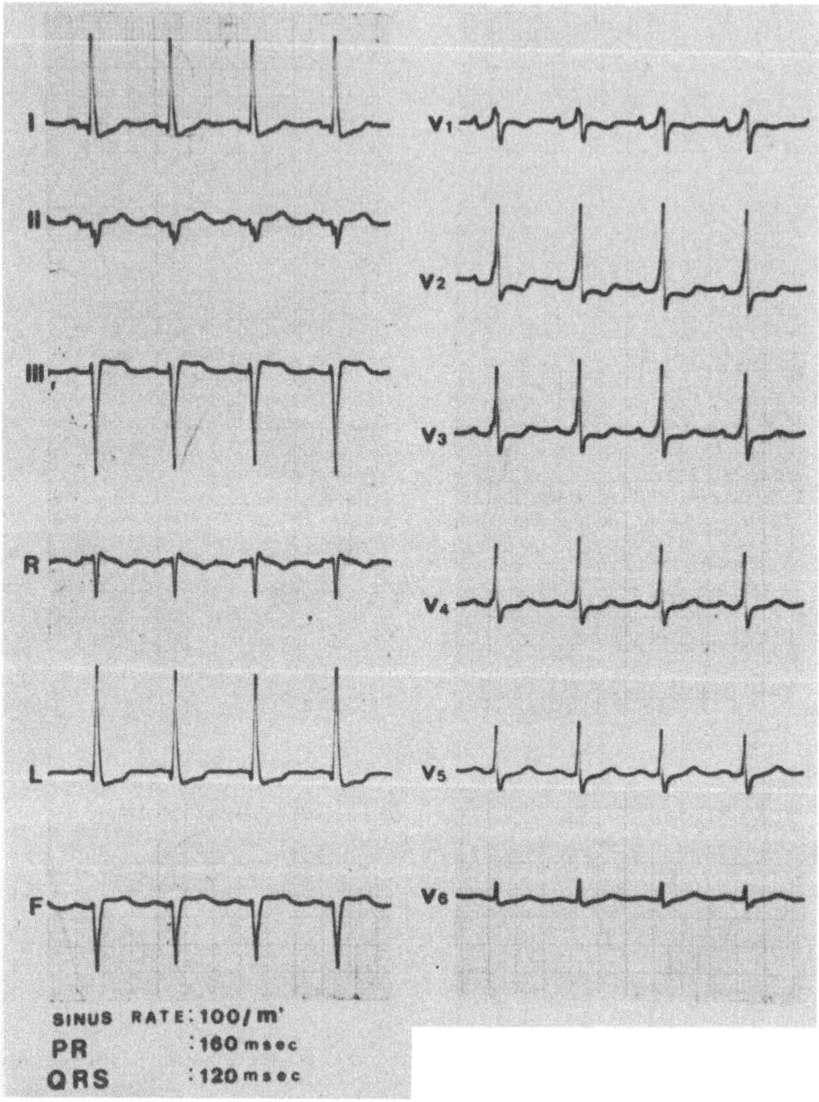

Figure 10. A rate-dependent anterior fascicular block appears, which cancels out the inferior myocardial infarction. The initial slurring in V_2-V_3 leads remains. (From Alboni, with permission of G Ital Cardiol [19])

RIGHT PERIPHERAL BLOCKS

A right peripheral block can be localized in the right ventricular walls (right ventricular peripheral block) or in the right part of the septum (right septal peripheral block).

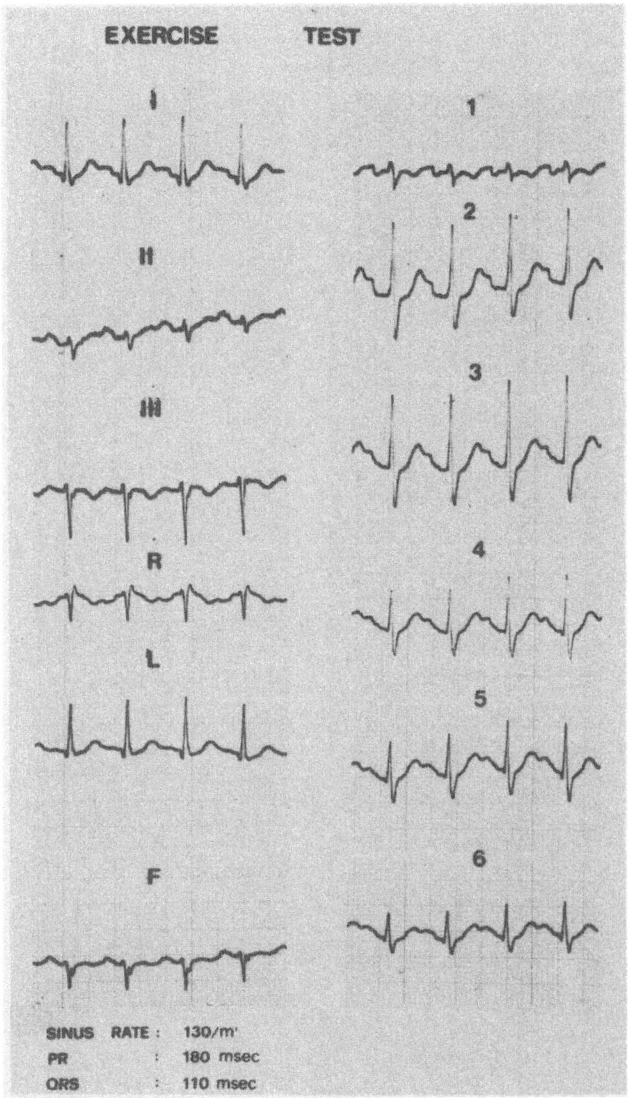

Figure 11. During exercise test sinus rate increases to 130/min, PR interval is prolonged to 180 msec and initial slurring in V_2-V_3 leads disappears. (From Alboni, with permission of G Ital Cardiol [19])

A right ventricular peripheral block can involve the postero-basal wall or the free anterior wall. It is more frequent in the postero-basal wall owing to the presence of the supraventricular crest [30].

In experimental blocks induced in such a wall [31-34] there was a slight increase in QRS duration, appearance or accentuation of a slurred S wave in the left-sided leads, and increase in amplitude of the terminal R wave in aVR. Sometimes in V_1 a

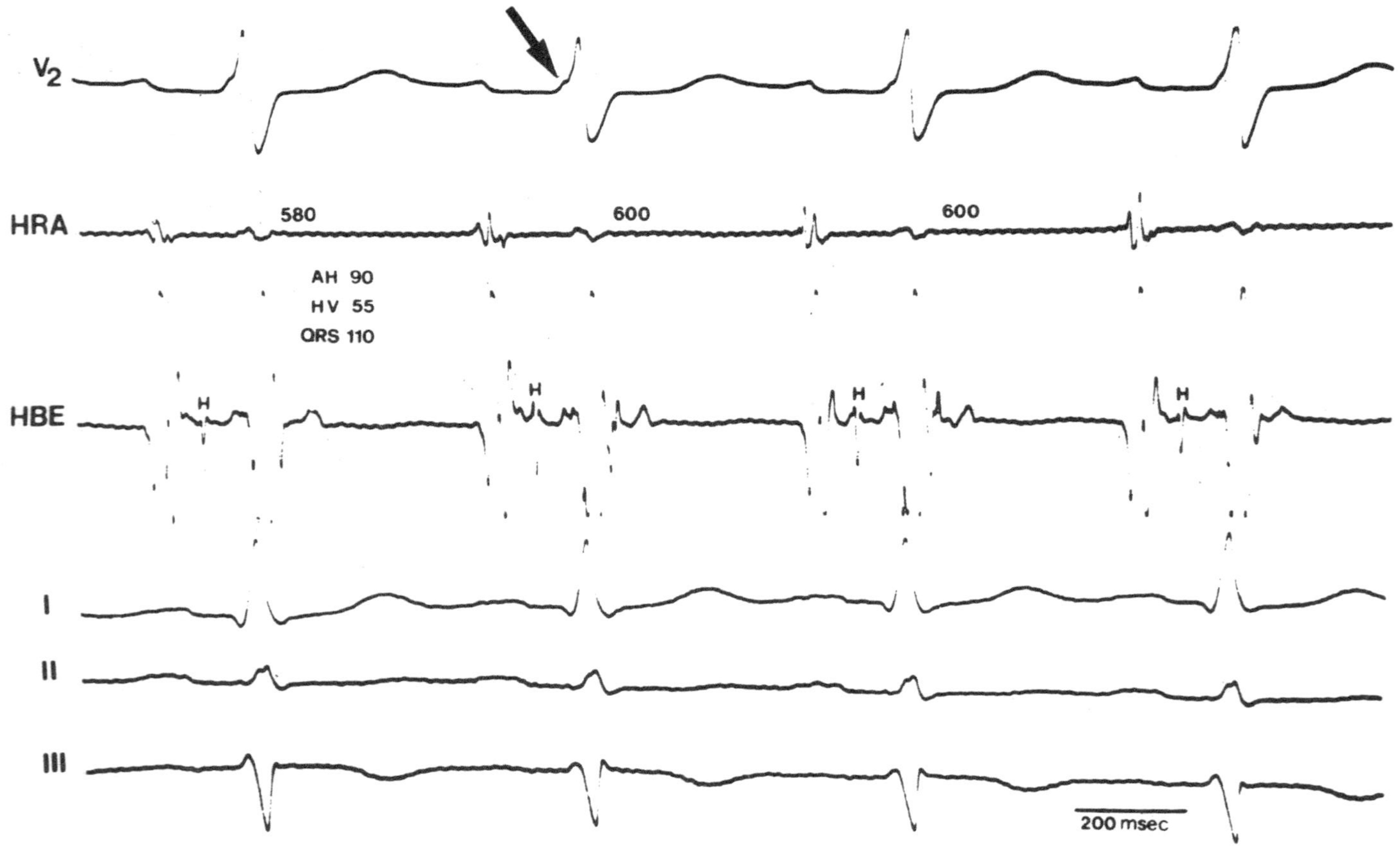

Fig. 12. During electrophysiological study the initial slurring in lead V_2 is present. HV and QRS intervals measure 55 and 110 msec, respectively. (From Alboni, with permission of G Ital Cardiol [19])

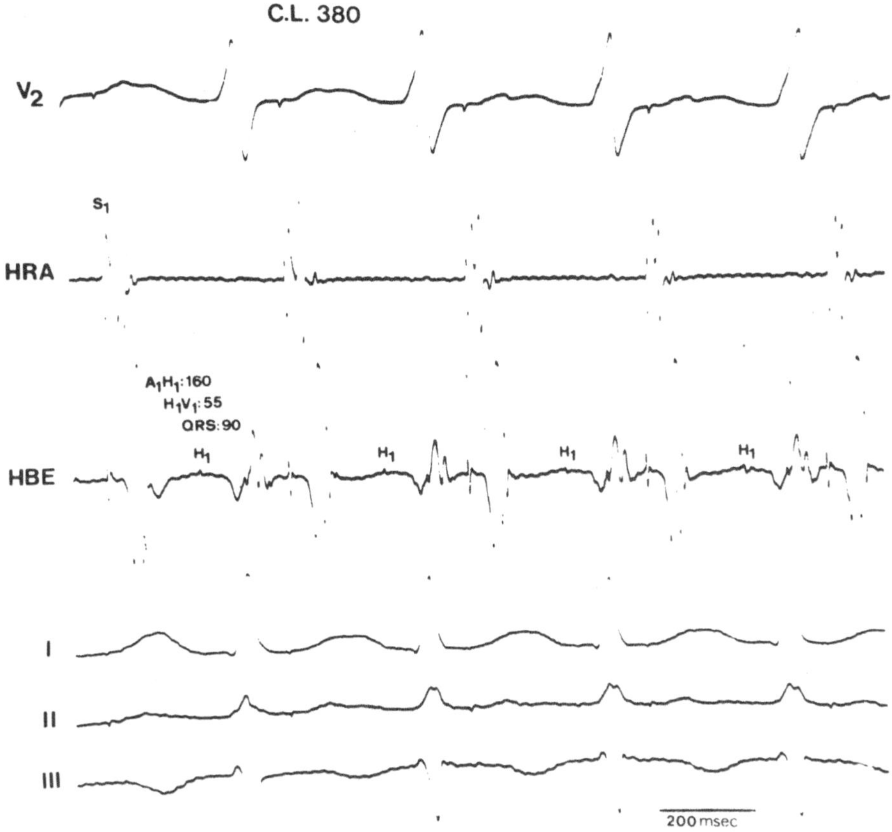

Figure 13. During atrial pacing (cycle length: 380 msec) the initial slurring in V_2 disappears. The HV interval does not change (55 msec) and the QRS interval decreases to 90 msec. (From Alboni, with permission of G Ital Cardiol [19])

terminal slurring on S wave or a small terminal r wave appeared. Electrical QRS axis at times shifted upward.

Moore et al. [32] also carried out vectorcardiographic recordings. The orientation of the first part of QRS loop was essentially unchanged, whereas the delayed terminal vectors shifted superiorly, posteriorly and to the right.

On the basis of such experimental data, a *peripheral block localized in the postero-basal wall of the right ventricle* can most likely be diagnosed in the presence of the following electrical signs:

- QRS complex of normal duration or slightly prolonged.
- rS morphology in V_1, often with a terminal slurring.
- Slurred S wave in left-sided leads.
- Slurred terminal R wave in aVR.

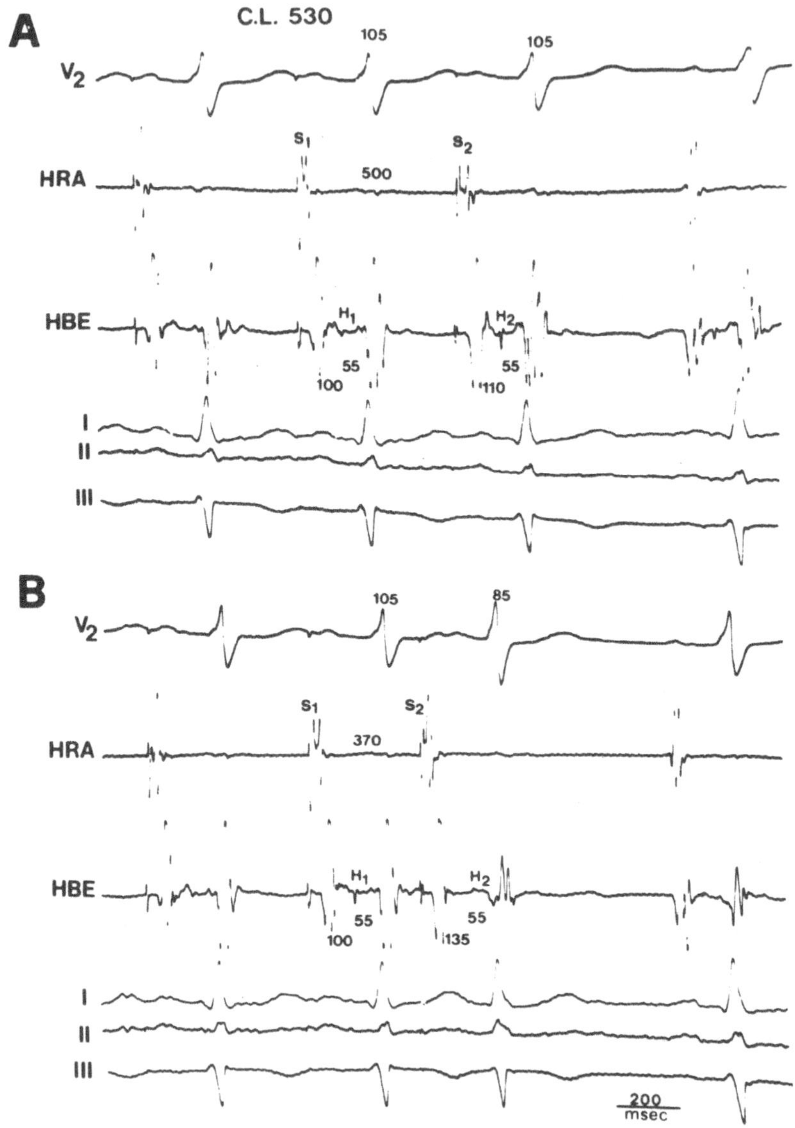

Figure 14. Driving cycle length is 530 msec. For an H_1H_2 of 510 msec, H_2V_2 and QRS intervals measure 55 and 105 msec, respectively. Initial slurring in V_2 lead is present. For an H_1H_2 of 405 msec, H_2V_2 interval does not change, whereas initial slurring in V_2 disappears and QRS duration decreases to 85 msec (see text for explanation). (From Alboni, with permission of G Ital Cardiol [19])

- Terminal vectors directed to the right, posteriorly, superiorly or, more rarely, inferiorly.
- Counterclockwise rotation in H plane and clockwise or counterclockwise rotation in F plane of VCG.

In some cases a small terminal r wave in V_1 is present, even if the terminal vectors are directed posteriorly [35].

Sometimes a pseudo left axis deviation is present, in so far as the mid-terminal vectors are directed superiorly as well as to the right. In such cases a differential diagnosis must be made with the anterior fascicular block. The presence of S wave in lead I is highly indicative of a right peripheral block. VCG recording is useful; if frontal QRS loop shows clockwise rotation, it excludes an AFB; if, on the other hand, it shows counterclockwise inscription, the maximum vector is generally oriented under 0° [36]. This pattern is contrary to the presence of an AFB (Figure 15) (see Chapter 4).

In cases where the terminal delay is oriented only slightly to the right (Figure 16) it is impossible to identify the ventricle affected by the peripheral block, since a part of the postero-basal region of the left ventricle may at times be displaced in the right hemithorax [37].

Recognition of peripheral block localized in the *anterior wall of the right ventricle* is more difficult, in that conduction delay in this wall — because of its anatomic position — shows terminal forces oriented anteriorly and to the right [5, 30, 38], thus evidencing an electric pattern identical to that of right bundle branch block (RBBB) (rSR morphology in lead V_1 and terminal delayed appendage in horizontal plane of VCG). In ECG and VCG recordings it is therefore impossible to differentiate whether the lesion responsible for the RBBB pattern is localized within the right bundle branch or the anterior wall of the right ventricle. A differential diagnosis may be possible within certain limits by introducing a catheter electrode in the right ventricular apex (RVA) for the recording of the V-RVA interval (see Chapter 3). If such an interval is normal ($\leq$30 msec), the block is most likely localized under the main bundle.

In our experience, and in that of other authors [39, 40] (see Chapter 3), in most all cases with a permanent RBBB pattern unrelated to surgery this interval is prolonged, thus indicating an involvement of the main right bundle branch. Different results were obtained in the surgically-induced RBBB (see Chapter 7).

A right septal peripheral block with normal conduction in the right bundle branch is an unknown electrical pattern. Such a block should not significantly alter the ventricular depolarization, due to the thinness of the right septal mass. However, there are no experimental data or anatomo-electrocardiographic correlations which allow us to define any diagnostic criteria.

INTRAPARIETAL LOCALIZATION

Either a subendocardial area with prevalent lesion of Purkinje network or a subepicardial area with prevalent lesion of muscular fibers can be affected. At present, in ECG and VCG recordings, it is impossible to assess whether the intraparietal

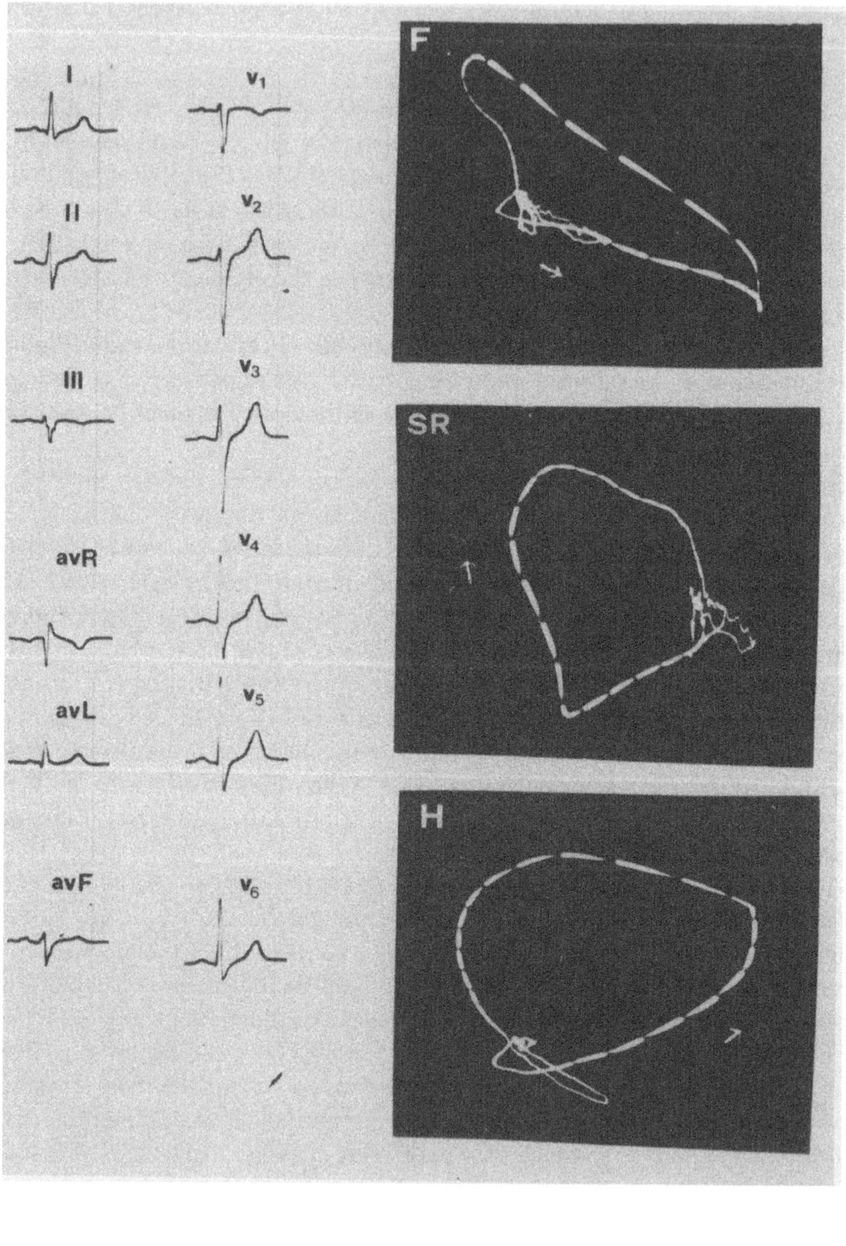

Figure 15. Right peripheral block localized in the postero-basal wall. ECG: QRS = 110 msec. Slurred S wave in I, II, III, aVF and V_1; slurred terminal R wave in aVR. Pseudo left axis deviation. VCG: Terminal delay lasting 40 msec, oriented to the right, posteriorly and superiorly. In F plane the rotation is counterclockwise, but the QRS loop shows a good development towards the left and the maximum vector is oriented at +20° (see text for explanation). (From Alboni et al., with permission of J Electrocardiol [18])

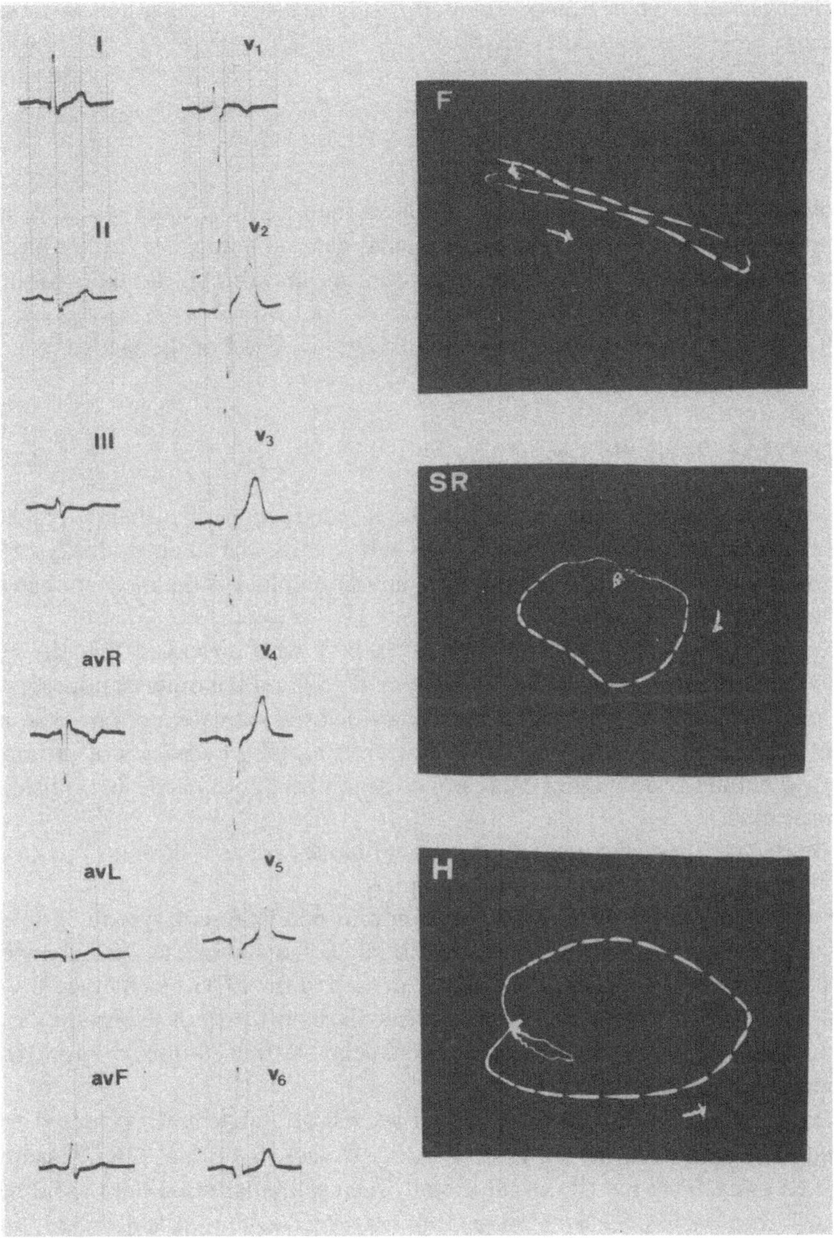

Figure 16. Terminal delay, lasting 30 msec, directed posteriorly, superiorly and slightly to the right. The ventricle affected by the peripheral block cannot be localized. (From Alboni et al., with permission of J Electrocardiol [18])

conduction delay has a subendocardial or subepicardial localization as these recordings only offer resultant vectors.

LEVEL OF THE BLOCK

Another still unanswered question is which anatomo-functional structure is affected in peripheral blocks. The experimental data on a dog's or sheep's heart 'in toto' at times suggest an affect within the Purkinje network [5], at others within the common myocardium [2, 7].

In a clinical setting it is not possible to assess the level of the block.

PERI-INFARCTION BLOCK

Peri-infarction block expresses a peripheral conduction disturbance related to acute myocardial infarction which does not involve the main pathways of the intraventricular conduction system. Peri-infarction block is the most studied peripheral block [41-51].

This term was introduced by First et al. [41], who presumed that the lesion surrounded the area of necrosis. Cabrera et al. [52], on the other hand, suggested the term intra-infarction block, postulating a delayed activation of not-dead muscular fibers inside the necrotic zone. Durrer et al. [43], by means of intramural electrodes, found conduction delay in not-dead fibers both inside and outside the necrotic area.

The electric characteristics of infarctional blocks are as follows:

- Widening, not constant, of QRS complex.
- Abnormality in the direction of initial and/or middle forces, typical of myocardial infarction, at times associated with initial slurring of the QRS complex.
- Alterations of the terminal vectors, evidenced in the ECG by enlarged S waves or by terminal slurring on R wave, particularly in the leads exploring the necrotic wall, and in the VCG by a terminal delay, lasting 30 msec or more, sometimes with irregularities.

Grant [53] observed that the terminal vectors are tangentially opposed to the initial ones with an angle of 120° or more. In fact, the initial QRS vectors are directed away from the site of infarction whereas the terminal ones are directed towards the necrosis. Such a feature is not however constant. According to Fischer et al. [51] the terminal vectors are opposed to the maximum vector of QRS loop more than to the initial vectors.

In anterolateral wall infarction the delayed terminal vectors are generally oriented to the left, superiorly and posteriorly, whereas in inferior wall infarction they are directed to the right, posteriorly, inferiorly or superiorly (Figure 17).

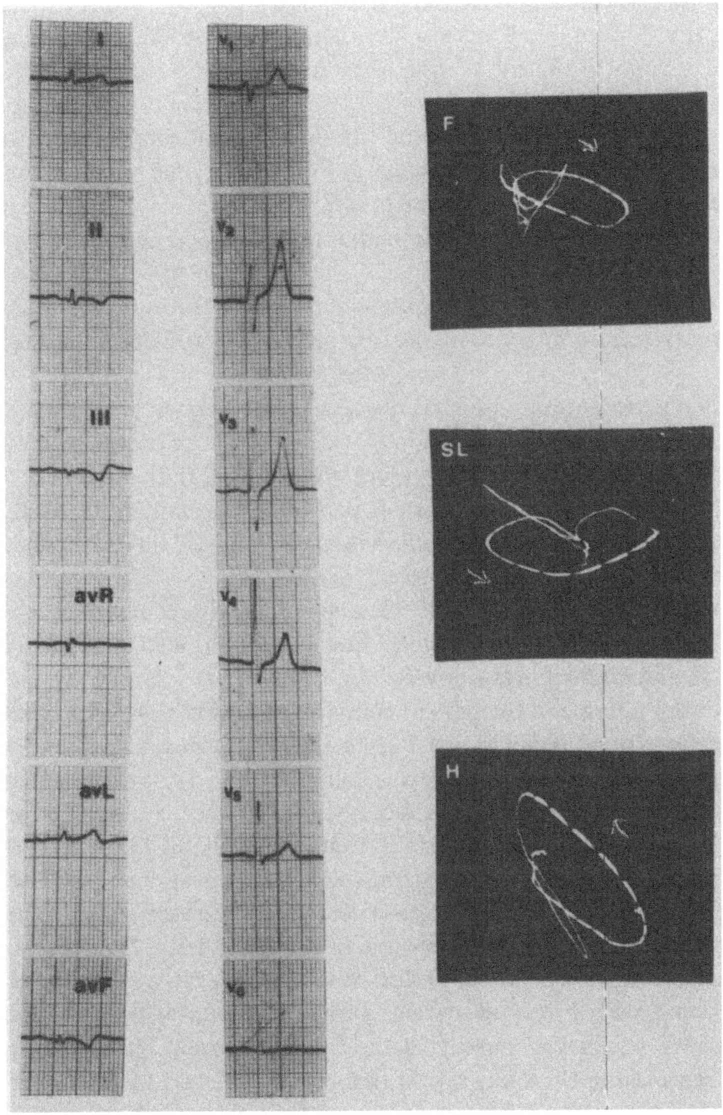

Figure 17. Postero-inferior myocardial infarction with peri-infarction block. ECG: QRS = 110 msec. Slurred S wave in I, II and V_5 leads. Terminal slurred r wave in aVR. QS morphology in III and aVF with terminal slurring. VCG: Terminal delay lasting 30 msec, oriented to the right, posteriorly and superiorly

The appearance of peri-infarction block did not differ significantly in the various ECG locations of the infarction [47, 49, 50]. It is rare in septal infarction, however, probably because of the close Purkinje network [47].

The majority of peri-infarction blocks appear during the first days following onset of acute myocardial infarction [47, 49, 50].

When peri-infarction block occurs several months after infarction it may be due to pressure atrophy of the conduction fibers in the scarred region of muscle, or to repeated bouts of ischemia [49].

Shadaksharappa et al. [49] observed that in most patients it tended to persist during the entire period of observation (3-4 years); in one third of the cases it disappeared or diminished during the first few months.

In rare cases the signs of myocardial infarction disappear, leaving only the peri-infarction block [47].

Very rarely does the peri-infarction block represent the only alteration of ventricular depolarization in acute myocardial infarction in ECG recording (Figure 18).

A transient peri-infarction block is observed quite frequently, whereas an intermittent, rate-dependent peri-infarction block represents an exceptional event, and only one case has been described by us [54] (Figures 19-23). In the case reported by Armenta [55], diagnosed as intermittent peri-infarction block, the evidence suggests an involvement of the left bundle branch because of the marked slurring of the middle portion of the QRS complex.

Figure 19 reports the admission ECG of a patient with acute inferior and antero-septal myocardial infarction. Sinus rate is 75/min, PR and QRS intervals measure 250 and 80 msec, respectively.

The day after admission the patient complained of dizziness. The ECG (Figure 20) showed sinus rhythm at a rate of 78/min and a 2:1 atrioventricular (AV) block. The PR interval of conducted beats was 280 msec. The alternate conducted QRS complexes exhibited a different morphology. The 1st, 3rd, 5th and 7th complexes of Figure 20 were of the same pattern as that seen in the ECG on admission. The 2nd, 4th, 6th and 8th QRS complexes showed a QRS duration of 120 msec and an aberrancy with the following features: 1) decrease in the amplitude of the R wave in I, aVL, V_4, V_5 and V_6 with rsr′ pattern in I, aVL and V_6; 2) increase in amplitude of terminal R wave in aVR; 3) slurred terminal negative waves in II, III and aVL; 4) deep S waves in V_1-V_4 with terminal slurring; 5) modifications of ST segment and T waves particularly in the right precordial leads. During a long period of observation the sinus rate varied between 72 and 85 beats/min and the PR interval of the conducted beats remained the same at 280 msec.

Figure 21A shows the vectorcardiogram of the nonaberrant complexes. The superior orientation of the first 27.5 msec vector in the F and RS planes indicates loss of inferior forces. Infarction of the anteroseptal wall is evidenced by the posterior displacement of the 10 msec vector in the H plane. Figure 21B shows the VCG loops of the aberrant ventricular complexes. The changes due to myocardial infarction were again seen. The orientation of the 10 msec vector was unchanged ($-30°$ in the F plane and $-55°$ in the H plane). However, the remaining QRS loop was modified and showed a marked rightward, superior and posterior orientation

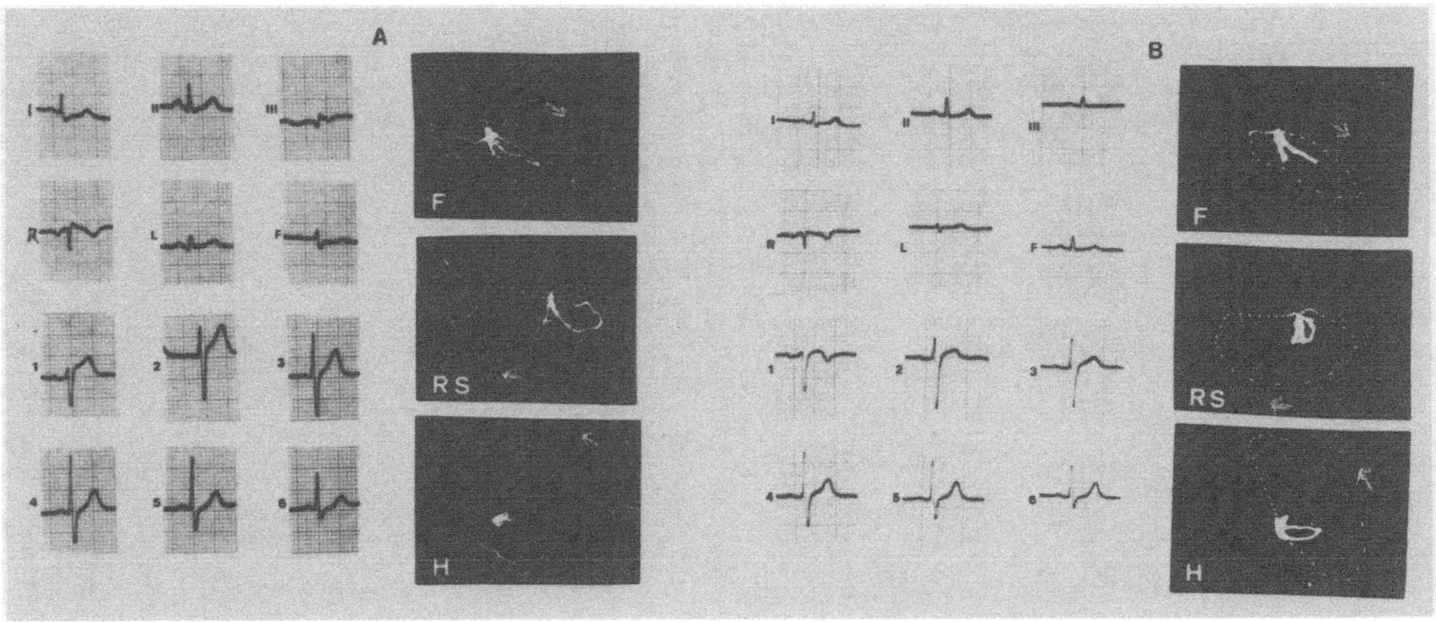

Figure 18. A patient, whose clinical and enzymatic data were typical of acute myocardial infarction. A: In ECG and VCG recordings an inferior can only be suspected. Slurred S wave in I, II, aVL and V_6; terminal slurred r wave in a VR. VCG: Terminal delay, lasting 40 msec, oriented to the right, superiorly and posteriorly. B: ECG and VCG recorded after 12 days. The terminal slurring remains. In this case the only expression of myocardial infarction is the peri-infarction block

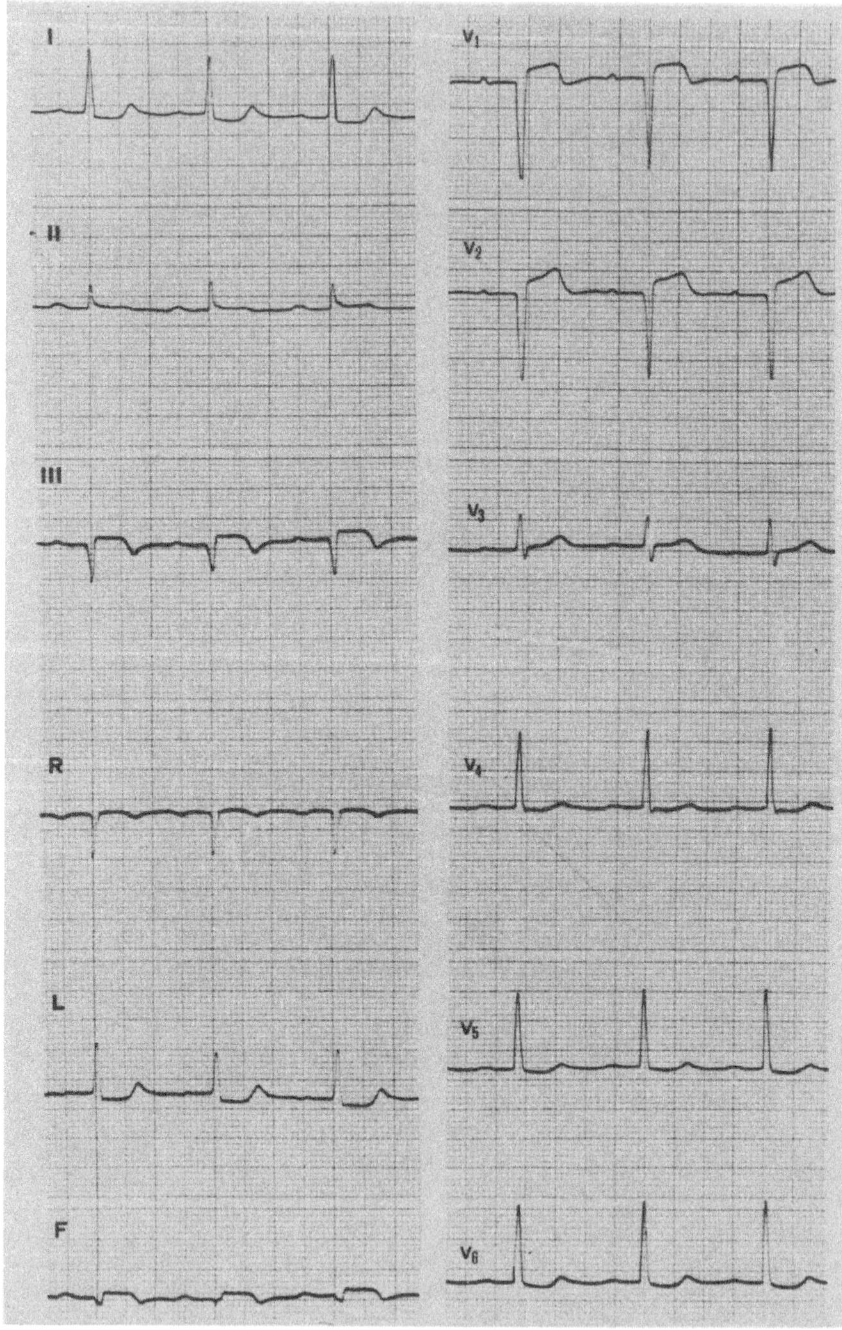

Figure 19. ECG at admission. A pattern of acute inferior and anteroseptal myocardial infarction is evident. The PR interval measures 250 msec. (From Alboni et al., with permission of Europ J Cardiol [54])

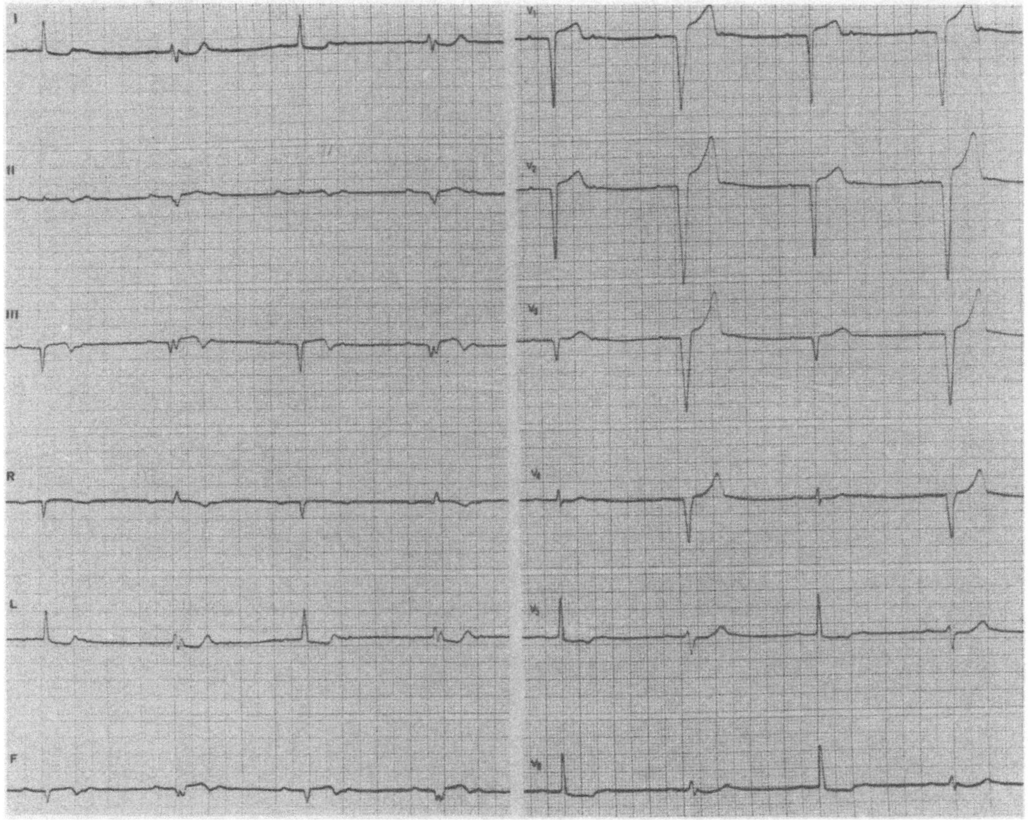

Figure 20. ECG on the day after admission. Sinus rate of 78/min with 2:1 atrioventricular block. The PR intervals of the conducted beats measure 280 msec. The alternate QRS complexes show a different morphology (see text for explanation). (From Alboni et al., with permission of Europ J Cardiol [54])

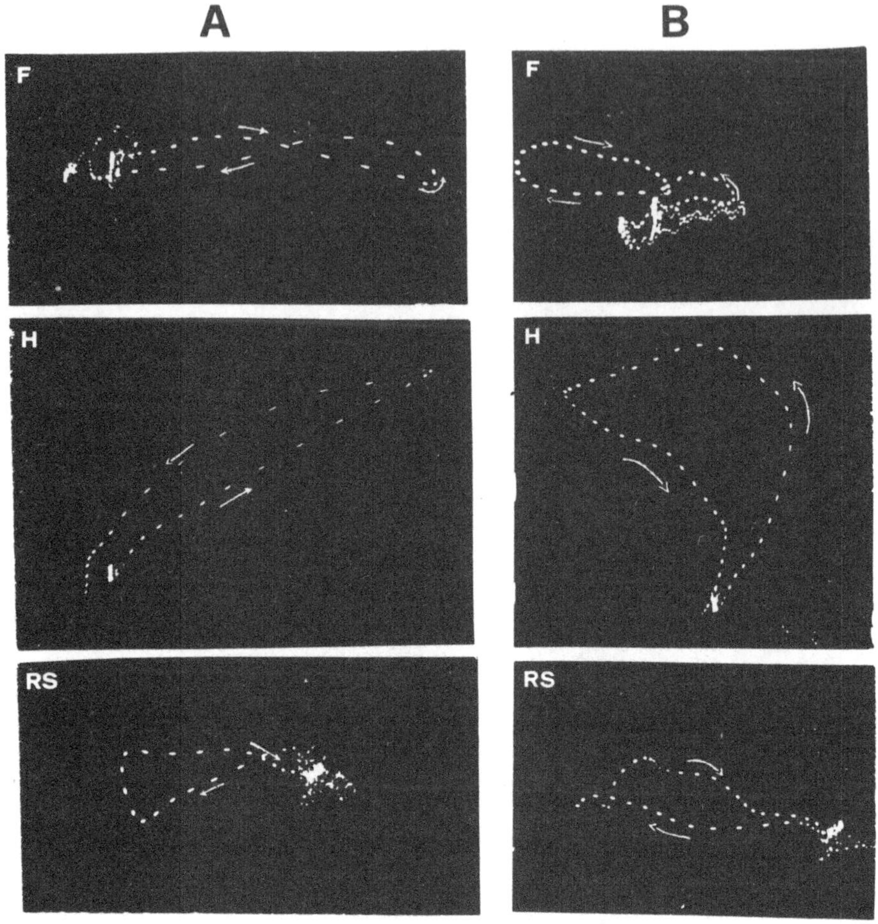

Figure 21. Vectorcardiographic recording. A: VCG of the ventricular complexes without aberrancy. B: VCG of the aberrant ventricular complexes (see text for explanation). (From Alboni et al., with permission of Europ J Cardiol [54])

of the middle and terminal vectors. The direction of the maximum vector shifted from $+5°$ to $-125°$ in the F plane and from $-35°$ to $-125°$ in the H plane. A terminal delay, lasting 40 msec, was evident.

In Figure 22 the His bundle electrocardiogram is reported. The AH and HV intervals of both aberrant and nonaberrant complexes were 155 and 45 msec, respectively. The site of the block during 2:1 AV conduction was localized above the His bundle.

Two days after admission, the ECG showed sinus rhythm with 1:1 AV conduction with a PR interval of 240 msec; aberrant ventricular complexes were absent. A Wenckebach-type 2nd degree AV block appeared for a short period of time, during which aberrant ventricular complexes, as seen in Figures 20 and 22, were

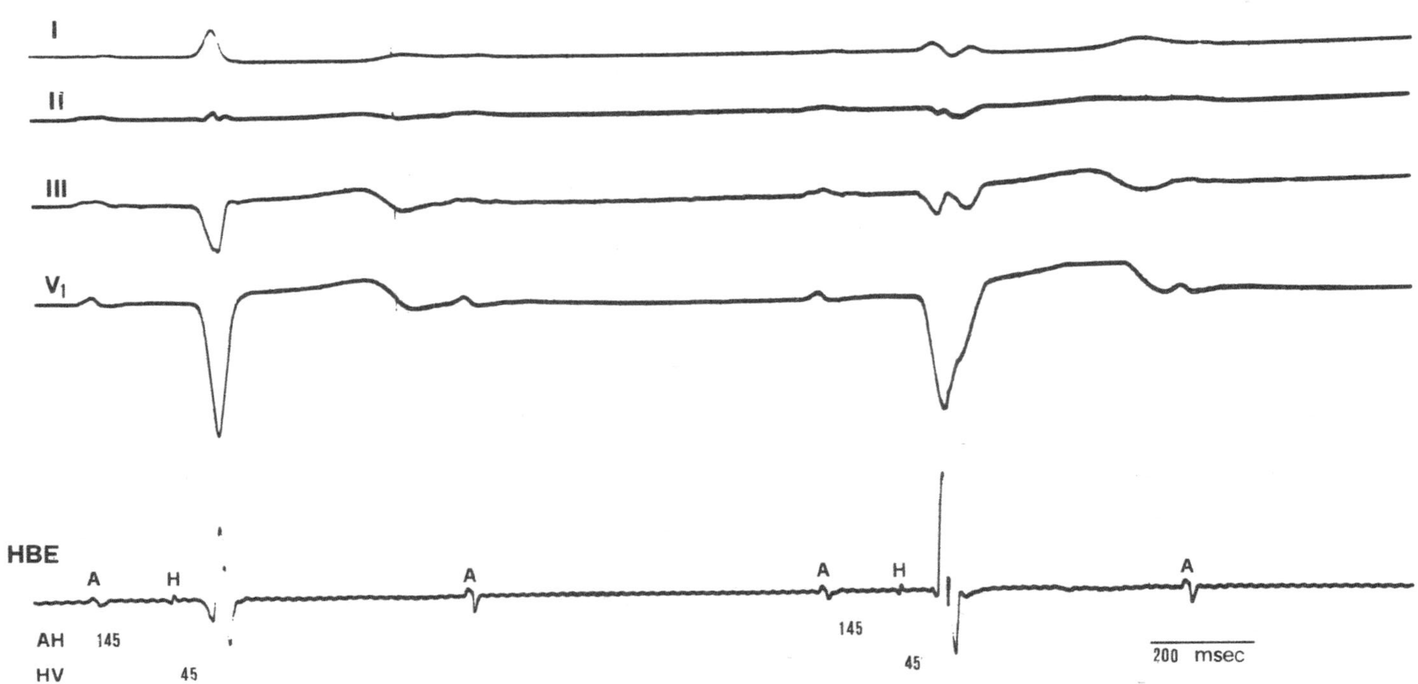

Figure 22. Intracardiac recording. QRS complexes with and without aberrancy are present. The blocked P waves are not followed by His deflection. The AH and HV intervals measure 155 and 45 msec, respectively. (From Alboni et al., with permission of Europ J Cardiol [54])

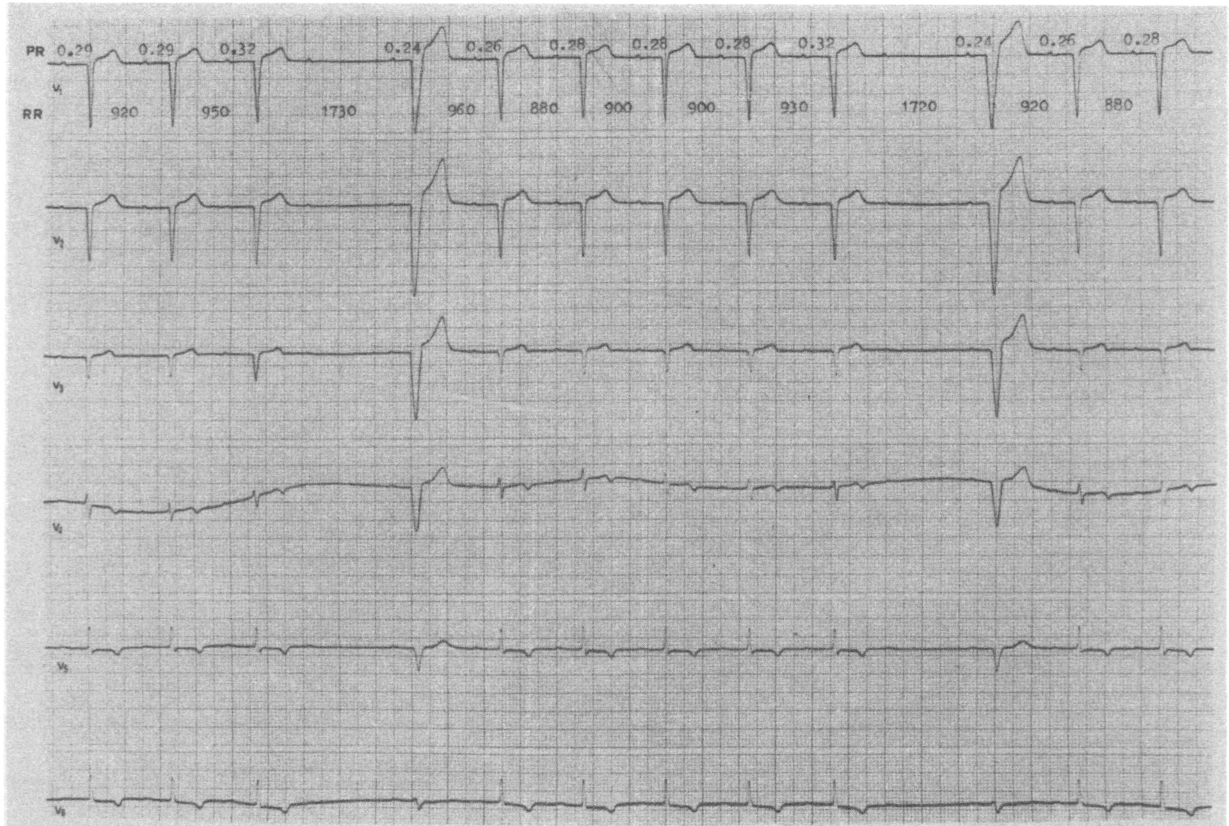

Figure 23. ECG two days after admission. Wenckebach AV block. After prolonged diastolic pauses the QRS complexes show an aberrancy like that of Figure 21. PR interval of such ventricular complexes measures 240 msec. (From Alboni et al., with permission of Europ J Cardiol [54])

seen at the end of the long diastolic pauses (over 1720 msec) caused by the blocked P wave (Figure 23). Subsequent ECGs did not show aberrancy of QRS complexes or 2nd degree AV block.

This case presents the following features: 1) acute inferior and anteroseptal infarction; 3) 2:1 AV block followed by Wenckebach-type 2nd degree AV block; 3) aberrant QRS complexes which were initially present alternately and later seen only after prolonged diastolic pauses.

We think that the aberrant ventricular complexes are conducted beats, and not escape beats, for the following reasons: a) HV intervals of both aberrant and nonaberrant ventricular complexes have the same duration, i.e. 45 msec; b) The wide QRS complexes, i.e. the aberrant ventricular complexes during 2:1 AV block, always appeared at a constant PR interval despite a significant change in the PR interval or sinus-cycle length during a 24-hr observation period; c) PR interval of the aberrant ventricular complexes during Wenckebach periodicity had a constant duration, i.e. 240 msec.

The aberrancy is therefore related to an intraventricular block. Analysis of ECG and VCG recordings showed that aberrancy is not related to: 1) Right bundle branch block, since there is no anterior displacement of the middle and terminal electrical forces, which in the ECG should produce a decrease in the depth of the S wave along with an R′/r′ wave in right precordial leads. On the contrary, in our case the S wave in these leads because deeper; 2) Left bundle branch block since the first vectors do not shift, the rotation in the H plane remains counterclockwise, a middle slurring does not appear, and middle and terminal electrical forces are directed markedly to the right, as is seen in the VCG and also in the ECG by the amplitude of the terminal R wave in aVR. It is, however, worth noting that in rare cases of LBBB the middle slurring may not be conspicuous, that the rotation in the H plane may remain unchanged and that the direction of the initial vectors may not change in the presence of septal infarction. Nevertheless, due to the absence of all the above-mentioned features, as well as the marked rightwards shifting of the middle-terminal forces (Figure 21), an LBBB is extremely unlikely; 3) Anterior fascicular block since R wave in I and aVL decreases in amplitude and there is no prolongation of the intrinsecoid deflection time in aVL (see Chapter 4); 4) Posterior fascicular block since the middle electrical forces are directed superiorly and to the right.

The aberrancy is therefore due to a peripheral intraventricular block, defined as peri-infarction block, because of its underlying etiology, which appears first as a 2:1 block and later as a phase 4 block.

As a result of the marked rightward orientation of the middle-terminal forces, in this case peri-infarction block could be localized in the postero-basal wall of the right ventricle. In fact, autopsy studies [56] showed frequent involvement of this wall, in association with inferior myocardial infarction.

Table 2. Clinical diagnosis of patients with left ventricular peripheral block

Clinical diagnosis	Cases
Coronary heart disease	24
Hypertensive heart disease	14
Aortic coarctation	2
Rheumatic mitral stenosis and regurgitation	2
Rheumatic aortic stenosis	2
Viral cardiomyopathy	2
Cardiomyopathy (Erb muscular dystrophy)	1
Rheumatic aortic regurgitation	1
Rheumatic aortic reguargitation and mitral stenosis	1
Primary non-obstructive cardiomyopathy	1
Cardiomyopathy in hypothyroidism	1
Normal heart	4
TOTAL	55

CLINICAL SIGNIFICANCE

Very little investigative work has been dedicated to the clinical significance of the peripheral blocks.

We studied 55 patients with left ventricular peripheral block diagnosed with ECG and VCG recordings. The clinical data are reported in Table 2. Most of these patients suffered from hypertensive and coronary heart disease and rheumatic valvular cardiopathy; only four patients (7.2 %) did not show underlying heart disease. This study was not performed on the general population and it is therefore possible that the actual incidence of heart disease in subjects with left ventricular block is lower; however our study suggests that in most cases this block coexists with heart disease.

To the best of our knowledge, there do not exist at present any studies on the clinical significance of the right peripheral block localized in the postero-basal wall.

In our experience it is frequent in young subjects without underlying heart disease. However, in some cases, it can represent the only ECG manifestation of right ventricular hypertrophy. Therefore we believe that patients with such an electric pattern must undergo clinical and radiological examinations.

The clinical meaning of peri-infarction block has been studied mostly by Shadaksharappa et al. [49]. Such a block has been encountered in 39 % of myocardial infarctions. Cabrera et al. [52] observed about the same incidence (33 %), whereas Laham [50] encountered a lower one (10 %). This discrepancy is not easy to explain.

The incidence is higher following recurrent myocardial infarction [49].

Mortality due to cardiovascular causes was clearly higher during the first year in patients with acute myocardial infarction and peri-infarction block (53.9 %) than in those without such a block (22.6 %). After the first year there was no difference in the mortality rate between the two groups [49]. Patients who manifested peri-infarction block had a mean serum glutamic-oxaloacetic transaminase (SGOT) higher than those without such a block (49). These data suggest that a peri-infarction block may be related to a larger area of myocardial necrosis.

COMMENT

The criteria we proposed for the diagnosis and localization of peripheral block were deduced by means of experimental and clinical data and theoretical considerations. We did not consider these criteria as definitive; further experimental studies and anatomo-electrocardiographic correlations are needed. However, it is extremely difficult and perhaps impossible, at present, to carry out a histological study of the entire Purkinje network.

It seems strange to us that so much time has been spent on the study of the main pathways of the intraventricular conduction system, while the so-called 'minor troubles' of intraventricular conduction have been practically ignored. Analysis of our clinical data suggests that peripheral blocks, if localized in the left ventricle, in most cases are associated with various types of underlying heart disease and sometimes they represent the only ECG alteration.

The peripheral blocks localized in the left part of the septum are of particular interest. It is likely that when the anatomo-functional lesion is slight, it is evidenced by an initial slurring of the QRS complex and when the lesion is more extended, it is evidenced by a loss of electrical forces, similar to or even indistinguishable from a healed myocardial infarction. In fact such a block superimposes, both from a morphological and pathophysiological point of view, the chronic myocardial infarction [59], of which it may represent an early expression.

REFERENCES

1. Oppenheimer BS, Rothschild MA: Abnormalities in the QRS group of the electrocardiogram associated with myocardial involvement. Proc Exp Biol Med 14: 57, 1916
2. Frau G: La pathogénie des troubles de la conduction ventriculaire. Contribution expérimentale. Cardiologia 19: 2, 1951
3. Alzamora Castro v, Abugattas R, Rubio C, Bouroncle J, Zapata C, Santa Maria E, Battilana C, Binder T, Subiria R, Paredes D: Parietal focal block: an experimental and electrocardiographic study. Circulation 7: 108, 1953
4. Dick HLH, McCawley EL, Voiss DV, Krueger JD: Electrocardiographic evaluation studies on quinidine induced changes of myocardial conduction. Am Heart J 56: 396, 1958
5. Noseda V, Santi A, Aguggini G, Filotto U, Bergamaschi M: Experimental focal block in the sheep and the dog. An electrocardiographic and histological study. Cardiologia

42: 243, 1963
6. Abitdskov JA, Boyle RS: Further studies of the electrocardiographic effects of experimental myocardial lesions. Am Heart J 69: 49, 1965
7. Ribeiro CS: Estudo da activação ventricular nos bloqueios intraventriculares esquerdos. (Contribução experimental para o seu diagnostico clinico). Arquivo de Patologia 41: 151, 1969
8. Weimberg HB, Katz LN: Two unusual types of electrocardiogram. Am Heart J 19: 519, 1940
9. Segers M: The different types of intraventricular block. Am Heart J 37: 92, 1949
10. Boyadjian N, Van Dooren FR: Etude de deux cas de bloc de branche bilatéral. Contribution à la localisation des blocs intraventriculaires. Acta Cardiol 5: 532, 1950
11. Piccolo E, Furlanello F, Crepaldi V: Studio elettrocardiografico dell'ipertrofia ventricolare sinistra nell'ipertensione arteriosa, con particolare riguardo alle alterazioni terminali del QRS. Cardiol Prat 16: 381, 1965
12. Testoni F, Narbone NB, Tommaselli A: Aspetti vectocardiografici nei blocchi focali sinistri con elettrocardiogramma tipo RI; SII; SIII. Mal Cardiovasc 3: 379, 1968
13. Fischer DM, Finzi C, Alboni P, Masoni A: La diagnosi vectocardiografica dei blocchi parietali ventricolar. G Ital Cardiol 3: 343, 1973
14. Alboni P: Diagnostic problems pertaining to the left parietal block. In: Electrocardiology I, Gandhi MJ, Metha AB, Pahlajani DB. Proceedings of World Congress on Electrocardiology. Bombay: Tata, 1975, p 118
15. Alboni P, Malacarne C, Masoni A: Diagnosis of left ventricular parietal block. 7th European Congress of Cardiology, Book II (Abstr.). Amsterdam, 1976, p 352
16. Alboni P, Malacarne C, Masoni A: Left ventricular parietal block: diagnostic and clinical study. J Electrocardiol 9: 139, 1976
17. Masoni A, Alboni P: Ipotesi fisiopatogenetiche nel blocco periferico. G Ital Cardiol 6: 812, 1976
18. Alboni P, Malacarne C, Masoni A: Physiopathological and diagnostic hypotheses in peripheral block. J Electrocardiol 10: 87, 1977
19. Alboni P: Il blocco periferico settale sinistro. Ipotesi fisiopatologica o nuovo elemento diagnostico? G Ital Cardiol 10: 365, 1980
20. Burch GE: An electrocardiographic syndrome characterized by absence of Q in leads I, V5 and V6. Am Heart J 51: 487, 1956
21. Horan L, Flowers N, Johnson J: Significance of the diagnostic Q wave of myocardial infarction. Circulation 43: 428, 1971
22. Gunnar RM, Pietras RJ, Blackaller J, Dadmun SE, Szanto PB, Tobin JR Jr: Correlation of vectorcardiographic criteria for myocardial infarction with autopsy findings. Circulation 35: 158, 1967
23. Gambetta M, Childers RW: Rate-dependent right precordial Q wave: septal focal block. Am J Cardiol 32: 196, 1973
24. Conde CA, Meller J, Espinoza J, Donoso E, Dack S: Disappearance of abnormal Q waves after aortocoronary bypass surgery. Am J Cardiol 36: 889, 1975
25. Zeft HJ, Freidberg HD, King JF, Manley JC, Huston JH, Johnson WD: Reappearance of anterior QRS forces after coronary bypass surgery. An electrovectocardiographic study. Am J Cardiol 36: 163, 1975
26 Alboni P, Malacarne C, De Lorenzi E, Pirani R, Baldassarri F, Masoni A: Right precordial q waves due to anterior fascicular block. Clinical and vectorcardiographic study. J Electrocardiol 12: 41, 1979
27. Pryor R, Blount SG: The clinical significance of true left axis deviation. Left intraventricular blocks. Am Heart J 72: 391, 1966

28. Rosenbaum MB, Elizari MV, Lazzari JG, Nari GJ, Levi RJ, Halpern MS: Intraventricular trifascicular blocks. I. Four cases of right bundle branch block with intermittent left anterior and posterior hemiblock. Am Heart J 78: 306, 1969
29. Rosenbaum MB: Types of right bundle branch block and their clinical significance. J Electrocardiol 1: 121, 1968
30. Lenegre J: Contribution à l'étude des blocs de branche comportant notamment les confrontations électriques et histologiques. Paris: JB Baillière et fils, 1958
31. Uhley HN, Rivkin L: Electrocardiographic patterns following interruption of main and peripheral branches of the canine right bundle of His. Am J Cardiol 7: 810, 1961
32. Moore N, Hoffman BF, Patterson DF, Stuckey JH: Electrocardiographic changes due to delayed activation of the wall of the right ventricle. Am Heart J 68: 347, 1964
33. Marquez-Montez J, Juffe A, Artaza-Andrade M, Castillo-Olivares JL: Bloqueo de rama izquierda troncular asociado a bloqueo periferico de rama derecha. Estudio experimental en perros. Rev Esp Cardiol 28: 399, 1975
34. Medrano GA, De Micheli A: Contribucion experimental al diagnostico de los bloqueos fasciculares derechos. Arch Inst Cardiol Mex 45: 704, 1975
35. Obiassi M, Neri G: Vettocardiografia clinica. Rome: Pensiero Scientifico Editore, 1969
36. Nava A, Rusconi L, Silvani S, Schivazappa L, Buja GF: I blocchi di branca destra con ansa dorsalizzata. G Ital Cardiol 6: 265, 1976
37. Grant RP: The relationship between the anatomic position of the heart and the electrocardiogram. A criticism of unipolar electrocardiography. Circulation 7: 890, 1953
38. Boineau JP, Spach MS, Ayers CS: Genesis of the electrocardiogram in atrial septal defect. Am Heart J 68: 637, 1964
39. Castellanos A Jr, Agna AS, Befeler B, Castillo CA, Berkovits BV: A study of arrival of excitation at selected ventricular sites during human bundle branch block using close bipolar catheter electrodes. Chest 63: 208, 1973
40. Kastor JA, Goldreyer BN, Moore EN, Shelburne JC, Manchester JH: Intraventricular conduction in man studied with an endocardial electrode catheter mapping technique. Patients with normal QRS and right bundle branch block. Circulation 51: 786, 1975
41. First SR, Bayley RH, Bedford DR: Peri-infarction block; electrocardiographic abnormality occasionally resembling bundle branch block and local ventricular block of other types. Circulation 2: 31, 1950
42. Mayer JW, Castellanos A Jr, Lemberg L: The apical vector-cardiogram in peri-infarction block. Am J Cardiol 11: 613, 1963
43. Durrer D, Van Lier AAW, Büller J: Epicardial and intramural excitation in chronic myocardial infarction. Am Heart J 68: 765, 1964
44. Libanoff AJ: Marked left axis deviation. Parietal and peri-infarction block. Am J Cardiol 14: 339, 1964
45. Castle CH, Keane WM: Electrocardiographic 'peri-infarction block'. A clinical and pathologic correlation. Circulation 31: 403, 1965
46. Corne RA, Parkin TW, Brandenburg RO, Brown AL Jr: Peri-infarction block: postmyocardial infarction intraventricular conduction disturbance. Am Heart J 69: 150, 1965
47. Piccolo E, Miori R, Furlanello F: Il blocco peri-infartuale nei suoi aspetti diagnostici. Folia Cardiol 24: 141, 1965
48. Castellanos A Jr, Lemberg L, Salhanick L: Le vectocardiogramme dans le bloc postinfarctus. Arch Mal Coeur 60: 712, 1967
49. Shadaksharappa KS, Kalbfleisch JM, Conrad LL, Sarkar NK: Recognition and significance of intraventricular block due to myocardial infarction (peri-infarction block). Circulation 37: 20, 1968

50. Laham J: Blocs peri-infarctus et blocs segmentaires. Arch Mal Coeur 66: 1267, 1973
51. Fischer DM, Scudelotti O, Finzi CM: I blocchi infartuali periferici. Analisi vettocardiografica ed ipotesi patogenetiche. G Ital Cardiol 6: 669, 1976
52. Cabrera E, Rocha JC, Flores G: El vectordiagrama de los infartos miocardios contrastornos de conduccion. Arch Inst Cardiol Mex 29: 625, 1959
53. Grant RP, Murray RH: The QRS complex deformity of myocardial infarction in the human subject. Am J Med 17: 587, 1954
54. Alboni P, Malacarne C, Pradella A, Masoni A: 2:1 and phase 4 peri-infarction block. Europ J Cardiol 10: 3, 1979
55. Armenta J: Bradycardia-dependent peri-infarction block. Br Heart J 39: 1386, 1977
56. Cohn JN, Guiha NH, Broper ME, Limas CJ: Right ventricular infarction. Am Heart J 33: 209, 1974
57. Piccolo E: Il vettocardiogramma del cuore polmonare cronico. Correlazione con l'elettrocardiogramma e rivalutazione dei problemi elettrofisiologici. Folia Cardiol 28: 121, 1969
58. Polu JM, Gilgenkrantz JM, Faivre G: Le diagnostic vectorcardiographique des hémiblocs de branche gauche isolés et associés à un bloc de branche droit ou à infarctus du myocarde. Arch Mal Coeur 65: 1041, 1972
59. Masoni A: Infarto cronico: questione terminologica o problema clinico? G Ital Cardiol 6: 185, 1976

7. INTRAVENTRICULAR CONDUCTION DISTURBANCES IN CONGENITAL HEART DISEASE AND FOLLOWING CARDIAC SURGERY

INTRAVENTRICULAR CONDUCTION DEFECTS IN CONGENITAL HEART DISEASES

In congenital heart diseases intraventricular conduction disturbances (IVCD) are not very frequent, but sometimes they are highly characteristic and their presence can suggest the clinical diagnosis.

Secundum atrial septal defect

In such congenital heart disease, as in others with volume overload of the right ventricle, there is often an 'incomplete right bundle branch block (RBBB) pattern' which Keith et al. [1] found in 58% of cases. The standard electrocardiogram shows an RSR′ pattern in the right precordial leads, with some widening of the S wave in I, aVL, and the left precordial leads. In most studies a correlation between the amplitude of the R′ wave in lead V_1 and the degree of left-to-right shunting has not been found [2-6] although a prominent R′ in V_1 has been described as being more commonly present in patients with large shunts [7-8].

In the frontal (F) plane of the vectorcardiogram (VCG), the QRS loop is generally narrow with clockwise rotation or figure-of-eight morphology. In the majority of cases, terminal delay is directed, rightward and superiorly (Figure 1). In a few cases the rotation is counterclockwise with the main forces oriented superiorly [9, 10] (Figure 2). The latter pattern is characteristically present in the endocardial cushion defects. In the horizontal (H) plane the majority show counterclockwise rotation. A clockwise figure of eight loop can be observed in patients with right ventricular pressure greater than 45 mmHg [10]. Terminal delay is directed posteriorly or slightly anteriorly. When marked right ventricular hypertrophy is present (RVH), such a delay is mostly directed forwards (Figure 3).

Experimental studies of ventricular depolarization in secundum atrial septal defect have shown a normal speed of conduction through the right bundle branch [7, 11]. Therefore the terminal delay of the QRS complex appears to be in relation to delayed activation of the high right ventricular free wall and crista supraventricularis. Ellison et al. [10] emphasize that such conduction delay is related to ventricular dilatation and hypertrophy. RSR′ morphology in lead V_1 in this con-

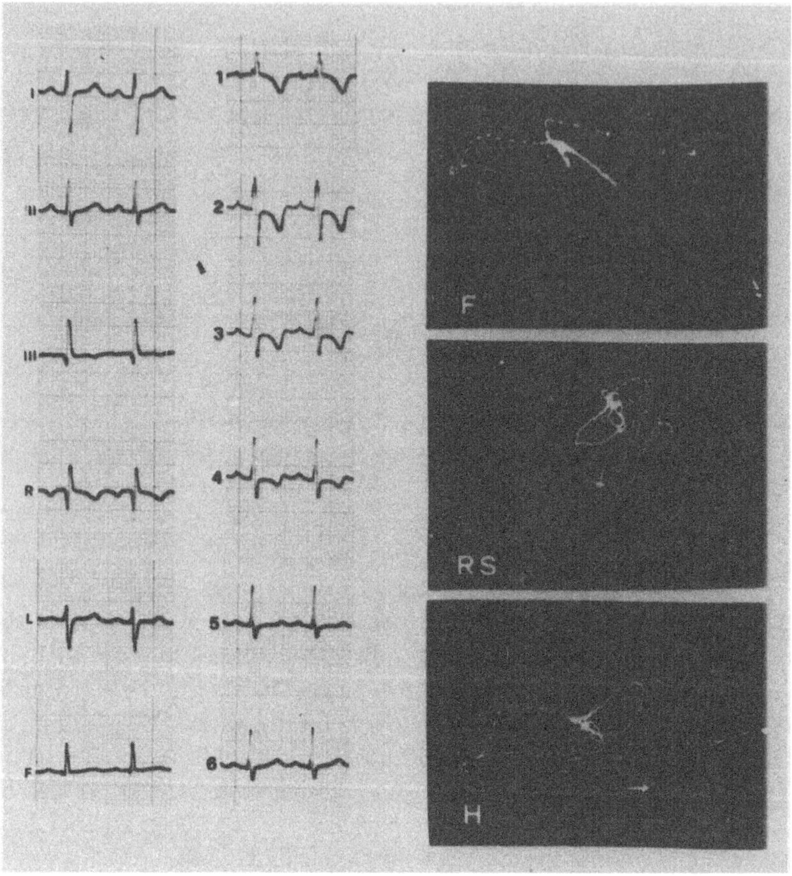

Figure 1. A 7-year-old patient with secundum atrial septal defect. QRS complex measures 85 msec. ECG and VCG tracings show an incomplete right bundle branch block pattern with vertical axis. The rotation of QRS complex is clockwise in the frontal plane and counterclockwise in the horizontal plane. A terminal delay is present, lasting 30 msec, oriented to the right, superiorly, partly anteriorly and partly posteriorly

genital heart disease therefore expresses a *right ventricular peripheral block* and not a true RBBB.

Endocardial cushion defects

Intraventricular conduction disturbances in this disorder are highly characteristic and useful in the differential diagnosis. An incomplete RBBB pattern associated with left axis deviation (LAD) is virtually constant. The exceptions to this feature are few. Liebman et al. [6] found it in 94% of cases and Pryor et al. [5] in 91%. Burchell et al. [12] found rare exceptions in the complete atrio-ventricular (AV)

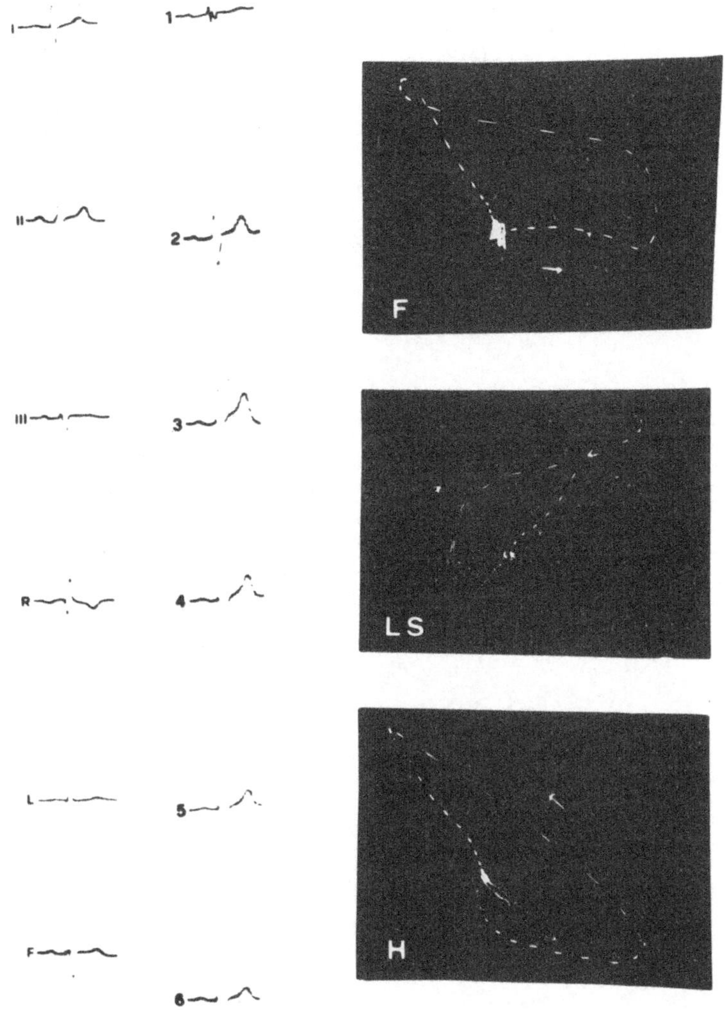

Figure 2. A 10-year-old patient with secundum atrial septal defect. QRS complex measures 80 msec. ECG shows an incomplete right bundle branch block with left axis deviation. The frontal and horizontal QRS loops rotate counterclockwise. A terminal delay is present, lasting 30 msec, oriented to the right, superiorly and posteriorly

canal. Other authors [8, 13, 14] found it in all cases.

In almost all patients the QRS duration is prolonged [10]. As in patients with secundum atrial defect, this QRS prolongation does not have the characteristics of complete RBBB, but suggests delayed conduction through a dilated right ventricle [10].

In the F plane the rotation of the QRS loop is counterclockwise (Figures 4 and 5). The first vectors are directed downward, rightward or leftward; the mid-ter-

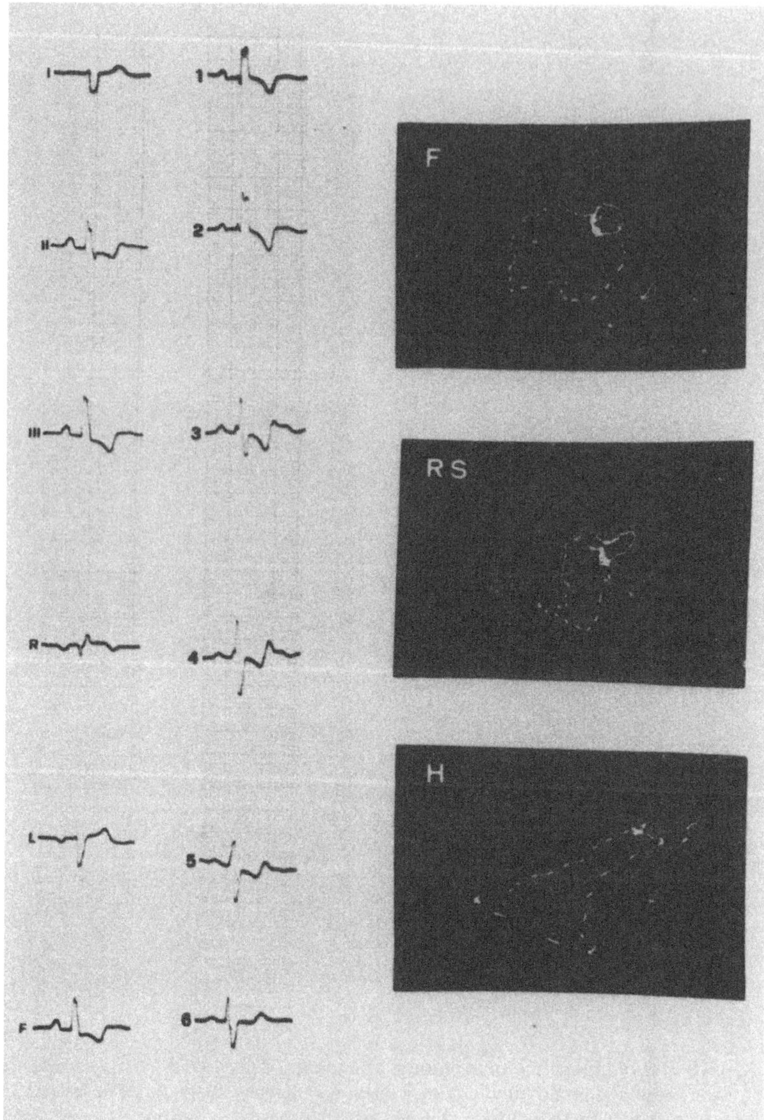

Figure 3. A 7-year-old patient with secundum atrial septal defect and very large left-to-right shunt. QRS complex measures 90 msec. Right bundle branch block pattern with vertical axis is present. The horizontal QRS loop rotates initially counterclockwise, then clockwise. The terminal delay lasting 35 msec, is directed anteriorly

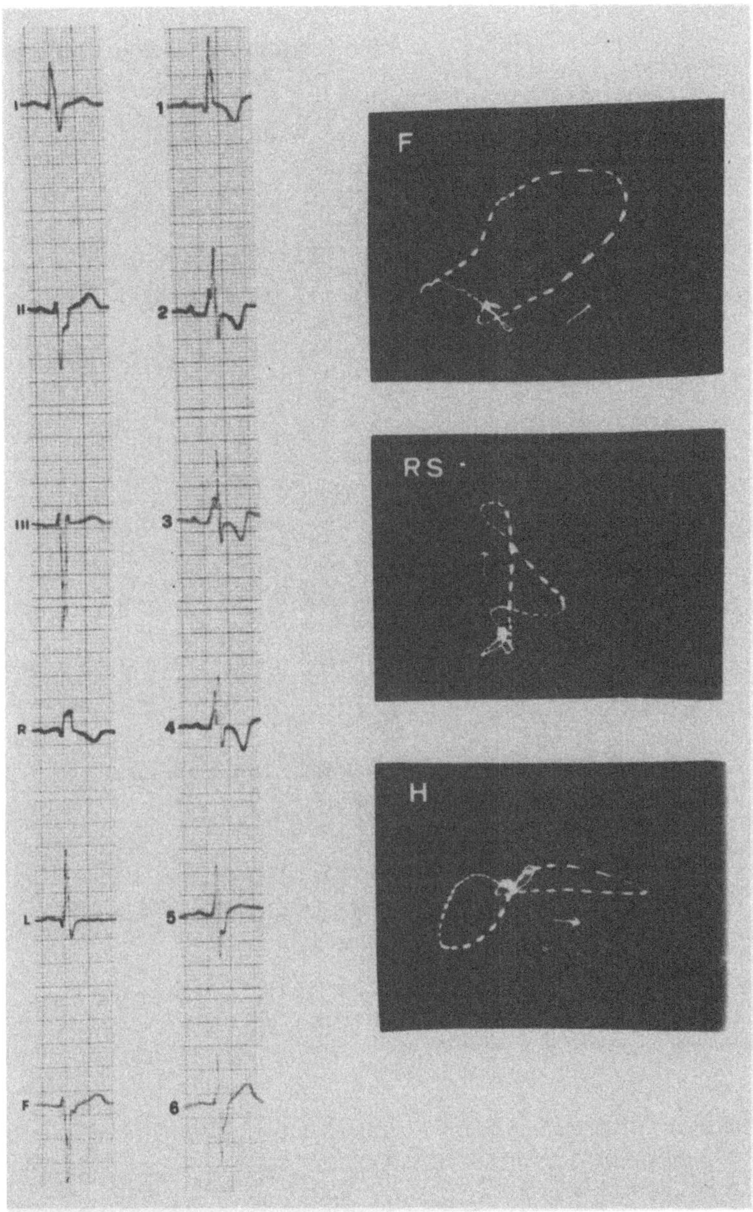

Figure 4. A 12-year-old patient with primum atrial septal defect. PR and QRS intervals measure 200 and 120 msec, respectively. ECG and VCG recordings show right bundle branch block and anterior fascicular block. The frontal QRS loop is inscribed counterclockwise and the horizontal loop shows a figure of eight. The delayed terminal appendage, oriented to the right and anteriorly, typical of right bundle branch block, is present in the horizontal plane

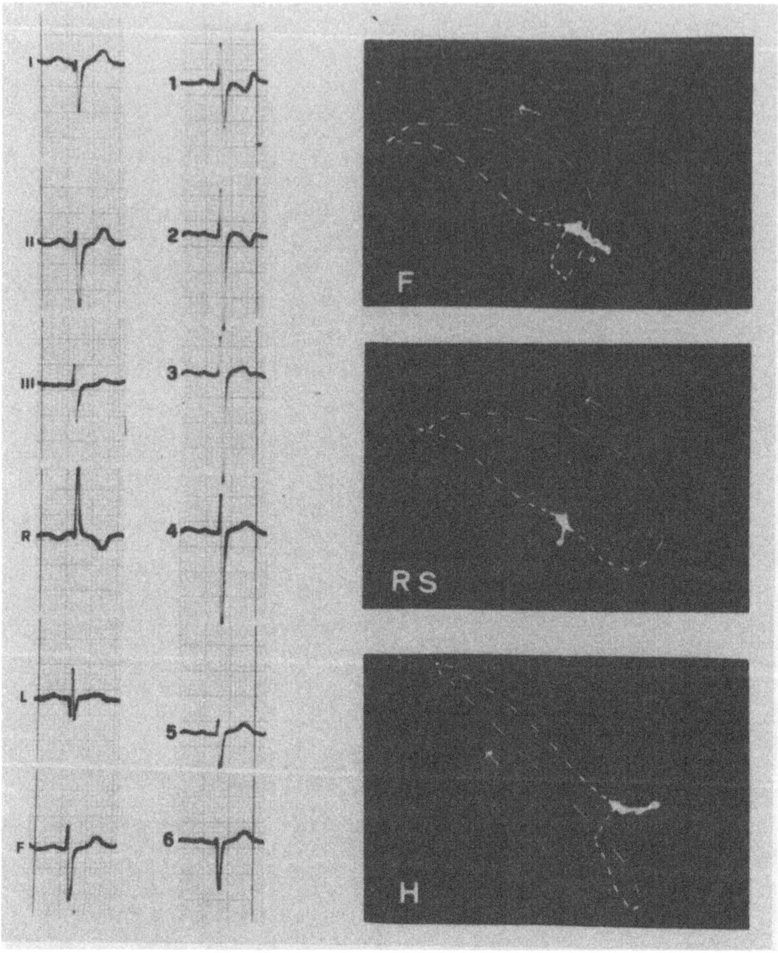

Figure 5. **A 3-year-old patient with complete atrioventricular canal. Marked right ventricular hypertrophy** is evident in ECG and VCG recordings. The frontal QRS loop is inscribed counterclockwise; such a rotation can be suspected in ECG tracing because of the presence of qRS morphology in lead aVL

minal forces are displaced mainly superiorly and rightward. The loop becomes superior at a mean of 36% of the QRS duration [10]. The terminal part of the loop is delayed. In the H plane the rotation of QRS loop reflects the right ventricular systolic pressure. In patients with low pressure the inscription is generally counterclockwise. However, with increasing right ventricular pressure, more and more patients develop figure-of-eight or clockwise loops.

The mechanisms of left axis deviation in endocardial cushion defects appear to be related to congenital alterations of conduction pathways into the ventricles. Anatomic studies of the AV conduction system in man and in dog have clarified this QRS pattern. Lev [15] demonstrated that the AV node is displaced posteriorly. The His bundle lies behind the lower margin of the defect and the left bundle branch has a very short posterior radiation. Feldt et al. [16] observed that the left bundle branch is abnormally displaced posteriorly and has a relatively early origin from the common bundle. Also, the anterior radiations of the left bundle branch were fewer in number than in normal hearts and had an increased length. These anatomic features have been confirmed by physiological studies using the technique of epicardial mapping. Durrer et al. [17] showed that the postero-basal portion of the left ventricle was activated earlier than in normal individuals. Similar findings were demonstrated by Boineau et al. [18] with epicardial mapping techniques in four patients and one dog with ostium primum atrial septal defect. These authors documented in the dog marked asynchrony in activation of the left ventricular endocardium with early posterior and delayed anterior depolarization. Thus, they concluded that the LAD resulted from asynchronous left ventricular activation secondary to a developmental asymmetry of the intraventricular conduction system. Normal or short HV intervals registered in patients with endocardial cushion defects are in accord with data showing early ventricular activation of the posterobasal wall.

Borkon et al. [19] observed that the degree of the right ventricular hypertrophy and/or biventricular hypertrophy influences the LAD. In fact the ÂQRS markedly diminished with the improvement of hemodynamic abnormalities of right ventricle or both ventricles after surgical correction.

Tricuspid atresia

A typical feature of this congenital heart disease is anterior fascicular block (AFB) pattern associated with left ventricular hypertrophy (LVH). Such a pattern was found in 84% of the cases by Donzelot et al. [20], in 86% by Brink et al. [21] and in 93% by Keith et al. [1].

In general, the presence of an inferior axis in tricuspid atresia denotes the presence of transposition of the great arteries or associated pulmonary atresia [22-24].

In the H plane of the VCG the QRS loop is oriented to the left and more posteriorly than normal. Rotation is usually counterclockwise, but occasionally it is figure-of-eight or even clockwise. Frequently there is a marked decrease of the anterior forces and sometimes the horizontal QRS loop has the appearance of an anterolateral myocardial infarction or left bundle branch block (LBBB) [22-24].

In the F plane the loop is usually counterclockwise and superior. However, on average the axis is not quite as superiorly shifted as is usually seen in patients with endocardial cushion defects [10]. Sometimes the first vectors are directed superiorly, an inferior myocardial infarction pattern being present in both the ECG and VCG recordings (Figure 6).

The genesis of LAD in tricuspid atresia is not completely clear.

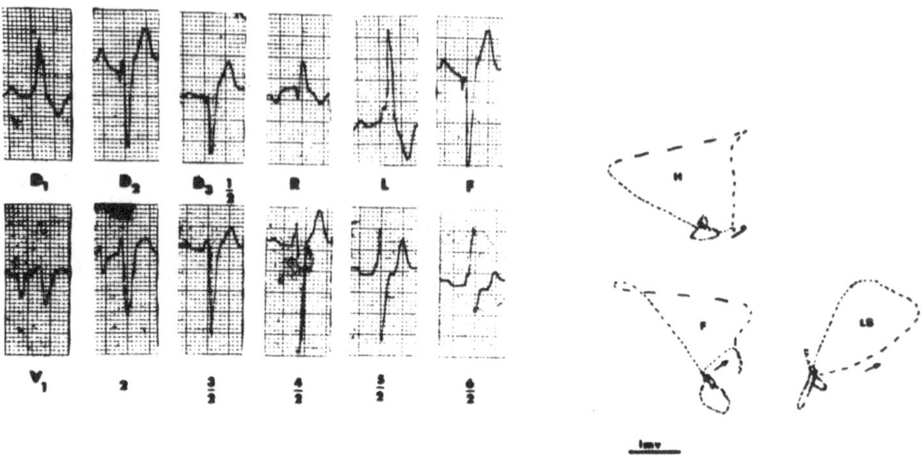

Figure 6. A 2-year-old patient with tricuspid atresia. ECG recording shows left atrial enlargement and a PR interval of 240 msec. The QRS complex evidences left axis deviation, left ventricular hypertrophy and an inferior myocardial infarction pattern. In the VCG, a reduction of inferior (frontal plane) and anteroseptal (horizontal plane) forces is evident. QRS loop rotates counterclockwise in F and H planes. In the three planes an initial slurring and a terminal one are evident

Several mechanisms have been suggested to explain the ECG pattern in these patients: lack of development of the right ventricle [25], increased left ventricular mass [26], fibrosis of the left bundle branch system [23], lesions of the antero-superior fibers of the left bundle branch [22] and unusual distribution of the conduction system resulting in asynchronous left ventricular activation [27]. The last hypothesis is strengthened by anatomic and electrophysiological data. In the study of the conduction system by Guller et al. [27] the AV node and His bundle were normally located, but the course of the bundle branches differed from normal in that the left bundle branch originated unusually close to the node/bundle junction (early arborization) and the right bundle branch was markedly elongated in its course to the right septal endocardium. In some cases studied by Bharati et al. [28], the posterior fibers of the left bundle branch gave off early and continuously, and the branch was shorter than normal. Moreover, in none of the cases studied by Guller et al. [27] and by Bharati et al. [28] was there any evidence of proximal disease in the bundle branches. Anomalous course of the bundle and early origin of the posterior fascicle can give rise to early activation of the posteroinferior part of the left ventricle, producing a pattern of LAD in the scalar electrocardiogram and counterclockwise superior QRS forces in the F plane. Serratto et al [29] performed electrophysiological studies in five patients with tricuspid atresia. The HV interval was short in three cases and normal in two. The pattern of LAD in the group with a short HV interval was thought to be due to early origin of the posterior branches of the left bundle branch from the His bundle and early activation of the posteroinferior parts of the left ventricle. In the two cases with normal HV interval, an early activation of the postero inferior part of the left ventricle was ruled out. In these cases the pattern of LAD may be due to the anomalous course of the common bundle and the bundle branches, which are situated in the posterior wall of the ventricular septal defect.

Schatz et al. [30] reported a case of tricuspid atresia in which the postoperative ECG pattern of LAD deviation changed to a pattern of posterior fascicular block (PFB) in the postoperative period. This alteration would exclude the possibility that the left axis deviation is due to AFB; in fact, in such an event an LBBB pattern would appear.

Ebstein's anomaly

A typical ECG pattern has been described in Ebstein's disease and frequently the diagnosis can be made from the electrocardiogram [31-33]. The typical feature is RBBB associated with prolonged PR interval and right atrial hypertrophy. R and S waves over right and transitional precordial leads are often abnormally low due to decreased right ventricular mass. Such a feature, associated with RBBB in congenital heart disease, should immediately arouse one's suspicion of Ebstein's anomaly. The electrical axis is directed inferiorly, seldom superiorly (Figure 7). Recently Anderson et al [34] studied histologically five hearts with Ebstein's

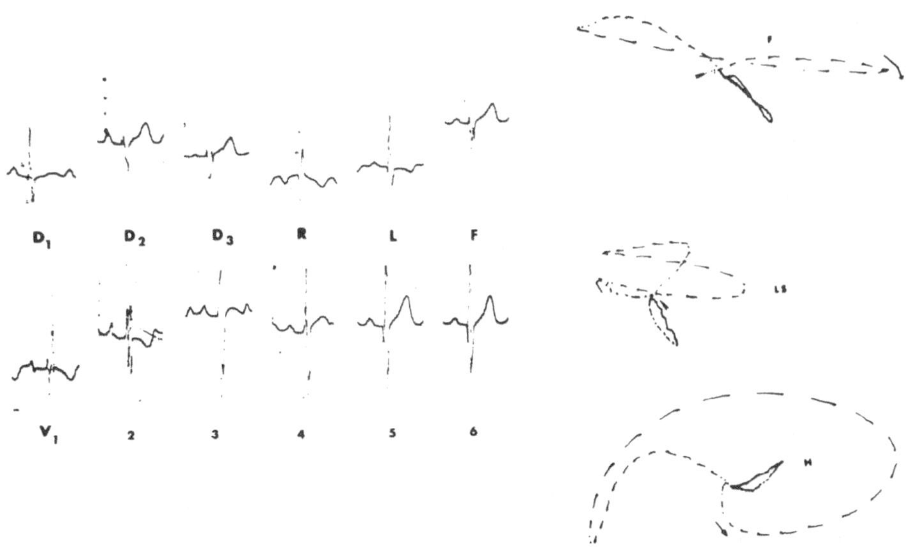

Figure 7. A 9-year-old patient with Ebstein's anomaly. ECG tracing shows right atrial enlargement, first degree AV block (PR: 200 msec) and incomplete right bundle branch block partern (QRS: 100 msec). In the VCG the frontal QRS loop is inscribed clockwise and the horizontal QRS loop counter-clockwise. A delayed appendage oriented to the right and anteriorly is present

anomaly. In two hearts there were abnormalities of the right bundle branch. In one, the proximal right bundle was unusually superficial and located in the subendocardium of the atrialized ventricle. In the others, the right bundle fanned out in a fashion reminiscent of a normal left bundle branch configuration. Minor abnormalities of the right bundle branch have been previously described [35]. Other types of conduction abnormalities, such as type B Wolff-Parkinson-White syndrome, may also be present [32].

Uhl's disease

Recently Bharati et al. [36] reported a case of Uhl's anomaly which developed complete AV block. His bundle electrocardiogram recorded before death showed H potentials following P waves, which is an expression of an infra-His block. Autopsy revealed absence of myocardium in most areas of the right ventricle and the right side of the ventricular septum with a normal tricuspid valve. Conduction system examination revealed total destruction of both bundle branches. In the electrocardiogram the escape rhythm was characterized by narrow QRS complexes which is strange when compared to the electrophysiological and histological data. According to these authors this probably reflects the absence of right ventricular forces, characteristic of this congenital heart disease.

Primary cardiomyopathies

Intraventricular conduction defects are frequently encountered in primary cardiomyopathies [37-40], which can also appear in pediatric age [41-43]. Any part of the conduction system may be affected. In a study by Forrester et al. [38], a bundle branch block was found to be far more common in patients with primary myocardial disease than in those with coronary heart disease. LBBB is a frequently observed conduction defect. The reported incidence of such a block varies between 10% and 40% [37, 39, 44-46]. Also, the AFB pattern has been frequently reported [39, 44-48]. Hamby et al. [48] found an incidence of 49%.

RBBB is less frequent and in almost all cases associated with LAD [48].

PFB pattern has been described but it is very rare [44, 46, 49]. Bizzarre intraventricular conduction defects not conforming to any recognizable pattern have been reported [49]. In our opinion, in some cases they represent right or left ventricular peripheral block.

It has been observed that in 83% of cases of idiopathic hypertrophic subaortic stenosis with narrow QRS complex, the HV interval is prolonged [50], expressing a lesion in the His bundle or in both bundle branches.

Miller et al. [51] described an infant affected by primary myocardial disease with complete AV block; the histological study of the conduction system showed both lack of connection between the atrial musculature and the intraventricular conduction system with absence of the AV node and destruction of the right bundle branch and the anterior fascicle of the left bundle branch.

Occasionally ECG features of WPW syndrome have been described, mostly in patients with obstructive cardiomyopathy [52-55].

Other congenital heart diseases

Right bundle branch block pattern can be observed in pulmonic stenosis (Figure 8), Fallot's tetralogy, simple ventricular septal defect, pulmonary valvular incompetence, and patent ductus arteriosus [1, 10, 56-58].

Anterior fascicular block pattern is rarely present in valvular pulmonic stenosis, secundum atrial septal defect, simple ventricular septal defect, Fallot's tetralogy (Figure 9), single ventricle, ventricular inversion (corrected transposition of the great arteries), or double outlet right ventricle [10, 59-62]. The reason for such an electric feature is not well known. It is possible that in some cases abnormalities or distortions of the interventricular pathways observed in endocardial cushion defect and in tricuspid atresia are present. The anatomy of the conduction system has been studied in single ventricle [63] but the variations from normal do not provide an explanation for LAD [64].

The conduction system has also been anatomically studied in ventricular inversion (corrected transposition of the great arteries) [65, 67] and though abnormal, does not clarify the mechanism of AFB pattern. In most cases, an anterior type of conduction system has been described by His bundle studies [68, 69] and pathologically [65, 70].

In ventricular inversion complete AV block [71-75] develops rather frequently in adult life. Electrophysiological studies have shown block proximal or distal to His bundle [75]. Pathologically, it is due either to lack of connection between the atria and the peripheral conduction system [75] or to fibrotic disruption of the His bundle in the anterior bundle [65, 70, 75].

COMMENT

Intraventricular conduction disturbances do not represent the most important ECG manifestations in congenital heart diseases, expressed on the other hand by atrial and ventricular hypertrophies. However, in some cases, the conduction defects may lead to clinical diagnosis. From the few anatomical data emerges the fact that in congenital heart diseases bundle branch and fascicular blocks pattern do not appear to be related, at least in most cases, to lesion of the main intraventricular pathways, but to an anomalous distribution of the conduction system. Incomplete RBBB pattern appears mainly to be related to a delayed conduction in the walls of the dilated right ventricle, particularly in congenital heart diseases with

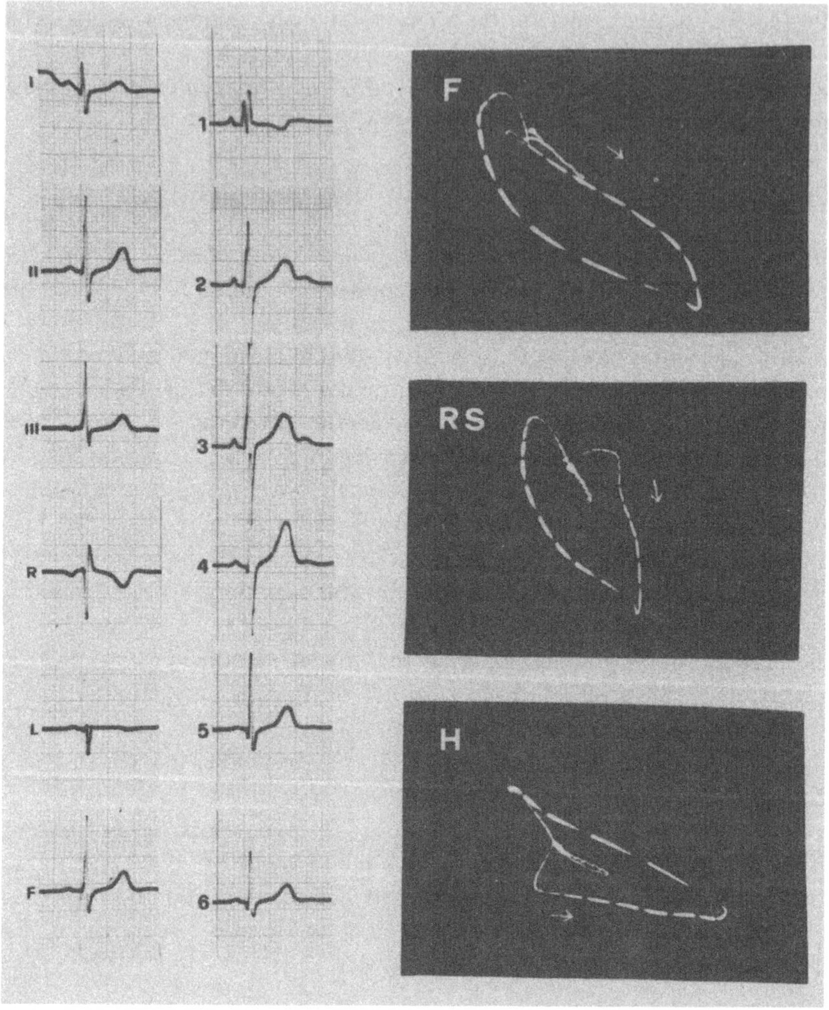

Figure 8. An 11-year-old patient with pulmonary valvular stenosis. QRS complex measures 90 msec. ECG and VCG tracings show an incomplete right bundle branch block pattern. The frontal QRS loop is inscribed clockwise and the horizontal QRS loop counterclockwise. A terminal delay, lasting 25 msec, oriented rightward, inferiorly and posteriorly is present

increased volume load. Such a pattern is not specific since it may be found in subjects without apparent heart disease. However, if incomplete RBBB pattern is associated with inferior electrical axis, slightly tall P wave and prolonged PR interval, secundum atrial septal defect must be suspected.

Characteristic, although nonspecific, is the fascicular block pattern, almost always present in endocardial cushion defect. In such an entity there is left asynchronous activation, as seen in true AFB. The latter, however, represents an

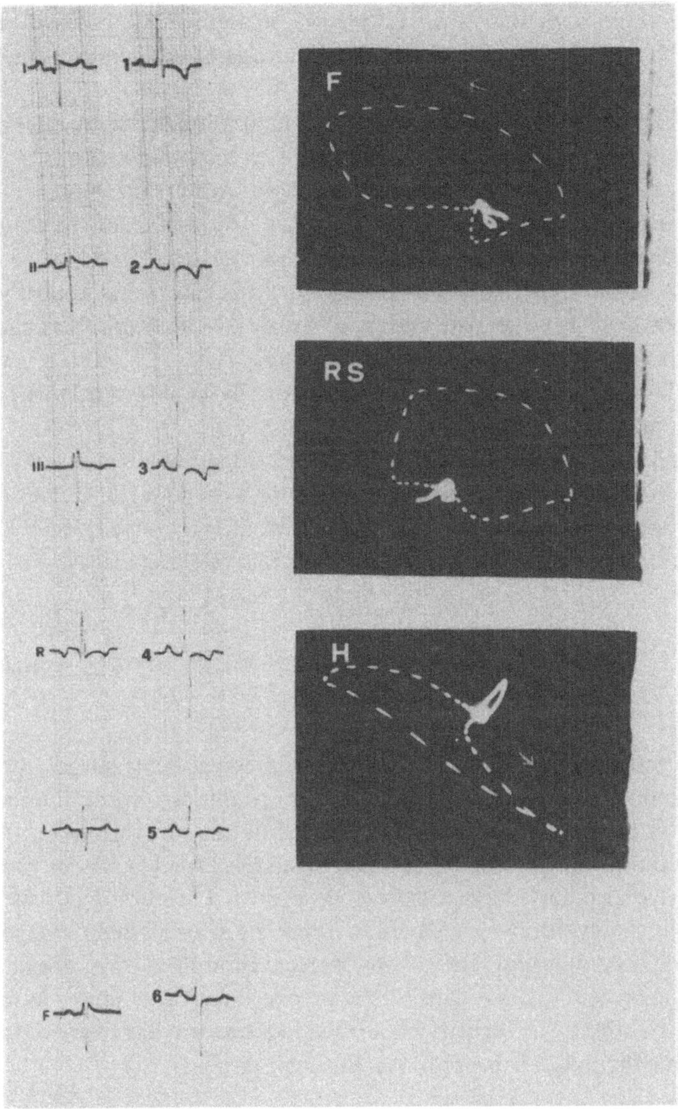

Figure 9. An 8-year-old patient with tetralogy of Fallot. ECG and VCG recordings show right ventricular hypertrophy. The frontal QRS loop is unusual for this congenital heart disease in that it is inscribed superiorly and counterclockwise

entirely different clinical entity in contrast to a superior ÂQRS resulting from a malpositioned and asymmetric left ventricular conduction system. The difference is exemplified by their natural history. While patients with true bifascicular block can develop progressive AV block, those with endocardial cushion defect remain asymptomatic. This distinction is important in the clinical management and follow-up of these patients. When RVH and prolonged PR interval are associated with the bifascicular block pattern, the diagnosis of endocardial cushion defect is almost certain.

An AFB pattern associated with left ventricular hypertrophy and with right and left atrial hypertrophy is highly suggestive of a tricuspid atresia.

In Ebstein's anomaly as well as in tricuspid atresia, the presence of the intraventricular conduction disturbances is particularly useful for the diagnosis. In the former, RBBB pattern associated with abnormally low R and S wave in precordial leads, right atrial hypertrophy and prolonged PR interval is almost pathognomic of such diseases. However, the finding of a normal QRS complex in an infant does not exclude the diagnosis of Ebstein's anomaly [10].

LBBB is rare in children and may occasionally be found in aortic stenosis and left ventricular myopathies.

Although the intraventricular conduction disturbances are nonspecific in the primary cardiomiopathies, when associated with deep and/or infarctional Q waves (Figure 10) and taken into consideration with the rest of the clinical picture, they may provide very helpful clues to the diagnosis of these diseases.

INTRAVENTRICULAR CONDUCTION DEFECTS FOLLOWING CARDIAC SURGERY

Intraventricular conduction disturbances after open heart surgery are a common event. In most cases such conduction abnormalities appear immediately upon termination of surgery and persist in almost all patients throughout their lifetime [76]. Late development [77, 78] and late disappearance [77, 79] of various types of intraventricular defects have also been described. The etiology of such blocks can be due to incision, suture placement, compression, small hemorrhages, small necrotic areas, inflammation, edema, myocardial infarction, or coronary embolism.

Controversy still exists regarding the precise location of injury in many of these patients, the ability to identify the exact location by electrocardiographic techniques, and the long-term prognosis for such patients.

Following repair of congenital heart diseases

Following heart surgery in congenital heart diseases all kinds of intraventricular blocks can be observed.

Right bundle branch block pattern. Right bundle branch block is the most common intraventricular conduction disturbance following open heart surgery in the pediatric population.

It has been observed in virtually all patients after repair of complete atrio-

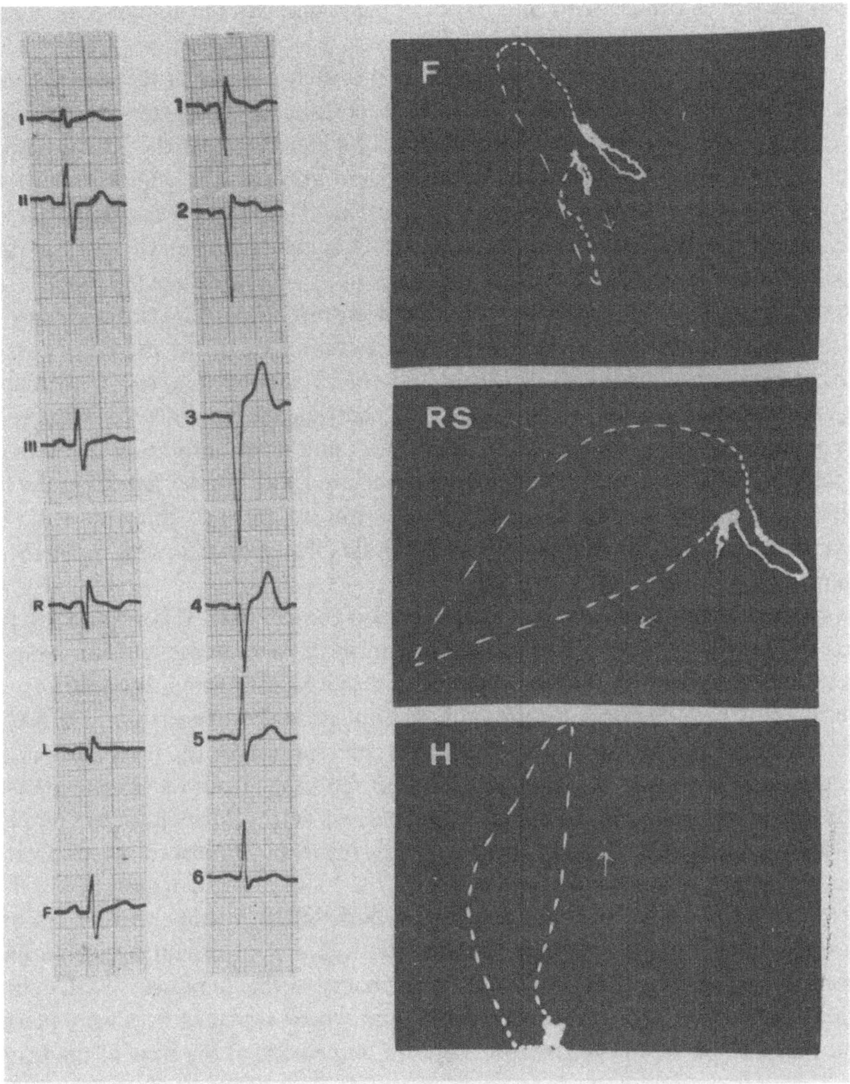

Figure 10. An 11-year-old patient with hypertrophic subaortic stenosis. An anteroseptal myocardial infarction pattern and an incomplete right bundle branch block are present. Such a feature in a young man is highly suggestive of primary cardiomyopathy

ventricular canal [80], in 60% to almost 100% following repair of Fallot's tetralogy [81-83], and in 60% to 81% of patients with ventricular septal defect repaired via a ventriculotomy [84, 85]. The incidence is lower in patients with the latter disease, repaired via the atrium (from 25% to 45%). Following repair of ostium primum defect [80] and following correction of intraventricular communications present in other forms of congenital heart diseases the incidence of RBBB is about 30%.

In most patients who had a right ventriculotomy for repair of their intraventricular defects, RBBB developed because of peripheral disruption of the right bundle branch [82, 86]. In fact, Gelband et al. [82] observed that the RBBB pattern appeared following the right ventricular incision and prior to the closure of the ventricular septal defect or pulmonary resection. This finding suggests that the postoperative RBBB pattern in those patients is related primarily to the right ventriculotomy. This has been shown to be equally true for dogs [87, 88].

Histologic studies have shown that RBBB pattern occuring during closure of the ventricular septal defect may also be due to an injury of the proximal part of the right bundle branch [81, 89-91]. In a study of 13 patients who succumbed after surgical correction of Fallot's tetralogy and ventricular septal defect, Titus et al. [89] encountered hemorrhage, suture placement and small infarction of the right bundle branch. These lesions were usually associated with similar lesions in the His bundle. Latham et al. [92] suggested that edema might also interfere with the proper function of the His bundle and bundle branches following open heart surgery.

In support of this interpretation there are also clinical data. Okoroma et al. [84] found that postoperative RBBB developed in 44% of patients with an isolated subaortic ventricular septal defect repaired through an atriotomy. Because none of these patients had a ventriculotomy, this finding strongly suggests that the RBBB pattern in these patients occurred because of interruption of the proximal part of the right bundle branch. Antar et al. [80] reported that 11 out of 13 patients with complete AV canal who had surgical repair of their defect through the atrium, had RBBB postoperatively. In all of these patients, sutures were placed on the crest of the interventricular septum during the operation. In addition, five out of 25 of their patients with an ostium primum defect also had RBBB postoperatively. All five had septal sutures placed through the interventricular septum during the surgical correction. In contrast, RBBB did not occur in any of the 20 patients with ostium primum defect who had surgical correction and whose septal sutures were placed, not at the crest of the interventricular septum, but rather at the base of the tricuspid valve.

Therefore the postoperative RBBB seen in patients with various forms of AV cushion defects in whom surgical repair was carried out through the atrium appears related to the use of sutures placed at the crest of the interventricular septum. These data indicate that all patients who require open heart surgery and whose right bundle branch is close to an interventricular septal defect are at risk of postsurgical RBBB. This group includes patients with Fallot's tetralogy, isolated subaortic ventricular septal defect, AV cushion defects and various other forms of congenital heart diseases with interventricular defects.

Quite recently Horowitz et al. [93] criticized some of these conclusions. These authors have done epicardial mapping during total surgical repair of Fallot's tetralogy through an atriotomy, thus avoiding the vertical ventriculotomy. It was observed that an RBBB pattern appeared during infundibular resection; in fact the activation was markedly delayed over the pulmonary outflow tract, but was unchanged over the body of the right ventricle. No further change in ventricular activation occurred after closure of the ventricular septal defect. This study shows that the RBBB pattern produced by ventricular resection expresses a peripheral block, and so bundle block observed after closure of the ventricular septal defect is not necessarily related to a lesion of the His bundle or the proximal part of the right bundle branch.

From anatomic and clinical data, it is therefore possible to deduce that RBBB pattern can represent a lesion in the His bundle, in the proximal part of the right bundle branch or in the peripheral divisions of such a branch.

Electrocardiogram and vectorcardiogram are not helpful in locating the site of this injury. Okoroma et al. [84] analyzed the VCG as well as scalar ECG taken at 50 mm/sec speed, and concluded that main right bundle injury, but not distal Purkinje fiber disruption, would induce an anterior-to-posterior shift of the initial 20 msec electrovectorcardiographic forces. Unfortunately, these changes, in general, are too subtle to be appreciated.

Within certain limits it is possible to evaluate if the RBBB pattern has a proximal or peripheral localization, by measuring the V-VRA interval (see Chapter 3).

This time was normal in 10 out of 11 patients with postoperative isolated RBBB, indicating a physiologically intact main RBBB, whereas it was abnormally lengthened (>30 msec) in all five patients with associated AFB [94].

The effect of the surgically created RBBB pattern on long-term prognosis is unknown. The prognosis is most likely related to the location of injury. The more proximal the lesion, the higher the likelihood that such patients will develop complete heart block distal to His bundle upon later development of LBBB. This event has been described recently in a patient who developed complete AV block upon subsequent injury to the left bundle branch [91].

Since the long-term prognosis is dependent on the site of injury to the right bundle branch, it can reasonably be assumed that two groups of patients with postoperative RBBB pattern will emerge: the first with peripheral RBBB in whom prognosis probably is not significantly affected, and the second with proximal right bundle branch lesions in whom the probability of complete AV block will be higher.

Fascicular and bifascicular blocks. In patients undergoing surgical correction of ventricular septal defect, whether isolated or associated with other malformations, RBBB with AFB pattern occurs in 8% to 22% of the cases [83, 95-98]. Such an electrical pattern can be related to [82, 86, 89, 99]: a) injury of right bundle branch fibers and of the anterior division of the left bundle branch; b) lesions of peripheral divisions of the bundle branches; or c) disruption of fibers within the common His bundle.

In fact Watt et al. [99] and Krongrad et al. [100] have shown in the canine heart that discrete lesions in the distal part of the His bundle produced an RBBB-AFB pattern and early activation of the inferior left ventricular wall.

Since the right bundle and the fibers of the anterior fascicle are adjacent structures, and are in proximity to the ventricular septal defect, there seems little doubt that a combined lesion of the proximal right bundle and of the anterior part of the left bundle branch can occur after repair of such defect.

On the other hand it is not possible to assess clinically whether the lesion involves the two separate conduction pathways or the common His bundle even when the V-VRA interval is measured. If a prolonged HV interval is associated with a prolonged V-VRA interval, it is more likely, but not certain, that the lesion is localized in the His bundle. Godman et al. [98] reporting on His bundle electrocardiographic findings in 17 patients after repair of ventricular septal defect or tetralogy of Fallot, found HV prolongation in five out of ten patients with bifascicular block; all five had transient complete AV block. Six patients with isolated RBBB had a normal HV interval. Pahlajani et al. [101] reported abnormal HV interval in four out of 18 patients who developed bifascicular block after repair of ventricular septal of Fallot's tetralogy. Two out of five patients with postoperative bifascicular block reported by Hougen et al. [102] showed prolonged HV interval, whereas 44 patients with RBBB had normal HV intervals. These data suggest that a lesion in the common His bundle is much more likely in the presence of bifascicular block than in an isolated RBBB.

The reported prognosis for patients who develop postoperative RBBB and AFB varies considerably. Some authors [97, 103, 104] have shown no increased incidence of late complications associated with this electrocardiographic pattern. This contrasts with the clinical follow-up data reported by others [83, 98, 105] for patients with a postoperative RBBB-AFB pattern.

Godman et al. [98] noted seven out of 11 patients who developed late complete AV block following repair of ventricular septal defect or tetralogy of Fallot acquired an RBBB-AFB pattern on their postoperative electrocardiograms. Among the patients reported by Wolff et al. [83], 41.7 % developed complete heart block and 12.5 % died suddenly from six months to two years after surgery. These complications far exceeded similar occurrences in a control group of postoperative patients. In a review of the literature, Krongrad [76] reported a total of 1856 patients followed from one month to 14 years. The cumulative incidence of RBBB and AFB patterns for the entire series was 11 %; over 4 % in these series were noted as having postoperative complete AV block and 3 % developed transient complete heart block and bifascicular block in the immediate postoperative period. Of the 204 patients who developed RBBB and AFB, one developed late complete AV block and two died suddenly, for total late complications of 1.5 %. Four of the 81 patients who developed transient complete AV block in the immediate postoperative period developed late complete AV block and 16 patients (29 %) who had transient complete heart block and bifascicular block either developed late complete AV block or died suddenly. These data strongly suggest that complete transient AV block is an indication of the development of late complete heart block or sudden death. Further, this author concludes that transient complete AV block in association with RBBB and AFB seems to be a better predictor of the possibility of development of late complete heart block or sudden death than either bifascicular block or transient complete AV block alone. Therefore, in children who undergo open heart surgery, it is important not only to achieve a good hemodynamic result but also to preserve normal AV conduction. In this regard the intraoperative electrophysiological identification of the specialized conduction system is important in order to avoid lesions of the His bundle and the right bundle branch [106-108].

The long-term prognosis of patients with postoperative RBBB-AFB pattern and prolonged HV interval was reported by Godman et al. [98], Pahlajani et al. [101] and Hougen et al. [102]. Their prognosis did not appear to be affected by the additional lesion. In particular there was no late permanent complete AV block or sudden death up to 20 years following surgery, although several of these patients had transient complete AV block in the early postoperative period. Thus, the limited available data suggest that the prognosis does not seem to be exacerbated by the added abnormality. However, only additional prospective studies of a large population of patients may allow definition of a high risk group.

Posterior fascicular block in children after open heart surgery is very rare; to the best of our knowledge only one such case has been reported [30] after repair of tricuspid atresia.

Following valvular replacement

There has been little investigation into intraventricular conduction disturbances after valve replacement [109-115].

After replacement of mitral and aortic valve, left conduction disturbances are more frequent, whereas after replacement of tricuspid valve right conduction disturbances occur more often [111]. Follath et al. [112] observed the appearance of intraventricular conduction abnormalities in about 25% of patients undergoing aortic valve replacement. In most cases an AFB associated with a RBBB pattern, or an LBBB was observed. The pathogenesis of the conduction defects is probably due to involvement of the conduction system during removal of the abnormal valve. Hemorrhagic lesions and necrosis of the intraventricular conduction system have been observed not infrequently after aortic valve replacement [116, 117]. Also myocardinal anoxia can often be responsible for intraventricular blocks. At times thromboemboli with microinfarcts have been seen to be responsible for conduction disturbances [118]. Posterior fascicular block, whether isolated or associated with RBBB, and isolated RBBB were less frequent. The frequency of such conduction defects was higher in calcified aortic stenosis than in aortic insufficiency [112].

When diagnosed immediately after operation, regression is common (50 %), especially of AFB. In patients with postoperative intraventricular conduction disturbances no hemodynamic complications were seen and the postoperative course was no different from those without electrocardiographic changes. The long-term prognosis looks good. In fact there was no long- or short-term mortality due to this cause [111, 112]. Nevertheless the possible risk of developing third degree AV block in later life is increased: Brodaty et al. [115] examined the ECG before and after mitral valve replacement in ten patients. The incidence of postoperative conduction disturbances was high (36 %), affecting patients with dominant stenosis and dominant incompetence equally. All types of intraventricular conduction defects were observed but the most frequent were AFB and LBBB. Regression was frequently observed.

Among the predisposing factors, statistically significant correlations were found with age, the hemodynamic changes caused by the cardiac lesion, and in patients with mitral valve incompetence.

After tricuspid valve replacement the appearance of RBBB pattern is frequent. Acar et al. [111] found it in 50 % of the cases. Such a block is due to the proximity of the right bundle branch to the tricuspid valve. In some cases Rosenbaum et al. [119] observed, after tricuspid valve replacement, the appearance of an AFB associated with RBBB. The authors believe that the anatomo-functional lesion is localized in the common His bindle.

Following coronary bypass surgery

Special attention has been given to the appearance of myocardinal infarction after coronary bypass surgery, but very little has been dedicated to the development of perioperative conduction disturbances. Selzer et al. [120] reported a potential 5 % to 15 % incidence rate of postoperative intraventricular conduction blocks. Zeldeis et al. [121] from an analysis of 200 patients, found an incidence rate of 20 %. Isolated RBBB and isolated AFB each developed in 6 % of cases. RBBB associated with AFB was the next most frequently observed disorder, affecting 4 % of the patients. LBBB developed in 3 % of cases and complete AV block in 2 %. Approximately one third of the disturbances were transient, lasting less than 24 hours. RBBB was most often persistent.

The prevalence of preoperative use of digitalis and of preoperative myocardial infarction was significantly greater among patients who had postoperative intraventricular conduction defects than among those who did not. On the other hand, the appearance of such disorders was not associated with the number of coronary bypass grafts performed or the extent of the preoperative coronary disease. These data suggest that patients with these defects have more extensive myocardial disease. It is likely that transient ischemia in the perioperative period affecting the conduction system is responsible for the intraventricular conduction disturbances noted. It is also likely that permanent conduction disturbances represent irreversible ischemic damage to the conduction system whereas transient disturbances may indicate reversible ischemia.

REFERENCES

1. Keith JD, Rowe RD, Vlad P: Heart disease in infancy and childhood. New York: Macmillan, 1958
2. Walker WJ, Mattingly TW, Pollock BE, Carmichael DB, Inmon TW, Forrester RH: Electrocardiographic and hemodynamic correlation in atrial septal defect. Am Heart J 52: 547, 1956
3. Milnor WR, Bertrand CA: The electrocardiogram in atrial septal defect. A study of twenty-four cases, with observations on the RSR′-V_1 pattern. Am J Med 22: 223, 1957
4. Toscano-Barboza E, Branderburg RO, Swan HJC: Atrial septal defect. The electrocardiogram and its hemodynamic correlation in 100 proved cases. Am J Cardiol 2: 698, 1958
5. Pryor R, Woodwark GM, Blount SG Jr: Electrocardiographic changes in atrial septal defects: ostium secundum defect versus ostium primum (endocardial cushion) defect. Am Heart J 58: 689, 1959
6. Liebman J, Nadas AS: The vectorcardiogram in the differential diagnosis of atrial septal defect in children. Circulation 22: 956, 1960
7. De Oliveira JM, Zimmerman HA: The electrocardiogram in interatrial septal defects and its correlation with hemodynamics. Am Heart J 55: 369, 1958
8. Lee YC, Scherlis L: Atrial septal defect. Electrocardiographic, vectorcardiographic and catheterization data. Circulation 25: 1024, 1962
9. Dushane JW, Weidman WH, Brandenburg RO, Kirklin JW: Differentiation of interatrial communications by clinical methods. Ostium secundum, ostium primum, common atrium and total anomalous pulmonary venous connection. Circulation 21: 363, 1960
10. Ellison RC, Restieaux NJ: Vectorcardiography in congenital heart disease: a method for estimating severity. Philadelphia: WB Saunders, 1972
11. Boineau JP, Spach MS, Ayers CR: Genesis of the electrocardiogram in atrial septal defect. Am Heart J 68: 637, 1964
12. Burchell HB, Dushane JW, Branderburg RO: The electrocardiogram of patients with atrioventricular cushion defects (defects of the atrioventricular canal). Am J Cardiol 6: 575, 1960
13. Burch GE, De Pasquale N: The electrocardiogram and ventricular gradient in atrial septal defect. Am Heart J 58: 190, 1959
14. Beregovich J, Bleifer S, Donoso E, Grishman A: The vectorcardiogram and electrocardiogram in persistent common atrioventricular canal. Circulation 21: 63, 1960
15. Lev M: The architecture of the conduction system in congenital heart disease. I. Common atrioventricular orifice. Arch Pathol 65: 174, 1958
16. Feldt R, Dushane JW, Titus JL: The atrioventricular conduction system in persistent common atrioventricular defect. Circulation 42: 437, 1970
17. Durrer D, Roos JP, Van Dam R Th: The genesis of the electrocardiogram of patients with ostium primum defects. Am Heart J 71: 642, 1966

18. Boineau JP, Moore EN, Patterson DF: Relationship between the ECG, ventricular activation and the ventricular conduction system in ostium primum ASD. Circulation 48: 556, 1973
19. Borkon AM, Pieroni DR, Varthese PJ, Ho CS, Rowe RD: The superior QRS axis in ostium primum ASD: a proposed mechanism. Am Heart J 90: 215, 1975
20. Donzelot E, Durand M, Metianu C, Vlad P: L'axe électrique normal ou dévié à gauche dans les cardiopathies congénitales cyanogènes. Etude de 29 cas personnels. Intérêt diagnostique. Arch Mal Coeur 43: 577, 1950
21. Brink AJ, Neil CA: The electrocardiogram in congenital heart disease, with special reference to left axis deviation. Circulation 12: 604, 1955
22. Gamboa R, Gersony WM, Nadas AS: The electrocardiogram in tricuspid atresia and pulmonary atresia with intact ventricular septum. Circulation 34: 24, 1966
23. Puri PS, Neill CA: Vectorcardiographic study in ten cases of tricuspid atresia. In: Electrocardiography in infants and children. New York: Grune & Stratton, 1966, p 268
24. Davachi F, Lucas RV Jr, Moller JH: The electrocardiogram and vectorcardiogram in tricuspid atresia. Correlation with pathologic anatomy. Am J Cardiol 25: 18, 1970
25. Taussing HB: The clinical and pathological findings in congenital malformations of the heart due to defective development of the right ventricle associated with tricuspid atresia or hypoplasia. Bull Johns Hopkins Hosp 59: 435, 1936
26. Somlyo AP, Halloran KR: Tricuspid atresia. An electrocardiographic study. Am Heart J 63: 171, 1962
27. Guller B, Dushane JW, Titus JL: The atrioventricular conduction system in two cases of tricuspid atresia. Circulation 40: 217, 1969
28. Bharati S, Lev M: The conduction system in tricuspid atresia with and without regular (d) transposition. Circulation 56: 423, 1977
29. Serratto M, Pahlajani DB: Electrophysiologic studies in tricuspid atresia. Am J Cardiol 42: 983, 1978
30. Schatz J, Krongrad E, Malm JR: Left anterior and left posterior hemiblock in tricuspid atresia and transposition of the great vessels. Observations and electrocardiographic nomenclature and electrophysiologic mechanisms. Circulation 54: 1010, 1976
31. Van Lingen B, Bauersfeld SR: The electrocardiogram in Ebstein's anomaly of the tricuspid valve. Am Heart J 50: 13, 1955
32. Lowe KG, Emslie-Smith D, Robertson PGC, Watson H: Scalar, vector, and intracardiac electrocardiograms in Ebstein's anomaly. Br Heart J 30: 617, 1968
33. Macruz R, Tranchesi J, Ebaid M, Pileggi F, Romero A, Decourt LV: Ebstein's disease. Electrocardiographic and radiologic correlations. Am J Cardiol 21: 653, 1968
34. Anderson KR, Zuberbuhler JR, Anderson RH, Becher AE, Lie JT: Morphologic spectrum of Ebstein's anomaly of the heart. A review. Mayo Clin Proc 54: 179, 1979
35. Yater WM, Shapiro MJ: Congenital displacement of the tricuspid valve (Ebstein's disease): review and report of a case with electrocardiographic abnormalities and detailed histologic study of the conduction system. Ann Intern Med 11: 1043, 1937
36. Bharati S, Cirauld DA, Bilitch M, Rosen KM, Lev M: Inexcitable right ventricle and bilateral bundle branch block in Uhl's disease. Circulation 57: 636, 1978
37 Marriott HJL: Electrocardiographic abnormalities, conduction disorders and arrhythmias in primary myocardial disease. Progr Cardiovasc Dis 7: 99, 1964
38. Forrester J, Kemp H, Gorlin R: Primary myocardial disease. Distinction from coronary heart disease. Circulation 40 (Suppl 4): 81, 1969
39. Stapleton JF, Segal JP, Harvey WP: The electrocardiogram of myocardiopathy. Progr Cardiovasc Dis 13: 217, 1970

40. Burch GE: Cardiomyopathy. Philadelphia: FA Davis, 1972
41. Tajik AJ, Giuliani ER, Weidman WH, McCoon DC, Branderburg RO, Ritter DG: Idiopathic hypertrophic subaortic stenosis (IHHS) in children. Circulation 47 (Suppl IV): 222, 1973
42. Maron BJ, Henry WL, Clark H, Redwood DR, Roberts WC, Epstein SE: Asymmetric septal hypertrophy in childhood. Circulation 53: 9, 1976
43. Romano A, Botti G: Le forme gravi e sintomatiche di cardiomiopatia ipertrofica ostruttiva dell'età pediatrica. A proposito di 5 casi operati. G Ital Cardiol 9: 1172, 1979
44. Dye CL, Rosenbaum D, Lowe JC, Behnke RH, Genovese PD: Primary myocardial disease. Ann Intern Med 58: 426, 1963
45. Banta DH, Estes EH: Electrocardiographic and vectorcardiographic findings in patients with idiopathic myocardial hypertrophy. Am J Cardiol 14: 218, 1964
46. Massumi RA, Rios JC, Gooch AS, Nutter D, De Vita VT, Datlow DW: Primary myocardial disease: report of fifty cases and review of the subject. Circulation 31: 19, 1965
47. Sanders V: Idiopathic disease of myocardium. Arch Intern Med 112: 661, 1963
48. Hamby RI, Raia F: Electrocardiographic aspects of primary myocardial disease in 60 patients. Am Heart J 76: 316, 1968
49. Bahl OP, Walsh TJ, Massie E: Electrocardiography and vectorcardiography in idiopathic hypertrophic subaortic stenosis. Am J Med Sci 259: 262, 1970
50. Ingram RE, Mason JW, Rossen RM, Goodman DJ, Harrison DC: Electrophysiologic findings in patients with idiopathic hypertrophic subaortic stenosis. Am J Cardiol 41: 811, 1978
51. Miller RA, Mehta AB, Rodriguez-Coronel A, Lev M: Congenital atrioventricular block with multiple ectopic pacemakers. Electrocardiographic and conduction system correlation. Am J Cardiol 30: 554, 1972
52. Schiebler GL, Adams P Jr, Anderson RC: Familial cardiomegaly in association with the Wolff-Parkinson-White syndrome. Am Heart J 58: 113, 1959
53. Schrader W, Pankley G, Davis R, Theologides A: Familial idiopathic cardiomegaly. Circulation 24: 599, 1961
54. Kariv I, Scherf L, Solomon M: Familial cardiomyopathy: with special consideration of electrocardiographic and vectorcardiographic findings. Am J Cardiol 13: 734, 1964
55. Frank S, Braunwald E: Idiopathic hypertrophic stenosis. Clinical analysis of 126 patients with emphasis on the natural history. Circulation 37: 759, 1968
56. Friedberg CK: Diseases of the heart. Philadelphia: WB Saunders, 1967
57. Fowler RS: Terminal QRS conduction delay in pulmonary stenosis in children. Am J Cardiol 21: 669, 1968
58. Watson H: Pediatric cardiology. London: Lloyd-Luke (Medical), 1968
59. Pileggi F, Bocanegra J, Tranchesi J, Macruz R, Borges S, Portugal O, Villarinho MG, Barbato E, Decourt LV: The electrocardiogram in tetralogy of Fallot: a study of 142 cases. Am Heart J 59: 667, 1960
60. Bender SR, Dreifus LS, Downing D: Anatomic and electrocardiographic correlation of Fallot's tetralogy. A study of 100 proved cases. Am J Cardiol 7: 475, 1961
61. Ongley PA, Dushane JW: Vectorcardiography in congenital heart disease: an introduction. In: Vectorcardiography I. Amsterdam: North-Holland, 1966, p 337
62. Perloff JK: Left axis deviation. A reassessment. Circulation 60: 12, 1979
63. Anderson RH, Arnold R, Thapar MK, Jones RS, Hamilton DI: Cardiac specialized tissue in hearts with an apparently single ventricular chamber (double inlet left ventricle). Am J Cardiol 33: 95, 1974

64. Perloff JK: The clinical recognition of congenital heart disease, 2nd edn. Philadelphia: WB Saunders, 1978
65. Anderson RH, Becker AE, Arnold R, Wilkinson JL: The conducting tissue in congenitally corrected transposition. Circulation 50: 911, 1974
66. Bharati S, Lev M: The course of the conduction system in single ventricle with inverted (L-) loop and inverted (L-) transposition. Circulation 51: 723, 1975
67. Lev M, Bharati S: The anatomy of the conduction system. In: Cardiac arrhythmias in the neonate, infant and child, Roberts NK, Gelband H, eds. New Work: Appleton-Century-Crofts, 1977, p 29
68. Stewart S, Manning J, Siegal L: Automated identification of cardiac conduction tissue in L-TGV and Ebstein's anomaly. Ann Thorac Surg 23: 215, 1977
69. Waldo AL, Maclean AN, James TN: Electrophysiologic delineation of the cardiac conduction system during open heart surgery. In: Cardiac arrhythmias in the neonate infant and child, Roberts NK, Gelband H, eds. New York: Appleton-Century-Crofts, 1977, p 373
70. Lev M, Fieloing RT, Zaeske D: Mixed levocardia with ventricular inversion (corrected transposition) with complete atrioventricular block. A histopathologic study of the conduction system. Am J Cardiol 12: 875, 1963
71. Wright FS, Adams P Jr, Anderson RC: Congenital atrioventricular dissociation due to complete or advanced atrioventricular heart block; clinical and cardiac catheterization findings in twelve children without cardiac malformations including three siblings. Am J Dis Child 98: 72, 1959
72. Berman DA, Adicoff A: Corrected transposition of the great arteries causing complete heart block in an adult. Am J Cardiol 24: 125, 1969
73. Hoffman JIE: Heart block in congenital heart disease. Bull NY Acad Med 47: 885, 1971
74. Michaelsson M, Engle MA: Congenital complete heart block: an international study of the natural history. Cardiovasc Clin 4: 85, 1972
75. Bharati S, McCue CN, Tingelstad JB, Mantakas M, Shiel F, Lev M: Lack of connection between the atria and the peripheral conduction system in a case of corrected transposition with congenital atrioventricular block. Am J Cardiol 42: 147, 1978
76. Krongrad EK: Prognosis for patients with congenital heart disease and postoperative intraventricular conduction defects. Circulation 57: 867, 1978
77. Quattlebaum TG, Varghese J, Neil CA, Donahoo JS: Sudden death among postoperative patients with tetralogy of Fallot. A follow-up study of 243 patients for an average of twelve years. Circulation 54: 289, 1976
78. Sonheimer HM, Izukawa T, Olley PM, Trusler GA, Mustard WT: Conduction disturbances after total correction of tetralogy of Fallot. Am Heart J 92: 278, 1976
79. Yabek SM, Jarmakani JM, Roberts N: Postoperative trifascicular block complicating tetralogy of Fallot repair. Pediatrics 58: 236, 1976
80. Antar RA, Krongrad E, Bowman FO Jr, Malm JR: Etiology of right bundle branch block pattern following surgical repair of AV cushion defects. Pediatr Res 10: 310, 1976
81. Kulbertus HE, Coyne JJ, Hollidie-Smith KA: Conduction disturbances before and after surgical closure of ventricular septal defect. Am Heart J 77: 123, 1969
82. Gelband H, Waldo AL, Kaiser GA, Bowman FO Jr, Malm JR, Hoffman BF: Etiology of right bundle branch block in patients undergoing total correction of tetralogy of Fallot. Circulation 44: 1022, 1971
83. Wolff GS, Rowland TW, Ellison RC: Surgically induced right bundle branch block with left anterior hemiblock. An ominous sign in postoperative tetralogy of Fallot.

Circulation 46: 587, 1972
84. Okoroma EO, Guller B, Maloney JD, Weidman WH: Etiology of right bundle branch block pattern after surgical closure of ventricular septal defects. Am Heart J 90: 14, 1975
85. Boxer R, Krongrad E, Bowman FO Jr, Malm JR, Gersony WM: Conduction defects following ventricular septal defect closure with and without a right ventriculotomy. Pediatr Res 11: 386, 1977
86. Krongrad E, Hefler SE, Bowman FO Jr, Malm JR, Hoffman BF: Further observations on the etiology of right bundle branch block pattern following right ventriculotomy. Circulation 50: 1105, 1974
87. Coggin CJ, Wareham EE, Selvester RH: Post ventriculotomy right bundle branch block: its etiology. Circulation (abstr) 22: 734, 1960
88. Genender LJ, Stuckey JH, Jomain SL, Hoffman BF: Effects of right ventriculotomy upon activation of the epicardial surface of the canine right ventricle. Circulation 27: 828, 1963
89. Titus JL, Daugherty GW, Kirklin JW, Edwards JE: Lesions of the atrioventricular conduction system after repair of ventricular septal defect: relation to heart block. Circulation 28: 82, 1963
90. Lev M, Fell EH, Arcilla R, Weinberg MH: Surgical injury to the conduction system in ventricular septal defect. Am J Cardiol 14: 464, 1964
91. Krongrad E, Bharati S, Steinfeld L, Lev M: Histologic observations of the cardiac conduction system in a heart with postoperative bilateral bundle branch block. Am J Cardiol 40: 635, 1977
92. Latham RA, Anderson RH: Anatomical variations in atrioventricular conduction system with reference to ventricular septal defects. Br Heart J 185: 34, 1972
93. Horowitz LN, Simson MB, Spear JF, Josephson ME, Moore EN, Alexander JA, Kastor JA, Edmunds LH Jr: The mechanism of apparent right bundle branch block after transatrial repair of tetralogy of Fallot. Circulation 59: 1241, 1979
94. Sung RJ, Tamer DM, Garcia OL, Castellanos A, Myerburg RJ, Gelband H: Analysis of surgically-induced right bundle branch block pattern using intracardiac recording techniques. Circulation 54: 442, 1976
95. Chesler E, Beck W, Schrire V: Left anterior hemiblock and right bundle branch block before and after surgical repair of tetralogy of Fallot. Am Heart J 84: 45, 1972
96. Downing JW, Kaplan S, Bore KE: Post surgical left anterior hemiblock and right bundle branch block. Br Heart J 34: 263, 1972
97. Cairns JA, Dobell ARC, Gibbons J, Tesseler I: Benign prognosis of right bundle branch block and left anterior hemiblock after intracardiac repair of tetralogy of Fallot. Am J Cardiol (abstr) 33: 129, 1974
98. Godman MJ, Roberts NK, Izukawa T: Late postoperative conduction disturbances after repair of ventricular septal defect and tetralogy of Fallot. Analysis of His bundle recordings. Circulation 49: 214, 1974
99. Watt TB Jr, Pruitt RD: Focal lesions in the canine bundle of His. Their effect on ventricular excitation. Circ Res 31: 531, 1972
100. Krongrad E, Rosen MR, Merker C, Hoffman BF: Creation of counterclockwise superiorly oriented frontal plane loops in isolated blood perfused canine hearts. Pediatr Res 7: 300, 1973
101. Pahlajani DB, Serratto M, Mehta A, Miller RA, Hastreiter A, Rosen KM: Surgical bifascicular block. Circulation 52: 82, 1975
102. Hougen TJ, Dick M, Freed MD, Keane JF: His bundle electrocardiogram after intracardiac repair of tetralogy of Fallot. Analysis of data in 59 patients. Am J Cardiol 41: 552, 1978

103. Bocala RR, Guller B, Danielson GK, Feldt RH: Left anterior hemiblock and complete repair of tetralogy of Fallot. Pediatr Res (abstr) 8: 347, 1974
104. Steeg CN, Krongrad E, Davachi F, Bowman FO Jr, Malm GR, Gersony WM: Postoperative left anterior hemiblock and right bundle branch block following repair of tetralogy of Fallot. Clinical and etiologic considerations. Circulation 51: 1026, 1975
105. Moss AJ, Klyman, G, Emmanouilides GC: Late onset complete heart block. Newly recognized sequela of cardiac surgery. Am J Cardiol 30: 884, 1972
106. Kaiser GA, Waldo AL, Beach PM, Bowman FO Jr, Hoffman BF, Malm JR: Specialized cardiac conduction system: improved electrophysiologic identification technique at surgery. Arch Surg 701: 673, 1970
107. Waldo AL, Pacifico AO, Bargeron LM, James TN, Kirklin JW: Electrophysiological delineation of the AV conduction system in patients with corrected transposition of the great vessels with ventricular septal defects. Circulation 52: 435, 1975
108. Dick M, Norwood WI, Chipman C, Castaneda AR: Intraoperative recording of specialized atrioventricular conduction tissue electrograms in 47 patients. Circulation 59: 150, 1979
109. Dreifus LS: Electrocardiographic alteration following prosthesis valve replacement. Circulation (Suppl III) 30: 70, 1964
110. Dubost CH, Chapelle M, Guery J, D'Allaines CL, Blondeau PH, Piwinica A, Cachera JP, Gilmet D, Vigand M: Etude des troubles du rythme chez les malades porteurs d'une prothèse post-opératoire intracardiaque, dans la période post-opératoire en milieu chirurgical. Arch Mal Coeur 61: 33, 1968
111. Acar J, Hanania G, Lancelin B, Fanjoux J, Auperin A, Krodonu J: Les modifications électrocardiographiques après chirurgie sous CEC pour replacement valvulaire. A propos de 95 cas observations. Arch Mal Coeur 64: 1160, 1971
112. Follath F, Ginks WR: Changes in the QRS complex after aortic valve replacement. Br Heart J 34: 553, 1972
113. Fukuda T, Hawley RL, Edwards JE: Lesions of conduction tissue complicating aortic valvular replacement. Chest 69: 605, 1976
114. Cannon PG, Sellers RD, Kanjuh VI, Edwards JE, Lillehei CW: Complete heart block following replacement of the aortic valve. Circulation (suppl) 33: 152, 1976
115. Brodaty D, Fournial JF, Terreau Y, Chomette G, Cabrol C, Acar J: Les troubles de conduction auriculo-ventriculaires et intraventriculaires après replacement valvulaire mitral. A props de 100 cas. Coeur et Med Int 48: 203, 1979
116. Hudson REB: Surgical pathology of the conducting system of the heart. Br Heart J 29: 646, 1967
117. Niles NR, Sandilands JR: Pathology of heart valve replacement surgery. Dis Chest 56: 373, 1969
118. Marchenese K, Schenk EA: Atrio-ventricular conductive system lesions following cardiac valve replacement. Circulation (abstr) 46: II-188, 1972
119. Rosenbaum MB, Elizari MU, Lazzari JO: The hemiblocks. Oldsmar: Tampa Tracing, 1970
120. Selzer A, Cohn K: Asymptomatic coronary artery disease and coronary bypass surgery. Am J Cardiol 39: 614, 1977
121. Zeldis SM, Morganroth J, Horowitz LN, Michelson EL, Josephson ME, Lozner EC, MacVaugh H, Kastor JA: Fascicular conduction disturbances after coronary bypass surgery. Am J Cardiol 41: 860, 1978

8. INTRAVENTRICULAR CONDUCTION DISTURBANCES IN ACUTE MYOCARDIAL INFARCTION. CLINICAL SIGNIFICANCE

For over 40 years it has been recognized that the prognosis in acute myocardial infarction (AMI) is affected adversely by the presence of intraventricular conduction disturbances (IVCD) [1]. In addition, the fact that the development of IVCD may be a precursor of high degree AV block is well known. However, contradictory data on the relationship between the incidence of IVCD, hospital, and late mortality rate may be related to the different criteria used for the diagnosis of the various IVCD, and to the subdivision in groups, often too small and not homogeneous, particularly with respect to infarct location and types and timing of onset of IVCD. Besides, blocks which occur in the terminal phases of shock have often been included with patients whose IVCD develops as a direct result of myocardial infarction. This does not seem logical as all the manifestations that appear only during the last moments preceding death should be considered apart.

Furthermore, groups of patients surviving the acute phase of myocardial infarction have been followed up for periods of time which are too different and often too brief to define the long-term effects of these conduction disturbances. It is for such reasons that the influence of IVCD on short- and long-term prognosis of AMI is still for the most part unclear.

INCIDENCE

The overall incidence of IVCD in AMI varied in several studies to between 7% and 28.8% [2-18]. In the patients who did not undergo continuous electrocardiographic monitoring the lowest incidences (7-13%) were observed [4, 9] in that in several cases the IVCD were transient, appearing for a short period of time. *In most of the studies in which the patients did undergo continuous monitoring the incidence of IVCD varied between 20% and 25%* (Table 1).

It is often difficult to evaluate whether an IVCD is preexistent to AMI or acquired, as in 40-83% of reported cases the IVCD was already present on admission and may have reflected a preexistent conduction disorder [4, 5, 15, 18, 19-21]. In a recent American Multicenter Project [22] in which 432 patients with AMI coexisting with IVCD were studied, 21% of the blocks were old, 37% were of indeterminate onset and 42% were observed to occur during infarction.

Table 1. Incidence of various_types of intraventricular conduction disturbances (IVCD) in patients with acute myocardial infarction

Authors	All No.	IVCD %	AFB %	PFB %	RBBB %	RBBB + AFB %	RBBB + PFB %	LBBB %
Atkins et al. [11]	77	(18)	4.5	1.1	0.7	7	0.2	4.2
Col et al. [6]	51	(24)	8	0.5	4.2	5.6	0.9	5.1
De Vita et al. [14]	181	(21.9)	5.8	0.5	6.3	5	0.1	3.8
Gann et al. [15]	324	(28.8)	6.3	–	2.3	3.3	1	5.7
Medrano [17]	120	(23)	3.2	4.8	5	4.2	1.5	3.9
Michalopoulos et al. [18]	104	(21.8)	4.4	0	3.7	8	0.4	4.8
Scheinman et al. [10]	96	(20)	4.2	0.2	3.7	4.8	0.8	6.4
Waugh et al. [12]	116	(21.5)	3.3	1.3	1.4	4.8	2.6	7.6

– = not reported

By evaluating only those cases in which the IVCD is definitely acquired, the frequency of occurrence varies between 5% and 10% [15, 23, 24].

The overall incidence of different types of IVCD varies considerably, as is evident in Table 1.

The most common abnormality observed is the association of right bundle branch block (RBBB) with anterior fascicular block (AFB), the incidence varying between 3.3 % and 8 %.

Isolated RBBB and left bundle branch block (LBBB) present a slightly lower incidence, the former varying between 2.3 % and 6.3 % and the latter between 3.8 % and 7.6 %.

In the studies by Atkins et al. [11] and Waugh et al. [12] the incidence of the isolated RBBB appears to be extraordinarily low: 0.7 % and 1.4 %, respectively.

AFB has often been evaluated in its totality, i.e. when it appeared both as an isolated manifestation or associated with RBBB, so it represents the most frequent IVCD during AMI. When it has been analyzed as an isolated block, its incidence is lower, varying between 3.2 % and 8 %.

The isolated posterior fascicular block (PFB) seems t be rare (0.2 %-1.3 %). Only in the study by Medrano et al. [17] was a high incidence encountered: 4.8 %. The discrepancy most probably lies in the different criteria employed, as the author diagnoses a PFB when the electric axis is directed between 60° and 90° and the signs of asynchronous left ventricular activation are present (see Chapters 4 and 9). Other authors use as their main diagnostic criterion a rightward axis deviation greater than 100°-120°.

RBBB associated with PFB is also a rare finding, its incidence varying between 0.1 % and 2.6 %.

Even more rare is the alternating bundle branch block, which has been reported only sporadically [12, 14, 17].

When AMI coexists with IVCD, the site of infarction is usually anteroseptal. In a total of 206 patients drawn from different series [11, 13, 25-32] in which the localization of the infarction was reported, anterior infarction was found in 83 %, inferior infarction in 9 % and both anterior and inferior infarction in 3 %; in 5 % the site of infarction was unrecognizable [33].

In almost all cases IVCD appears within the first 4 days of hospitalization [11, 18].

The manner in which a bundle branch block appears during the acute phase of myocardial infarction is not well known. Only Lie et al. [21] have registered in 10 patients the ways in which RBBB appears during continuous tape recordings. Five patients developed incomplete RBBB over periods ranging from several minutes to 2 hours. This was followed by the occurrence of sudden onset (within one beat) of complete RBBB without a change in the preceding R-R intervals. The other five patients abruptly (within one beat) developed complete RBBB without either passing through a phase of incomplete RBBB or a change in the preceding cycle length.

Regarding the disappearance of IVCD during hospitalization, precise data are lacking. In the study by Hindam et al. [22], 72 out of 303 patients (33 %) discharged from hospital had normal intraventricular conduction. De Vita et al. [14] observed that an IVCD was no longer present on discharge in 45 % of the cases.

ATRIO-VENTRICULAR BLOCK

In patients with AMI and IVCD, the reported incidence of progression to high degree AV block* varies in different studies between 8 % and 47 % [5, 7, 10-12, 18-20, 25-27, 31, 34].

This diversity in results is possibly related to factors such as type of population, sample size and method of observation. From an analysis of ten series [5, 7, 10, 12, 19, 25-27, 31, 34] *an average incidence of high degree AV block of 24% was observed* [22].

It must be underlined that the high degree AV block does not represent a homogeneous finding in that, although in most cases of AMI with IVCD such AV block is distal to His bundle, in a few rare cases it can be localized in the AV nodes [21, 35].

Infarct location did not appear to influence the risk of high degree AV block. According to Hindam et al. [36], such a block was as common with inferior or posterior infarction (20 %) as with anterior infarction (25 %) or with anterior and indeterminately located infarcts considered together (22 %). However, the anterior infarction group and the inferior infarction group are not easily comparable because of the different number of patients studied, which was much higher in the first group.

* Mobitz II AV block and complete AV block are reported in this term because they are considered together in most papers.

Conversely, in AMI without IVCD, the inferior infarction is about three times the more common cause of high degree AV block than anterior infarction [37-44].

Isolated anterior and posterior fascicular blocks

In the papers [6, 10, 19, 20, 25, 27, 32, 34, 36, 45] where the incidence of progression of the various types of IVCD has been analyzed (Table 2) it came to light that the patients with isolated AFB or PFB present a risk of progression which is not greater than that of patients with AMI without IVCD, evaluated between 2 and 12 % [9, 46-49]. In only one patient out of 32 (3.1 %) with AMI and AFB, reported by Gould et al. [50], a transient 2:1 AV block appeared.

Table 2. Incidence of progression to high degree AV block in various types of intraventricular conduction disturbances

Authors	RBBB		RBBB + AFB		RBBB + PFB		LBBB	
	No.	%	No.	%	No.	%	No.	%
Basualdo et al. [45]		–	2/7	(28.5)		–	1/5	(20)
Blanc et al. [20]	2/13	(15.3)	6/16	(37.5)	0/1	(0	2/14	(14.2)
Godman et al. [27]		–	15/51	(29)	9/20	(45)		–
Hindam et al. [22]	6/48	(14)	40/149	(27)	13/45	(29)	21/163	(13)
Lie et al. [34]		–	7/18	(38)	7/14	(50)		–
Marriot et al. [6]		–	1/10	(10)	1/2	(50)		–
Roos et al. [25]		–	4/10	(40)	1/1	(100)		–
Scheidt et al. [19]	6/19	(32)		–		–	2/20	(10)
Scheinman et al. [10]	3/18	(17)	3/23	(13)	1/4	(25)	3/31	(10)
Stephens et al. [32]		–	9/25	(36)	8/12	(67)		–

Bifascicular blocks

The highest incidence of progression was observed in patients with bifascicular block. Such incidence varied between 25 % and 67 % in patients with RBBB and PFB and between 13 % and 40 % in those with RBBB and AFB (Table 2).

Considering only the acquired bifascicular blocks, the incidence of progression was 50 % in RBBB with PFB and 38 % in RBBB with AFB [34].

Isolated bundle branch blocks

In patients with isolated RBBB and in those with LBBB there is less tendency toward progression; in the former a high degree AV block was observed in 14-32 % of the cases, in the latter in 10-20 % (Table 2).

In patients with RBBB, Lie et al. [21] always observed the appearance of an anterior or posterior fascicular block before the development of a high degree AV block.

The same authors, analyzing separately the patients with preexisting and those with acquired RBBB, observed that out of 42 patients with preexistent RBBB, only one progressed to high degree AV block; they concluded that only the patients with acquired RBBB are at a high risk of progression.

Also Nimetz et al. [31] reported that none of the seven patients with preexistent isolated RBBB presented progression to high degree AV block. Moreover, out of nine patients with acquired LBBB, five (55%) developed high degree AV block and out of seven with preexistent LBBB, two (28.5%) showed progression. These data are not sufficient to draw definite conclusions, but it does seem that old LBBB has less tendency towards AV block complication than new LBBB.

These considerations stress the importance of evaluating those factors which may help in the early identification of patients with an acquired bundle branch block (BBB) by distinguishing them from those with a preexistent BBB.

The QRS configuration in V_1 appears helpful in differentiating acquired from preexistent RBBB. It was observed that 90% of patients with acquired RBBB and acute anteroseptal infarction showed a QR complex in V_1 during the first 24 hours of admission, whereas 90% of the patients with preexistent RBBB showed either a qR or a trifasic QRS pattern in V_1. Two patients with a preexistent RBBB also showed QR pattern in V_1 and each had had a previous anteroseptal infarction. Therefore, the QRS configuration in lead V_1 is probably more valuable in patients with a first attack than in those with a recurrent infarction [21].

Other factors, besides the type of IVCD and the preexistence or otherwise of the intraventricular block, seem to condition the progression to high degree AV block. Lie et al. [34] observed that 14 out of 39 patients (36%) in which a BBB appeared within 24 hours after onset of infarction, developed complete heart block (CHB), whereas none of the 11 patients who developed BBB later than 24 hours after onset of infarction developed CHB. The same authors studied 15 patients with transient BBB and noted that no patient with BBB of short duration (1-6 hours) developed CHB. For a duration of BBB of any time between 6 hours and 6 days, a CHB appeared in 42% of cases.

First degree AV block

Contrasting views are to be found regarding the problem of whether a first degree AV block in patients with AMI and IVCD represents a predictive factor for the development of high degree AV block. Some authors [12, 14, 51] hold that a lengthening of the PR interval represents a sensitive discriminator whereas this is denied by others [21, 22, 25, 31].

In several studies in which this aspect has been analyzed in patients with first degree AV block, a progression in 25-50% of the cases was observed [12, 14, 36, 41, 49, 51]. In the study by Hindam et al. [36] the presence of first degree AV block was associated with a 25% incidence of progression compared to a 19% incidence in patients without first degree AV block.

These different views, in our opinion, do not depend on the varyious results obtained, but on a different interpretation of the data. In fact some authors [12, 14, 51] stress the relatively greater incidence of progression in patients with first degree AV, whereas others stress that the appearance of a high degree AV block in over one third of cases is abrupt, i.e. not preceded by a lengthening of the PR interval or by type I second degree AV block [21, 22, 25, 31].

HEART FAILURE

A greater incidence of severe heart failure in patients with AMI and IVCD compared to those without intraventricular block has been reported in almost all papers. However, few papers [5, 11, 14, 17, 22, 31, 34, 52] have reported precise data. The incidence of severe heart failure, as manifested by pulmonary edema and cardiogenic shock, varied between 24% and 58.9% (Table 3).

De Vita et al. [14] and Hindam et al. [22] encountered an incidence of severe heart failure almost twice as high in patients with BBB compared to those without intraventricular block (45% vs 25% and 46% vs 21%, respectively) (Table 3).

Literature offers very few precise data on the incidence of heart failure in the various types of IVCD. In the study by Hindam et al. [22], the patients with isolated RBBB had a 35% rate of severe heart failure compared to an average incidence of 47% with other intraventricular blocks. In the study by De Vita et al. [14] the incidence of severe heart failure in the presence of RBBB, LBBB and of bifascicular block varied from 40% to 50%.

In patients with isolated AFB the incidence of severe heart failure appeared only

Table 3. Incidence of severe heart failure in patients with and without intraventricular conduction disturbances

Authors	No. of patients with IVCD	Percentage of severe heart disease in patients with IVCD	Percentage of severe heart disease in patients without IVCD
Atkins et al. [11]	77	24	–
De Vita et al. [14]	181	45	25
Fazzini et al. [52]	39	58.9	–
Godman et al. [5]	68	58.8	–
Hindam et al. [22]	432	34* 46**	21
Lie et al. [34]	170	30	–
Medrano [17]	120	26.6	–
Nimetz et al. [31]	71	35	–

– = not reported
* = preexistent IVCD
** = indeterminate onset and acquired IVCD

slightly increased compared to patients without IVCD [12, 14, 50]. At present, precise data on the incidence of heart failure in the presence of PFB are not available.

The incidence of severe heart failure appears only slightly higher in patients with anterior or indeterminately located infarcts (48 %) compared to those with inferior or posterior infarctions (39 %) [22].

Several authors [7, 14, 22, 53, 54] encountered a very high incidence of pulmonary edema and cardiogenic shock in patients with IVCD and high degree AV block.

HOSPITAL MORTALITY

In studies in which the hospital mortality rate of patients with IVCD was compared with that of patients without intraventricular block, the differences were statistically significant [8, 10-14, 17, 18, 20, 22].

In patients with IVCD the mortality rate varied between 24 % and 55.5 %, whereas in those without intraventricular blocks it was between 11 % and 22 % (Table 4).

Table 5 reports the mortality rate of several types of IVCD [8, 10, 11, 13, 14, 17, 18, 21, 22, 27, 31, 50, 51, 55].

Isolated anterior and posterior fascicular blocks

In the presence of isolated AFB the mortality rate appears only slightly higher (10.8-35 %) compared to that observed in the absence of IVCD.

In patients with PFB it appears higher (25-40 %). The cases reported are, however, too few to draw any conclusions. Furthermore, this block, if not intermittent,

Table 4. Hospital mortality of patients with and without intraventricular conduction disturbances

Authors	No. of patients with IVCD	Hospital mortality of patients with IVCD, %	Hospital mortality of patients without IVCD, %
Atkins et al. [11]	77	30	14
Blanc et al. [20]	45	55.5	15.5
Col et al. [8]	51	47	13.6
De Vita et al. [14]	181	41	22
Hindman et al. [22]	432	28	12
Medrano [17]	120	35.8	12.7
Michalopoulos et al. [18]	104	28	19
Rizzon et al. [13]	81	24	11
Scheinman et al. [10]	96	40	17
Waugh et al. [12]	116	29	16

Table 5. Hospital mortality in various types of intraventricular conduction disturbances

Authors	No. of patients with IVCD	Hospital mortality					
		AFB %	PFB %	RBBB %	RBBB + AFB %	RBBB + PFB %	LBBB %
Atkins et al. [11]	77	30	40	33	33	0 (0*)	22
Col et al. [8]	51	25	0(1*)	42	55.5	100 (2*)	63.5
De Vita et al. [14]	181	25	25	42.3	53.6	–	46.8
Folli et al. [55]	60	10.8	–	–	42.2	–	–
Gould et al. [50]	32	12	–	–	–	–	–
				x xx xxx	x xx xxx	x xx xxx	x xx xxx
Hindam et al. [22]	432	–	–	19 25 25	18 34 28	28 29 43	30 24 21
					x xxx		
Levy et al. [51]	33	–	–	–	50 52.6	–	–
				xxx	xxx	xxx	
Lie et al. [21]	108	–	–	69	70	90	–
Medrano [17]	120	23.5	28	23	54.5	50	44
Michalopoulos et al. [18]	104	14	0 (0*)	25	37	50 (2*)	30
Nimetz et al. [31]	71	–	–	15	34	66	25
Rizzon et al. [13]	81	12	–	18	36	75	33
Scanlon et al. [26]	28	–	–	–	36	–	–
Scheinman et al. [10]	96	35	100 (1*)	44	35	50	42

* = absolute number of patients
– = not reported
x = preexistent IVCD
xx = indeterminate onset IVCD
xxx = acquired IVCD

is difficult to recognize in the presence of myocardial infarction (see Chapter 9) and a different patient selection is extremely probable in the various studies.

Bifascicular blocks

The highest hospital mortality rate is observed in patients with AMI and bifascicular block; in RBBB associated with PFB it varies between 43 % and 90 % and in RBBB associated with AFB between 28 % and 70 % (Table 5).

Isolated bundle branch blocks

In patients with isolated BBB the mortaility rate is slightly lower; in those with RBBB it varies between 15 % and 69 % and in those with LBBB between 21 % and 63.5 % (Table 5).

Owing to the marked variability in the mortality rate in the several studies, these results are not very reliable.

In almost all studies preexistent and acquired BBB have been included. Some authors [21, 22] considered them separately and observed a higher mortality rate in the patients with acquired BBB (Table 5).

Hospital mortality appears directly related to the degree of heart failure. In about two thirds of the patients dying from AMI complicated by IVCD, the primary cause of death was severe heart disease [4, 7, 8, 10, 11, 13-15, 19, 22, 31, 33, 34, 45, 52, 53, 55].

In a prospective study of 100 unselected patients with AMI, Julian et al. [56] found that pump failure was twice as often the main cause of death in intraventricular block as it was in patients without such block.

Severe heart failure appears more frequently in patients with IVCD and anteroseptal myocardial infarction than those with IVCD and inferior infarction (Hindam et al. [22]: 31% vs 17%; Constans et al. [57]: 32% vs 11%).

Patients with IVCD and documented previous infarctions had a significantly higher hospital mortality rate than patients with IVCD, but without previous infarction (42% vs 25%). In patients without IVCD the mortality rate was lower: 14% in patients with prior infarction compared to 10% in patients without prior infarction [22].

Some authors [15, 25, 28, 30, 34, 58] have analyzed the hospital mortality rate in patients with persistent BBB and those with transient BBB and in most of the studies it appeared higher in the former. Lie et al. [34] reported a 12.5% mortality (one out of eight patients) with BBB lasting less than 6 hours, a 50% mortality rate (two out of four patients) at 6-24 hours, and no survivors (three out of three patients) when BBB lasted for 24 hours or longer. There also appeared to be a higher risk of sudden death in patients who developed IVCD within 24 hours (32 out of 39 patients, 82%) than those who did not (five out of eleven patients, 45%).

However, in our opinion, the cases studied are too few to draw any conclusions regarding this problem.

The hospital mortality rate related to abrupt development of CHB varied in several studies between 3.4% and 9% [11, 18, 22]. The authors, naturally, only refer to the cases in which the cause of death has been documented, since in patients discharged from coronary care units (CCU) it is not always possible to demonstrate whether sudden death is related to abrupt CHB, ventricular fibrillation or to other causes. It is therefore probable that the hospital mortality rate related to abrupt CHB in patients with IVCD is higher than has been reported so far, as is also suggested by the continuous Holter monitoring of patients with bifascicular block complicating anterior wall myocardial infarction [59]. However, a high incidence of hospital sudden death has been demonstrated as being due to ventricular fibrillation. It has been observed that more than one-third of hospitalized CCU survivors with BBB and anteroseptal infarction developed late ventricular fibrillation 1-6 weeks after the onset of infarction [60].

In patients with documented high degree AV block during AMI the prognosis is very poor, with a varying mortality rate of between 70% and 90% [21, 27, 34, 39, 43,

53, 54, 57]. It is generally accepted that the poor prognosis of these patients is mainly due to extensive myocardial damage as temporary pacing does not seem to affect the immediate prognosis significantly (see Chapter 14).

Calculations based on the series of Kostuk et al. [70], Rosen et al. [35] and Friedberg et al. [39] show mortality with narrow QRS complexes, i.e. without IVCD (usually caused by inferior infarction), to be 35%, a finding which stresses the quite different clinical significance of complete AV nodal block and complete His-Purkinje block in AMI.

The relationship between AV block and hospital mortality in patients with AMI and IVCD has been carefully studied by Hindam et al. [22]. These authors observed that first degree AV block was not associated with increased mortality. The patients who developed type 1 second degree AV block or third degree block preceded by type I block also presented a slight increase in the hospital mortality rate (29%). However, a subgroup of patients with anterior infarctions and third degree AV block, who presented a greatly increased mortality rate (83%), has been signled out. The patients who progressed to high degree AV block had more than twice the hospital mortality rate than patients who never progressed beyond first degree AV block (47% vs 23%). In these patients mortality was increased whether the AV block was isolated type II second degree AV block (43%), third degree AV block preceded by type II block (50%) or third degree AV block without preceding second degree AV block (55%) or whether the infarction was inferior or posterior (41%) or anterior or indeterminate (55%). In these patients hospital mortality was mainly related to severe heart failure.

LATE MORTALITY

Scarce and contradictory data are available about late mortality in patients with AMI and IVCD. In the few studies [18, 20, 36, 57, 62] in which late mortality in patients with IVCD has been compared to that of patients without IVCD, it appeared slightly higher in the former (Table 6). In patients with IVCD, such

Table 6. Late mortality of patients with and without intraventricular conduction disturbances

Authors	No. of patients with IVCD	Deaths No.	Deaths %	Percentage of sudden death	No. of patients without IVCD	Deaths No.	Deaths %	Percentage of sudden deaths	Follow-up period
Blanc et al. [20]	20	11	(55)	15	38	12	(32)	13.1	26 months
Constans et al. [57]	72	32	(44.4)	23.6	82	29	(35.3)	12.1	48 months
Domenighetti et al. [62]	36	9	(25)	55.5	100	8	(8)	–	19 months
Hindam et al. [36]	309	87	(28.1)	51.7	–	–	(15)	–	12 months
Michalopoulos et al. [18]	75	16	(21.3)	25	75	11	(14.6)	36.3	18 months

mortality varied between 21.3% and 55% and in those without IVCD between 14.6% and 35.3% for follow up periods varying between 12 and 48 months. The two groups of patients present a difference in late mortality which is less marked than in hospital mortality.

Two subgroups of patients at higher risk of late sudden death have been singled out: 1) patients with anterior or indeterminately located infarcts and power failure during hospitalization and, 2) patients with documented prior myocardial infarction and acute anterior or indeterminately located infarcts without power failure [36].

Regarding the relationship between the type of intraventricular block and late mortality, the latter appears higher in patients with bifascicular block. De Vita et al. [14] for a follow-up period of one year, observed a mortality rate of 42% in the presence of RBBB associated with AFB, and of 26% and 29% in the presence of RBBB and LBBB, respectively. In patients with isolated AFB, mortality rate was only 16%. Very similar data have been reported in the study by Hindam et al. [36] in which the mortality rate was 37% in bifascicular blocks, 33% in LBBB, 24% in isolated RBBB and only 14% in isolated AFB and PFB.

Late mortality is higher in patients with IVCD and anterior myocardial infarction compared to those with inferior infarction [36, 57]. On the other hand this difference has also been observed in patients with AMI without IVCD.

Some authors have observed a higher mortality rate in patients with persistent IVCD compared to those with transient IVCD [36], whereas others did not encounter any significant difference between the two groups [14].

Recently a subgroup of patients has been defined that are at very high risk from late sudden death. Patients who developed IVCD during an AMI and who proceeded to complete heart block (CHB), but recovered from this block before discharge, showed a marked propensity to late sudden death (42.8-100%) in the first year after the infarction [11, 12, 26, 63] (Table 7). In these patients a dramatic reduction in late sudden deaths was documented after the institution of permanent demand ventricular pacing (see Chapter 14).

Scanlon et al. [26] found that five out of eight unpaced patients died suddenly

Table 7. Follow-up of non-paced patients showing transient high degree AV block during acute myocardial infarction

Authors	No. of patients	Deaths No.	Deaths %	Percentage of sudden deaths	Follow-up period
Atkins et al. [11]	6	5	(83.3)	100	6 months
Ginks et al. [64]	21	7	(33.3)	42.8	49 months
Marchi et al. [65]	9	5	(55.5)	40	6 months
Nimetz et al. [31]	13	4	(30.7)	100	21 months
Ritter et al. [63]	5	5	(100)	100	18 months
Scanlon et al. [26]	8	5	(62)	100	8 months
Waugh et al. [12]	10	5	(50)	100	12 months

within 8 months of initial hospital discharge. Atkins et al. [11] reported that five of six such patients died suddenly within 6 months and in the study by Waugh et al. [12] five out of ten patients not treated with permanent pacing died suddenly within a 12-month follow-up period. Ritter et al. [63] found that all five unpaced patients with IVCD and transient CHB during AMI died within a 20-month follow-up period.

Different results were reported by Nimetz et al. [31], Ginks et al. [64] and Marchi et al. [65].

However, the analysis of seven series [11, 12, 26, 29, 31, 63, 64] in which the patients reported by Nimetz and Ginks were also included, revealed a late mortality of 51 % (21 out of 41 patients) in the nonpaced groups, and of 12 % (3 out of 26 patients) in the paced group [57]. In a recent American Multicenter Project [36], it was revealed that patients who were not continuously paced had a higher incidence of sudden death or recurrent AV block than patients who were continuously paced (65 % vs 10 %).

COMMENT

In most studies in which patients with AMI underwent continuous electrocardiographic monitoring the incidence of IVCD varied between 20% and 25%. There is, however, no way of determining the true incidence of IVCD since many patients die outside hospital before they can be admitted. Moreover, identification of fascicular blocks is particularly difficult in the presence of myocardial infarction if the block is not intermittent (see Chapter 9). In fact the diagnosis of such blocks is mainly based on the presence of a marked axis deviation which may be related to the infarct itself. It is therefore possible that in the various studies several patients have been included who do not have a true fascicular block. It must also be noted that, if perinfarction block is present, a posterior myocardial infarction may simulate an RBBB and an anteroseptal infarction an LBBB. For a more precise definition of the incidence of IVCD, greater precision in diagnostic criteria of various intraventricular blocks coexisting with myocardial infarction would be desirable.

In studies which classified BBB by the timing of onset, the average frequency of occurrence of old, indeterminate and new onset blocks is approximately 33 % for each group [4, 5, 15, 19, 22, 31].

The most common IVCD observed is the association of RBBB with AFB; isolated RBBB, LBBB and AFB present a slightly lower incidence whereas the isolated PFB and the RBBB associated with PFB represent a rare complication.

Incidence and mechanism of IVCD following AMI are closely related to the blood supply of the specific conduction system and the site of infarction [7, 40, 66]. Since in almost all cases an IVCD complicates an anterior infarction [5, 13, 16, 22,

24, 25, 27, 28, 31, 53, 61] the high incidence of RBBB associated with AFB is easily understandable. In fact the anterior division of the left bundle branch is longer and thinner than the posterior division and consequently more vulnerable to ischemia or necrosis. In addition, the anterior division of the left bundle branch and the right bundle branch are usually supplied only by septal branches of the anterior descending coronary artery [67]. Therefore interruption of blood supply via these vessels would be expected to cause damage in both conducting tissue. Instead, the inferior division is supplied by branches from either the right coronary artery or the circumflex branch of the left coronary artery and sometimes from both. Because of the more diffuse nature of its blood supply compared to that of the superior division, the inferior radiation would rarely be ischemic. Also because of their different sources of blood supply, the right bundle and the inferior division would less often be diseased concomitantly. When RBBB does occur with PFB, a more significant disease should be suspected, since presumably more of the vascular supply to the heart is diseased. In fact in a high percentage of cases this bifascicular block is observed in patients with coexisting inferior and anterior wall infarctions [14, 51].

A small number of patients with IVCD shows inferior myocardial infarction [10, 14, 18, 26, 54]. This can be attributed, in the case of AFB, to preexisting left coronary disease which can produce a fascicular block if collaterals from the right coronary artery are interrupted [10, 13, 68]. In the case of RBBB alone, its association with inferior wall infarction could also be explained on the basis of some anatomical findings showing that in 20% of normal hearts the proximal part of the right bundle branch receives the blood supply only from the AV node artery, which in 90% of patients arises from the right coronary artery [69].

Clinicopathological studies also indicate the relationship between the site of infarction and the involvement of the conduction system [7, 40, 66, 70].

However, it is still unclear whether the focal necrosis, often evident in the intraventricular conducting tissues in the presence of acute anteroseptal infarction, is sufficient to cause the interruption of impulse conduction [71, 72]. A recent clinicopathological study [70] has revealed that hydrophic cell swelling together with an infiltration of polymorphonuclear leukocytes, is present in those cases exhibiting IVCD, whereas it is absent in a control group without conduction disturbances but with the same site of infarction. These data also account for the common transient nature of conduction disorders associated with AMI.

According to Hackel et al. [73], reversible IVCD are caused by the effect of increased extracellular potassium released by necrotic myocardial cells on viable conducting fibers. The potassium released from necrotic myofibers is at its greatest level 24 hours after the AMI and the necrotic area gradually loses potassium until the fourth day after the AMI. The IVCD, if transient, may also be explained on the basis of this pathophysiological mechanism and, therefore, they may be considered as metabolic blocks.

In patients with AMI and IVCD the reported incidence of progression to high degree AV block in most cases distal to His bundle, varies between 8% and 47%. Hindam et al. [22], from an analysis of ten series [5, 7, 10, 12, 19, 25-27, 31, 34], observed an average incidence of progression of 24%. The incidence of high degree AV block in AMI without IVCD is lower, varying between 2% and 12% [9, 46-49].

Several factors seem to condition the progression to high degree AV block in patients with IVCD.

First of all, the type of intraventricular block: the highest incidence is observed in fascicular blocks and the lowest, similar to those of AMI without IVCD, in isolated fascicular blocks.

Of particular importance appears to be the time of appearance of IVCD in relation to onset of AMI; in fact it has come to light that the acquired BBB have a higher incidence of progression compared to preexistent BBB [21, 31, 34, 36].

Lie et al. [21] have reported that the duration of a BBB also conditions the progression to high degree AV block; no patient with BBB of short duration (1-6 hours) developed CHB, whereas for such blocks varying in duration between 6 hours and 6 days, a CHB appeared in 42.8% of cases. This analysis was, however, carried out in 15 cases, too few in order to draw any conclusions.

Infarct location and PR interval duration do not seem to influence significantly the progression to high degree AV block.

Recording the HV interval would seem to define with greater precision the risk of progression, but further studies are required (see Chapter 11).

It has been stressed that patients with AMI complicated by BBB have a high incidence of severe heart failure and die as a result of progressive and irreversible deterioration [3, 4, 7, 8, 12-19, 21-28, 31, 52, 53, 61, 74, 75]. Such incidence is about 45% and almost twice that of patients without BBB [14, 22]; this seems due to extensive myocardial damage, necessary to cause involvement of the intraventricular conduction system when the BBB is new; and to the presence of underlying myocardial and/or coronary artery involvement when the block is old. In this connection Carvalho et al. [76] – who compared coronary arteriographic and ventriculographic aspects in patients with and without IVCD – found that the incidence of total obstruction of the left anterior descending and of circumflex arteries was greater in patients with IVCD than in those without it. In addition, the incidence of akinesis and aneurysm was statistically higher among patients with IVCD than among those without intraventricular block.

Autoptic studies revealed very extensive myocardial infarctions, generally involving the anterior wall of the left ventricle and most of the interventricular septum in patients with BBB [20, 25].

The large extent of infarction necessary to involve the bundle branches is responsible for the greater incidence of severe heart failure, which in its turn induces an increased mortality rate in patients with BBB [3, 4, 7, 8, 10-18, 21-28, 31, 52, 61, 75].

In an American Multicenter Project [22], the 28% mortality rate in 432 patients with BBB is significantly higher than the 12% mortality for a control group of patients without BBB. This mortality rate is almost comparable to those observed in other studies [11, 12, 17, 18], but it is lower than the 47% mortality reported by Col et al. [8] and the 55.8% mortality reported by Blanc et al. [20]. These differences probably reflect different CCU populations.

The highest hospital mortality rate is observed in patients with bifascicular block. Recently Sclarovsky et al. [77] reported 30 cases in which transient AFB obscured in right precordial leads the diagnosis of RBBB appearing during the first days of an AMI. The electrocardiogram was characterized by an AFB with wide QRS complexes; RBBB was diagnosed in the ECG on the appearance of rSr′ morphology by recording high V_1 lead and in the vectorcardiogram by a slight displacement to the right of the terminal forces. The clinical course of this type of bifascicular block was benign, with an in-hospital mortality rate of 6.7%. In our opinion, however, this electrical pattern may express a peri-infarction block or an incomplete RBBB coexisting with AFB and not a true bifascicular block.

As yet it is not clear whether the mortality rate is significantly higher in patients with acquired BBB compared to those with preexistent BBB as the data available in literature are contradictory [21, 22, 51]. If severe heart failure represents the most frequent cause of death in patients with IVCD, above all if the AMI has an anteroseptal location, other causes, particularly ventricular fibrillation, are often responsible for in-hospital mortality, even if the exact incidence has not been clearly defined. Lie et al. [60] observed that more than one-third of CCU survivors with BBB developed late in-hospital ventricular fibrillation, from 1 to 6 weeks after onset of infarction. These authors suggest keeping all CCU survivors with acquired BBB and anteroseptal infarction in the monitoring area for 6 weeks.

Other authors [7, 8, 29] mentioned ventricular fibrilation as a frequent complication in these patients and noted that this arrhythmia was often repetitive and fatal.

Abrupt development of CHB has been reported as the cause of hospital mortality in 3.4-9% of cases [11, 18, 22]. However, in patients discharged from CCU it is often impossible to document the cause of sudden death; therefore the actual incidence of such a complication is unknown. But it has been demonstrated that in-hospital mortality of AMI with IVCD complicated by documented high degree AV block is very high (60-80%), due to the large size of infarction; in fact a temporary pace-maker does not seem to affect the immediate prognosis in these patients (see Chapter 14).

Hospital survivors of myocardial infarction complicated by IVCD have an increased risk of dying during the first years following infarction compared to patients who survive AMI which is not complicated by intraventricular block [18, 20, 36, 57, 62]. The highest incidence of late mortality is observed in patients with bifascicular block, the lowest in those with isolated AFB; in the latter the mortality rate is similar to that of patients without IVCD [14, 18, 22].

These date suggest the importance of permanent and extensive myocardial damage in determining the long-term prognosis after AMI complicated by BBB.

The percentage of late sudden deaths is higher in patients with IVCD compared to those without, even if it does not appear in all studies [18, 20]. Various factors suggest that ventricular fibrillation is the major cause of such sudden deaths. In patients with coronary heart disease, serious ventricular arrhythmias have been correlated with multivessel disease and left ventricular disfunction [78, 79]. In addition, depressed left ventricular ejection fraction [80, 81], and persistent ST segment displacement [82] are associated with ventricular arrhythmias and sudden death after AMI. However, the mechanism of late suddden death, and in particular the role of the abrupt development of CHB in patients with AMI and IVCD, remains speculative. At present it is not known whether the institution of permanent demand pacing reduces the sudden mortality rate in these patients.

Several authors [5, 11, 12, 26, 36, 63] have noted an extraordinarily high incidence of late sudden death in patients with AMI and BBB who developed transient CHB and who were subsequently discharged from hospital with normal AV conduction. Even in such cases the mechanism of late sudden death remains speculative; however, several authors have observed a dramatic reduction of sudden death with the institution of permanent demand pacing (see Chapter 14). It is however most likely that in these patients the abrupt development of CHB plays an important role in the genesis of sudden death.

REFERENCES

1. Masters AM, Dack S, Jaffe HL: Bundle branch and intraventricular block in acute coronary occlusion. Am Heart J 16: 285, 1938
2. Killip T III, Kimball JT: Treatment of myocardial infarction in a coronary care unit: a two year experience with 250 patients. Am J Cardiol 20: 457, 1967
3. Stock RJ, Macken DL: Observations on heart block during continuous electrocardiographic monitoring in myocardial infarction. Circulation 38: 993, 1968
4. Hunt D, Sloman G: Bundle branch block in acute myocardial infarction. Br Med J 1: 85, 1969
5. Godman MJ, Lassers BW, Julian DG: Complete bundle branch block complicating acute myocardial infarction. N Engl J Med 282: 237, 1970
6. Marriot HJL, Hogan P: Hemiblock in acute myocardial infarction. Dis Chest 58: 342, 1970
7. Norris RM, Croxsen MS: Bundle branch block in acute myocardial infarction. Am Heart J 79: 728, 1970
8. Coll JJ, Weinberg SL: Incidence and mortality of intraventricular conduction defects in acute myocardial infarction. Am J Cardiol 29: 344, 1972
9. Malpartida F, Froute J, Nadal B: Bloqueo auriculo-ventricular de segundo y tercer grado en el infarto agudo del miocardio tratado con marcapaso transitorio. Arch Inst Cardiol Mex 42: 402, 1972

10. Scheinman M, Brenman B: Clinical and anatomic implications of intraventricular conduction block in acute myocardial infarction. Circulation 46: 753, 1972
11. Atkins JM, Leshen SJ, Blomqvist G, Mullins CB: Ventricular conduction blocks and sudden death in acute myocardial infarction: potential indications for pacing. N Engl J Med 288: 281, 1973
12. Waugh RA, Wagner GS, Haney TL, Rosati RA, Morris JJ: Immediate and remote prognostic significance of a fascicular block during acute myocardial infarction. Circulation 48: 765, 1973
13. Rizzon P, Di Biase M, Baissus C: Intraventricular conduction defects in acute myocardial infarction. Br Heart J 36: 660, 1974
14. De Vita C, De Ponti C, Pioselli D, Bossi M: I disturbi di conduzione intraventriculare in corso di infarto miocardico acuto. Prognosi immediata e a distanza. G Ital Cardiol 5: 513, 1975
15. Gann D, Balachandran PK, Sherif NE, Somet P: Prognostic significance of chronic versus acute bundle branch block in acute myocardial infarction. Chest 67: 298, 1975
16. Mullins CB, Atkins JM: Prognosis and management of ventricular conduction blocks in acute myocardial infarction. Mod Conc Cardiovasc Dis 45: 129, 1976
17. Medrano GA: Bloqueos fasciculares y de ramas del haz de His en el infarto del miocardio. Arch Inst Cardiol Mex 47: 750, 1977
18. Michalopoulos A, Athanasopoulos C, Lekakis J: The fate of patients with intraventricular conduction disturbance complicating acute myocardial infarction. Acta Cardiol 34: 189, 1979
19. Scheidt S, Killip T: Bundle branch block complicating acute myocardial infarction. JAMA 222: 919, 1972
20. Blanc JJ, Boschat J, Granatelli D, Morin JF, Germa D, Penther PH: Bloc de branche complet et infarctus du myocarde. Histoire naturelle. Etude comparative. Arch Mal Coeur 71: 43, 1978
21. Lie KI, Durrer D: Conduction disturbances in acute myocardial infarction. In: Cardiac arrhythmias. Electrophysiology, diagnosis and management, Narula OS. Baltimore: Williams & Wilkins, 1978, p 140
22. Hindam MC, Wagner GS, Jaro M, Atkins JM, Scheinman MM, De Sanctis R, Hutter AH Jr, Yeatman L, Rubenfire M, Pujura C, Rubin M, Morris JJ: The clinical significance of bundle branch block complicating acute myocardial infarction. 1. Clinical characteristics, hospital mortality and one-year follow-up. Circulation 58: 679, 1978
23. Bouvrain Y, Bouchet PF, Motte G, Roche P: Les blocs de branche de la phase aiguë de l'infarctus du myocarde. Arch Mal Coeur 65: 649, 1972
24. Lie KI, Wellens HJ, Schuilenburg RM: Bundle branch block and acute myocardial infarction. In: The conduction system of the heart: structure, function and clinical implications, Wellens HJJ, Lie KI, Janse MJ, eds. Philadelphia: Lea & Febiger, 1976, pp 662-672
25. Roos JC, Dunning AJ: Right bundle branch block and left axis deviation in acute myocardial infarction. Br Heart J 32: 847, 1970
26. Scanlon PJ, Pryor R, Blount SG: Right bundle branch block associated with left superior or inferior intraventricular block: associated with acute myocardial infarction. Circulation 42: 1135, 1970
27. Godman MJ, Alpert BA, Julian DG: Bilateral bundle branch block complicating acute myocardial infarction. Lancet 2: 345, 1971
28. Lichstein E, Gupta PK, Chadda KD, Liu HM, Sayeed M: Findings of prognostic value in patients with incomplete bilateral bundle branch block complicating acute myocardial infarction. Am J Cardiol 32: 913, 1973

29. Waters DD, Mizgala HF: Long-term prognosis of patients with incomplete bilateral bundle branch block complicating acute myocardial infarction. Am J Cardiol 34: 1, 1974
30. Lichstein E, Gupta PK, Chadda KD: Long term survival of patients with incomplete bundle branch block complicating acute myocardial infarction. Br Heart J 83: 928, 1975
31. Nimetz AA, Shubrooks SJ, Hutter AM, De Sanctis RW: The significance of bundle branch block during acute myocardial infarction. Am Heart J 90: 439, 1975
32. Stephens MR, Fadayomi MO, Davies GJ, Muir JR: The clinical features and significance of bifascicular block complicating acute myocardial infarction. Europ J Cardiol 3: 289, 1975
33. Roos JC, Dunning AJ: Bundle branch block in acute myocardial infarction. Europ J Cardiol 6: 403, 1978
34. Lie KI, Wellens HJ, Schuilenburg RM, Becher AE, Durrer E: Factors influencing prognosis of bundle branch block complicating acute anteroseptal infarction: the value of His bundle recordings. Circulation 50: 935, 1974
35. Rosen KM, Loeb HS, Chuquimia R, Zaid Sinno M, Rahimtoola SH: Site of block in acute myocardial infarction. Circulation 42: 925, 1970
36. Hindam MC, Wagner GS, Jaro M, Atkins JM, Scheinman MM, De Sanctis RW, Hutter AH, Yeatman L, Rubenfire M, Pujura C, Rubin M, Morris JJ: The clinical significance of bundle branch block complicating acute myocardial infarction. 2. Indications for temporary and permanent pacemaker insertion. Circulation 58: 689, 1978
37. Cohen DB, Doctor L, Pick A: The significance of atrioventricular block complicating acute myocardial infarction. Am Heart J 55: 215, 1958
38. Paulk EA Jr, Hurst JW: Complete heart block in acute myocardial infarction. A clinical evaluation of the intracardiac bipolar catheter pacemaker. Am J Cardiol 17: 695, 1966
39. Friendberg CK, Cohen H, Donoso E: Advanced heart block as a complication of acute myocardial infarction. Role of pacemaker therapy. Prog Cardiovasc Dis 10: 466, 1968
40. Sutton R, Chatterjee K, Leatham A: Heart block following acute myocardial infarction. Treatment with demand and fixed rate pacemakers. Lancet 2: 645, 1968
41. Brown RW, Hunt D, Sloman JG: The natural history of atrioventricular conduction defects in acute myocardial infarction. Am Heart J 78: 460, 1969
42. Chatterjee K, Harris A, Leatham A: The risk of pacing after infarction and current recommendations. Lancet 2: 1061, 1969
43. Norris RM: Heart block in posterior and anterior myocardial infarction. Br Heart J 31: 352, 1969
44. McNally EM, Benchimol A: Medical and physiological considerations in the use of artificial cardiac pacing. I. Am Heart J 75: 380, 1975
45. Basualdo CAE, Haraphongse M, Rossal RE: Intraventricular blocks in acute myocardial infarction. Chest 67: 75, 1975
46. Lown B: Treatment of acute heart block associated with acute myocardial infarction. Drug therapy. In: Proceedings of the Symposium on Cardiac Pacing and Cardioversion. New York: Charless, 1967
47. Gregory JJ, Grace WJ: The management of sinus bradycardia nodal rhythm and heart block for the prevention of cardiac arrest in acute myocardial infarction. Progr Cardiovasc Dis 10: 505, 1968
48. Julian DG, Oliver MF: Acute myocardial infarction. Baltimore: Williams & Wilkins, 1968

49. Resnekov L, Lip H: Pacemaking and acute myocardial infarction. Progr Cardiovasc Dis 14: 475, 1972
50. Gould L, Riedel J, Reddy R, Gomprecht RF: Prognosis of left anterior hemiblock in acute myocardial infarction. J Electrocardiol 8: 333, 1975
51. Levy S, Castellanos A Jr, Arcebal A, Lemberg L: Le bloc de branche droit avec hémibloc gauche à la phase aiguë de l'infarctus du myocarde. Pronostic et rôle de l'entraînement électrosistolique. Arch Mal Coeur 68: 497, 1975
52. Fazzini PF, Marchi F, Pucci P: Il significato prognostico dei blocchi intraventricolari nell'infarto miocardico acuto. G Ital Cardiol 5: 526, 1975
53. Fenig S, Lichstein E: Incomplete bilateral bundle branch block and A-V block complicating acute anterior wall myocardial infarction. Am Heart J 84: 38, 1972
54. Voridis E, Plessas M, Mallios K, Cokkinos O: Blocs complets droits et bifasciculaires au cours de la phase aiguë de l'infarctus du myocarde. Arch Mal Coeur 66: 1193, 1973
55. Folli G, Rumolo R, Graziina A, Vitolo E, Lotto A: Emiblocchi ed infarto del miocardio. G Ital Cardiol 3: 329, 1973
56. Julian DG, Valentine PA, Miller GG: Disturbances of rate, rhythm and conduction in acute myocardial infarction. Am J Med 37: 915, 1964
57. Constans R, Marco J, Berthoumiev H, Alibelli MJ, Daroenne P: Devenir des infarctus du myocarde compliqués en phase aiguë de troubles de la conduction. Arch Mal Coeur 72: 957, 1979
58. Bauer GE, Julian DG, Valentine PA: Bundle branch block in acute myocardial infarction. Br Heart J 27: 724, 1965
59. Lichstein E, Letafati A, Gupta PM, Chadda KD: Continuous Halter monitoring of patients with bifascicular block complicating anterior wall myocardial infarction. Am J Cardiol 40: 860, 1977
60. Lie KI, Liem KL, Schuilenburg RM, David GK, Durrer D: Early identification of patients developing late in-hospital ventricular fibrillation after discharge from the coronary care unit. A $5\frac{1}{2}$ year retrospective and prospective study of 1,897 patients. Am J Cardiol 41: 674, 1978
61. Kostuk WJ, Benlands DS: Complete heart block with acute myocardial infarction. Am J Cardiol 26: 380, 1970
62. Domenighetti G, Perret C: Intraventricular conduction disturbances in acute myocardial infarction: short and long-term prognosis. Europ J Cardiol 11: 51, 1980
63. Ritter WS, Atkins JM, Blomquist CG, Mullins CB: Permanent pacing in patients with transient trifascicular block during acute myocardial infarction. Am J Cardiol 38: 205, 1976
64. Ginks WR, Sutton R, Oh W, Leatham A: Long-term prognosis after acute anterior infarction with atrioventricular block. Br Heart J 39: 186, 1977
65. Marchi F, Pucci P, Santoro M, Zerauscher M, Fazzini PF: La prognosi a distanza dell'infarto anteriore complicato da blocco atrio-ventricolare totale. G Ital Cardiol 9: 182, 1979
66. James TN, Burch GE: Blood supply of the human interventricular septum. Circulation 17: 391, 1958
67. Lasser P, Haft J, Friedberg C: Relationship of right bundle branch block to marked left axis deviation (with left parietal or peri-infarction block) to complete heart block and syncope. Circulation 37: 429, 1968
68. Rosenbaum MB, Elizari MV, Lazzari JO: Los hemibloqueos. Buenos Aires: Paidos, 1968
69. Frink RJ, James TN: Normal blood supply to the human His bundle and proximal bundle branches. Circulation 47: 8, 1973

70. Becker AE, Anderson B, Lie KI: Bundle branch block and anteroseptal infarction. Clinicopathologic correlations. Br Heart J 40: 773, 1978
71. Blondeau M, Rizzon P, Lenegre J: Les troubles de la conduction auriculo-ventriculaire dans l'infarctus du myocarde récent. Arch Mal Coeur 54: 1104, 1961
72. Rotman M, Wagner GS, Wallace AG: Bradyarrhythmias in acute myocardial infarction. Circulation 45: 703, 1972
73. Hackel DB, Wagner G, Ratlif NB, Cies A, Estes EH Jr: Anatomic studies of the cardiac conduction system in acute myocardial infarction. Am Heart J 83: 77, 1972
74. Gould L, Venkataraman K, Mohammad N, Gomprecht RF: Prognosis of right bundle branch block in acute myocardial infarction. JAMA 219: 502, 1972
75. Gould L, Ramana CV, Gomprecht RF: Left bundle branch block: prognosis in acute myocardial infarction. JAMA 225: 625, 1973
76. Carvalho ET, Tranchesi J, Moffa PJ, Netto MP, Pileggi F, Marrara JP, Pasini U, Azul LGS: Estudo cinecoronarografico e cineventriculografico em pacientes com enfarte do miocardio associato a bloqueo divisional e troncular. Arq Bras Cardiol 28: 55, 1975
77. Sclarovsky S, Lewin RF, Strasberg B, Agmon J: Left anterior hemiblock obscuring the diagnosis of right bundle branch block in acute myocardial infarction. Circulation 60: 26, 1979
78. Calvert A, Lown B, Gorlin R: Ventricular premature beats and anatomically defined coronary heart disease. Am J Cardiol 39: 627, 1977
79. Califf RM, Burke JM, Behar VS, Margolis JR, Wagner GS: Relationships among ventricular arrhythmias, coronary artery disease and angiographic and electrocardiographic indicators of myocardial fibrosis. Circulation 57: 725, 1978
80. Vismara LA, Amsterdam EA, Mason DT: Relation of ventricular arrhythmias in the late hospital phase of acute myocardial infarction to sudden death after hospital discharge. Am J Med 59: 6, 1975
81. Schulze RA, Humphries JO, Griffith LSS, Ducci H, Achuff S, Baird MG, Mellits ED, Pitta B: Left ventricular and coronary angiographic anatomy: relationship to ventricular irritability in the late hospital phase of acute myocardial infarction. Circulation 55: 839, 1977
82. Wilson C, Pantridge JF: ST segment displacement and early hospital discharge in acute myocardial infarction. Lancet 2: 1284, 1973

9. INTRAVENTRICULAR CONDUCTION DISTURBANCES COEXISTING WITH HEALED MYOCARDIAL INFARCTION. DIAGNOSTIC PROBLEMS

Intraventricular conduction disturbances induce alterations of the ventricular depolarization to a more or less advanced degree and consequently also alter the QRS complex.

These blocks may either mask or mimic a myocardial infarction. Thus the electrocardiographic and vectorcardiographic (VCG) diagnosis of a healed myocardial infarction in the presence of intraventricular block may sometimes be difficult. The more marked the alteration of the ventricular depolarization induced by the block, the more difficult it is to recognize a coexisting myocardial infarction.

RIGHT BUNDLE BRANCH BLOCK

In right bundle branch block (RBBB), the initial phases of ventricular depolarization, apart from rare exceptions, are not significantly affected whereas the middle phases, as opposed to what is quite unanimously reported in literature, are often affected, being shifted anteriorly or more rarely posteriorly.

On the other hand the terminal vectors are always displaced by the RBBB because of the presence of a delayed terminal appendix oriented rightward and anteriorly.

In most cases the changes in the ventricular depolarization related to RBBB do not cancel out the alterations of the initial-middle phases, typical of myocardial infarction. On the other hand, myocardial infarction induces only moderate changes in the electric forces produced late in the QRS complex. Therefore it is usually possible to diagnose coexisting myocardial infarction and RBBB; the former on the basis of the initial 40 msec vectors deformity, the latter on the basis of the terminal QRS vectors changes.

In the anteroseptal wall infarction (Figure 1) pathologic Q waves are, however, present in right and transitional precordial leads; in the lateral infarction, in the left-sided leads and in the inferior infarction (Figure 2) in the diaphragmatic leads. One exception to this rule is the RBBB with posterior myocardial infarction. This type of necrosis typically affects the mid-terminal instantaneous QRS vectors

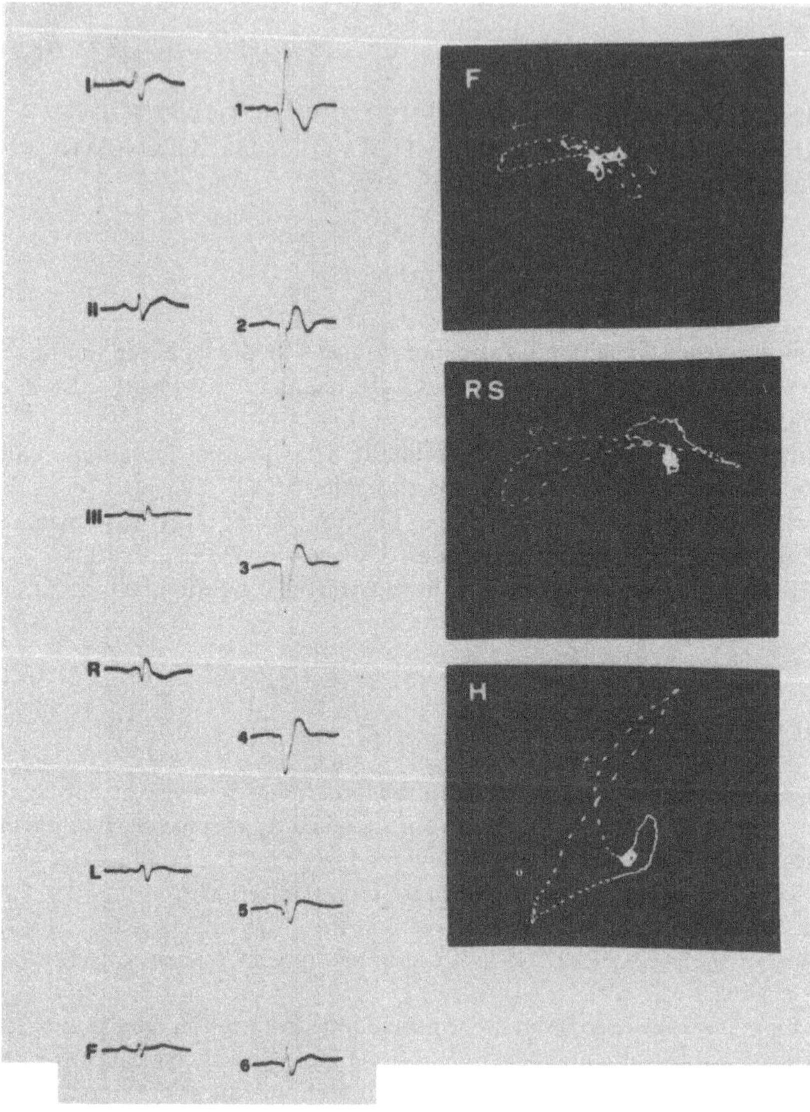

Figure 1. Right bundle branch block coexisting with healed anteroseptal and lateral myocardial infarction. The RBBB is evident in lead V_1 by the tall R′ wave and in the horizontal plane of the vectorcardiogram by the delayed terminal appendix oriented rightward and anteriorly. Infarctional Q waves are present in V_2-V_5. In the horizontal plane the first vectors are directed rightward and posteriorly with clockwise rotation, an expression of anteroseptal and lateral myocardial infarction

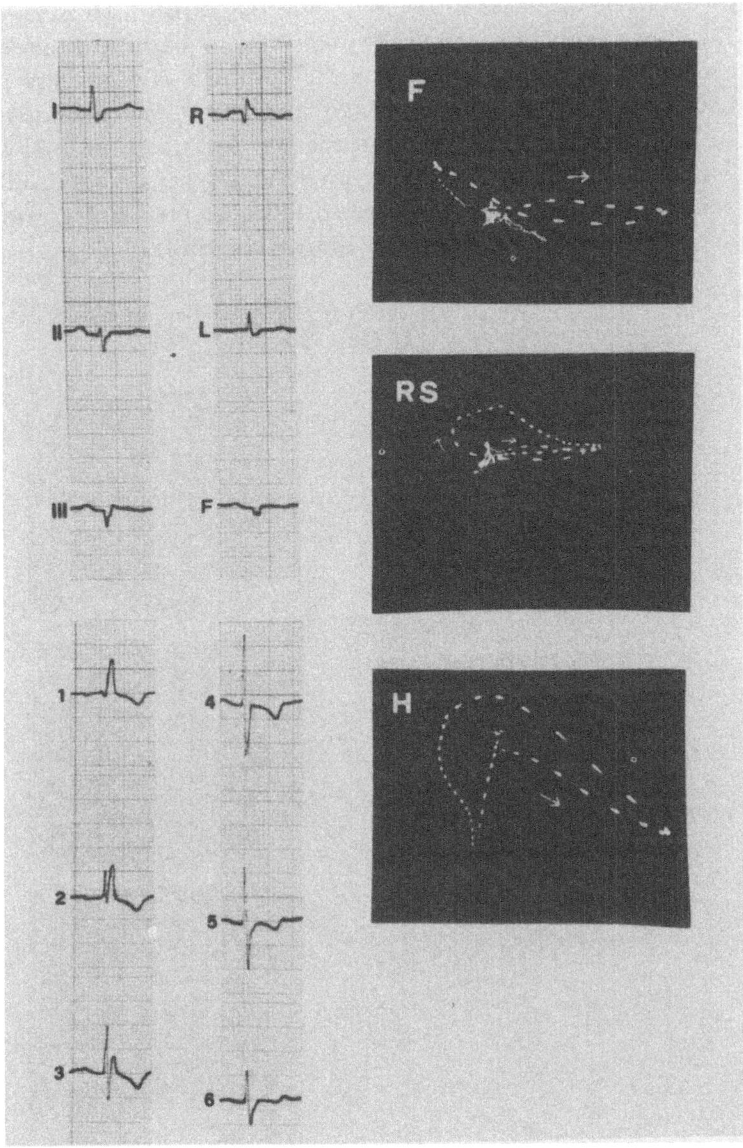

Figure 2. Right bundle branch block coexisting with healed inferior myocardial infarction. RBBB is clearly evident in V_1-V_2 leads and in the H plane of the vectorcardiogram. QS morphology in III and aVF leads and a large initial deflection of the frontal QRS loop, oriented superiorly with clockwise rotation, are diagnostic of inferior myocardial infarction

causing them to be displaced anteriorly. Since the RBBB itself often shifts the middle forces anteriorly, it is practically impossible to diagnose a coexisting posterior myocardial infarction (Figure 3) in the ECG and VCG tracings.

In rare cases in which the initial forces are markedly shifted anteriorly from the RBBB, an anteroseptal myocardial infarction may be partially or totally canceled out (Figures 4 and 5). Some authors [1], even though they do not proffer pathophysiological explanations, have encountered difficulties in several cases in diagnosing a healed anteroseptal infarction coexisting with RBBB.

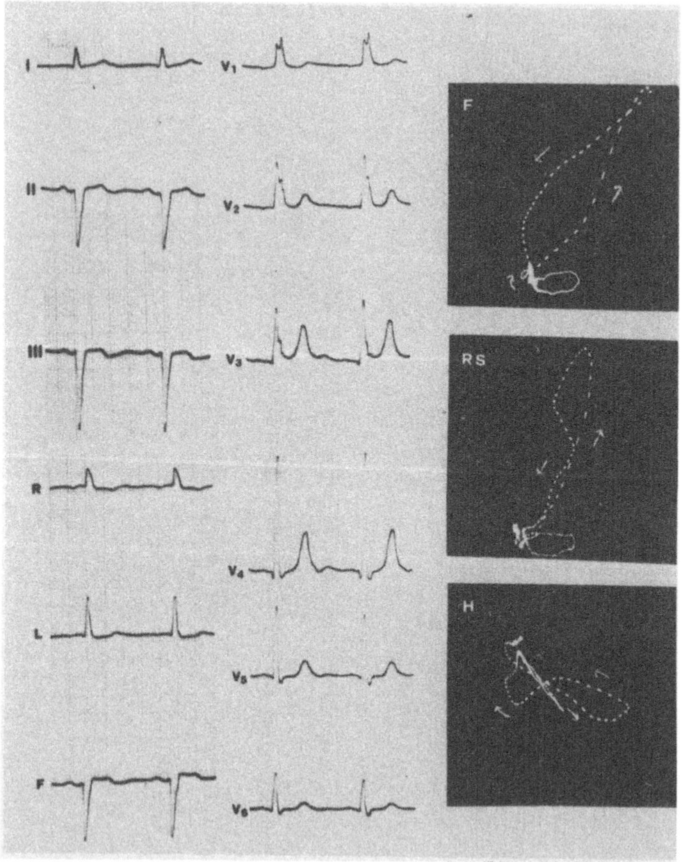

Figure 3. Electrocardiogram shows anterior fascicular block and right bundle branch block pattern. However the S wave in lead V_6 – which is generally deep in the presence of these two blocks – is very small. In the frontal plane of the vectorcardiogram the first part of the QRS loop shows clockwise rotation. Such an element in the presence of AFB is suggestive of coexisting inferior myocardial infarction. In the horizontal plane the middle forces are displaced markedly anteriorly, but only slightly rightward; the latter, together with the small S wave in lead V_6, contrasts with an RBBB. Coronary arteriograms and ventricular angiograms showed an inferior and posterobasal myocardial akinesis. On the basis of the above-mentioned electrical and radiological data, we may diagnose an AFB, a posterior and inferior infarction with peri-infarction block

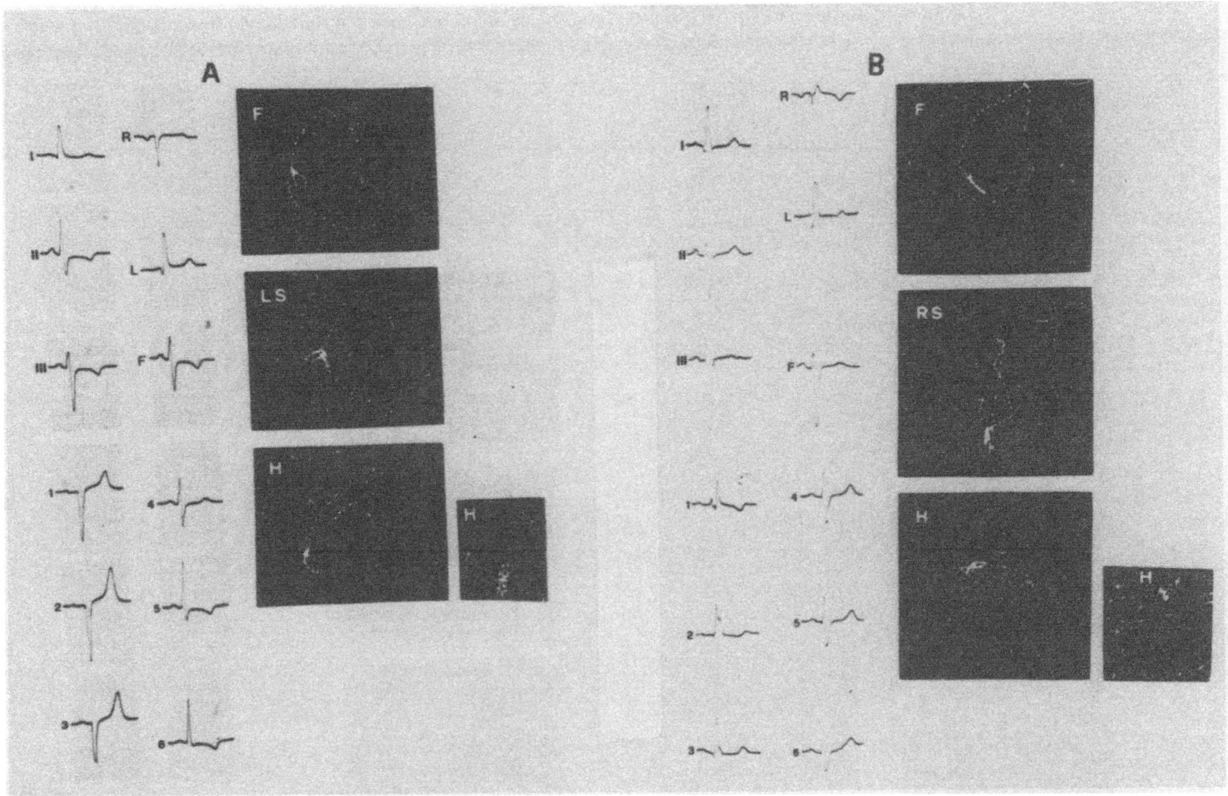

Figure 4. A: A healed anteroseptal infarction is evident in both electrocardiographic and vectorcardiographic tracings. A left axis deviation is present (ÂQRS: −20°) probably related to an incomplete anterior fascicular block. B: ECG and VCG tracing registered 7 months later. The appearance of RBBB and AFB is observed. Owing to marked anterior shifting of the initial-middle forces of the QRS complex, as is evident in the horizontal plane of the VCG, the anteroseptal necrosis is canceled out. Only a small q wave in V_2-V_3 leads persists, on the other hand, frequently in the presence of AFB

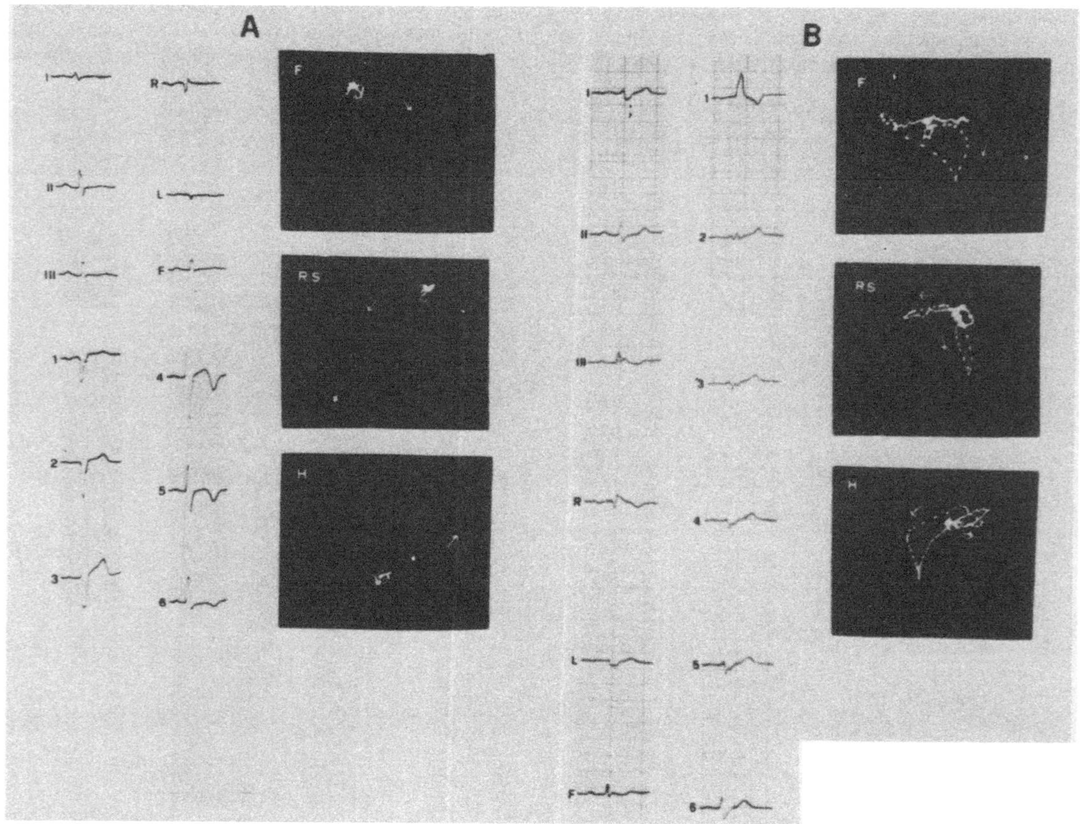

Figure 5. A: An old anteroseptal myocardial infarction is evident in the electrocardiogram and vectorcardiogram. B: Tracings registered 3 years later. The appearance of an RBBB is observed, which shifting anteriorly the initial-middle forces partially cancels out the myocardial infarction

In other cases, RBBB may simulate antero-septal or inferior wall infarction. In fact non-infarctional QR complexes may occur in leads V_1-V_2 and sometimes in leads III and aVF. Horan et al. [2] noted pathologic Q waves in 10 out of 40 cases of RBBB without anatomic evidence of infarction. This pattern was particularly common in acute right ventricular overload, probably in so far as the QR complexes reflect epicardial potentials from leads overlying the dilated right atrium [3]. However, QR complexes seen in the right precordial leads differ in several aspects from the infarctional Q waves. In pure RBBB, the right precordial QR complexes rarely extend beyond V_2, whereas in anteroseptal infarction coexisting with RBBB, Q waves are often seen in the mid to lateral precordial leads as well [4].

Although RBBB may be associated with non-infarctional QR complexes in leads III and aVF, it does not generally produce a significant Q wave in lead II. Therefore the presence of QR complexes in leads II, III and aVF suggests inferior wall infarction.

The Q waves in uncomplicated RBBB are usually sharply inscribed without notching or slurring. Conversely, in the majority of cases myocardial infarction deforms the initial forces to produce a characteristically notched or W-shaped Q wave.

LEFT BUNDLE BRANCH BLOCK

In the presence of left bundle branch block (LBBB) it is difficult and often impossible to detect a healed myocardial infarction. The main reasons are:

1) Septal depolarization occurs in a right-to-left direction and requires over 40 msec for completion [5]. As a result, the instantaneous QRS vectors during the first 20 msec of the QRS complex are oriented toward the left ventricle rather than away from it; the instantaneous QRS vectors appearing during the next 20 msec are also directed to the left and posteriorly, whether the left ventricular free wall happens to be infarcted or not.
2) Since activation of left ventricle free wall does not commence in LBBB until about the second half of the QRS interval [5], the electrical effects of a free wall infarction likwise do not appear until this portion of the QRS interval. The diagnostic signs of infarction can thus be lost. In other words, abnormal Q waves cannot appear in the left precordial or extremity leads in LBBB even in the presence of infarction.

   The electrocardiographic and vectorcardiographic signs suggestive of LBBB coexisting with healed myocardial infarction are reported in Table 1.

Septal myocardial infarction

Septal myocardial infarction in the left part of the septum usually abolishes the

Table 1. Electrocardiographic and vectorcardiographic signs, suggestive of healed myocardial infarction coexisting with left bundle branch block

ELECTROCARDIOGRAM	VECTORCARDIOGRAM
Anteroseptal infarction	
– Q waves in leads I, aVL, and V_6 – QS, qrS or QrS patterns in leads V_3 and V_4 – Progressive diminution in amplitude of the r wave from leads V_1 to V_4	– First vectors of the horizontal QRS loop oriented rightward, anteriorly or posteriorly
Infarction of the left ventricular free wall	
– RS morphology in left-sided leads – W-shaped deflection in leads V_4 and V_5 – Decrease in the middle slurring in the left-sided leads	– Displacement to the right of the efferent limbs of the horizontal QRS loop – Counterclockwise rotation of the horizontal QRS loop – Irregularities of the horizontal QRS loop – Decrease in the middle slurring in the three planes
Inferior infarction	
– QR morphology in the inferior leads – rSr morphology in leads III and aVF – qRS morphology in the inferior leads – Initial r wave in lead aVR	– Clockwise inscription of the first part of the frontal QRS loop – Superior displacement of the frontal QRS loop – Irregularities of the frontal QRS loop

electric forces caused by right-to-left septal depolarization, therefore allowing electric forces, presumably arising in the right ventricle, to dominate the electric field of the heart. Consequently, the initial and early leftward-directed vectors characteristic of LBBB are shifted to the right and can project Q waves of varying depth and width on leads I, aVL and V_6 [5, 6].

In lead V_1 these vectors produce an initial R wave which is maximal in this lead and diminishes in amplitude from right to left across most of the precordium (Figures 6 and 7). The reversal in the R wave transition is related to the fact that as a result of the infarction, the vectors of the first 40 msec of the QRS complex are oriented to the right, while subsequent vectors develop to the left and posteriorly, i.e. away from the other precordial leads. When after considerable delay left ventricular activation commences, the vectors appearing after 40 msec are oriented toward the left ventricle, just as in uncomplicated LBBB, and these vectors project terminal R waves on leads I, aVL and V_6.

Experimental studies suggest that when the necrosis extends to the right part of the septum, the first QRS vectors are oriented to the right and posteriorly due to the prevalence of the electric forces of the free wall of the right ventricle on the

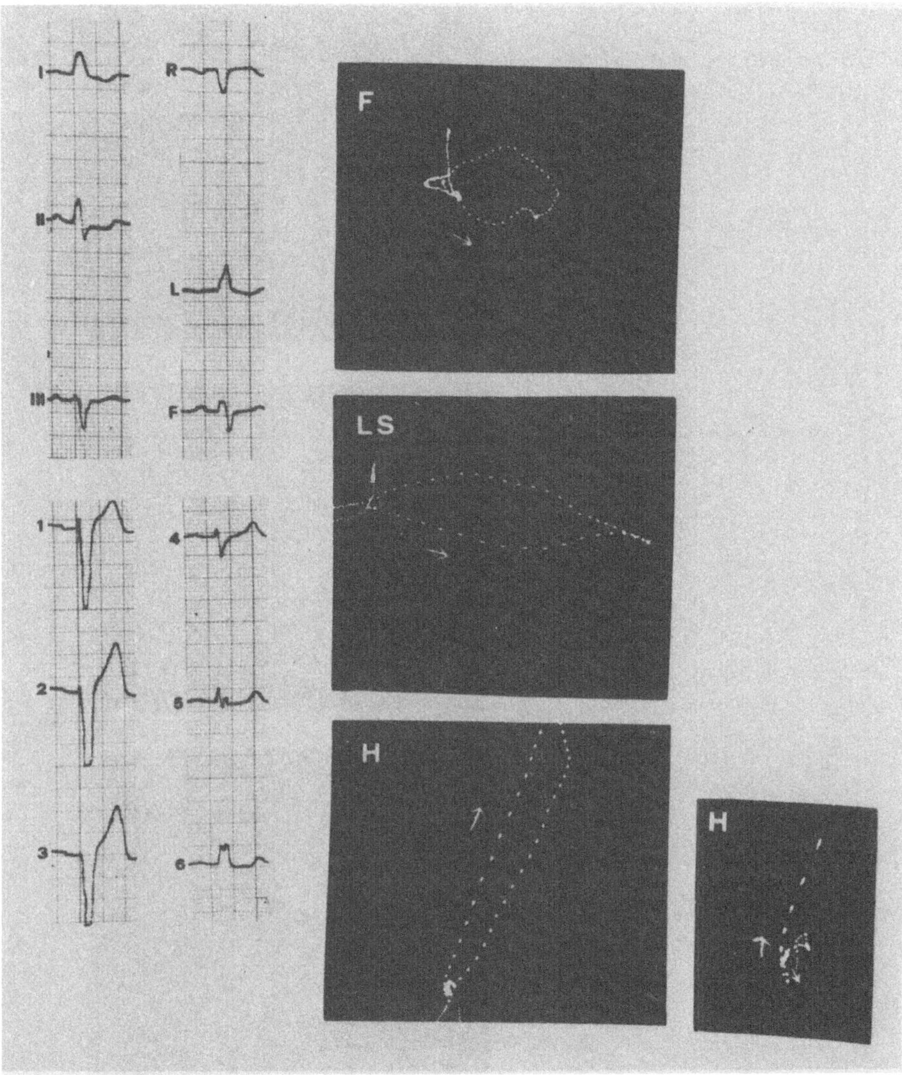

Figure 6. **Left bundle branch block complicated by septal myocardial infarction. Patient with a typical** history of acute myocardial infarction. QRS complex measures 130 msec and its configuration is compatible with LBBB. In the electrocardiogram the initial r wave diminishes in amplitude from V_1 to V_3 and in the vectorcardiogram the first vectors are oriented rightward and anteriorly. These findings are indicative of coexisting septal myocardial infarction. After this abnormality, the remainder of the QRS loop displays the usual features of LBBB

septal ones and of the posterior forces on the anterior ones [7]. In such cases a QS morphology in V_1-V_2 and the appearance of Q waves in the left precordial leads are observed.

In some cases isolated LBBB can simulate a septal myocardial infarction.

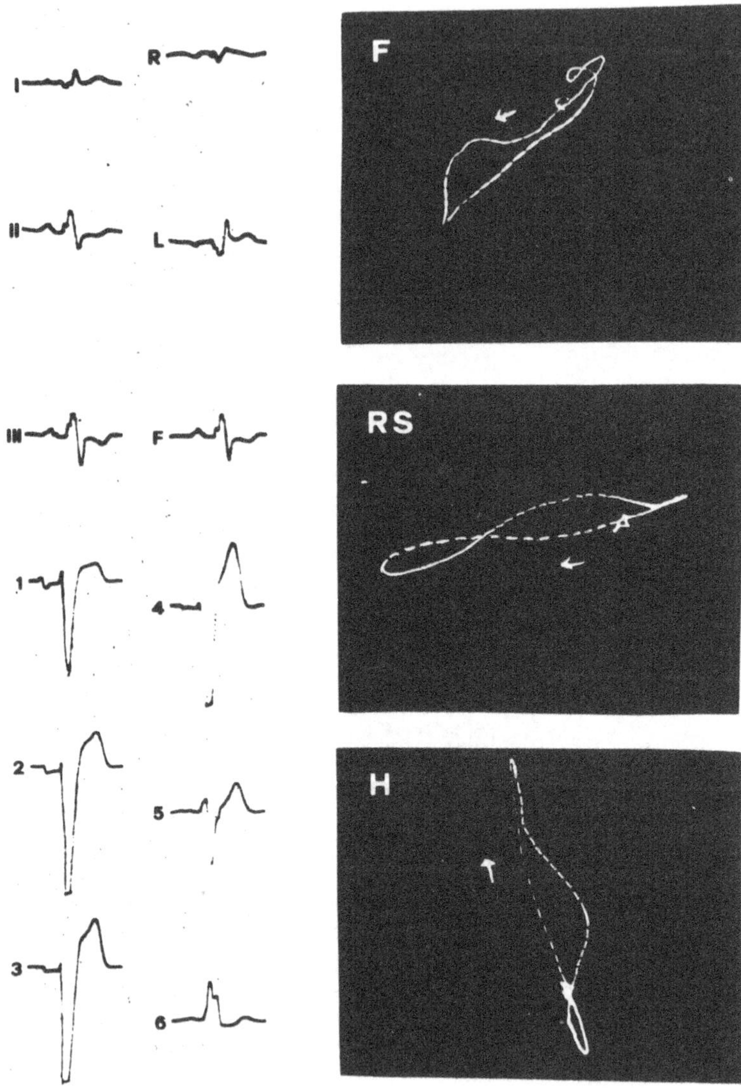

Figure 7. Electrocardiographic and vectorcardiographic findings of left bundle branch block complicated by anteroseptal myocardial infarction. Patient with a typical history of acute myocardial infarction. QRS complex measures 160 msec; its configuration is compatible with LBBB. In the electrocardiogram a slurred Q wave is evident in leads I and aVL. The initial r wave diminishes in amplitude from V_1 to V_4. In the horizontal plane of the vectorcardiogram the first vectors are oriented rightward and posteriorly. These findings are indicative of coexisting anteroseptal infarction. In the frontal and horizontal planes the middle forces of the QRS loop are displaced to the right, which is probably an expression of an extension of the myocardial infarction to lateral wall

Abnormal Q waves in left-sided leads, particularly in lead I are sometimes present in LBBB without myocardial infarction [8, 9] (Figure 8). Such waves have been observed above all in the presence of marked left or right axis deviation or of right ventricular enlargement (see Chapter 3). Such Q waves do not usually last 40 msec. The pathophysiology has not been clearly defined so far.

Even diminution in R wave amplitude from lead V_1 to the midprecordial leads [10] may be noted in the presence of septal infarction.

In rarer instances a non-infarctional QS complex may extend from lead V_1 as far left as lead V_5 or V_6 [10, 11] in relation to a concomitant marked right ventricular dilatation [4].

An opposite occurrence is not infrequent; that is, an LBBB can cancel out a healed septal infarction (Figure 9). The appearance of small r waves in right precordial leads may be related to unbalanced forces originating in the trabecular zone of the right ventricle [12].

The vectorcardiographic changes of LBBB coexisting with septal infarction appear in the horizontal plane, where the first QRS vectors are oriented to the right, anteriorly (Figure 6) or posteriorly (Figure 7) [5, 13]. After this abnormality, the remainder of the QRS loop displays the usual features of LBBB. The presence of first vectors oriented to the left and posteriorly may express a septal infarction, but this finding is frequent also in patients without such a necrosis and therefore has no diagnostic value (see Chapter 3).

The frontal QRS loop presents the same morphology as the uncomplicated LBBB.

Infarction of the left ventricular free wall

This infarction manifests after 30-40 msec from the onset of the QRS complex since the free wall of the left ventricle in the LBBB is activated tardily. The failure of the infarcted portion of the free wall to generate QRS potentials during the 40-80 msec of the QRS interval allows opposing forces to become dominant so that the late vectors are displaced away from the effective electrical site of the infarction. Therefore the displacement of the terminal vectors can only be recognized on the leads which, in the presence of LBBB, would be expected to register terminal positivity.

For this reason, free wall infarction in LBBB can usually be detected only if it produces terminal S waves in leads I, aVL, V_5 and V_6 (Figure 10). In free wall infarction such leads, which prior to infarction had recorded the wide R waves typical of LBBB, afterwards typically display RS morphology, the initial R wave resulting from undisturbed right-to-left septal depolarization and the terminal S wave reflecting the lateral wall infarction [14].

Due to reduction in the excitable left ventricular mass the middle slurring of the QRS may decrease in both the leftsided leads of the ECG and in the three planes of

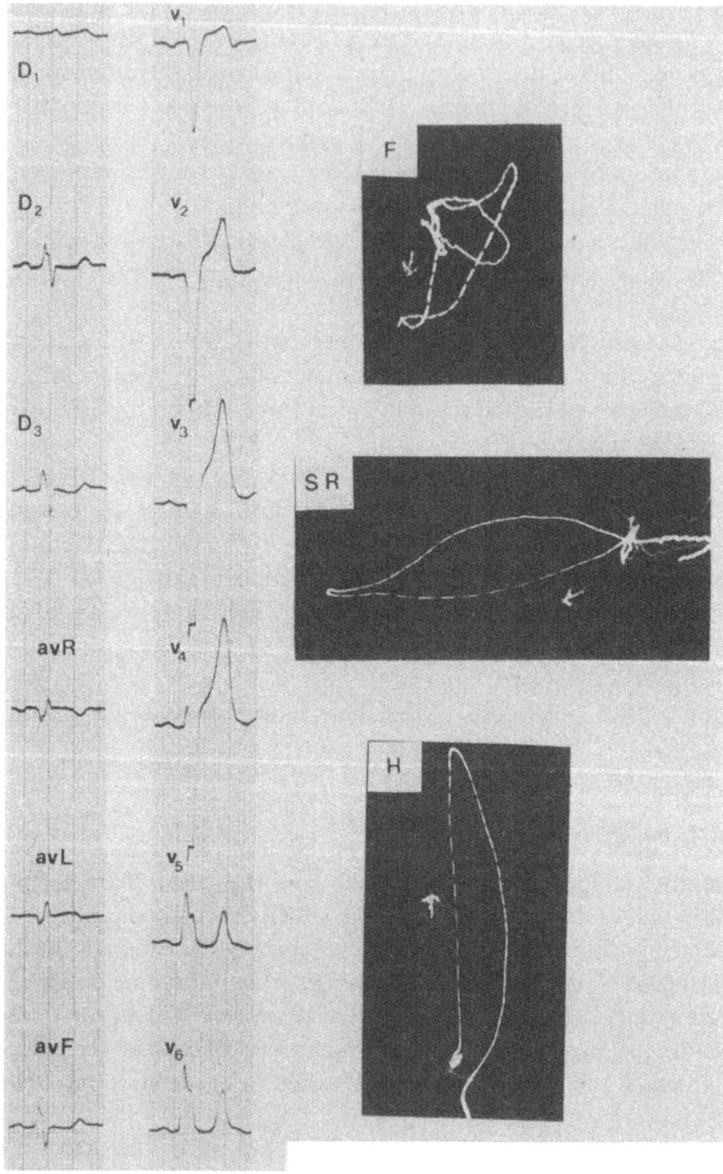

Figure 8. Left bundle branch block with Q wave in lead aVL without healed myocardial infarction. QRS complex measures 130 msec and its configuration is compatible with LBBB. In lead aVL, a QR morphology is present. In the horizontal plane of the vectorcardiogram the first vectors are directed rightward and posteriorly and the middle forces of the QRS loop are displaced rightward. Coronary arteriograms did not show critical stenosis and ventricular angiograms did not show any segmental abnormalities. Pulmonary emphysema and right ventricular enlargement were present

the VCG [7]. In some cases, however, the presence of an LBBB coexisting with anterolateral myocardial infarction may be doubtful.

In several cases S waves in left-sided leads may appear in uncomplicated LBBB [9, 10] (Figure 11). There are various reasons for this:

a) In patients with right ventricular enlargement a displacement of the transition zone between V_6 and V_7, with subsequent persistence of the S wave in V_6 was frequently observed [9]. A displacement towards the left of the transition zone is in fact frequent in subjects with LBBB and acute pulmonary embolism. For this reason precordial leads should be recorded farther to the left of lead V_6 to confirm or refute this possibility.

b) In the presence of LBBB with left axis deviation (LAD), the terminal forces are directed markedly superiorly and the lead V_6, exploring the latero-inferior wall of the left ventricle, can record terminal negative deflections.

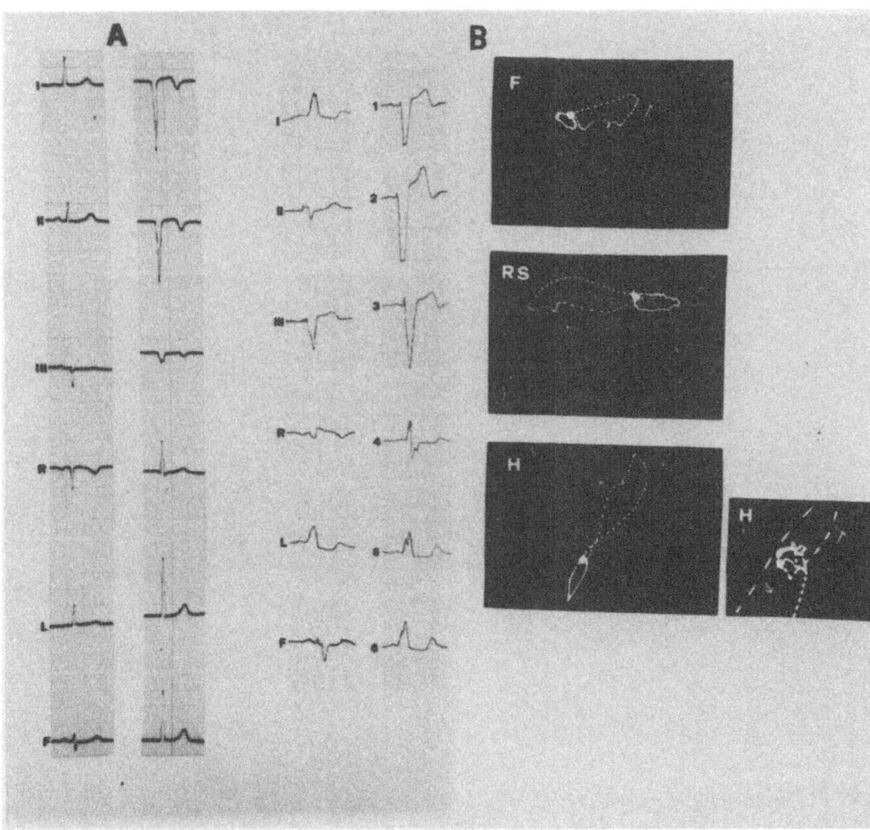

Figure 9. **A: Electrocardiogram shows a healed anteroseptal myocardial infarction. B: Electrocardiogram and vectorcardiogram registered 18 months later.** The appearance of a left bundle branch block is evident. The signs of septal infarction are no longer evident. In both tracings, in fact, the QRS complex is typical of an uncomplicated LBBB

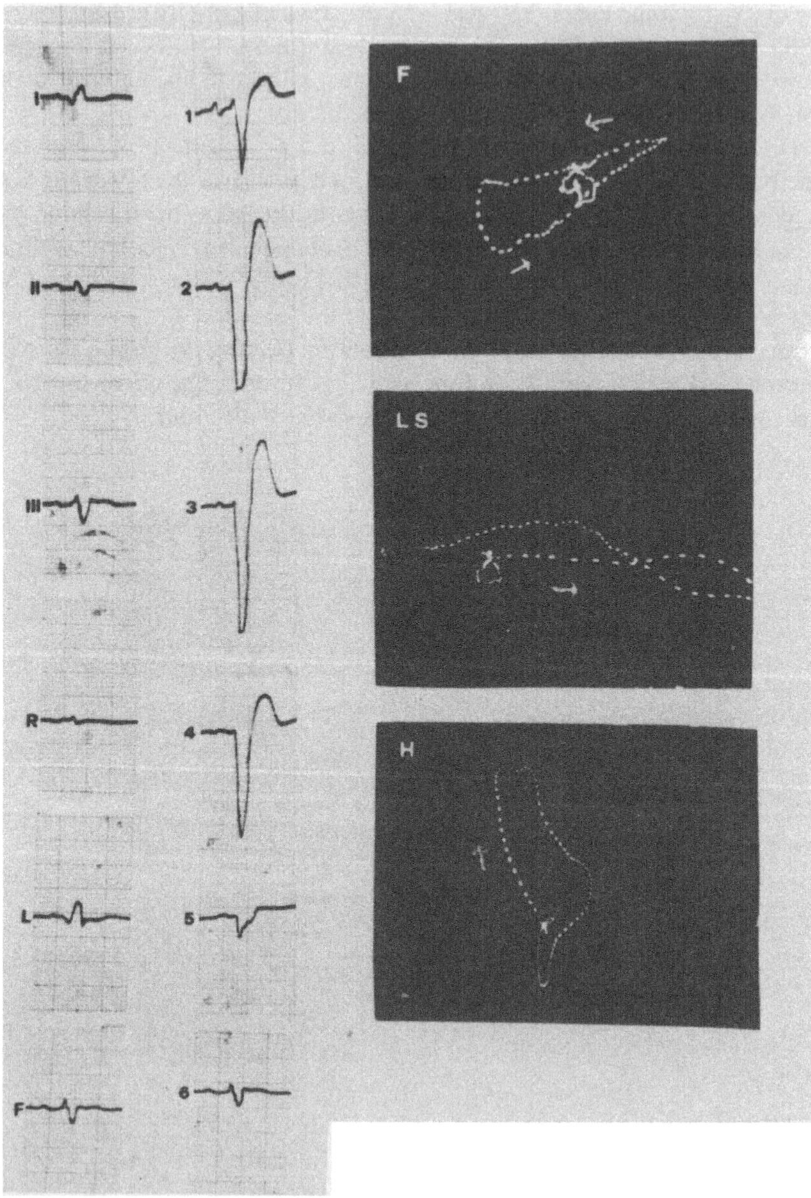

Figure 10. Left bundle branch block coexisting with myocardial infarction of the left ventricular free wall. Patient with a typical history of acute myocardial infarction. In electrocardiographic and vectorcardiographic tracings, QRS complex measures 150 msec and shows LBBB. In lead aVL, an S wave is present and in lead V_6 an rS morphology. In the frontal and horizontal planes of the VCG the middle QRS forces are displaced to the right. These findings are indicative of coexisting free wall infarction. Owing to the presence in the ECG of Q waves in leads I and aVL and the reduction of the r wave from V_1 to V_5, an anteroseptal necrotic area is also likely

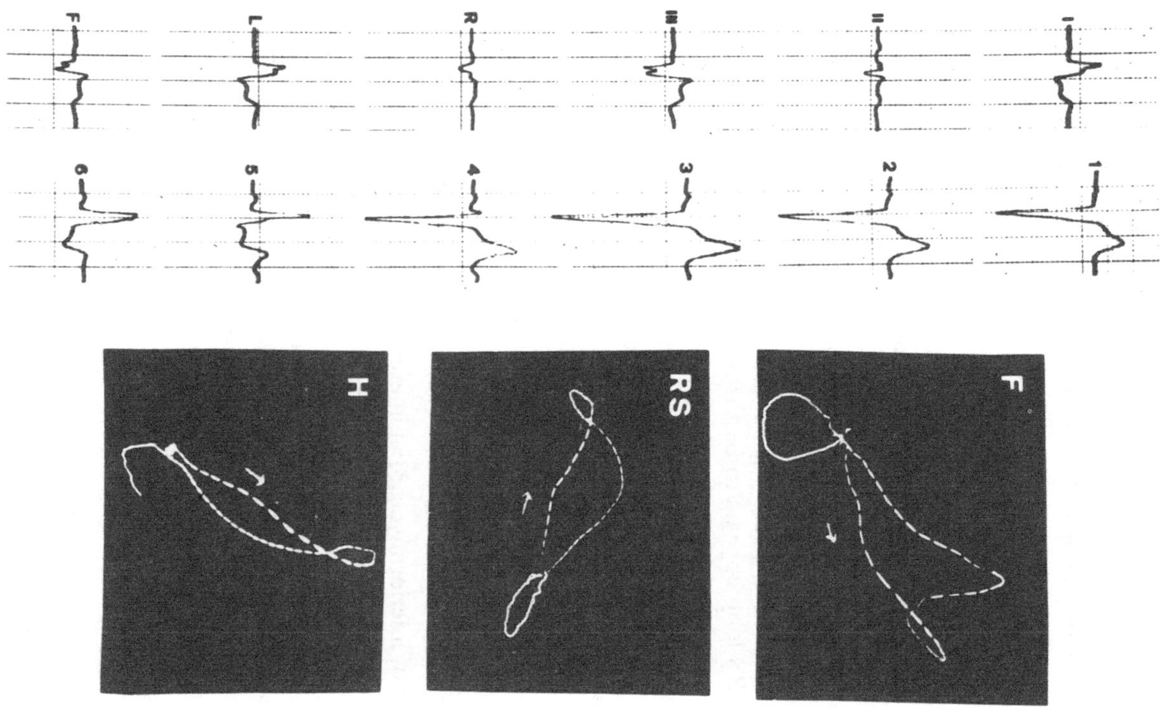

Figure 11. QRS complex in electrocardiographic and vectorcardiographic recordings measures 160 msec and shows left bundle branch block pattern. A myo-cardial infarction localized in free wall and in inferior wall is suspicious, the former because of the presence of S wave in leads I and aVL, the latter because of a QR morphology in lead III and aVF and because of a completely superior displacement of the frontal QRS loop. Coronary arteriograms did not show critical stenosis and ventricular angiograms did not show any segmental abnormalities

c) Often the exploring electrode of lead V_6 is more or less routinely applied below the transverse plane through the cardiac dipole center. Since the indifferent electrode of lead V_6 is at the central terminal or, in effect, at the electrical center of the heart, the low position of the chest electrode causes the axis of the lead V_6 to be tilted downward. This in turn may cause the portion of the QRS loop in LBBB to project on the negative rather than the positive half of the axis of lead V_6. To determine whether this factor is responsible for the presence of a terminal S wave in lead V_6, the latter lead can be recorded one intercostal space higher.

The vectorcardiographic changes are best appreciated in the horizontal plane. The first vectors of the QRS loop are oriented as in the uncomplicated LBBB but the afferent limb is displaced to the right and the efferent limb can present marked irregularities.

Such a displacement to the right of the efferent limbs in the presence of LBBB is not, however, specific since it can be observed in patients with pulmonary embolism or right ventricular hypertrophy [15] (see Chapter 3). A counterclockwise horizontal QRS loop appears to be the most specific VCG sign of the left ventricular free wall infarction in the presence of LBBB pattern [14] (Figure 12).

If there is septal as well as free wall infarction, leads I, aVL and V_6 may display notched QR, qR or qrS complexes. In addition, W-shaped deflections may appear in leads V_4 and V_5 [1, 5] (Figure 13).

In the vectorcardiogram both the first vectors and the efferent limb of the horizontal QRS loop can be displaced to the right.

Inferior myocardial infarction

The diagnosis of inferior myocardial infarction coexisting with LBBB remains an unresolved problem. Various authors [2, 8, 16] think that a QS morphology in leads II, III or aVF is highly suggestive of an inferior wall infarction. Other authors do not attribute any diagnostic value to such a morphology [11, 17-19]. Five patients reported by Timmis et al. [18] demonstrated disappearance of Q waves in inferior leads on spontaneous reversal of LBBB to normal conduction. These authors think that these Q waves represent a postdivisional conduction variant most closely equivalent to anterior fascicular block (AFB) coexisting with predivisional LBBB. However, at present this explanation still remains speculative.

Recently Izumi et al. [19] compared ECGs and VCGs of 12 patients with LBBB and inferior infarction to ECGs and VCGs of 10 patients with LBBB and no infarction. Inferior infarction was diagnosed on the basis of a typical history and inferior surface perfusion defect on thallium-201 imaging. The presence of QR complex in II, III or aVF, irrespective of the size of the Q wave, appeared specific for infarction, but identified only five out of 12 (42%).

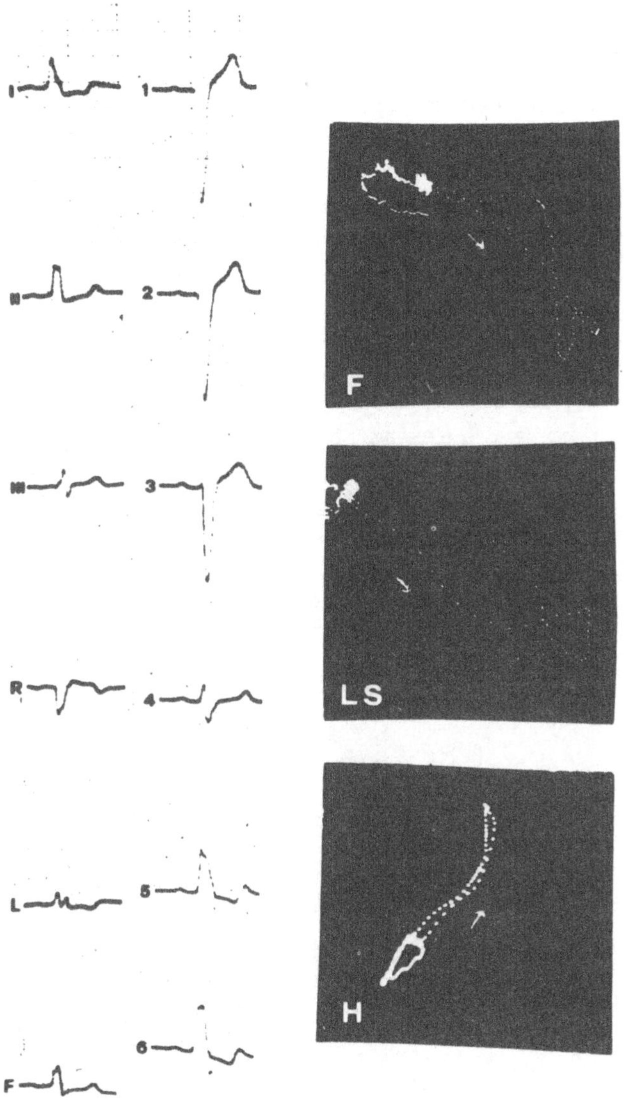

Figure 12. Electrocardiogram shows an uncomplicated left bundle branch block pattern (QRS: 160 msec). In the horizontal plane of the vectorcardiogram the QRS loop shows counterclockwise rotation. Such a pattern is indicative of coexisting myocardial infarction of the free wall. Ventricular angiograms evidenced a lateral dyskinesis

According to our experience a QR morphology in the diaphragmatic leads is not specific since it can be found also in the absence of inferior infarction (Figure 11). In some patients in whom LBBB appeared after the acute inferior myocardial infarction and in others in whom the inferior infarction was diagnosed after coronarographic and angiographic examinations, we observed an rSr morphology in leads III and/or aVF (Figures 14, 15 and 16). We have never observed such a pattern in patients with LBBB without a history of myocardial infarction.

When such an ECG pattern is present, in the frontal plane of the VCG one observes a marked QRS loop irregularity (Figures 14, 15 and 16). We believe this ECG finding is highly characteristic of the inferior myocardial infarction coexisting with LBBB even if at present its exact specificity and sensitivity is not known.

In our experience a qrS morphology in the diaphragmatic leads is also highly suggestive of inferior myocardial infarction coexisting with LBBB (Figure 17).

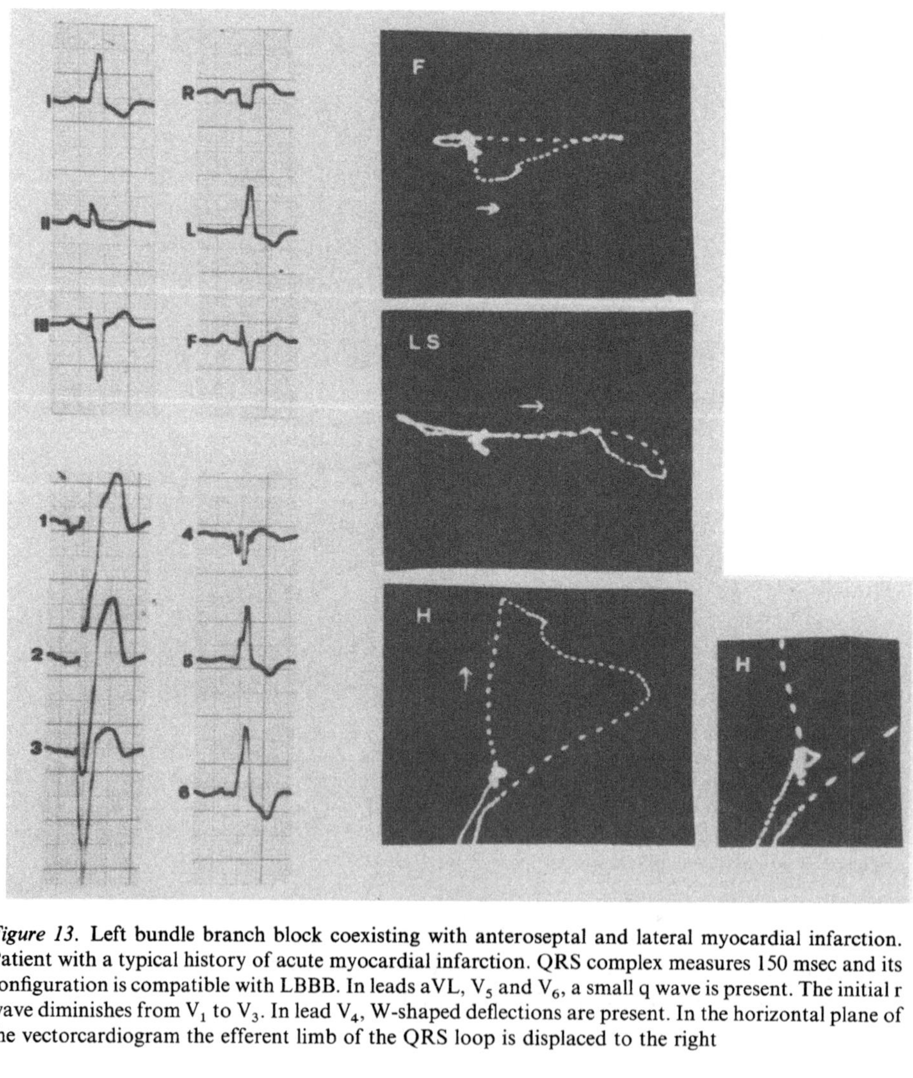

Figure 13. Left bundle branch block coexisting with anteroseptal and lateral myocardial infarction. Patient with a typical history of acute myocardial infarction. QRS complex measures 150 msec and its configuration is compatible with LBBB. In leads aVL, V_5 and V_6, a small q wave is present. The initial r wave diminishes from V_1 to V_3. In lead V_4, W-shaped deflections are present. In the horizontal plane of the vectorcardiogram the efferent limb of the QRS loop is displaced to the right

Particular importance was attributed to the presence of an initial r wave in aVR.

In some cases LBBB may mask the Q waves of a true inferior myocardial infarction [16], since it can induce an r wave in the diaphragmatic leads, shifting inferiorly the first vectors.

The vectorcardiographic changes are best appreciated in the frontal plane. A

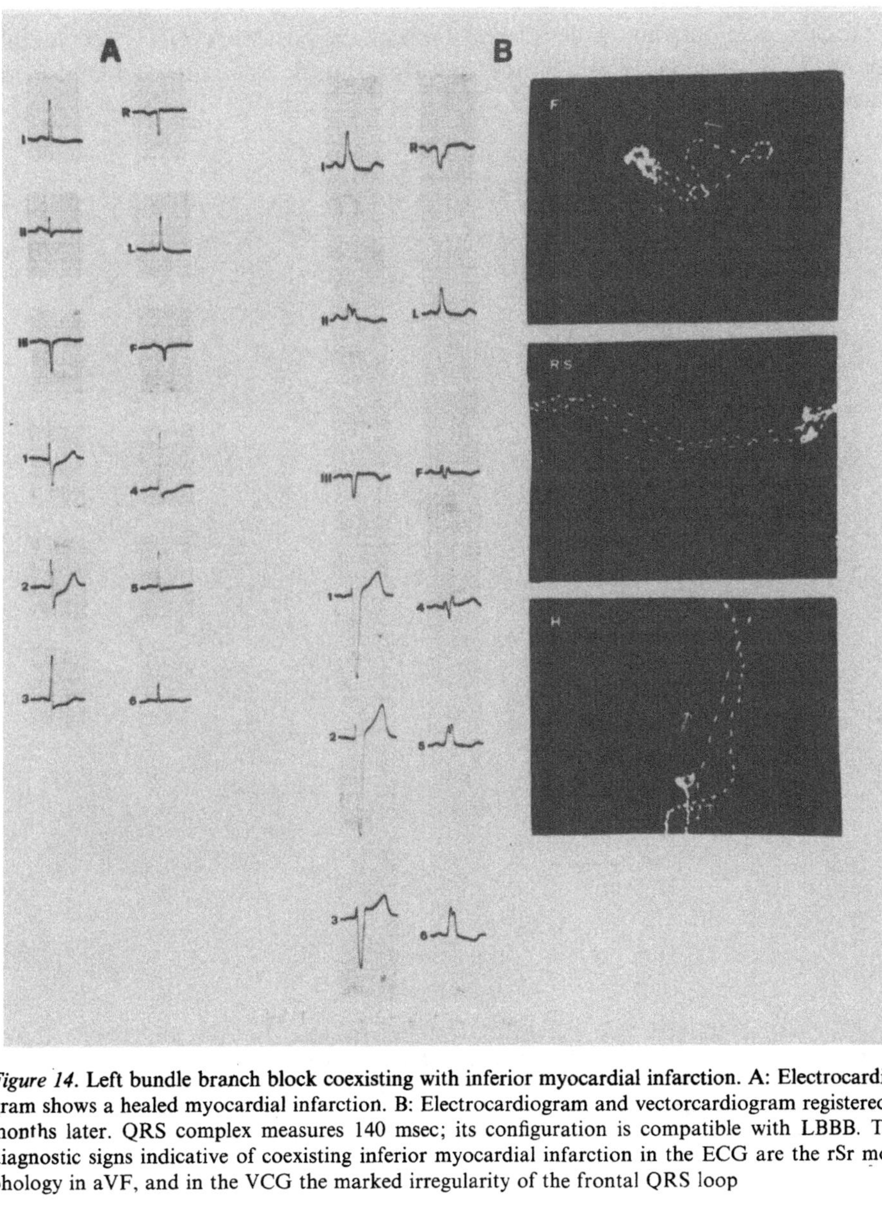

Figure 14. **Left bundle branch block coexisting with inferior myocardial infarction.** A: Electrocardiogram shows a healed myocardial infarction. B: Electrocardiogram and vectorcardiogram registered 4 months later. QRS complex measures 140 msec; its configuration is compatible with LBBB. The diagnostic signs indicative of coexisting inferior myocardial infarction in the ECG are the rSr morphology in aVF, and in the VCG the marked irregularity of the frontal QRS loop

clockwise rotation of the first part of the QRS loop with or without superior orientation of the 10, 20 and 30 msec vectors has been suggested as a highly suspicious sign [20] (Figures 16, 17 and 18). Irregular inscriptions of the frontal QRS loop is often present [6] (Figures 14, 15, 16 and 17). A significant reduction has been observed in the magnitude of the instantaneous 10, 20, 30, 40 and maximum QRS vectors [19].

When the myocardial infarction extends to the postero-basal wall of the left ventricle a delay of the whole afferent limb of the horizontal QRS loop may be observed [7]. This VCG sign is not, however, specific as it can be found in the uncomplicated LBBB.

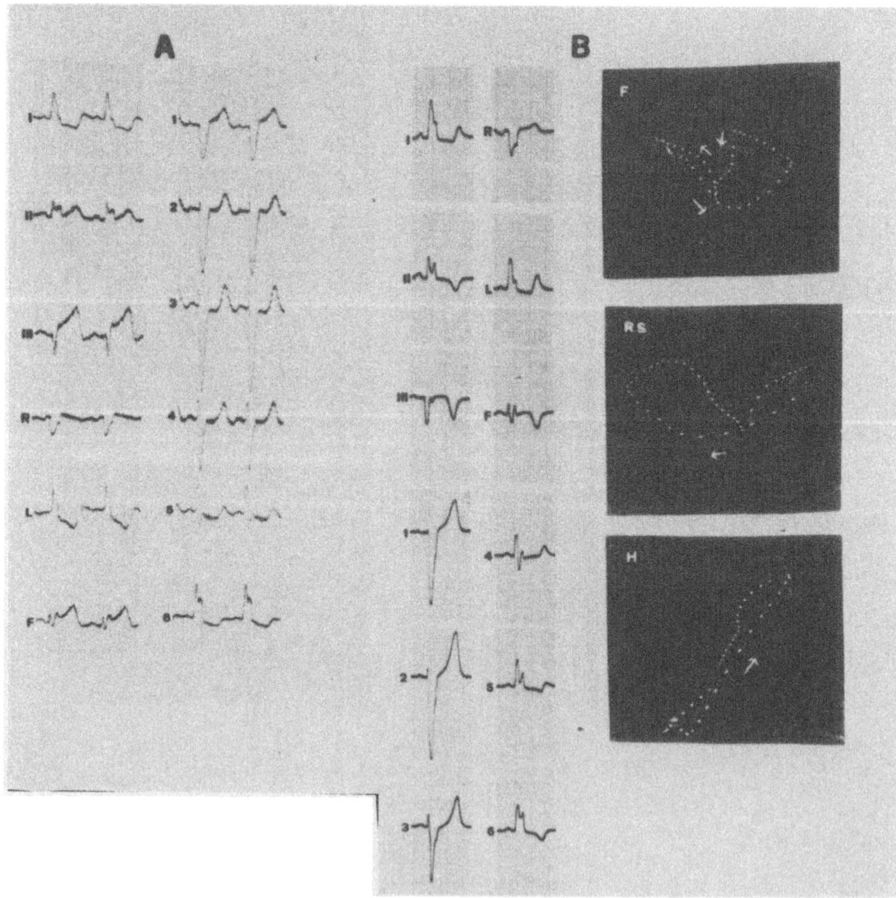

Figure 15. Left bundle branch block coexisting with inferior myocardial infarction. QRS complex shows LBBB. In leads III and aVF elevated ST segment is evident. B: Electrocardiogram and vectorcardiogram registered after two days. In lead III the r wave disappears and the T wave becomes negative. The myocardial infarction can therefore be located in the inferior wall. In lead aVF an rSr morphology is present and in the VCG the frontal QRS loop shows marked irregularities. Horizontal QRS loop shows clockwise rotation: this finding is indicative of coexisting lateral wall infarction

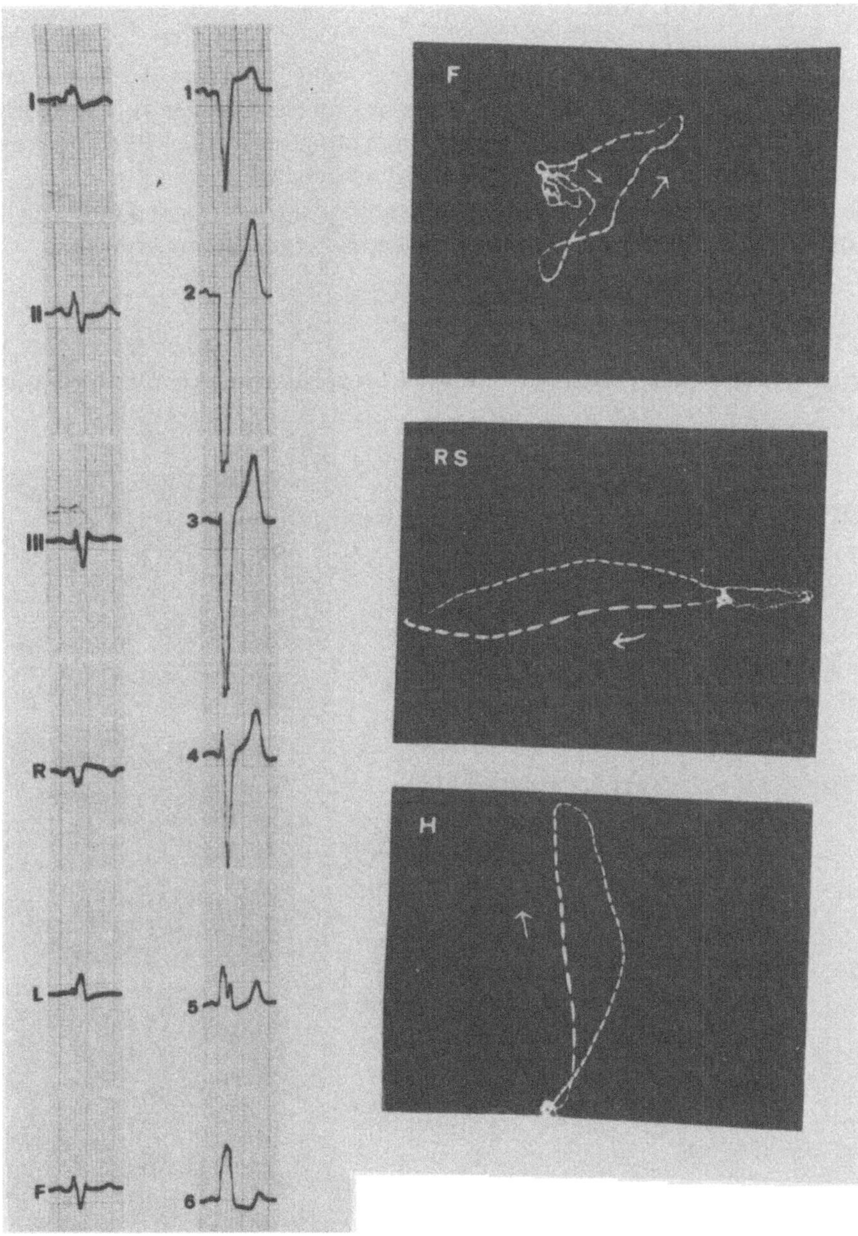

Figure 16. **Left bundle branch block coexisting with inferior myocardial infarction. Patient with a** typical history of acute myocardial infarction. QRS complex measures 130 msec and its configuration is compatible with LBBB. In leads III and aVF, rSr morphology is present. In the vectorcardiogram the frontal QRS loop evidences marked irregularities; the first part of such a loop shows clockwise rotation. These findings are highly indicative of coexisting inferior infarction, documented by coronary arteriograms and ventricular angiograms

ANTERIOR FASCICULAR BLOCK

The anterior fascicular block causes an asynchronous left ventricular activation due to delayed excitation of the antero-superior wall (see Chapter 4). This block induces QRS alterations more modest than those produced by the LBBB and only rarely can it obscure or simulate a myocardial infarction.

The AFB coexisting with healed myocardial infarction has received little attention and consequently various diagnostic problems remain unresolved so far.

Anteroseptal myocardial infarction

In reported cases of intermittent AFB, R wave progression in precordial leads was

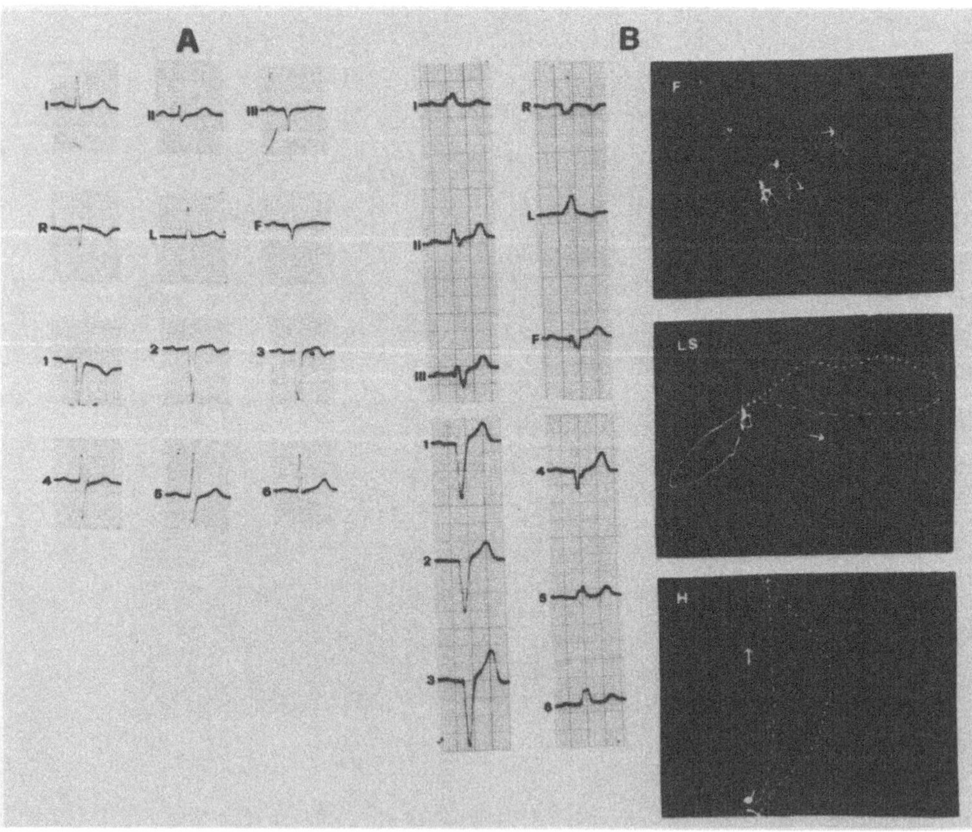

Figure 17. **Left bundle branch block coexisting with inferior myocardial infarction. A: The electrocardiogram shows a healed inferior wall infarction.** B: Electrocardiogram and vectorcardiogram registered 8 months later. The appearance of an LBBB is observed (QRS = 160 msec). The signs indicative of the myocardial infarction are, in the ECG, the qrS morphology in leads III and aFV and in the VCG the frontal QRS loop, which shows marked irregularities and clockwise rotation of its first part

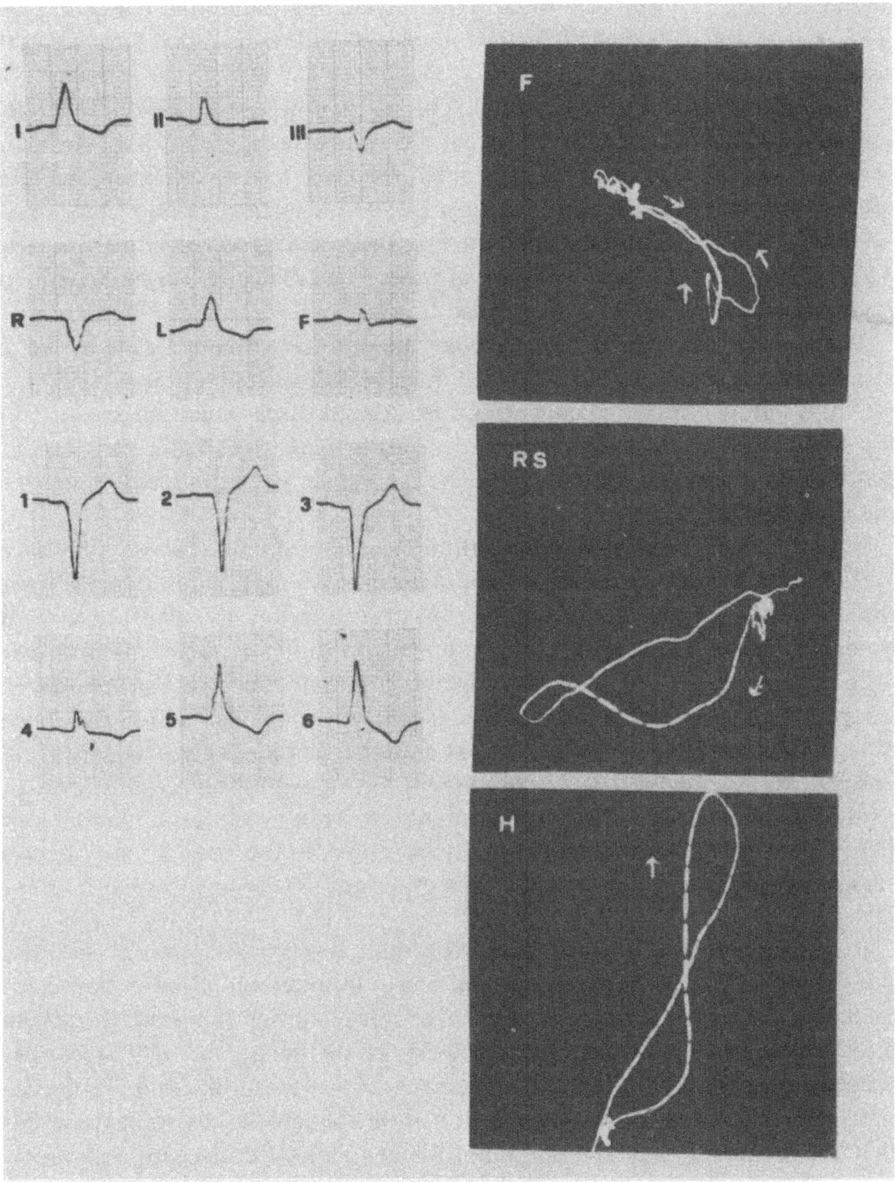

Figure 18. Left bundle branch block coexisting with inferior myocardial infarction. Patient without history of acute myocardial infarction. Electrocardiogram shows an uncomplicated LBBB. In the vectorcardiogram the clockwise rotation on the first part of the frontal QRS loop suggests a coexisting inferior infarction, documented by coronary arteriograms and ventricular angiograms

unaffected [21, 22]. Thus an anteroseptal myocardial infarction coexisting with AFB is generally recognizable by the presence of wide and slurred Q waves in the right and transitional precordial leads (Figures 19 and 20).

There is one recent case reported [23] of a patient whose scalar electrocardiogram showed anterior fascicular block and QS complexes in leads V_2-V_3. Normal R wave progression was recorded only when the chest leads were taken one interspace lower than usual. A vectorcardiogram showed normal anterior forces in the horizontal plane. The authors attributed the precordial Q waves in this case to the AFB. However, until more substantial proof is available, QS complexes in the right chest leads should not be ascribed to AFB.

The anterior fascicular block is recognizable in the extremity leads by the left axis deviation, together with a delayed intrinsecoid deflection time in aVL ($>$ 50 msec). A left axis deviation coexisting with AFB is of particular diagnostic value for AFB, since in most cases, anterior necrosis tends to shift the electrical axis downwards due to loss of left forces and consequently electric predominance of the right ventricle.

In 13.7% of cases an AFB induces the appearance of small q waves in leads V_2-V_3 [24], which could simulate an anteroseptal myocardial infarction. However, these q waves are thpically small and of short duration (20 msec or less). We observed that AFB represents a facilitating but not sufficient factor for the appearance of q waves in V_2-V_3 leads if a concomitant septal fibrosis is not present (see Chapter 4). Theoretically such fibrosis, if marked, could also induce the appearance of infarctional Q waves in the right and/or transitional precordial leads. It is possible that various tracings, considered to be an expression of AFB coexisting with healed anteroseptal myocardial infarction, actually express a marked septal fibrosis. In fact, no clearcut limit exists from the electric point of view between septal fibrosis, chronic myocardial infarction and healed myocardial infarction [25].

Rosenbaum et al. [21] believe that when those q waves disappear in chest leads one interspace below the conventional level, an anteroseptal infarction can be excluded,.whereas when they can also be recorded in lower chest leads they express a real anteroseptal infarction. In our experience the smaller the right precordial q waves, the more likely it is that they disappear in low precordial leads. In the cases in which those waves do not disappear it is not possible to discriminate whether they are related to a marked septal fibrosis or to a healed myocardial infarction.

In very rare cases an AFB can produce r waves in the right precordial leads on a previous QS pattern, thus concealing the signs of healed septal infarction [21, 26, 27]. The explanation is not simple. One interpretation was offered by Horwitz et al. [27]. The first normal septal vectors originate within the left mid septal mass. In the event of necrosis of the left septal portion, this vector diminishes or disappears on the ECG and VCG and QS complexes are registered on the right precordial leads. If the infarction extends to the antero-inferior portion of the right septal

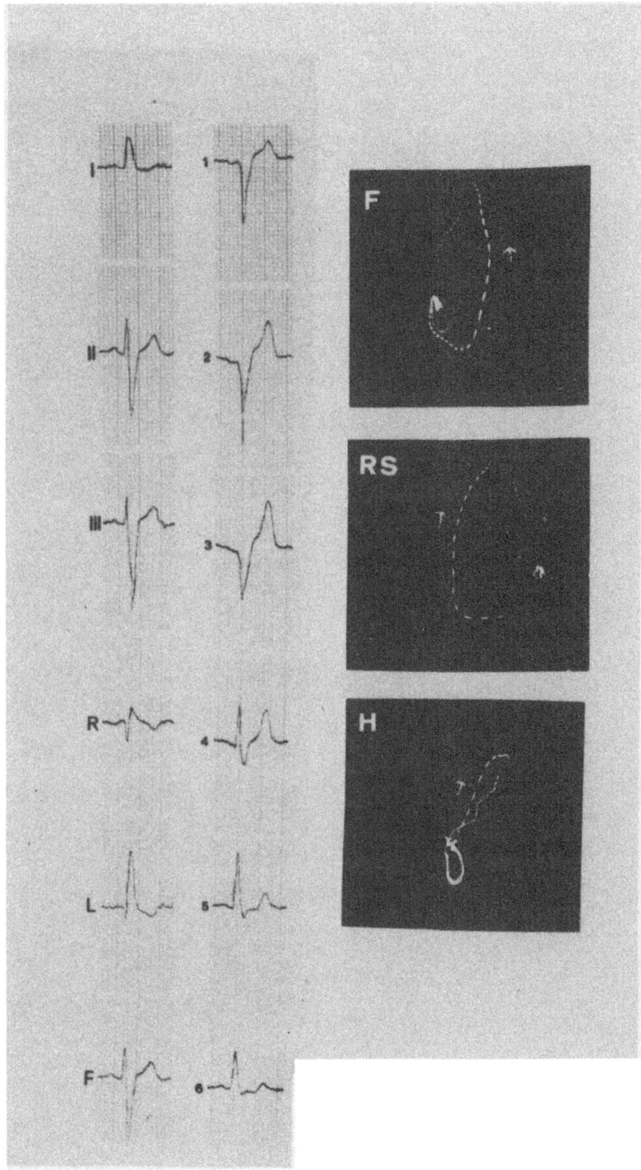

Figure 19. Anterior fascicular block coexisting with anteroseptal myocardial infarction. AFB is recognizable in the electrocardiogram by the marked left axis deviation together with a delayed intrinsecoid deflection time (55 msec) in aVL and in the vectorcardiogram by frontal QRS loop, inscribed superiorly and to the left in a counterclockwise fashion. Anteroseptal myocardial infarction is evident in the ECG by the QS morphology in V_1-V_3 and in the VCG by the posterior orientation of the first vectors

mass the small vector originating in these portions will also disappear, thus producing either QS complexes or a diminished voltage of the r waves from V_1 to V_3.

Under normal conditions the r wave in V_1 and V_2 and the q wave in V_5 and V_6 are generated by the sum of the vectors resulting from the midseptal activation process (directed anteriorly and to the right) and the small forces produced by the

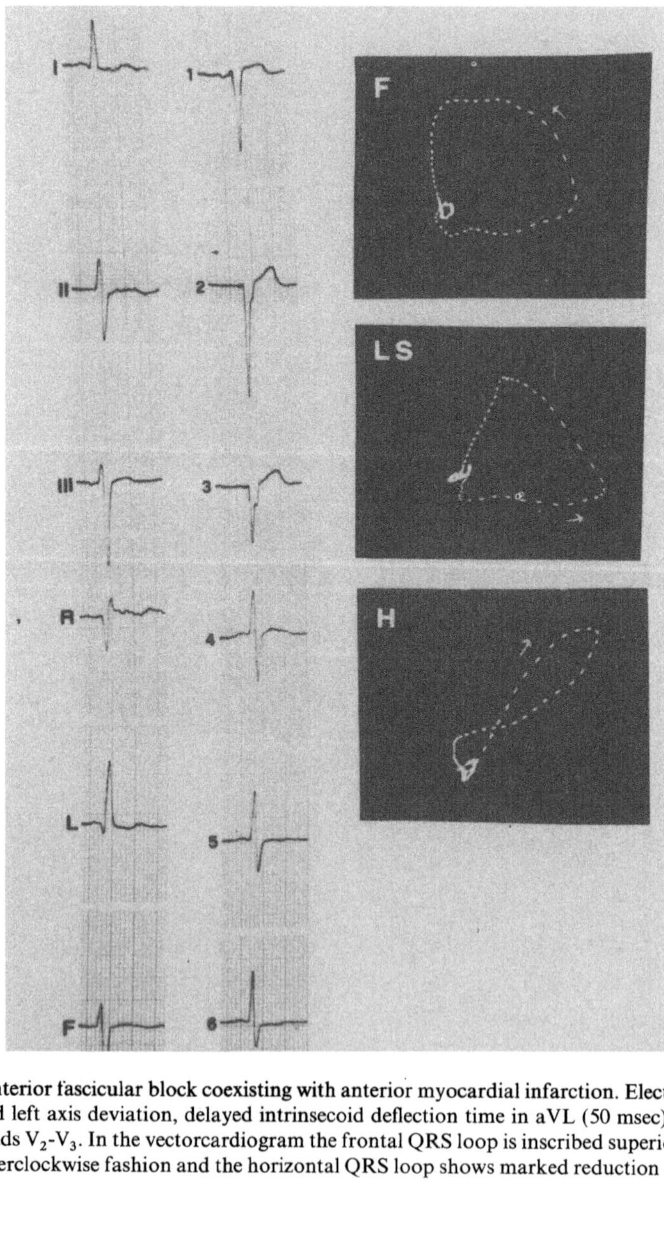

Figure 20. Anterior fascicular block coexisting with anterior myocardial infarction. Electrocardiogram shows marked left axis deviation, delayed intrinsecoid deflection time in aVL (50 msec) and QS morphology in leads V_2-V_3. In the vectorcardiogram the frontal QRS loop is inscribed superiorly and to the left in a counterclockwise fashion and the horizontal QRS loop shows marked reduction of the anterior forces

activation of the trabecular zone of the right ventricular wall. In anteroseptal infarction, as in this case, the area of necrosis would usually involve the anterior middle third of the septum while the posterior portions remain unaffected. Under these circumstances, most of the mid third septal forces are destroyed but the small vectors arising from the right ventricular trabecular zone remain intact. This could become apparent as a focal vector in V_1 determining a small r wave. When an AFB appears, the activation of the antero-superior portions of the left septal mass is delayed about 30 msec. Thus, an early activation process does not originate in the postero-inferior portions of the septum; a new vector is therefore directed forwards and to the right. This septal vector occurs simultaneously with, and is added to, the vector from the trabecular zone in the presence of anteroseptal infarction. The resulting vector deviates more anteriorly and an r wave becomes apparent in the right precordial leads. Hence, the signs of septal necrosis may be concealed. This explanation, even if highly suggestive, needs experimental confirmation. It is not clear because such an eventuality so rarely occurs as in most cases the anteroseptal infarction is not obscured by the AFB.

Few studies deal with vectorcardiographic findings of AFB coexisting with anteroseptal myocardial infarction [28-30].

In the frontal plane the QRS loop is very similar to that of an uncomplicated AFB, with the exception of the first vectors which are often directed to the left instead of to the right (Figures 19 and 20). The remaining portion of the loop is directed superiorly and is inscribed in a counterclockwise fashion or more rarely in a figure of eight. However, with regard to the uncomplicated fascicular block, QRS irregularities and a shifting to the right of the afferent limb are more frequent. The anteroseptal wall infarction is recognizable in the horizontal plane. In most cases the QRS loop moves immediately to the left and posteriorly and usually remains in this quadrant during its counterclockwise rotation. Sometimes the first 10-20 msec vectors are inscribed anteriorly, leftward or more rarely rightward, in a counterclockwise or clockwise fashion. In general the long axis of the horizontal QRS loop tends to lie markedly posteriorly but it does not significantly differ from the one observed in the isolated anterior myocardial infarction.

Lateral myocardial infarction

To the best of our knowledge there are no ECG or VCG studies of AFB coexisting with lateral myocardial infarction; only a few experimental (Medrano 74) and clinical cases have been reported [20, 21, 30-32].

The lateral wall infarction in most cases is easily recognizable in the ECG by the presence of wide and slurred Q waves in the left-sided leads (Figures 21 and 22).

The anterior fascicular block is recognizable by the left axis deviation. Under such circumstances the latter is of particular diagnostic value for AFB, as the lateral infarction shifts downward the electric axis.

In very rare cases AFB may mask a lateral inferior wall. In Figure 23 a healed anteroseptal and lateral infarction is present. The appearance of a transient AFB reduces the infarctional Q waves in leads I and aVL. The AFB, shifting superiorly the middle forces of the ventricular depolarization, decreases such Q waves substituting them with positive deflections.

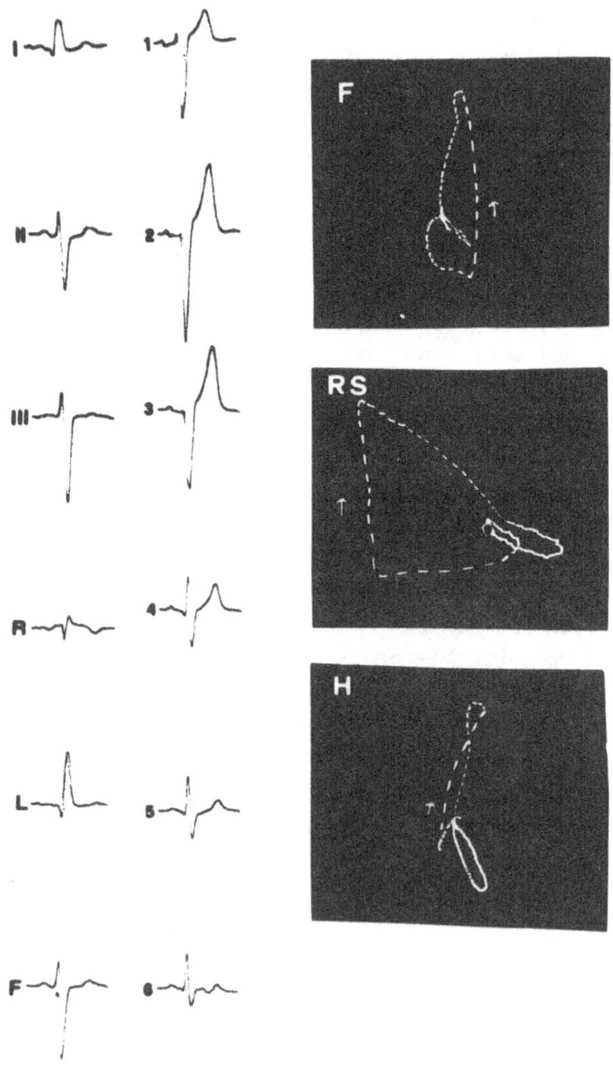

Figure 21. Anterior fascicular block coexisting with anterolateral myocardial infarction. Electrocardiogram shows left axis deviation and slurred Q waves in leads aVL, V_4, V_5 and V_6. The vectorcardiogram evidences a frontal QRS loop mainly inscribed superiorly and to the left in a counterclockwise fashion. In the horizontal plane, the first vectors are directed rightward and anteriorly; then the QRS loop is inscribed posteriorly in a clockwise fashion. This finding expresses lateral infarction

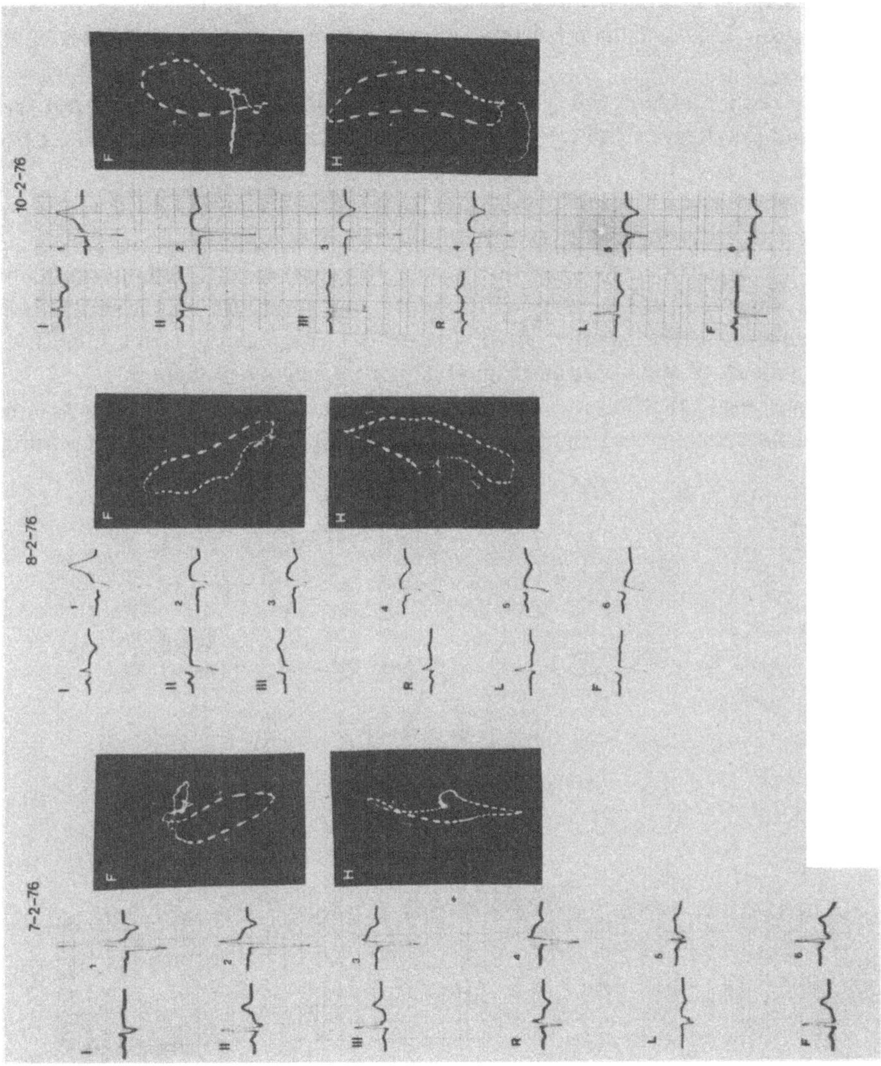

Figure 22. Anterior fascicular block coexisting with anterolateral myocardial infarction. A: Electrocardiogram and vectorcardiogram of a patient with acute anterolateral wall infarction, recorded on admission. Infarctional Q waves are evident in leads V_1-V_5; V_1 lead and horizontal QRS loop evidence right bundle branch block pattern. The frontal QRS loop shows clockwise rotation. B: The ECG of the day after admission shows left axis deviation and the frontal QRS loop is inscribed superiorly in a counterclockwise fashion, an expression of anterior fascicular block. C: Three days after admission, extension of the myocardial infarction is observed (QS morphology appears in lead V_5) and the frontal QRS loop is still superiorly inscribed, but in a clockwise fashion

At times an AFB eliciting a deep q wave in aVL may simulate a lateral myocardial infarction. However such q waves are generally not slurred and narrow (< 40 msec).

In a few cases, however, the Q wave is borderline, the left axis deviation not very marked and the diagnosis of lateral myocardial infarction coexisting with AFB is difficult.

We have little knowledge of the vectorcardiographic findings of AFB associated with lateral or anterolateral myocardial infarction [28-30].

In most cases the first vectors of the frontal QRS loop are directed inferiorly and rightward; then the loop is inscribed to the left and superiorly in a counterclockwise fashion, as in the isolated AFB (Figure 21). Very rarely is the QRS loop inscribed in a clockwise rotation (Figure 22) or in a figure of eight.

The horizontal QRS loop shows increased magnitude of the 20 msec vectors located in the anterior and rightward quadrant, indicative of lateral myocardial

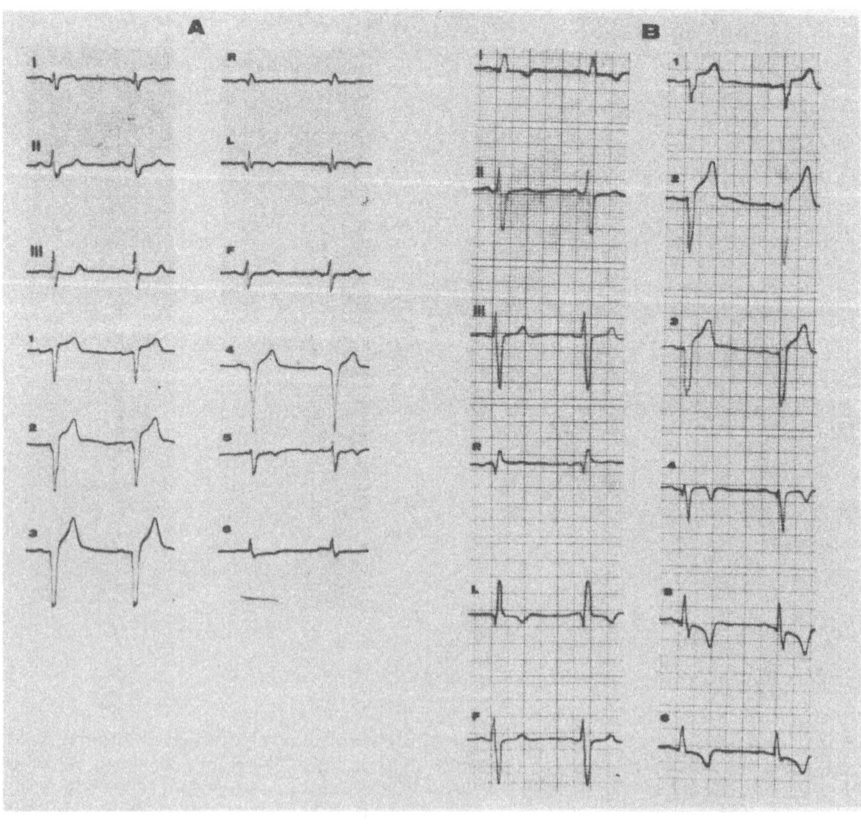

Figure 23. A: Anteroseptal and lateral myocardial infarction is evident. B: One can observe the appearance of an anterior fascicular block, which reduces Q waves in leads I and aVL, thus masking the lateral wall infarction

infarction. The loop is then directed posteriorly towards the left and is inscribed in a counterclockwise direction or in a figure of eight. The AFB tends to shift the midterminal forces towards the left, generally displaced to the right in the isolated lateral wall infarction [12].

Inferior myocardial infarction

In most cases an inferior myocardial infarction coexisting with AFB is recognizable in the ECG tracing. Cosin et al. [32], in 32 patients with healed myocardial infarction, performed synchronized right atrial stimulation in order to obtain supraventricular beats with aberrant intraventricular conduction. When an AFB appeared in the presence of an inferior myocardial infarction, the following patterns were observed: QS in II and III (33 %), QS in II and rS in III (44 %) and rS in II and III with r II $<$ r III (22 %). Thus the inferior wall infarction was recognizable in the ECG in 78 % of cases and was doubtful in 22 %. In fact an r II $<$ r III represents only a suspicious sign of inferior myocardial infarction. However, as we observed, an AFB block inducing the appearance of small r waves in the diaphragmatic leads can mask both partially and at times completely, an inferior infarction.

The appearance of these r waves is related to a modification of septal activation induced by the fascicular block. In fact, the excitation of the postero-inferior region in the interventricular septum occurs earlier and results in dominant electric forces. Accordingly, the initial vectors can be shifted inferiorly, changing the QS complexes in rS complexes [21, 26, 32-34].

Rosenbaum et al. [21] suggest that in the presence of AFB, even minimal changes of the QRS complex in leads II, III and aVF should be minutely scrutinized for possible manifestations of inferior infarction. In fact, sometimes we can observe in only one of the diaphragmatic leads a qrS morphology with a very small q wave or a small bifid or notched initial r wave.

The inferior wall infarction, shifting the first vectors superiorly, can partially or totally cancel out in leads I and aVL the q waves related to AFB. Such behavior was observed by Cosin [32] in 66 % of cases. In the absence of these characteristic q waves the anterior fascicular block can therefore be difficult to recognize and its presence in the ECG recording is doubtful. The two tracings tend therefore to cancel each other out. In general, recognition of the AFB is more difficult. Medrano et al. [35] attribute particular diagnostic value to the delayed intrinsecoid deflection time in aVL ($>$ 50 msec). However, in our experience such time is often within the limits of normality when the q waves in aVL are canceled out by an inferior infarction.

Other authors consider important the presence of a deep S wave in lead II and of a terminal r wave in a VR [36], without a terminal positive deflection (r wave) in lead II [36-38].

AFB coexisting with inferior wall infarction may be mimicked by chronic obstructive pulmonary disease in which a QS morphology may be present in the inferior leads, together with a pseudo left axis deviation. In such cases, however, a low voltage of the extremity and precordial leads and S wave in lead I are generally present.

The vectorcardiogram has proved to be more helpful than the ECG in evaluating patients with AFB associated with inferior infarction [37, 39-42].

The simultaneous presence of these two abnormalities can be diagnosed in the frontal plane. The initial 30 msec QRS vectors are inscribed superiorly in a clockwise fashion. This initial rotation is different from that of isolated AFB, which results in counterclockwise rotation of these vectors. The balance of the QRS loop beyond the inscription of the 40 msec vectors rotates counterclockwise (Figures 24 and 25) and this reversal in rotation results in a figure-of-eight configuration (Figure 26) in 56% of cases [40]. Beyond the inscription of the 40 msec vectors, the rotation was similar to that in isolated AFB. This change in rotation is useful in differentiating coexisting AFB and inferior infarction from isolated inferior wall infarction which results in a completely clockwise rotation in the frontal plane [43]. Furthermore, the 20 and 30 msec vectors are directed superiorly; this contrasts with isolated AFB which results in inferiorly directed 20 msec vectors.

The maximal QRS deflection vector is located in the left superior quadrant and the major area of the QRS loop is above the X axis.

In some cases we have observed a frontal QRS loop completely inscribed superiorly in counterclockwise fashion (Figure 27).

In about 50% of cases the initial 10-15 msec vectors are directed inferiorly [40]. This is important in terms of electrocardiographic recognition of coexisting AFB and inferior wall infarction. In a few of these cases a small r wave is present in leads II, III and aVF, thus masking the myocardial infarction.

In the right sagittal plane, one can observe superior inscription of the 20 to 30 msec vectors, deviation of the maximal QRS deflection superiorly and posteriorly and figure-of-eight or clockwise rotation of the QRS loop.

In the horizontal plane there are no characteristic alterations.

When a posterior myocardial infarction also ceoxists, the horizontal QRS loop is abnormally displaced anteriorly. There are, however, no reliable VCG criteria for diagnosing such a wall infarction [44, 45] unless a series of tracings are available (Figure 28).

If an RBBB is associated with the AFB, the diagnostic problems for recognition of a healed myocardial infarction do not vary greatly (Figures 29 and 30).

POSTERIOR FASCICULAR BLOCK

The posterior fascicular block (PFB) induces an asynchronous left ventricular de-

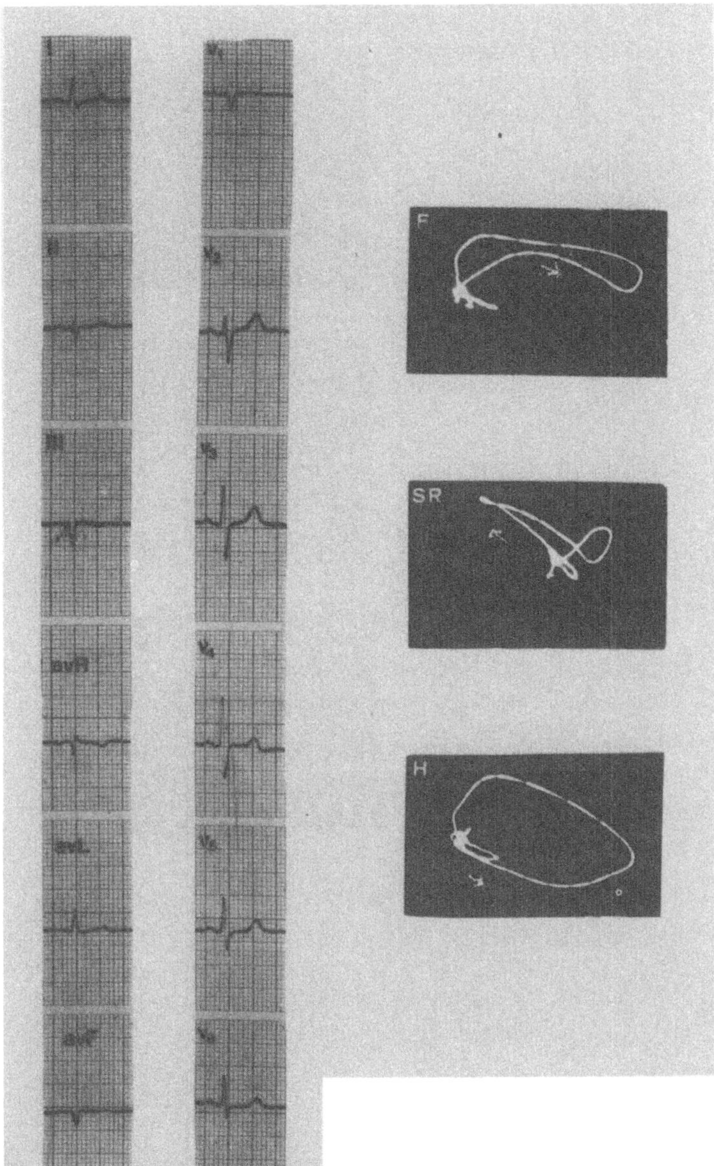

Figure 24. Anterior fascicular block coexisting with inferior myocardial infarction. Electrocardiogram shows qrS morphology in lead II and QS morphology in leads III and aVF. In leads I and aVL, q wave is absent and the intrinsecoid deflection time in aVL measures 40 msec. An anterior fascicular block can only be suspected in the electrocardiogram by left axis deviation. In the frontal plane of the vectorcardiogram the first 40 msec vectors rotate clockwise and the second part of the QRS loop, counterclockwise. The loop is completely displaced superiorly. This finding is highly suggestive of AFB coexisting with inferior myocardial infarction

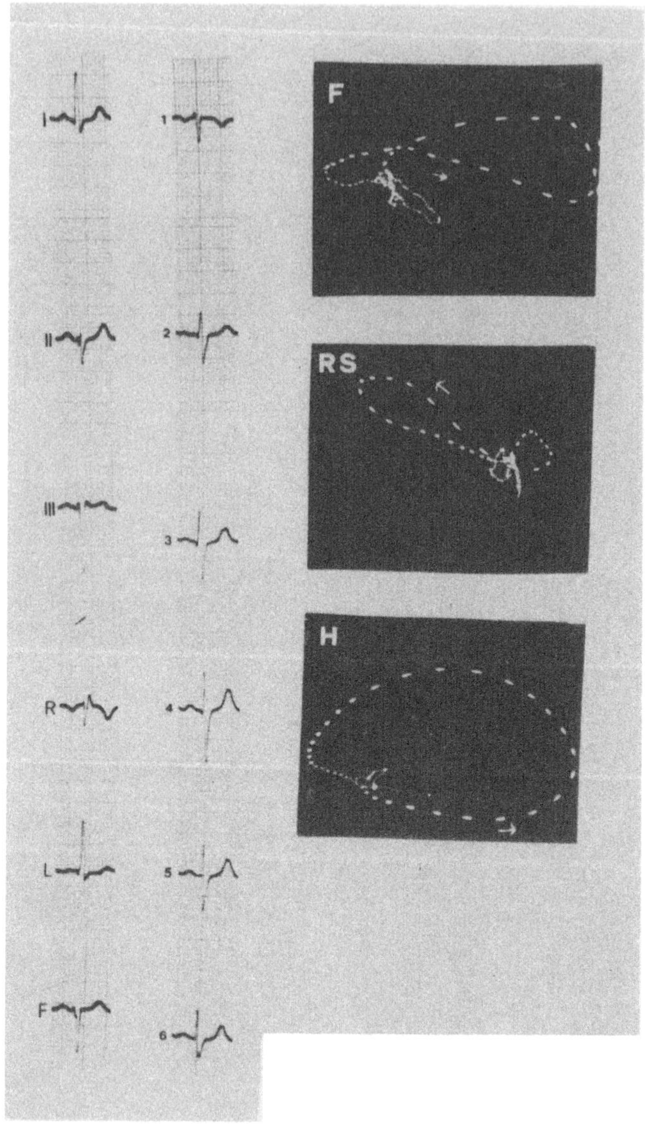

Figure 25. Anterior fascicular block coexisting with inferior myocardial infarction. Patient with typical history of acute myocardial infarction. In the electrocardiogram the only sign suggestive of a healed myocardial infarction is a qrS pattern in lead II. A coexisting anterior fascicular block may be suspected as a result of the left axis deviation. In the frontal plane of the vectorcardiogram the first 30 msec vectors are displaced superiorly and rotate clockwise, whereas the remaining part of the QRS loop rotates counterclockwise

polarization due to delayed excitation of the postero-inferior wall (see Chapter 4). The modification of the ventricular depolarization induced by this fascicular block is not important enough to mask, in most cases, a coexisting myocardial infarction. However, due to the difficult detection of this fascicular block, very little is known regarding the association of the two affections.

Anteroseptal and lateral myocardial infarction

Anteroseptal and lateral myocardial infarction coexisting with PFB are generally

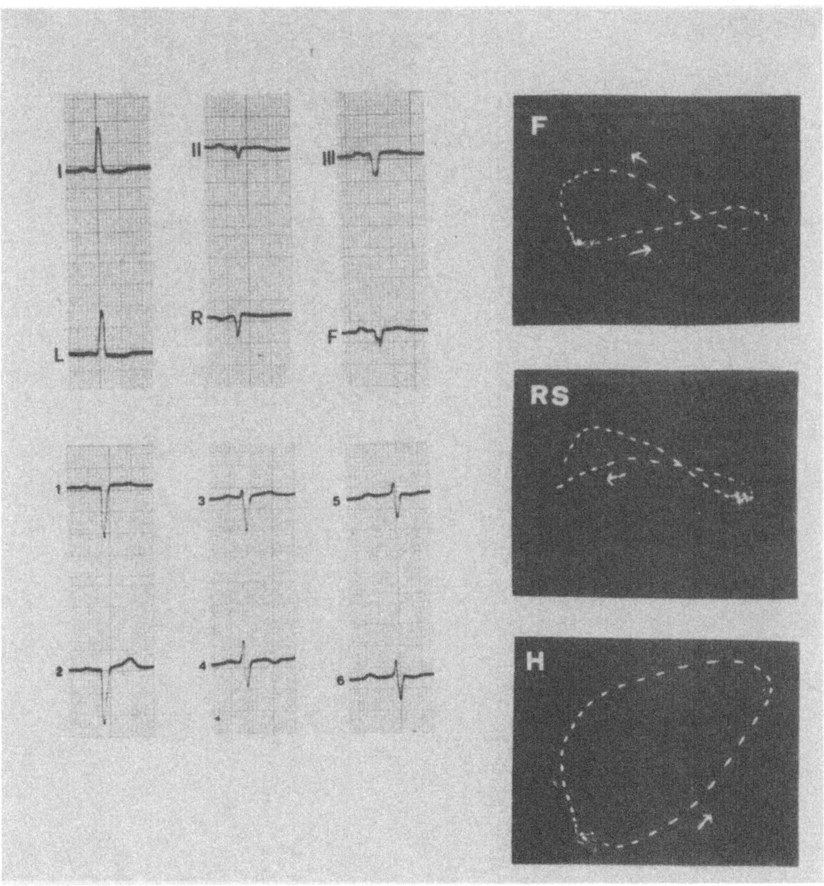

Figure 26. Anterior fascicular block coexisting with septal and inferior myocardial infarction. Patient with a typical history of acute myocardial infarction. Electrocardiogram shows qrS morphology in lead II and QS morphology in leads III and aVF. Q waves are not evident in leads I and aVL. An anterior fascicular block may only be suspected as a result of the axis deviation. In the vectorcardiogram the frontal QRS loop is completely displaced superiorly and shows figure-of-eight morphology with first part of the loop inscribed in a clockwise fashion. This finding is highly suggestive of an anterior fascicular block coexisting with inferior myocardial infarction

easily recognizable in the precordial leads by means of the pathologic Q wave.

On the other hand, in most cases the presence of PFB is doubtful as the antero-lateral infarction itself induces right axis deviation due to the loss of left electric forces and consequently electric prevalence of the right ventricle. Moreover, the

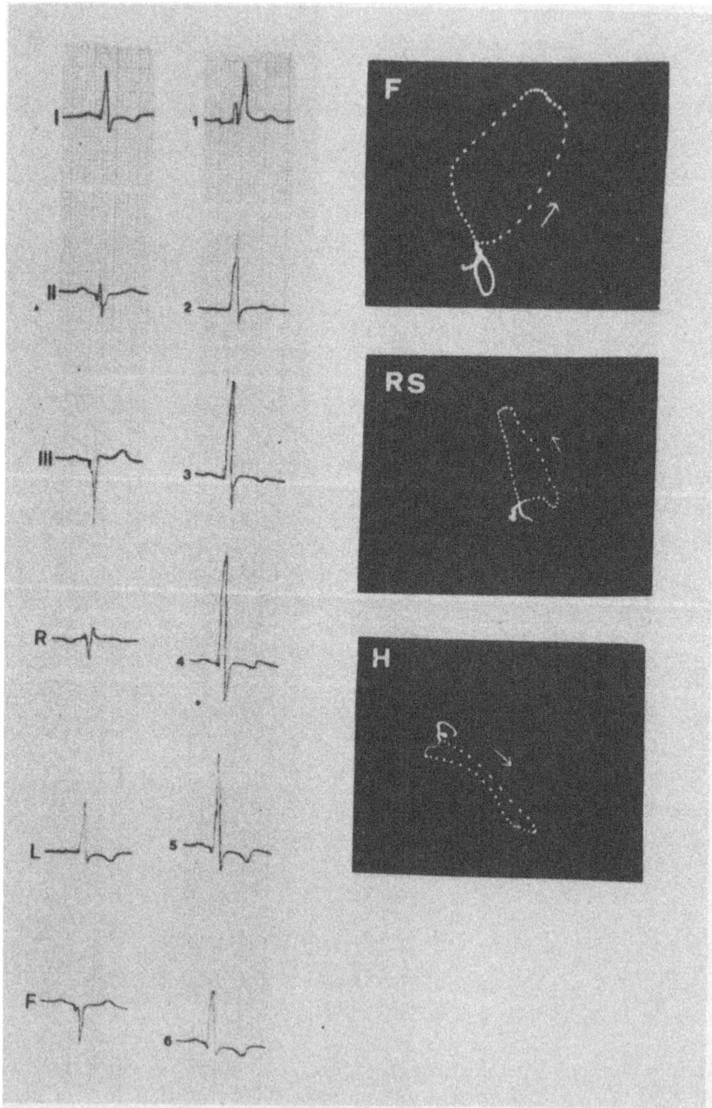

Figure 27. **Anterior fascicular block, right bundle branch block and inferior myocardial infarction.** In the electrocardiogram the inferior wall infarction is evidenced by a qrS pattern in lead II and by a QS morphology in leads III and aVF. In the vectorcardiogram the frontal QRS loop is inscribed superiorly in a counterclockwise fashion

lateral infarction may partially or completely cancel out the q waves in leads II, III and aVF typical of the PFB, as is evident in a few cases so far published [46-49].

The reason for such behavior is not clear at present. Lemberg et al. [47] believe that the infarction extends somewhat into the free left ventricular wall affecting the areas first depolarized by the impulse emerging from the unblocked antero-superior division; therefore, the initial vectors will not be directed superiorly. According to the amount of muscle affected they will point inferiorly and either to the right or to the left.

In the presence of anterolateral myocardial infarction, a PFB, if it is not intermittent, can therefore only be suspected when there are tall R waves in the diaphragmatic leads (Figures 31 and 32).

In lateral wall infarction a terminal r wave in aVL is frequent. According to Castellanos et al. [49] its absence, together with a vertical axis, is indicative of PFB.

Cases were described of anterolateral myocardial infarction in which the superimposition of PFB resulted in small r waves in leads I and aVL in place of the Q waves, most likely for a greater conditioning of the PFB than of the lateral wall infarction on orientation of the first vectors [33]. However, in these cases the precordial leads continued to show unequivocal evidence of the infarction and were not changed by the PFB.

In the few cases of PFB coexisting with anterolateral myocardial infarction registered by vectorcardiogram [28, 30], the frontal QRS loop showed clockwise rotation. However, the first 20 msec QRS vectors can be inscribed inferiorly, unlike the isolated PFB [30]. The maximum vector is oriented inferiorly and to the left and the delayed terminal vectors rightward and downward. The QRS loop in the horizontal plane shows the typical finding of the anterolateral myocardial infarction and does not appear significantly conditioned by the PFB even if a QRS counterclockwise rotation is more frequent than in isolated anterolateral infarction.

Inferior myocardial infarction

The posterior fascicular block, in the majority of cases is secondary to an inferior wall infarction.

In fact it is very rarely observed as an isolated electric manifestation or related to other wall infarctions. The diagnosis of the two coexisting pathologies would therefore appear to be particularly important.

In most cases the inferior infarction is recognizable by the deep and slurred Q waves in the diaphragmatic leads (Figures 33 and 34).

Recognition of coexisting PFB is always difficult if not impossible. The main reasons, in our opinion, are the following:

1) We observed that an inferior infarction which appears on a vertical heart can induce in the diaphragmatic leads a QR morphology with tall R waves com-

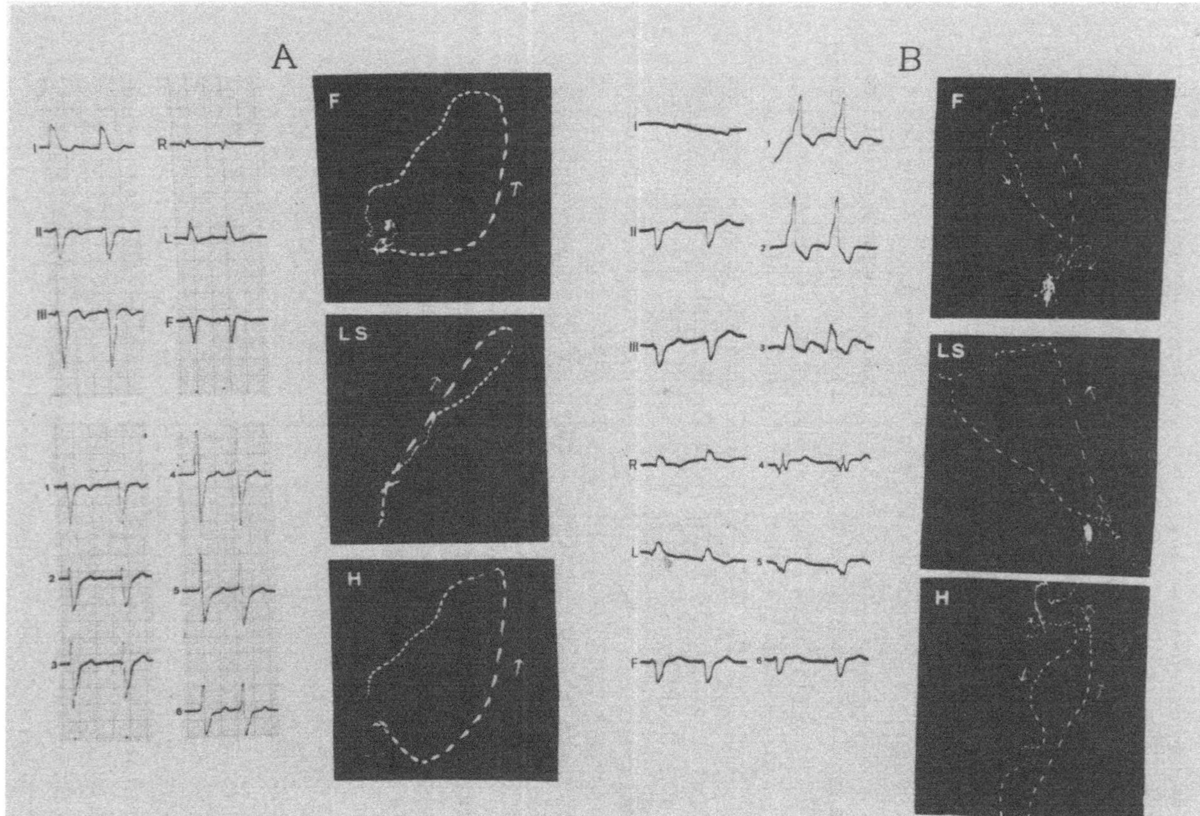

Figure 28. Anterior fascicular block coexisting with postero-inferior and anterolateral myocardial infarction. A: Patient with atrial fibrillation. Electrocardiographic and vectorcardiographic pattern of anterior fascicular block with marked terminal delay of the QRS complex. The first vectors are oriented leftward, probably related to septal fibrosis. B: ECG and VCG recorded after two years. The ECG is highly suggestive of the appearance of a right bundle branch block and an anterolateral myocardial infarction. The presence of an inferior wall infarction is doubtful. In the frontal plane of the VCG the first 15 msec vectors are oriented inferiorly; then the QRS loop is inscribed superiorly in a counterclockwise fashion. This finding is highly suggestive of an anterior fascicular block coexisting with inferior wall infarction. In the horizontal plane the first 20 msec vectors are oriented posteriorly; then the QRS loop is inscribed to the right and anteriorly in a counterclockwise fashion. The afferent limb is oriented to the left, without a terminal delay. The latter finding tends to exclude right bundle branch block. Horizontal QRS loop morphology is suggestive of anterolateral and posterior myocardial infarction

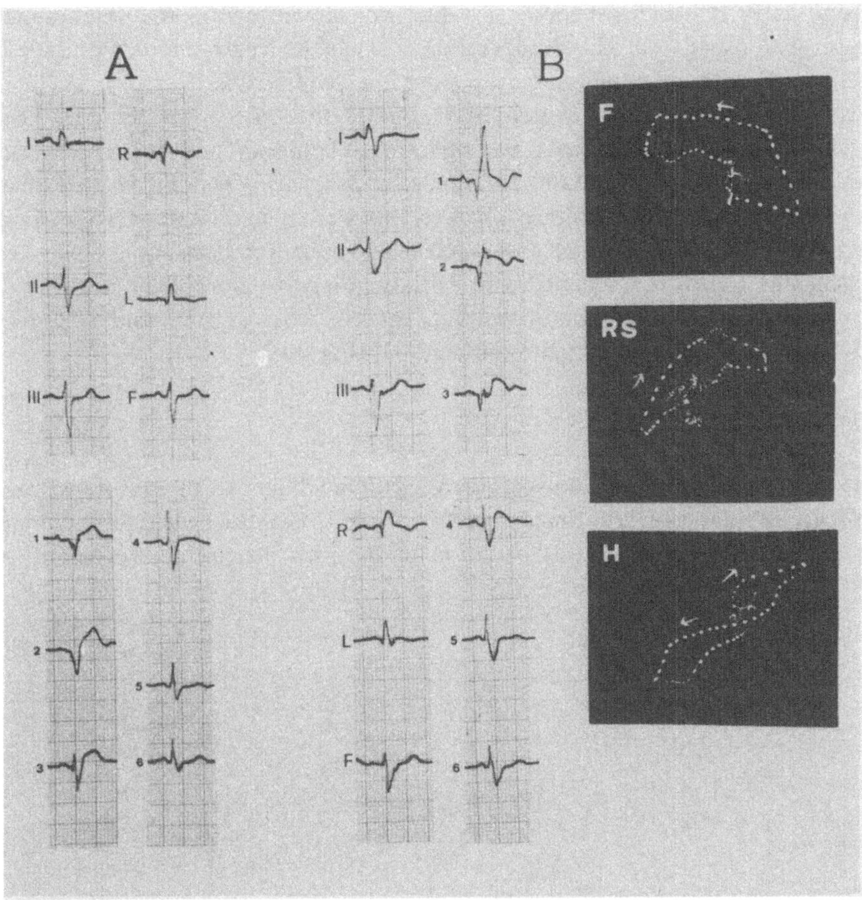

Figure 29. A: Electrocardiogram typical of an anterior fascicular block coexisting with healed antero-septal myocardial infarction. B: Electrocardiogram and vectorcardiogram recorded after 7 months. One can observe the appearance of a right bundle branch block which does not cancel out the myocardial infarction pattern

pletely superimposable to the one observed in the inferior infarction coexisting with PFB (Figure 35).

2) Due to the loss of inferior electric forces there is a reduction in the ventricular mass excited tardily and so the effects of the PFB are partially or completely canceled out. In fact the electric axis tends to normalize and the S waves in leads I and aVL decrease [32].

On the basis of these data we believe that, if a series of tracings are not available or if the PFB is not intermittent, recognition of the fascicular block is practically impossible (Figure 36). In some cases the PFB may mask the inferior infarction [12, 31, 32, 50] (Figure 37). Due to the delayed activation of the left inferior wall related to PFB, the main forces are displaced downward in the diaphragmatic leads. Accordingly, in the diaphragmatic leads the ventricular complexes can become qR with small and narrow q waves, instead of QR.

In vectorcardiographic experimental studies the QRS loop [35, 51] showed clockwise rotation in the frontal and right sagittal planes. The first part of the loop was directed superiorly and the duration of such a part depended on the extent of the necrotic area. The middle terminal vectors were then directed downward. The horizontal QRS loop did not present characteristic alterations.

When an RBBB is associated with PFB, the diagnostic problems relative to the healed myocardial infarction do not vary greatly, whereas ECG and VCG recognition of the PFB is much more difficult [52] (Figure 38).

COMMENT

The electrocardiographic and vectorcardiographic diagnosis of an isolated healed myocardial infarction is at times a great problem in that the healed infarction may be simulated by other causes: rotation of the heart, atrial enlargements, ven-

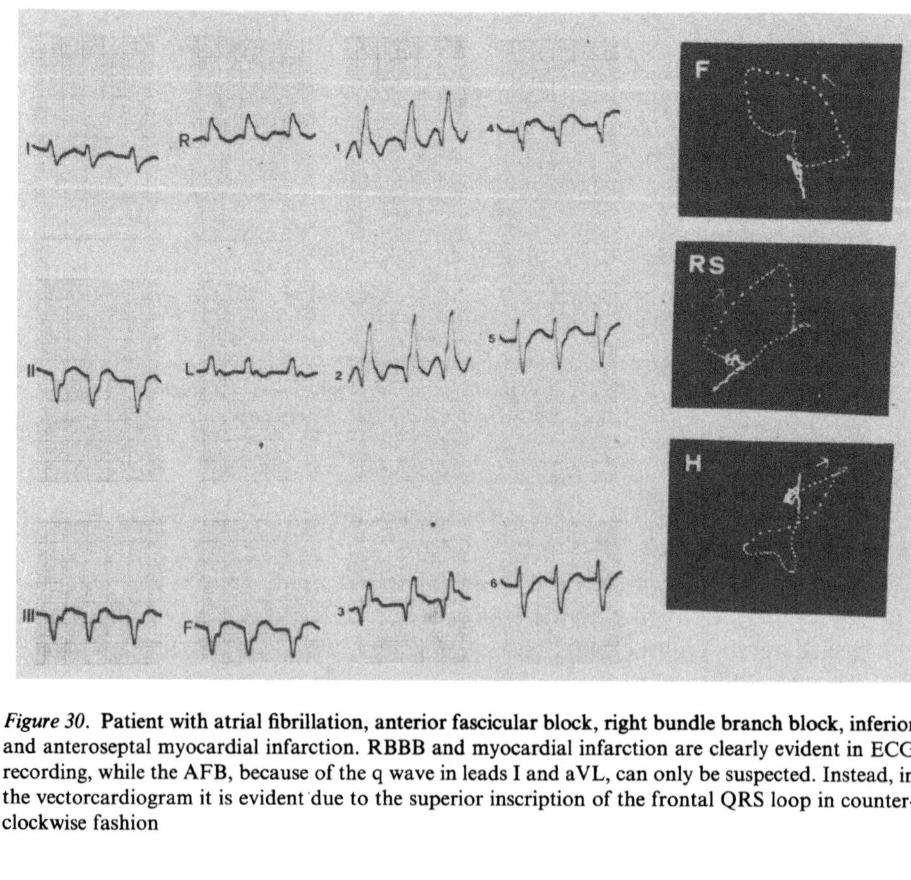

Figure 30. Patient with atrial fibrillation, anterior fascicular block, right bundle branch block, inferior and anteroseptal myocardial infarction. RBBB and myocardial infarction are clearly evident in ECG recording, while the AFB, because of the q wave in leads I and aVL, can only be suspected. Instead, in the vectorcardiogram it is evident due to the superior inscription of the frontal QRS loop in counter-clockwise fashion

tricular hypertrophies and dilatations, pulmonary emphysema, pneumothorax, thoracic deformities, idiopathic cardiomyopathies, metabolic and immunologic injuries, muscular dystrophies, cardiac tumors, chronic myocarditis, endocardial fibroelastosis, cardiac echinococcosis, constrictive pericarditis, myocardial fibrosis not related to acute infarction. Any of these conditions may induce Q waves

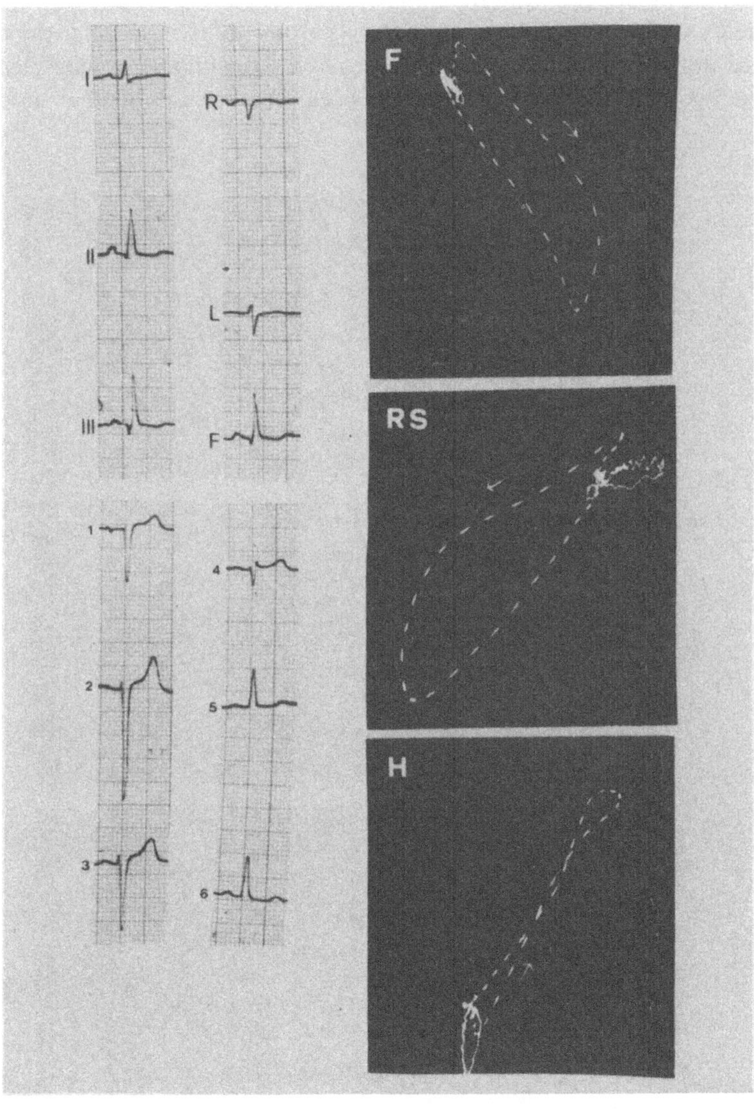

Figure 31. Anterior myocardial infarction with doubtful posterior fascicular block. Infarction is well evident in the precordial leads and in the horizontal plane of the vectorcardiogram. In leads II, III and aVF, tall R waves are present, the frontal QRS loop is inscribed downward and leftward in a clockwise fashion; these data are only suggestive of coexisting posterior fascicular block

simulating a healed myocardial infarction. When intraventricular conduction disturbances are present, the diagnostic problem is more complex since such conduction defects, modifying the ventricular activation, make recognition of a coexisting myocardial infarction more difficult. Furthermore, the ventricular depolarization changes induced by the intraventricular blocks may at times mask, and at others simulate, a healed wall infarction. Such a problem exists particularly for the left ventricular conduction defects as the myocardial infarctions in most cases are localized in the left ventricle. For this reason a right bundle branch block rarely masks a myocardial infarction. This may occur in rare cases of small anteroseptal

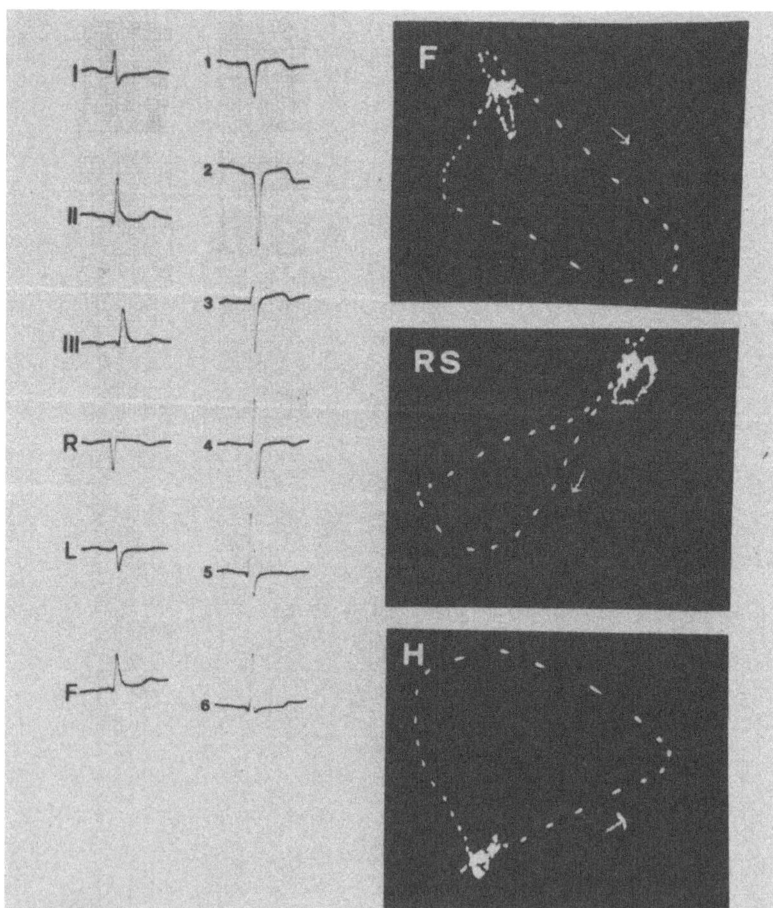

Figure 32. Anteroseptal myocardial infarction with doubtful posterior fascicular block. The infarction is clearly evident in electrocardiogram and vectorcardiogram. The electrical axis is oriented downward. Tall R waves in diaphragmatic leads and a frontal QRS loop inscribed inferiorly in a clockwise fashion represent suggestive signs of coexisting posterior fascicular block

necrosis in which the initial-middle forces are markedly shifted anteriorly by the block.

Moreover, in the presence of RBBB, recognition of a strictly posterior myocardial infarction is impossible as the middle electric forces are often displaced anteriorly by the right intraventricular block. On the other hand, a healed posterior wall infarction can never be diagnosed with any certainty in the ECG and VCG recordings even in the absence of RBBB [44, 45] as an anatomic displacement of

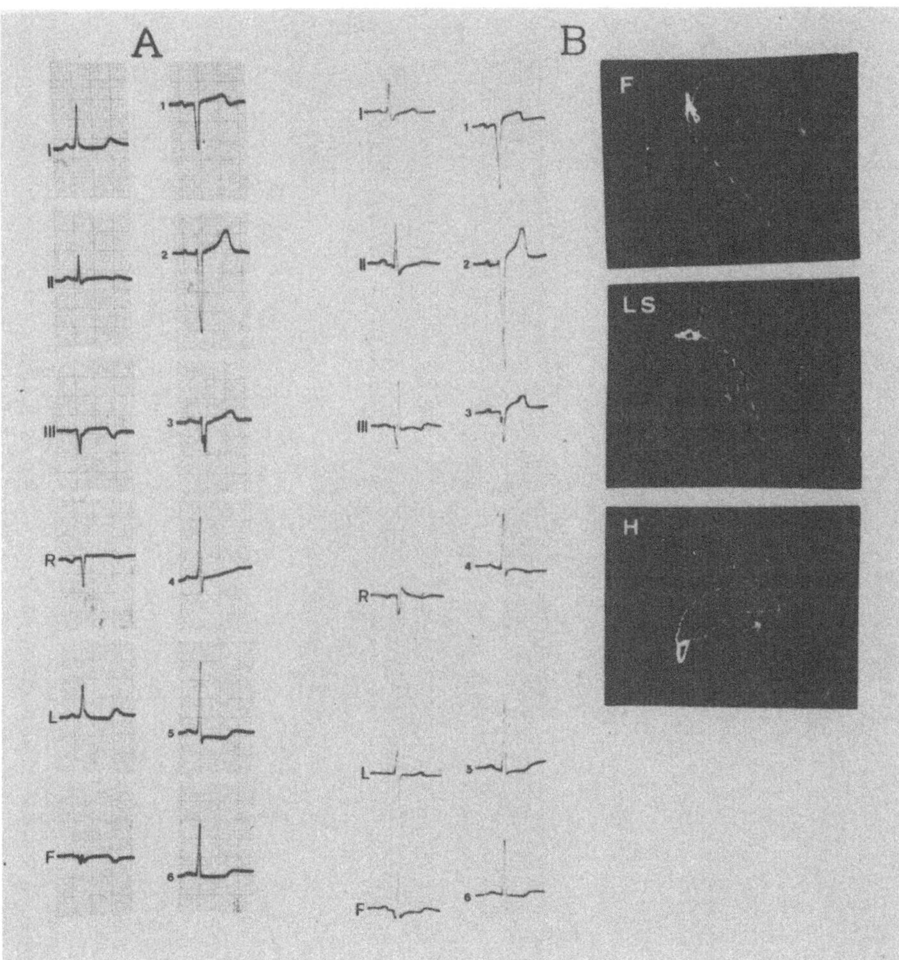

Figure 33. A: Electrocardiogram shows acute inferior and septal myocardial infarction. B: Electrocardiogram and vectorcardiogram recorded 40 days later. The infarction is still evident, but the appearance of tall R waves in leads III and aVF is observed. In the frontal plane of the VCG the first 35 msec vectors are oriented superiorly, then the QRS loop is inscribed inferiorly and to the left in a clockwise fashion; these data express the appearance of posterior fascicular block

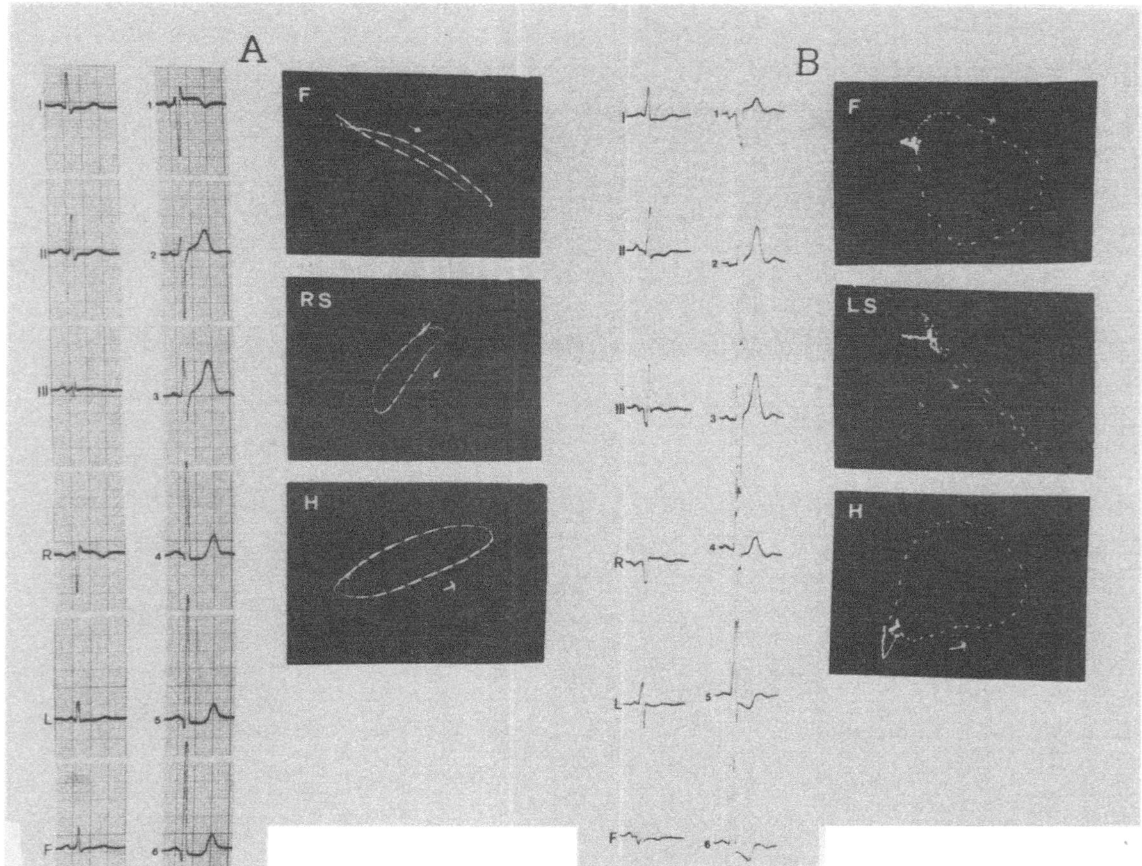

Figure 34. A: Electrocardiogram and vectorcardiogram show left ventricular hypertrophy. B: Electrocardiogram and vectorcardiogram recorded one year later. One can observe infarctional Q wave in leads III and aVF and a downward shifting of the electrical axis. The first 35 msec vectors of the frontal QRS loop are oriented superiorly; then the loop is inscribed inferiorly in a clockwise fashion. These data express the appearance of an inferior myocardial infarction coexisting with posterior fascicular block

the heart to the right or an initial and atypical RBBB [53] can induce the same electric pattern.

At times an RBBB, if coexisting with marked right atrial enlargement, may simulate an anteroseptal infarction. In these cases, however, the Q waves of non infarctional genesis are not slurred and do not extend beyond lead V_2.

Far more difficult is recognition of a healed myocardial infarction in the presence of LBBB, because such a block induces marked changes in the left ventricular depolarization. ECG and VCG criteria reported in the literature are not specific and present a high incidence of false positive diagnoses. Pietras et al. [54]

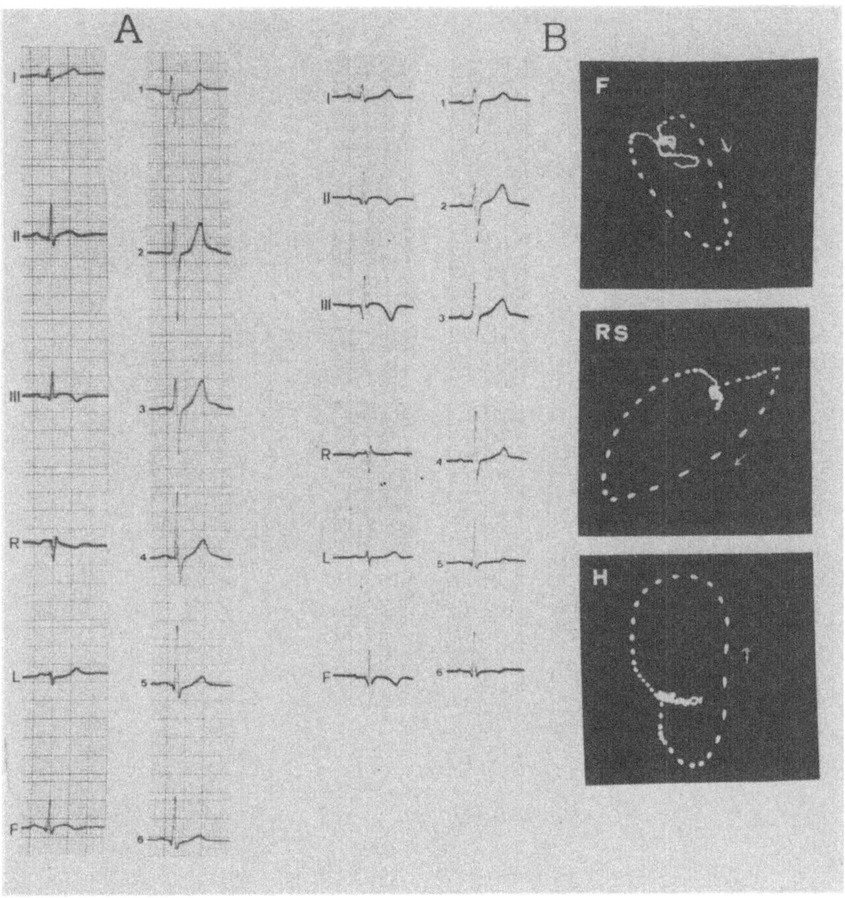

Figure 35. A: Electrocardiogram at admission of a patient with acute myocardial infarction. Only inverted T waves in leads III and aVF are present. The electrical axis is vertical. B: Electrocardiogram and vectorcardiogram recorded 10 days later. The appearance of infarctional Q waves in leads III and aVF is observed. As a result of tall R wave in the diaphragmatic leads and the characteristic frontal QRS loop morphology, ECG and VCG recordings simulate posterior fascicular block coexisting with inferior myocardial infarction

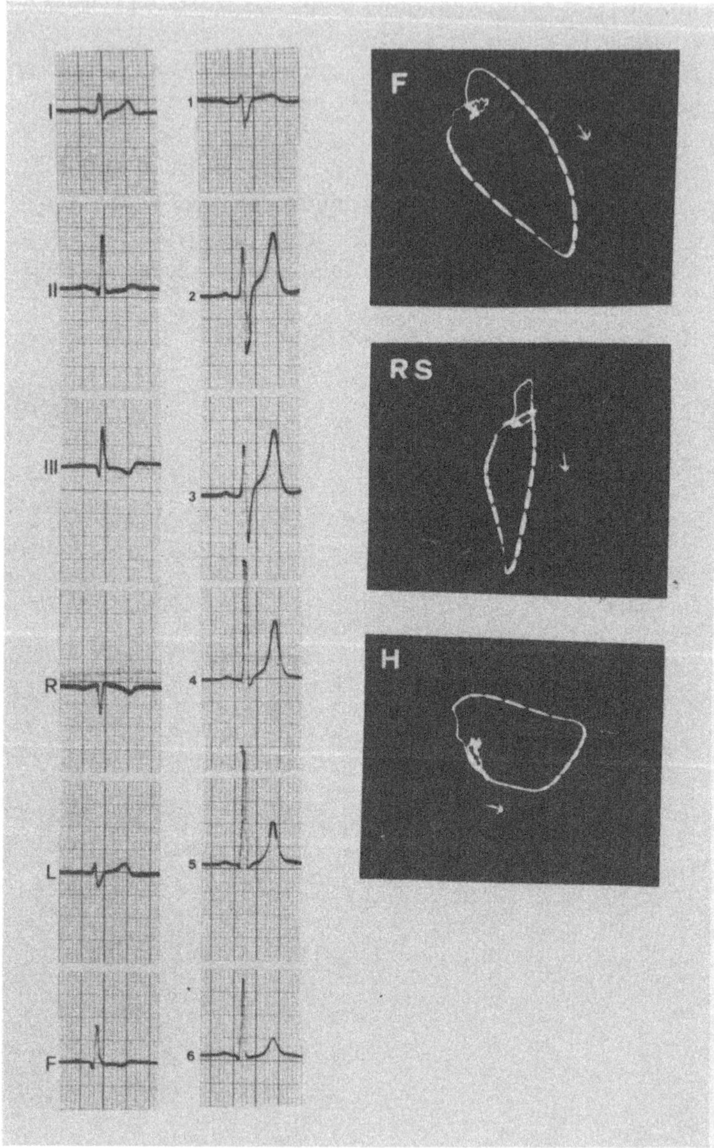

Figure 36. Patient with a typical history of acute myocardial infarction. In leads III and aVF infarctional Q waves and tall R waves are present. The first 30 msec vectors of the frontal QRS loop are directed superiorly, then the loop is inscribed inferiorly in a clockwise fashion. It is not possible to discriminate, in the absence of a series of tracings, whether the inferior myocardial infarction coexists with posterior fascicular block or with anatomic vertical heart

correlated the autopsy findings with the ECG and VCG recordings of 33 patients with LBBB. Twenty-eight had myocardial infarction at necroscopy. Using all VCG criteria, myocardial infarction was correctly localized in 21 hearts. In three hearts (11 %) it could not be identified. There were 12 (35 %) false positive diagnoses. Comparing the ECG to the VCG criteria, fewer infarcts were predicted and localized by the ECG, but the number of false positive diagnoses was no different. These data suggest that in the absence of a reliable clinical and enzymatic pattern, the diagnosis of healed myocardial infarction can never be posited with absolute certainty in the presence of LBBB; only from the ECG and VCG do there exist signs that suggest, but by no means with certainty, coexisting myocardial infarc-

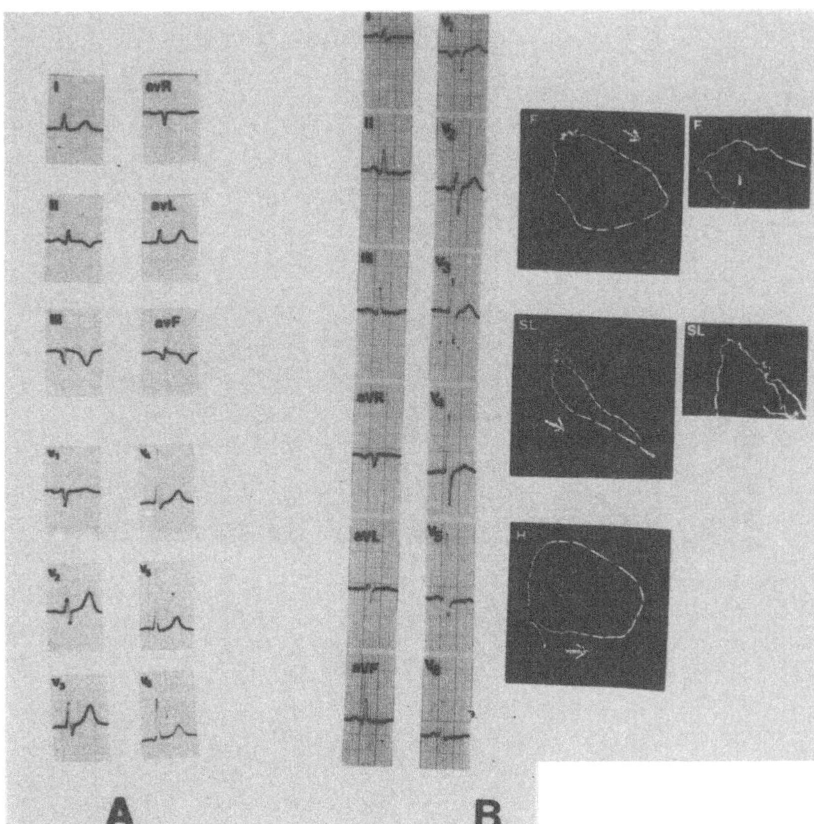

Figure 37. A: Electrocardiogram shows inferior myocardial infarction. B: Electrocardiogram and vectorcardiogram recorded one year later. One can observe the appearance of a posterior fascicular block, evidenced by tall R wave in leads III and aVF, which mask in the ECG the inferior infarction. Such infarction may only be suspected in the VCG since the first 27.5 msec vectors of the frontal QRS loop are oriented superiorly

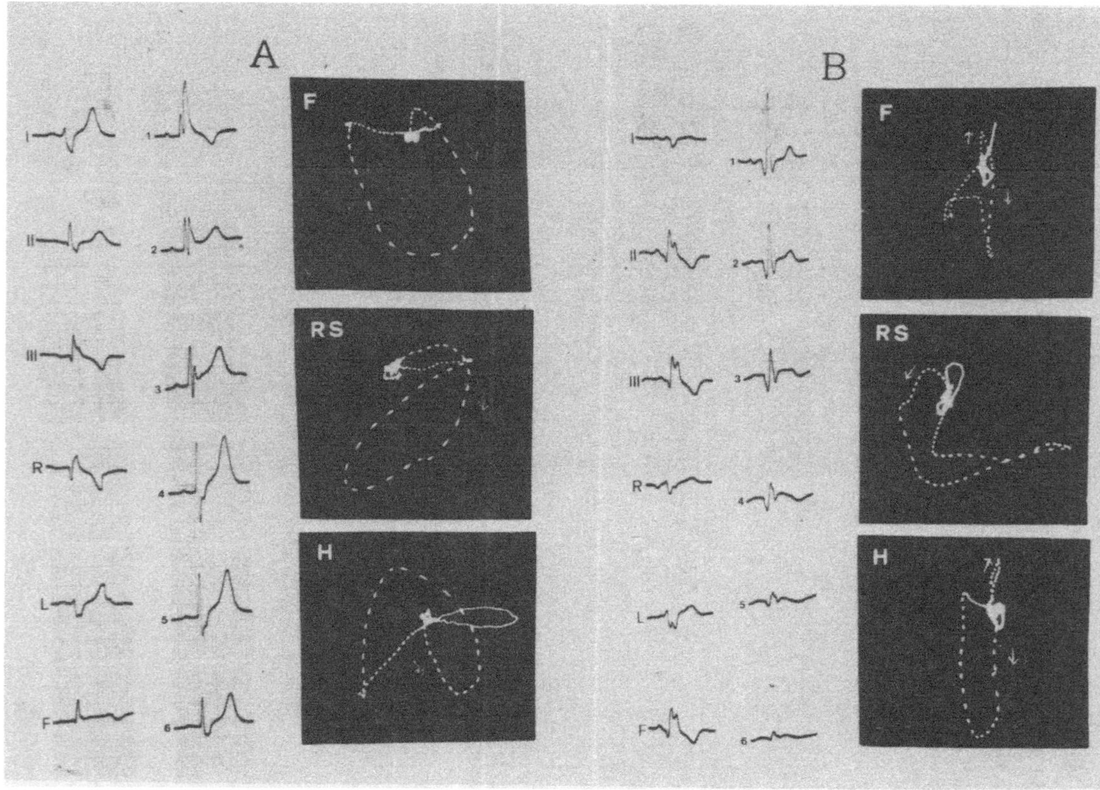

Figure 38. **A: Right bundle branch block. A coexisting posterior fascicular block is likely, due to the marked right axis deviation and to the characteristic frontal QRS loop** morphology. B: Electrocardiogram and vectorcardiogram recorded 5 years later. One can observe an anterolateral myocardial infarction which does not cancel out the intraventricular conduction disturbances.

tion. This represents a serious limit in that the isolated LBBB and the LBBB coexisting with myocardial infarction have a very different clinical-prognostic value [55].

The main factors responsible for false positive diagnoses are the right ventricular enlargement and the pulmonary emphysema [56-58].

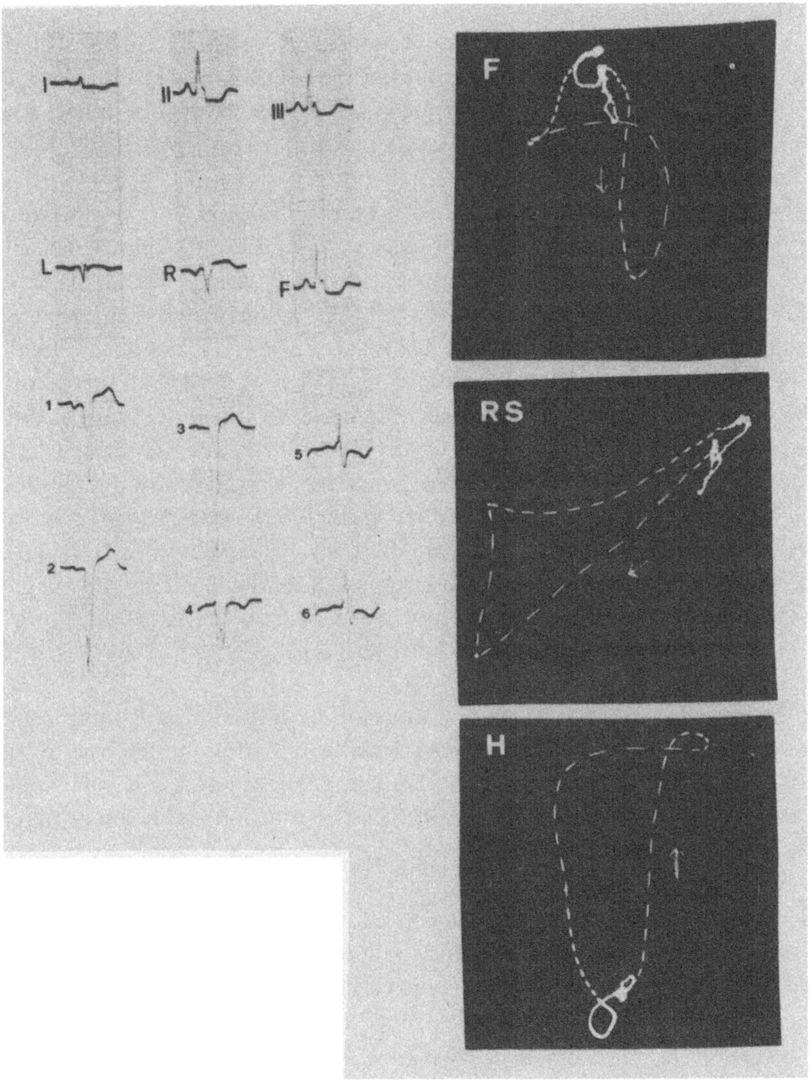

Figure 39. An anteroseptal myocardial infarction is evident. The tall R wave in leads II, III and aVF are highly suspicious of a coexisting posterior fascicular block. A frontal QRS loop inscribed counterclockwise excludes such a block.

Body surface maps provide more precise information on healed myocardial infarction coexisting with LBBB [59]. However, this technique requires over one hundred precordial electrodes and computerized analysis of the data and at present is utilized only in a few research centers.

Criteria for the diagnosis of the fascicular blocks in the presence of healed myocardial infarction are poorly documented and relatively few reports have appeared.

It has, however, been reported that in most cases, unlike in LBBB, recognition of the fascicular block is more difficult than the coexisting infarction. In fact, the latter is only rarely masked, whereas recognition of the fascicular block, which is often already problematic in the absence of necrotic areas, is particularly difficult when a myocardial infarction coexists.

Actually, the diagnosis of such blocks is mostly based on the axis deviation and on asynchronous left ventricular activation. A myocardial infarction itself can induce marked axis deviation and by canceling out ventricular forces, it makes recognition of an asynchronism of the left ventricular depolarization extremely difficult. In most cases, therefore, the fascicular block, if it is not intermittent, may only be suspected in the ECG recording,

The vectorcardiogram offers, in our opinion, data which are more useful than those of the electrocardiogram, but unfortunately, they are not always decisive.

Since a peri-infarction block is often associated with myocardial infarction, the ECG, which is extremely sensitive in intercepting local electric forces, can record S waves both in leads I and aVL in the presence of AFB, and in leads II, III and aVF in the presence of PFB. Under such circumstances the electrical axis is indeterminate and consequently recognition of a fascicular block is extremely difficult. The vectorcardiogram offers a clearer pattern on the development of ventricular depolarization.

In the presence of an anterolateral myocardial infarction, a frontal QRS loop oriented mainly superiorly with counterclockwise rotation, on the basis of experimental data [12] is highly suggestive of a coexisting anterior fascicular block. In rare cases the frontal QRS loop shows clockwise rotation, as shown in Figure 22, unlike the isolated AFB in which it is always counterclockwise.

Even the diagnosis of AFB coexisting with inferior myocardial infarction is particularly difficult in the ECG tracing as such an infarction itself may induce marked left axis deviation; moreover the inferior necrosis may mask the AFB, canceling out the typical q waves in leads I and aVL. The vectorcardiogram shows instead a characteristic pattern: in the frontal plane the first 30-40 msec vectors are inscribed superiorly in a clockwise fashion; then the afferent limb deviates superiorly with counterclockwise rotation [37, 40]. However, at present we do not known the specificity of such morphology. Theoretically a peripheral block localized in the postero-superior wall of the right ventricle coexisting with inferior myocardial infarction may also induce the same frontal QRS morphology. Further experimental and clinical studies are necessary.

The vectorcardiogram does not appear particularly useful for recognizing a posterior fascicular block coexisting with myocardial infarction.

When such a block is suspected in the ECG recording, we believe that the vectorcardiogram does not confirm the presence of the fascicular block. In fact, a downward orientation with clockwise rotation of the frontal QRS loop may be related to an isolated anterolateral myocardial infarction. A downward shifting of the mid-terminal electric forces in the presence of inferior wall infarction may be related not only to a PFB, but also to a vertical position of the heart.

However in some cases the vectorcardiogram may exclude a PFB, dubious in ECG recording. In Figure 39, an antero-septal myocardial infarction is evident. The tall R waves in leads II, III and aVF are highly suspicious of a coexisting PFB. A counterclockwise rotation in the frontal QRS loop, on the basis of experimental data [12], excludes such a block.

However, we believe that the diagnostic criteria of a fascicular block coexisting with myocardial infarction may be perfected by means of: 1) Multicenter studies of the intermittent fascicular blocks, unfortunately rare in patients with myocardial infarction; 2) Induction by means of synchronized atrial stimulation, which can evidence fascicular block [32, 60, 61], mainly after atropine administration. In fact this drug improves AV nodal conduction and facilitates the appearance of functional intraventricular blocks during extrastimuli induction.

At times the differential diagnosis lies between a fascicular block and a peri-infarction block, which involves the Purkinje-muscular fibers of the ventricular walls. The latter in fact causes alteration of the terminal vectors, clearly evident on the VCG, which can simulate in the ECG a marked axis deviation [62] (see Chapter 6).

REFERENCES

1. Goldman MJ, Pipberg HV: Analysis of the orthogonal electrocardiogram and vectorcardiogram in ventricular conduction defects with and without myocardial infarction. Circulation 39: 243, 1969
2. Horan LG, Flowers NC, Johnson JC: Significance of the diagnostic Q wave of myocardial infarction. Circulation 43: 428, 1971
3. Sodi-Pallares D, Bisteni A, Herrmann GR: Some views on the significance of qR and QR type complexes in right precordial leads in the absence of myocardial infarction. Am Heart J 43: 716, 1952
4. Goldberger AL: Myocardial infarction. Electrographic differential diagnosis. St Louis: CV Mosby, 1979
5. Sodi-Pallares D, Cisneros F, Medrano GA, Bisteni A, Testelli MR, De Micheli A: Electrocardiographic diagnosis of myocardial infarction in the presence of bundle branch block (right and left), ventricular premature beats and Wolff-Parkinson-White syndrome. Prog Cardiovasc Dis 6: 107, 1963

6. Doucet P, Walsh TJ, Massie A: A vectorcardiographic and electrocardiographic study of left bundle branch block with myocardial infarction. Am J Cardiol 17: 171, 1966
7. De Micheli A, Medrano GA: Electrocardiograma y vectorcardiograma en el infarto del miocardio. Mexico: La Prensa Medica Mexicana, 1971
8. Rhoads DV, Edward JE, Pruitt R: The electrocardiogram in the presence of myocardial infarction and intraventricular block of the left bundle-branch block type. A clinical pathologic study. Am Heart J 62: 735, 1961
9. Laham J, Gerbaux A: Les blocs de branche gauche atypiques. Ann Cardiol Angeiol 23: 1, 1974
10. Scott RC: Left bundle branch block: a clinical assessment (II). Am Heart J 70: 691, 1965
11. Myers GB: QRS-T patterns in multiple precordial leads that may be mistaken for myocardial infarction. III. Bundle branch block. Circulation 2: 60, 1950
12. Medrano GA, De Micheli A, Sodi-Pallares D: Necrosis anterolateral complicada con bloqueo bifascicular y trifascicular. Arch Inst Cardiol Mex 44: 63, 1974
13. Neuman J, Blackaller J, Tobin JR, Szanto PB, Gunnar RM: The spatial vectorcardiogram in left bundle branch block. Am J Cardiol 16: 352, 1965
14. Cooksey JD, Dunn M, Massie E: Clinical vectorcardiography and electrocardiography. Chicago: Medical Year Book, 1977
15. Alboni P, Longhini C, Malacarne C, Giovannini G: Il blocco di branca sinistro con asse elettrico deviato a destra. Studio clinico ed elettro-vettocardiografico. G Ital Cardiol 5: 543, 1975
16. Luy G, Bahl OP, Massie E: Intermittent left bundle branch block. A study of the effects of left bundle branch block on the electrocardiographic patterns of myocardial infarction and ischemia. Am Heart J 85: 332, 1973
17. Wasserburger RH, White DH, Lindsay ER: Noninfarctional QS, II, III, aVF complexes as seen in the Wolff-Parkinson-White syndrome and left bundle branch block. Am Heart J 64: 617, 1962
18. Timmis GC, Gangadnaran V, Ramos RG, Gordon S: Reassessment of Q waves in left bundle branch block. J Electrocardiol 9: 109, 1976
19. Izumi K, Goldstein S, Stein PD: Vectorcardiographic and electrocardiographic diagnosis of diaphragmatic myocardial infarction in patients with left bundle branch block. Jap Circ J 43: 49, 1979
20. Benchimol A: Vectorcardiography. Baltimore: Williams & Wilkins, 1973
21. Rosenbaum MB, Elizari MD, Lazzari JO: The hemiblocks. Oldsmar, Fla.: Tampa Tracings, 1970
22. Alboni P: Revisione del concetto di emiblocco. IX Congresso Nazionale ANMCO. Firenze, 1978, p 205
23. Farnam DJ, Shah PM: Left anterior hemiblock simulating anteroseptal myocardial infarction. Am Heart J 92: 363, 1976
24. Alboni P, Malacarne C, De Lorenzi E, Pirani R, Baldassarri F, Masoni A: Right precordial q waves due to anterior fascicular block. Clinical and vectorcardiographic study. J Electrocardiol 12: 41, 1979
25. Masoni A: Infarto cronico: questione terminologica o problema clinico? G Ital Cardiol 6: 185, 1976
26. Altieri P, Schaal S: Inferior and anteroseptal myocardial infarction concealed by transient left anterior hemiblock. J Electrocardiol 6: 257, 1973
27. Horwitz S, Medrano GA, Salazar E: Left anterior fascicular block concealing anteroseptal infarction. Arch Inst Cardiol Mex 46: 35, 1976
28. Polu JM, Gilgenkrantz JM, Faiure G: Le diagnostic vectocardiographique des hémi-

blocs de branche gauche isolés et associés à un bloc de branche droite ou à un infarctus du myocarde. Arch Mal Coeur 65: 1041, 1972
29. Mate I, Sobrino JA, codina J, Suarez DE, Lezo J, Fuster M: Vectocardiografia de los trastornos de la conduccion intraventricular en el infarto de miocardio. Rev Esp Cardiol 27: 297, 1974
30. Valentin V, Peris L, Cervera M, Valls F, Tormo C, Arnau A: Los hemibloqueos en el infarto agudo de miocardio de localizacion anterior y anterolateral. Estudio evolutivo electrovectocardiografico. Rev Esp Cardiol 32: 41, 1979
31. Castellanos A, Myerburg RJ: The hemiblock in myocardial infarction. New York: Appleton-Century-Crofts, 1976
32. Cosin J, Olague J, Beltram M, Salvador A: Hemibloqueo asociado a infarto de miocardio. Patrones electrocardiograficos diagnosticos. Rev Esp Cardiol 30: 141, 1977
33. Leachman RD, Angelini P, Lufschandwsky R: Electrocardiographic signs of infarction masked by coexistent controlateral hemiblock. Chest 62: 542, 1972
34. Schamroth L, Friedberg HD, De Kock J: Studies of acute myocardial infarction with intermittent bundle branch and hemiblock. J Electrocardiol 11: 165, 1978
35. Medrano GA, De Micheli A, Brenes C, Alatriste VM, Sodi-Pallares D: Necrosis posterior complicado con bloqueo bifascicular y trifascicular. Arch Inst Cardiol Mex 42: 375, 1972
36. Fisher ML, Mugmon MA, Carliner NH, De Felice CE, Plotnick GD: Left anterior fascicular block: electrocardiographic criteria for its recognition in the presence of inferior myocardial infarction. Am J Cardiol 44: 645, 1979
37. Castellanos A: Diagnosis of left anterior hemiblock in the presence of inferior wall myocardial infarction. Chest 60: 533, 1971
38. Valentin V, Cervera M, Peris I, Vall S, Paricio V, Bertolin V: Diagnostico electrocardiografico del hemibloqueo anterior izquierdo en presencia de infarto agudo de miocardio de localizacion inferior. Rev Esp Cardiol 33: 35, 1980
39. Kulbertus HE, Collignon P, Humblet L, Deleval-Rutten F: Left axis deviation inferior infarction. Vectorcardiographic recognition of concomitant left anterior hemiblock. Chest 60: 362, 1971
40. Benchimol A, Desser KB: Co-existing left anterior hemiblock and inferior wall myocardial infarction. Am J Cardiol 29: 7, 1972
41. Libretti A, Gregorini L, Valentini R: Studio vettocardiografico del complesso QRS negli emiblocchi associati ad infarto miocardico. G Ital Cardiol 2: 856, 1972
42. Khair GZ, Tristani FE, Brooks HL: Recognition of myocardial infarction complicated by left anterior hemiblock. J Electrocardiol 13: 93, 1980
43. Benchimol A, Barreto EC: Serial vectorcardiograms with the Frank system in patients with acute inferior wall myocardial infarction. J Electrocardiol 2: 159, 1969
44. Ha D, Kraft DI, Stein PD: The anteriorly oriented horizontal vector loop: the problem of distinction between direct posterior myocardial infarction and normal variation. Am Heart J 88: 408, 1974
45. Fischer DM, Benini A, Scudelotti O, Pirazzini L, Finzi CM: Valutazione statica dei criteri vettocardiografici per la diagnosi di necrosi miocardica posteriore. G Ital Cardiol 7: 1075, 1977
46. Wagner R, Rosenbaum MB: Transient left posterior hemiblock. Association with acute lateral myocardial infarction. Am J Cardiol 29: 558, 1972
47. Lemberg L, Castellanos A Jr: Vectorcardiography. A programmed induction, 2nd edn. New York: Appleton-Century-Crofts, 1975.
48. Ogawa S, Kimura M, Okada M, Ogino T, Katayama K: A case of acute anterolateral infarction complicated with left posterior hemiblock. Jap Heart J 17: 123, 1976

49. Castellanos A Jr, Portillo B, Lemberg L, Myerburg RJ: Diagnostic de l'hémibloc postérieur gauche à la phase aiguë de l'infarctus du myocarde. Coeur et Med Int 41: 493, 1977
50. Schamroth L, Ziady F, Kock J: Acute inferior wall myocardial infarction associated with complete atrioventricular block and left posterior hemiblock. Br Heart J 37: 471, 1975
51. Medrano GA, Brenes C, Sodi-Pallares D: Necrosis postero-inferior del ventriculo izquierdo aislada y asociada a bloqueo de la subdivision posterior de la rama izquierda del haz de His. Arch Inst Cardiol Mex 40: 645, 1970
52. Gandhi MJ, Desai JM, Pahlajani DB, Mehta AB: Problems in diagnosis of left posterior hemiblock in acute myocardial infarction. In: Electrocardiology I. Proceedings of World Congress on Electrocardiology, Gandhi MJ, Mehta AB, Pahlajani DB. Bombay: Tata, 1975 p 110
53. Piccolo E, Raviele A, Delise P, Dainese F, Pascotto P, Totaro G, Sartori F, D'Este D: The role of left ventricular conduction in the electrogenesis of left ventricular hypertrophy. An electrophysiologic study in man. Circulation 59: 1044, 1979
54. Pietras RJ, Winslow EBJ, Boswell J, Szanto PB, Gunnar RM: The spatial vectorcardiogram in left bundle-branch block. Correlation of autopsy findings with the vectorcardiogram. In: Vectorcardiography 2, Hoffman I, Hamby RI, Glassman E. Amsterdam: North-Holland, 1971, p 277
55. Carvalho ET, Tranchesi J, Moffa PJ, Netto MP, Pileggi F, Marrara JP, Pasini U, Serro Azul LG: Estudo cinecoronarografico e cineventriculografico em pacientes com enfarte do miocardio associato a bloqueio divisional e troncular. Arq Bras Cardiol 28: 55, 1975
56. Chou TC, Helm RA: The diagnosis of right ventricular hypertrophy in the presence of left bundle branch block. In: Vectorcardiography 2, Hoffman I, Hamby RI, Glassman E. Amsterdam: North-Holland, 1971, p 289
57. Tranchesi J, Moffa P, Ebaid M: Right axis deviation in left bundle branch block: an electrovectorcardiographic study. In: Vectorcardiography 2, Hoffman I, Hamby RI, Glassman E. Amsterdam: North-Holland, 1971, p 283
58. Alboni P, Malacarne C: Problemi di asincronismo fascicolare nel blocco di branca sinistro avanzato con marcata deviazione assiale sinistra. G Ital Cardiol 6: 255, 1976
59. Musso E, Stilli D, Taccardi B, Rolli A, Aurier E, Favaro L, Botti G: Body surface maps in left bundle branch block. XX Symposium Electrocardiologicum (Abstr). Yalta, 1979, p 156
60. Befeler B, Gomez J, Agma AS, Castellanos A, Myerburg RJ: Changes in the pattern of old inferior wall myocardial infarction produced by acute left bundle branch block and hemiblock. Chest 63: 18, 1973
61. Chawla NPS, Wolf R: The utilization of atrial premature beats in the diagnosis of myocardial infarction in a patient with left bundle branch block. In: Electrocardiology I. Proceedings of World Congress on Electrocardiology, Gandhi MJ, Mehta AB, Pahlajani DB. Bombay: Tata, 1975, p 234
62. Alboni P, Malacarne C, Pradella A, Masoni A: 2:1 and phase 4 peri-infarction block. Europ J Cardiol 10: 205, 1979

10. INTERMITTENT INTRAVENTRICULAR BLOCKS

Intraventricular conduction disturbances (IVCD) in most cases are *permanent*. At times they persist for a variable period, generally secondary to acute affections and independent of cardiac rate, and then disappear. Such a type of IVCD is therefore defined as *transient*. The appearance and the disappearance of IVCD may also occur from one beat to another, usually in relation to changes in cardiac rate. In these cases the IVCD is defined as *intermittent*. If the aberrancy occurs during very early beats in relation to physiologic dishomogeneous refractoriness of the main intraventricular pathways it is defined as *functional*. Considering the longest duration of the His-Purkinje system (HPS) recovery time is approximately 400 msec [1, 2] (Figure 1), an IVCD which appears after longer cardiac cycles should be considered pathologic.

Intermittent IVCD can be observed in the main bundle branches and in the fascicles of the left bundle branch; recently they have been described also in the periphery of the intraventricular conduction system [3, 4] (see Chapter 6).

In most cases IVCD are rate-dependent; two types have been described. In one, IVCD occurs when the heart rate accelerates or after short diastolic intervals; in the other type it appears when cardiac rate decelerates or after long diastolic

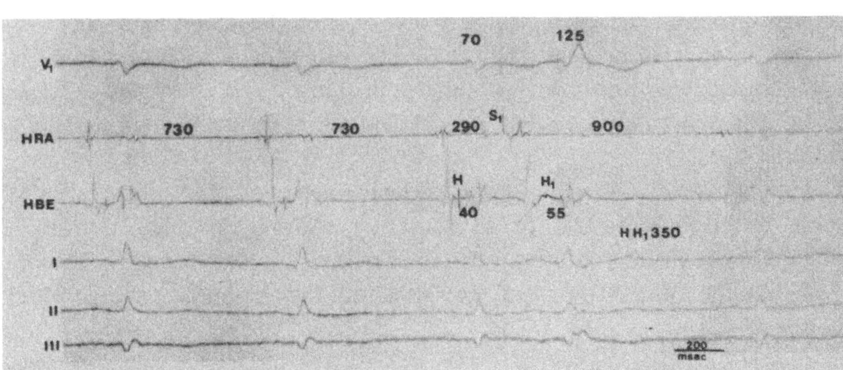

Figure 1. **Premature atrial beat is introduced during spontaneous sinus rhythm. HH_1 interval measures 350 msec and right bundle branch block appears. Due to the short duration of the HH_1 interval (<400 msec), right bundle branch block can be considered functional.** HRA: high right atrium; HBE: His bundle electrocardiogram

intervals. The former, tachycardia-dependent, is attributed to a prolonged refractoriness [5-15]; the latter, bradycardia-dependent, to enhanced spontaneous diastolic depolarization [6-8, 16-18].

In some cases, tachycardia- and bradycardia-dependent IVCD coexist in the same affected bundle [10, 11, 17, 19-22]; thus, intermittent IVCD tends to occur at both rapid and slow rates with an intermediate normal conduction range.

Tachycardia-dependent IVCD is also termed phase 3 block [10, 17, 19, 22-24], assuming that the block occurs when an impulse reaches the diseased bundle during phase 3 of the preceding action potential. Bradycardia-dependent BBB, possibly related to enhanced spontaneous diastolic depolarization, is also termed phase 4 block [10, 17, 22-24].

In rare cases an intermittent IVCD is rate-independent.

Phase 3 intraventricular block

Phase 3 or tachycardia-dependent intraventricular block represents the most common type of intermittent intraventricular blocks. In order for bundle branch block (BBB) to appear the controlateral bundle branch must function normally or less abnormally than the ipsilateral one.

The extension of the phase 3 block range varies from case to case and at times in the same subject from day to day or even from hour to hour. Tavazzi et al. [13], in a study of 31 cases, observed that phase 3 block range varied from 450 to 1390 msec. The duration of this range conditions the form of IVCD. If the recovery time of a fascicle is only slightly prolonged, aberrancy will be observed sporadically, whereas if this time is very prolonged, the IVCD will be almost always be present.

Phase 3 block is more likely to occur in the presence of affections inducing fluctuations of cardiac cycle, such as atrial or ventricular premature beats (Figure 2), 2° sino-atrial or atrio-ventricular block, or atrial fibrillation.

In the absence of an electrophysiological investigation, however, it is not possible to define with certainty whether a prolonged QRS complex expresses an aberrant intraventricular conduction or a ventricular escape beat, in cases of atrial fibrillation.

The introduction in clinical setting of electrophysiological studies, especially of the programmed premature atrial stimulation, showed that phase 3 intraventricular blocks are much more frequent than was commonly thought. They are in fact encountered quite often in subjects in whom they had not appeared in several standard ECG.

In Figure 3, as the A_1A_2 and H_1H_2 intervals progressively decrease, one can observe QRS complexes conducted with right bundle branch block (RBBB) whose duration progressively increases. In Figure 4, as the H_1H_2 interval shortens to 490 msec, a QRS complex appears conducted with left bundle branch block (LBBB), which had never been manifested in standard electrocardiograms.

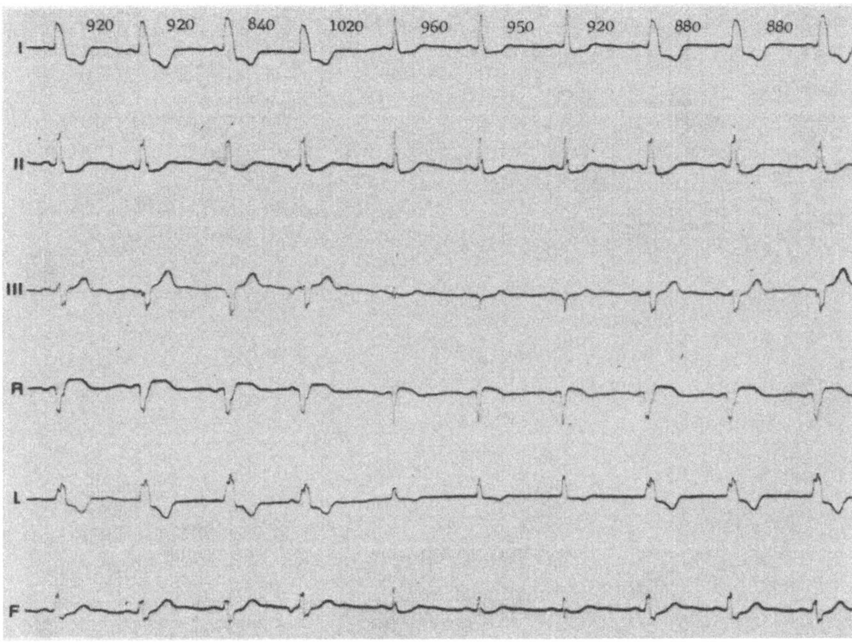

Figure 2. **Left bundle branch block was considered permanent since it was constantly present in all the** electrocardiograms recorded. Premature atrial beat induces prolonged post-extrasystolic pauses and left bundle branch block disappears

Phase 4 intraventricular block

Phase 4 or bradycardia-dependent intraventricular block is much rarer than phase 3 block. Like tachycardia-dependent block, it occurs if the controlateral bundle branch functions normally or less abnormally than the ipsilateral branch.

It has also been termed paradoxical [16], since it appears only during slowing of cardiac rate or after prolonged R-R intervals. In phase 4 block, in contrast with phase 3 block, LBBB is more frequently observed than RBBB [25, 26].

The extension of the phase 4 block range varies from case to case and at times in the same subject from day to day or even from hour to hour.

In a study of 16 cases [13] the phase 4 block range varied from 480 to 5200 msec. The last datum is very important in that it is not always possible to obtain such a marked cardiac cycle prolongation, even during carotid sinus massage; therefore it may be that several patients with normal intraventricular conduction or with phase 3 IVCD present an undetected phase 4 block as well.

The beginning of phase 4 block range conditions the form of the intraventricular conduction. If the phase 4 block appears after short RR intervals, the IVCD will almost always be present, thus simulating a permanent block, whereas if it appears only after prolonged RR intervals, it will be observed sporadically.

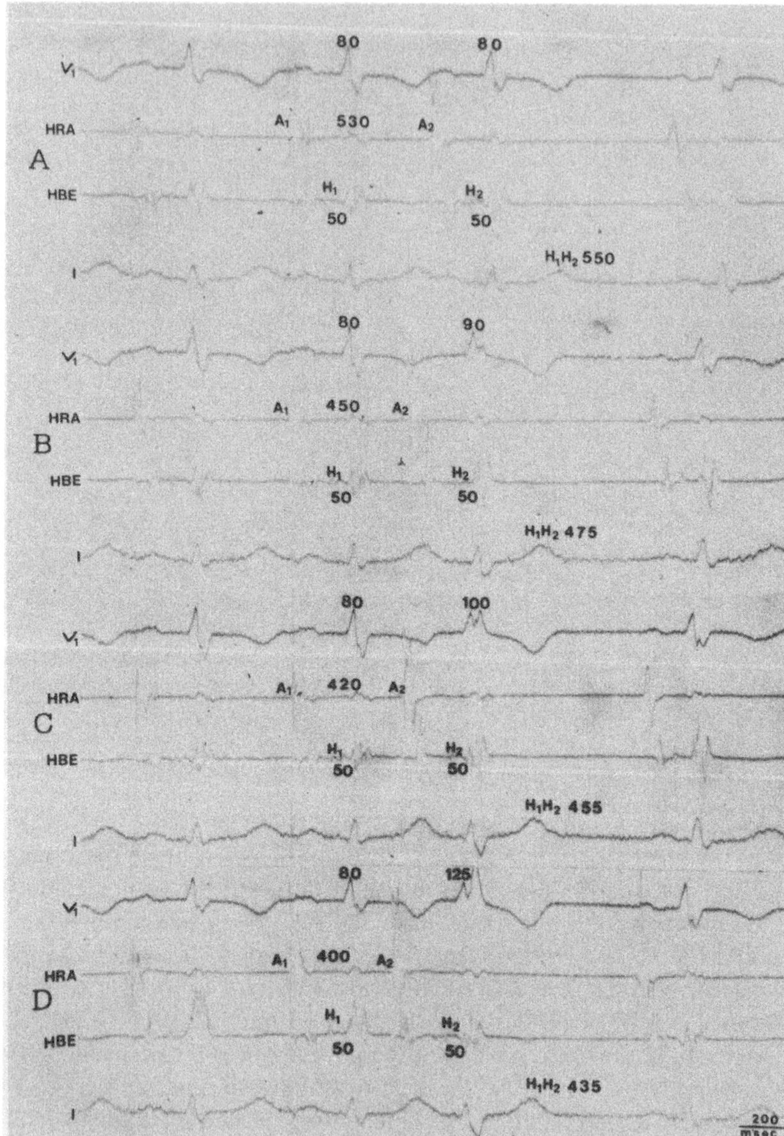

Figure 3. Phase 3 right bundle branch block. Programmed premature atrial stimulation. As A_1A_2 and H_1H_2 intervals progressively decrease, one can observe QRS complexes conducted with right bundle branch block pattern whose duration progressively increases

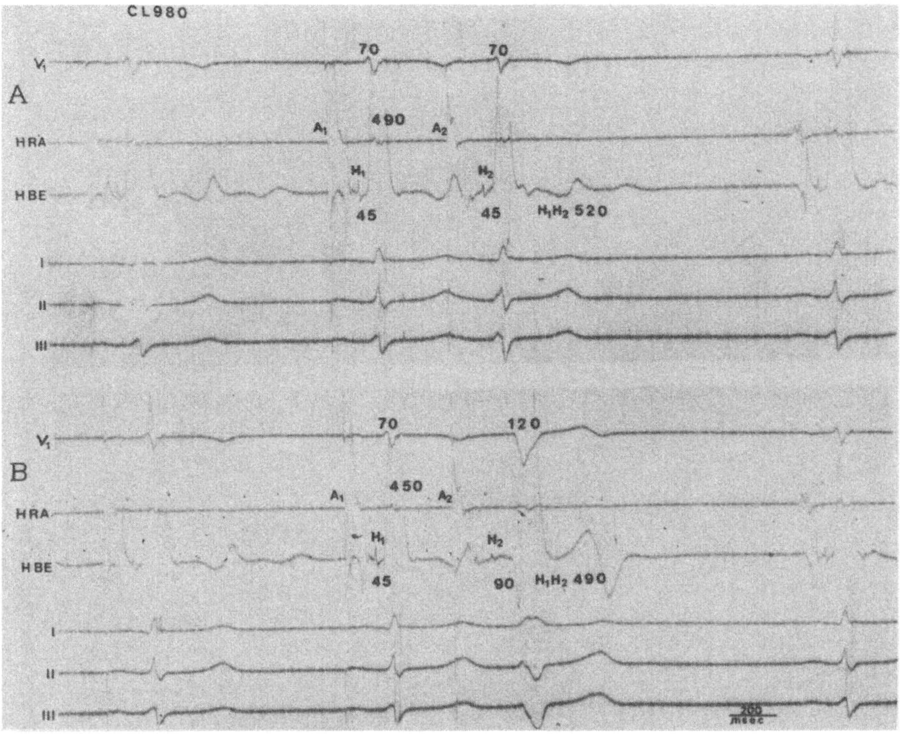

Figure 4. **Phase 3 left bundle branch block manifested only during electrophysiological study.** Programmed premature atrial stimulation. As the H_1H_2 interval shortens to 490 msec, a QRS complex conducted with left bundle branch block appears

In Figure 5 a typical pattern of phase 4 block is described. Atrial escape beats are present and RR intervals show marked fluctuations. The ventriculograms following RR intervals of 870 msec or shorter provide evidence for normal intraventricular conduction, whereas those following longer RR intervals are conducted with LBBB pattern.

In Figure 6 a case of acute inferior myocardial infarction is reported. During Wenckebach AV block there appear prolonged RR intervals, showing phase 4 anterior fascicular block (AFB).

Coexisting phase 3 and phase 4 intraventricular block

Most cases of phase 4 IVCD also show a coexisting phase 3 block [13, 27]. In such cases an intermediate normal conduction range is therefore present. Outside this range, whether there is an increase or a decrease of the cardiac cycle length, an intraventricular block is observed. Rosenbaum et al. [10] introduced the term 'accordion effect', meaning that the two blocks' ranges seem to compress more or

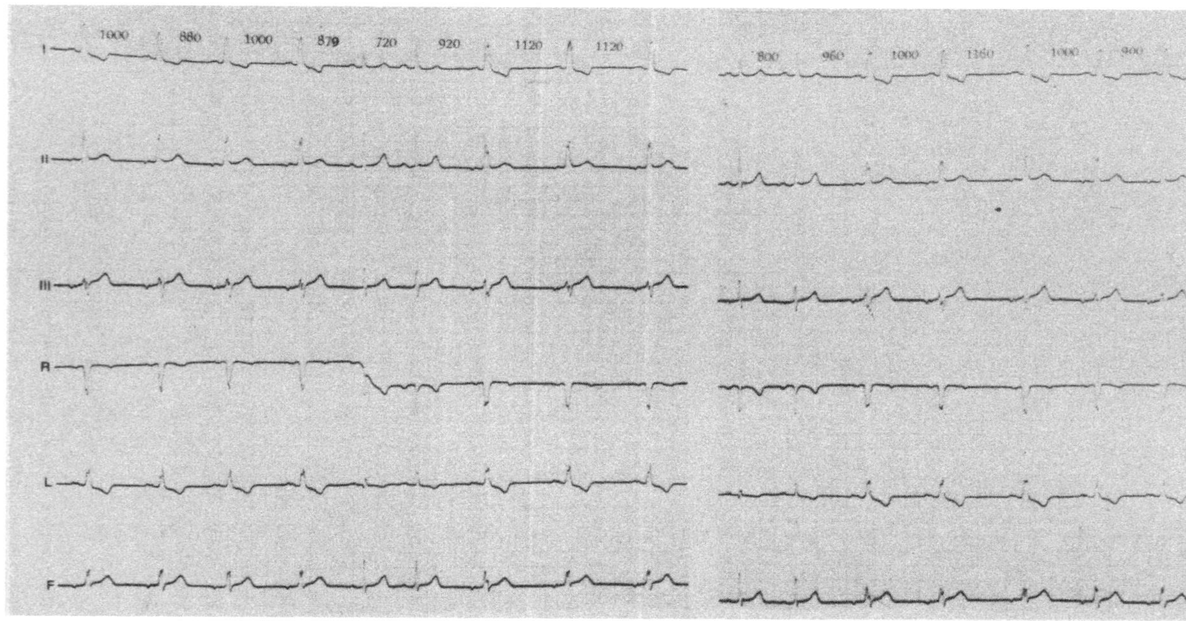

Figure 5. Phase 4 left bundle branch block in a patient with acute myocarditis. Atrial escape beats are evident. The beats following RR intervals of 870 msec or shorter show normal intraventricular conduction, whereas those following longer RR intervals are conducted with left bundle branch block pattern

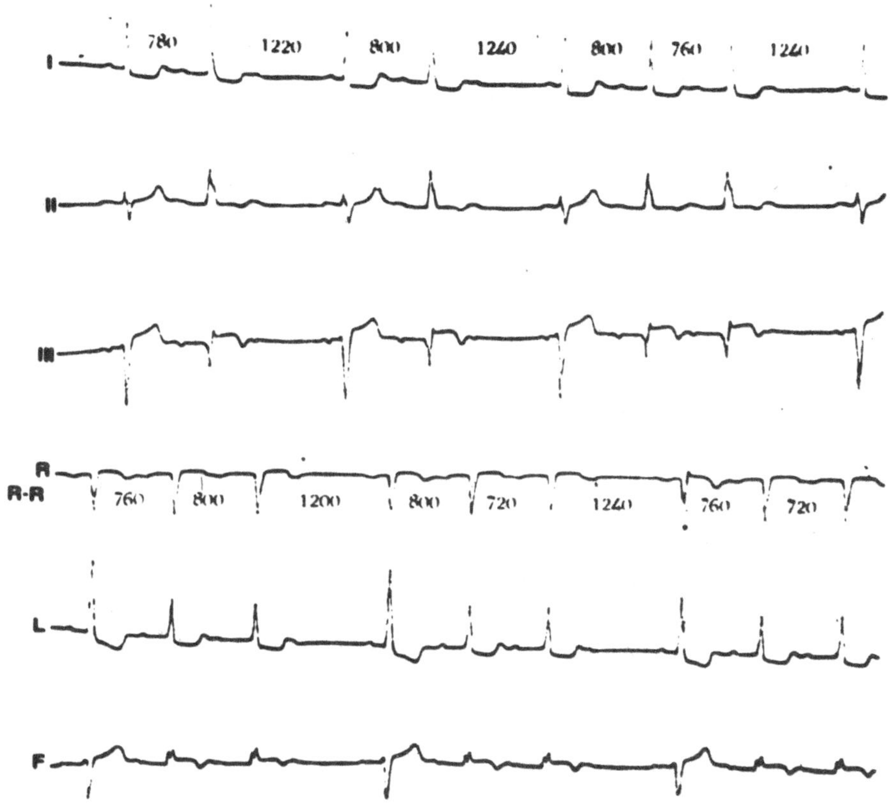

Figure 6. Phase 4 anterior fascicular block in patient with acute inferior myocardial infarction. For a short time a Wenckebach AV block appeared, which inducing prolonged RR intervals, evidenced phase 4 anterior fascicular block

less the intermediate normal conduction range.

When patients with intermittent BBB are electrophysiologically explored, it is rather easy to demonstrate the existence of phase 3 BBB, but it may be extremely difficult to uncover the presence of phase 4 BBB. Obviously the demonstration of the latter depends on the possibility of provoking, by means of carotid sinus pressure or other maneuvers, long enough diastolic intervals, which in many patients may not be feasible or safe. Some authors [13, 28], through the systematic use of vagal stimulation, demonstrated that phase 4 BBB coexisting with phase 3 BBB is rather frequent.

The intermediate normal conduction range varied from 40 to 4700 msec in 17 patients with coexisting phase 3 and phase 4 BBB reported by Tavazzi et al. [13] and from 50 to 4800 msec in 14 patients described by Rosenbaum et al. [28].

Figure 7 illustrates a phase 3 LBBB with a critical shortening of RR interval to 570 msec in a patient with anterior fascicular block. Phase 4 LBBB was dem-

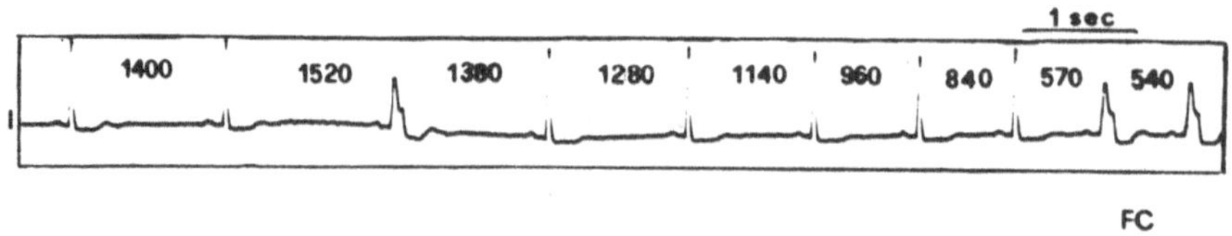

Figure 7. Phase 3 and phase 4 left bundle branch block in a patient with anterior fascicular block. Phase 3 LBBB appears with a critical shortening of RR intervals to 570 msec. During carotid sinus massage, phase 4 LBBB is evident with a critical cycle length of 1520 msec

onstrated in the same ECG tracing during carotid sinus compression.

In Figure 8 a patient with RBBB and left axis deviation (LAD) (−30°) is reported. During atrial pacing at high rate and during carotid sinus massage, a marked accentuation of LAD (−75°) appeared. This case, therefore, shows an incomplete AFB, which becomes complete both in phase 3 and in phase 4.

In a few rare cases the simultaneous presence of phase 3 block in a main bundle branch and phase 4 block in the controlateral bundle branch has been described [13]. Girotti et al. [29] reported a patient with acute myocardial infarction, showing coexisting phase 3 and phase 4 blocks in both the main bundle branches and phase 4 block in the posterior fascicle. Most of these changes were, of course, not simultaneous and their successive appearance was related to day-to-day variations in the degree and quality of the multifascicular injury caused by the infarct.

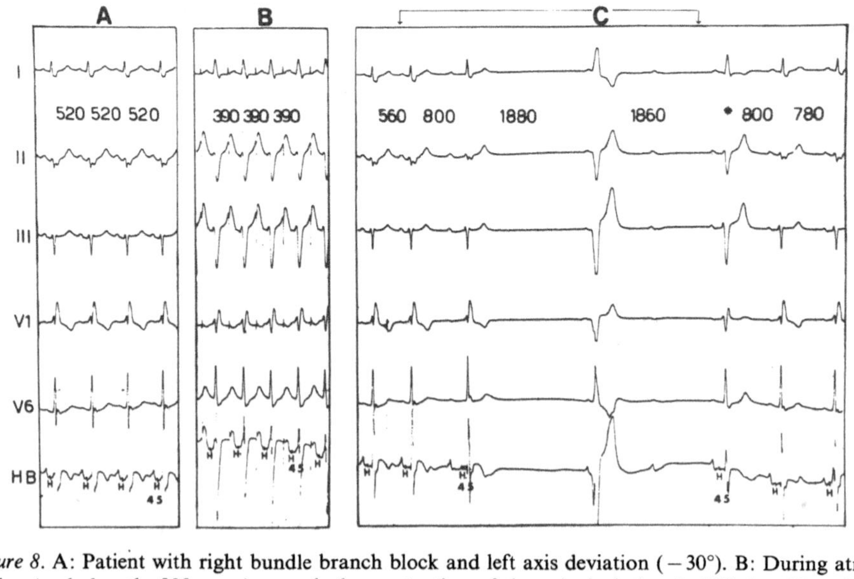

Figure 8. A: Patient with right bundle branch block and left axis deviation (−30°). B: During atrial pacing (cycle length: 390 msec) a marked accentuation of the axis deviation (−75°) is evident. The same behavior is observed during carotid sinus massage in the QRS complex subsequent to ventricular escape beat. HV interval does not change. This case evidences therefore an incomplete AFB which becomes complete in phase 3 and in phase 4

Rate-independent intraventricular block

Rate-independent intermittent intraventricular blocks are very rare and extremely unstable. Only two such cases out of 63 intermittent BBB have been observed whose change from not rate-related to rate-dependent was very rapid [13]. Most probably it is for this reason that, as far as we know, they have not been investigated either from a pathophysiologic or a clinical point of view.

In Figure 9 a case of rate-independent RBBB in a patient with ischemic heart disease is reported. In all the subsequent ECG recordings the RBBB was permanent.

Incomplete intermittent intraventricular block

An intermittent IVCD is often expressed with an incomplete intraventricular block. In 34 (55 %) out of 63 cases of intermittent BBB [13], it was incomplete in 14 cases in phase 3, in 10 in phase 4 and in 10 both in phase 3 and phase 4. All the phase 4 incomplete BBB were observed during acute myocardial infarction. The extension of the block range in a few cases was short, i.e. a few tens of milliseconds, in other cases relatively wide.

In some patients incomplete BBB is persistent and increases in degree in phase 3 or in phase 4; this behavior is frequently observed during programmed premature atrial stimulation (Figure 10).

2:1 intraventricular block

Sometimes in patients with phase 3 or phase 4 BBB, a 2:1 BBB in the injured fascicle appears for a short time. It has been observed in seven out of 63 cases of intermittent BBB [13].

Cohen et al. [29, 30] subdivided 2:1 BBB, or BBB alternans, into two main types: 'tachycardia-dependent alternans' and 'bradycardia-dependent alternans'.

Tachycardia-dependent BBB alternans was shown to occur when persistently normal or almost normal conduction changed to a pattern of BBB in alternate beats, beginning with the QRS complex which ends the first short cycle associated with an increase in cardiac rate. Bradycardia-dependent BBB alternans occurred when persistently normal or almost normal intraventricular conduction changed

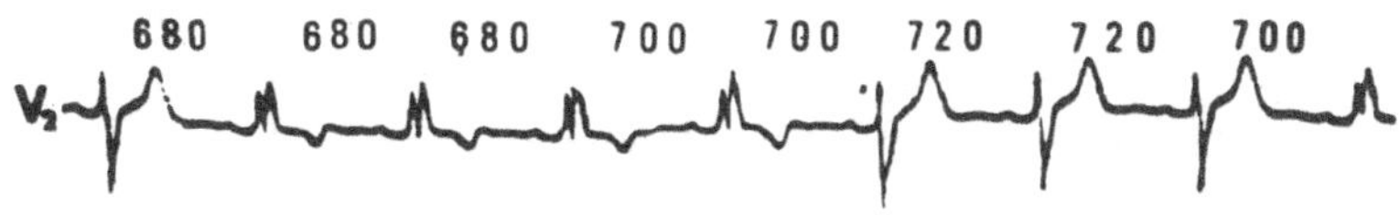

Figure 9. Rate-independent right bundle branch block in patient with ischemic heart disease. In all the subsequent ECG recordings right bundle branch block was permanent

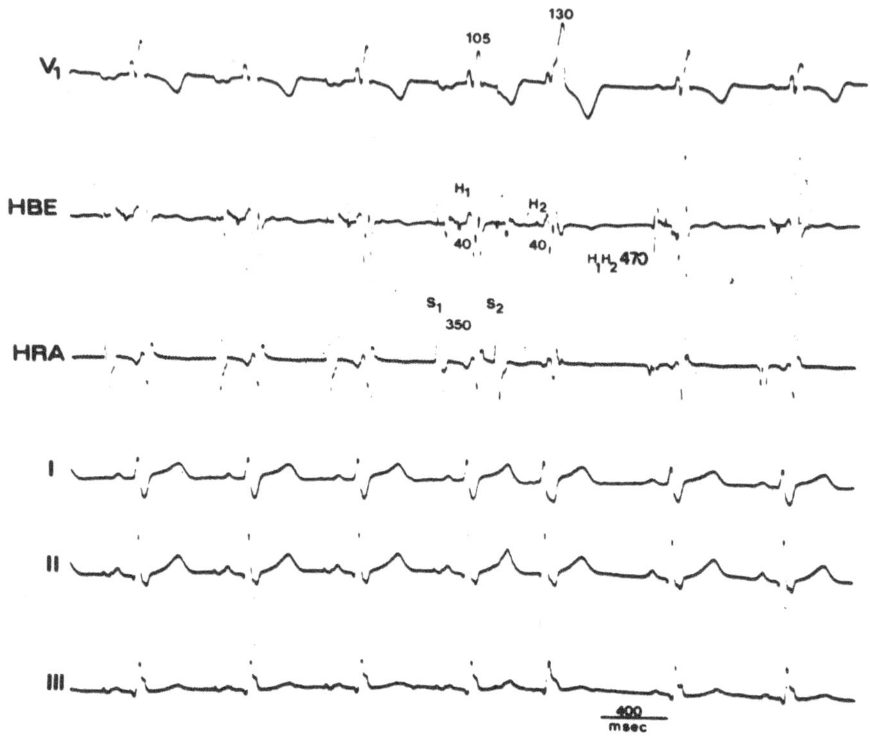

Figure 10. A permanent incomplete right bundle branch block is present (QRS: 105 msec). During programmed premature atrial stimulation right bundle branch block (QRS: 130 msec) appears (H_1H_2: 470 msec)

to a pattern of BBB on alternate beats beginning with the QRS complex which ends a long pause. A variation of tachycardia-dependent BBB alternans, 'pseudo-bradycardia-dependent BBB alternans' was also described, in which BBB on alternate beats changed to persistent BBB with slowing of cardiac rate. However, with further slowing, normal conduction supervened. The latter suggests that the block is actually tachycardia-dependent.

In Figure 11 alternans between RBBB and incomplete RBBB is present. The RR intervals measure 520 msec. A few minutes later, sinus cycle length showed marked fluctuations between 620 and 980 msec. Alternans is converted to persistent RBBB, apparently of the bradycardia-dependent type. However, the beat following the most prolonged RR interval (980 msec) showed an incomplete RBBB pattern. The latter indicates that RBBB is tachycardia-dependent or rather pseudo-bradycardia-dependent even though initially persistent RBBB appears with slowing of the rate.

Another type of 2:1 BBB has been described attributed to an intraventricular conduction in supernormal phase; when the cardiac cycle coincides with conduc-

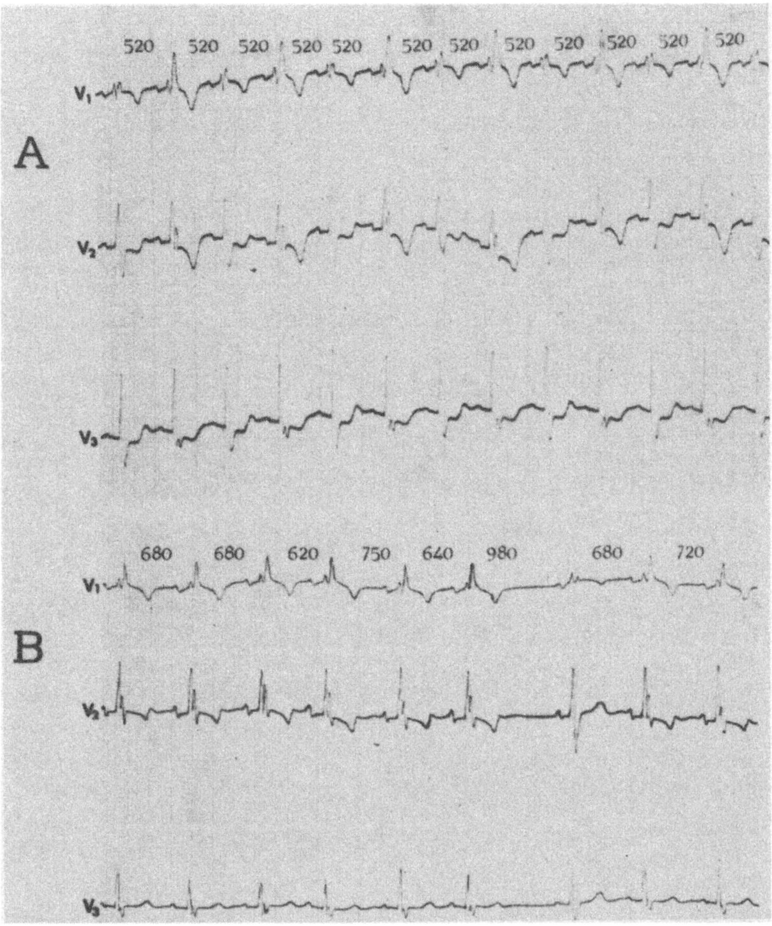

Figure 11. **Pseudo-bradycardia-dependent 2:1 right bundle branch block. A: Alternans between right** bundle branch block and incomplete right bundle branch block is present. Cardiac cycle length measures 520 msec. B: ECG recorded a few minutes later. Cardiac cycle length increases and shows marked fluctuations. Alternans is converted to persistent right bundle branch block. However, the beat following the most prolonged RR interval (980 msec) shows an incomplete right bundle branch block pattern. Thus this tracing is suggestive of pseudo-bradycardia-dependent alternans. (For details see text)

tion zone in supernormal phase a BBB alternans may occur [13].

In Figure 12 a patient with persistent LBBB is reported. Such a block is constantly present during slowing of the sinus cycle length induced by carotid sinus massage and during programmed premature atrial stimulation. When atria are being paced at a constant cycle length of 420 msec, LBBB patttern alternates with narrow QRS complex. It is very likely that such alternating aberrancy expresses conduction in supernormal phase.

The electrophysiological mechanisms of the 2:1 BBB will be discussed later.

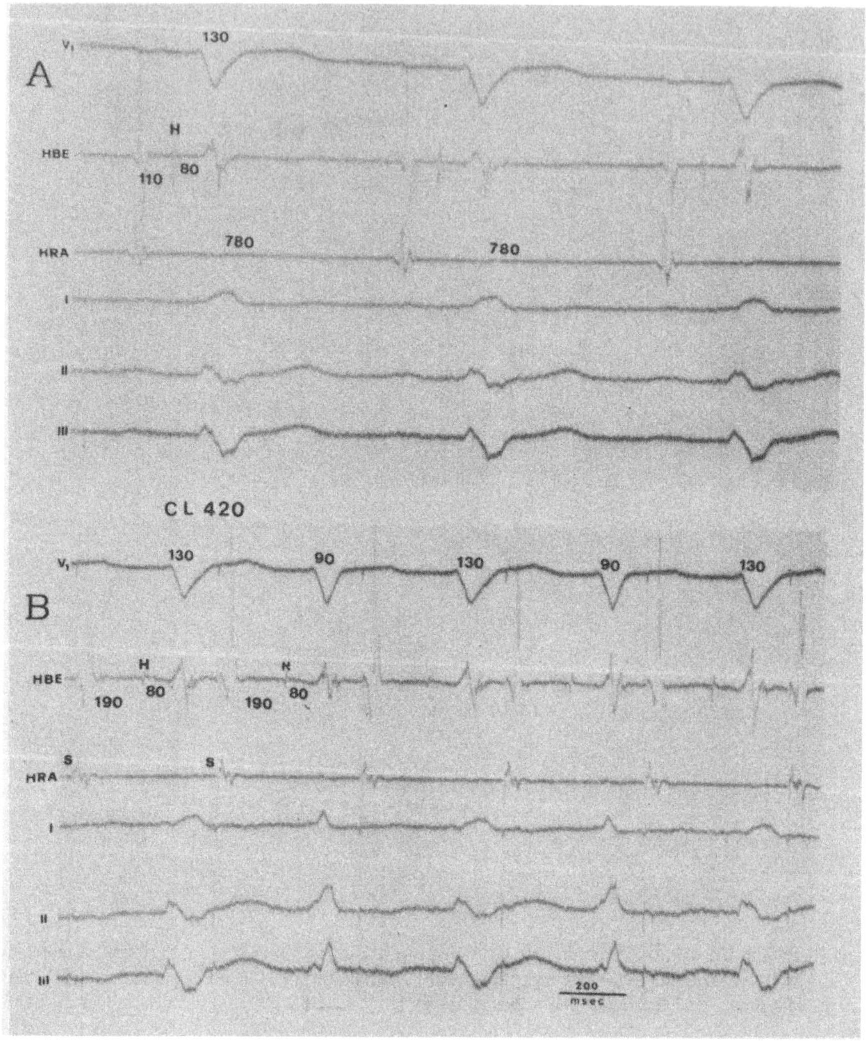

Figure 12. 2:1 left bundle branch block probably related to conduction in supernormal phase. Left bundle branch block is constantly present in several standard electrocardiograms and in the basic recording during electrophysiological study (A). Such a block persists during programmed premature atrial stimulation and continuous atrial pacing at a cycle length of 600-440 msec. At a cycle length of 420 msec left bundle branch block alternates with normal QRS complex (90 msec). HV interval does not change. This finding is suggestive of 2:1 left bundle branch block related to conduction in supernormal phase

Normal electrophysiological properties of the His-Purkinje system

When a microelectrode is positioned in the extracellular fluid adjacent to a cell, a level of zero potential is recorded. As the electrode is inserted into a cell of HPS, a change from zero to an electronegative potential occurs and a transmembrane potential of about −95 mV is recorded. The basis for the maintenance of a large electronegative potential is the active transport of ions across the cell membrane, a process requiring energy expenditure by the cell [31, 32]. As a result of active transport, the ratio of the intracellular to the extracellular potassium concentration is large (approximately 30:1). Similarly, there is a high concentration of extracellular sodium in relation to that within the cell [5].

The resting membrane potential is the transmembrane potential recorded during electrical quiescence. Any increase in extracellular potassium will result in hyperpolarization, whereas increases in extracellular potassium will depolarize.

Application of an electrical stimulus of sufficient magnitude to the resting cell induces *an action potential* (Figure 13). The first phase of the action potential is a rapid depolarization (phase 0). This is related to a sudden increase in the membrane permeability to sodium ion.

The rate of change of membrane potential during phase 0 depends on the ratio

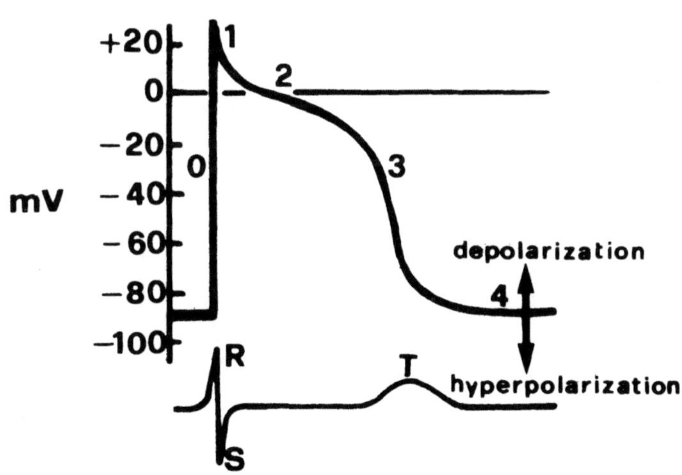

Figure 13. Diagram of the action potential of a Purkinje fiber. When the cell is quiescent the resting potential is negative (about −90 mV). At the peak of the action potential the interior of the cell becomes positive (about +30 mV) with respect to the outside, so that there is an overshoot. The upstroke is referred to as phase 1, the plateau or period of persisting depolarization as phase 2, and the period of more rapid repolarization as phase 3. The subsequent period of electrical diastole is referred to as phase 4. A change in membrane potential away from the resting potential towards zero is a depolarization; a change in the membrane potential that makes the inside of the cell more negative is a hyperpolarization

of extracellular to intracellular sodium concentration. As extracellular sodium increases or intracellular sodium decreases, the rate of rise in phase 0 is increased [33]. Phase 0 depolarization in the cells of the HPS terminates in an overshoot during which transmembrane potential is positive (about +30 mV) compared to extracellular environment. The magnitude of the overshoot is related to the ratio between extracellular and intracellular Na^+ concentration. After phase 0 three repolarization phases appear: phase 1 is a rapid reversal of membrane potential, phase 2 a plateau and phase 3 a return to the resting membrane potential. During phase 2, a decreasing inward sodium current and a slow inward calcium current appear to maintain membrane potential at a fairly steady level, thereby accounting for the plateau [34]. During phase 3, permeability to potassium ion increases and an outward potassium current is accompanied by a return of membrane potential to the resting level [35]. The subsequent period of electrical diastole is referred to as phase 4.

The events which occur during the course of the cardiac action and resting potentials are interdependent. When the resting potential increases, there is also a rise in the action potential amplitude (reflected in the magnitude of the phase 0 overshoot) and the rate of change of membrane potential during phase 0 [36]. The relationship between membrane potential, the action potential overshoot and the maximum rate of change of membrane potential during phase 0 (Vmax) is expressed by a sigmoid curve [36] (Figure 14). It is evident that over a wide range of membrane voltages there is a readily definable relationship between membrane potential and the Vmax and overshoot magnitude. The relationship between the Vmax of phase 0 and the level of membrane potential at which the action potential is initiated is referred to as the *membrane responsiveness* [36].

The sigmoid membrane responsiveness curve is a good indicator of ability of a

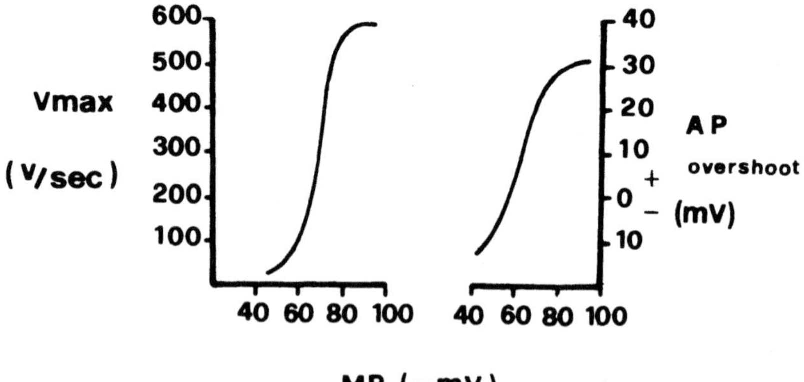

Figure 14. Sigmoid membrane responsiveness curve of a Purkinje fiber. Relationship of membrane potential (MP) to masimum rate of change of membrane potential during Vmax of the phase 0 and action potential overshoot. For details see text. (Modified from Rosen [38])

cell to respond to an electrical stimulus. In the fibers of the HPS at membrane potentials less than −55 to −50 mV there is no response; at membrane potential greater than −85 mV responsiveness is maximal.

The fibers of the HPS present, besides the excitability characteristic of all electrophysiologically functional cardiac cells, an *automaticity*. The latter refers to the ability of a cell to undergo spontaneous phase 4 depolarization until threshold potential is attained and an action potential is elicited (Figure 15). The ionic basis for spontaneous phase 4 depolarization and resultant automaticity is not fully understood. A small inward sodium current which would tend to induce depolarization persists during spontaneous phase 4. immediately following repolarization there is large outward potassium current [37]. If maintained, this would hold membranc potential at a steady resting level. However, in automatic cells membrane permeability to potassium decreases during phase 4 and the outward potassium current steadily decreases. As a result, the cell gradually depolarizes during phase 4 until threshold potential is attained and an action potential is initiated.

The spontaneous rate of impulse initiation by an automatic cell is not only related to phase 4 depolarization but also to the level of threshold potential and the *maximum diastolic potential* (the maximum transmembrane potential attained on termination of repolarization). Those last factors which favor acceleration of spontaneous rate include an increase in the slope of phase 4 depolarization, an increase in threshold potential and/or a decrease in maximum diastolic potential. In instances where threshold potential or the slope of phase 4 decrease or the maximum diastolic potential increases, spontaneous rate tends to decelerate. In normal hearts the fibers of the HPS present less automaticity than the cells of the sinus node, the atrial specialized conduction system and the lower AV node margin. Therefore they present a pacemaker function only when higher pacemakers are nonfunctional.

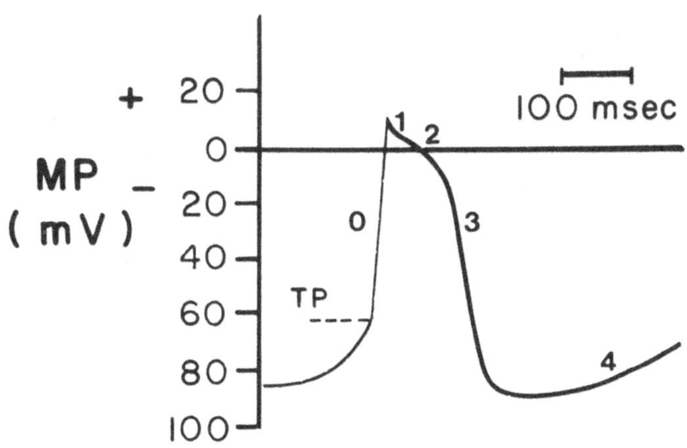

Figure 15. Spontaneous phase 4 depolarization of a Purkinje fiber resulting in attainment of threshold potential (TP)

The propagation of the cardiac impulse is conditioned by various interrelated factors; of particular importance are the passive properties of the cardiac cells [38]. Both the cellular cytoplasm and the extracellular fluid are good conductors of electrical current. Interposed between them is a membrane which introduces a resistance to current flow. Because the membrane resistance is greater than that of the extracellular or intracellular fluid, the current tends to flow longitudinally along any fiber of the conducting system from any point of excitation. As the current advances along the membrane it reduces membrane potential from the resting level to threshold resulting in regeneration of the action potential and further propagation of activation through the conducting system [5].

Conduction velocity depends on the cellular resting membrane potential, threshold potential, action potential amplitude and Vmax of phase o [5]. Resting membrane potential conditions above all the conduction velocity because, as it increases, so do action potential amplitude and Vmax. These changes would result in an acceleration of conduction. Also threshold potential can condition the conduction velocity; when threshold potential and resting membrane potential approach each other, excitability is increased and conduction would tend to be accelerated; as they diverge, excitability would decrease and conduction would slow [39].

In order for a cell to elicit an action potential, it must be excited after its membrane potential has returned to at least from -55 to -50 mV. Thus from phase 0 through a portion of phase 3 repolarization, a stimulus applied to a cell will not initiate an action potential. Once the cell has repolarized beyond this level of membrane potential, a stimulus can induce an inward sodium current resulting in phase 0 depolarization and an action potential capable of further propagation [5].

Brooks et al. [40] found: 1) *an effective refractory period* during which a response cannot be elicited by an electrical stimulus; 2) *a relative refractory period* during which only stimuli of large magnitude can elicit responses; and 3) *a supernormal period* during which the stimulus required to induce an action potential is of lesser magnitude than that needed when the cell is fully recovered. Effective refractory period is measured from the onset of the earliest premature depolarization that can propagate further in the conducting system. In the HPS the effective refractory period is longer in the distal fibers than in more proximal ones [38]. Thus in the area of maximum action potential duration or 'gate' the effective refractory period limits the extent to which a premature depolarization may be propagated.

In the normal conducting system there is a gate for each Purkinje fiber ramification into the myocardium, and all gates are of approximately equal action potential duration. The result is that at all gates the effective refractory period tends to be uniform. In depressed tissues, however, gates may be of unequal duration [5] and a premature depolarization can therefore initiate in a re-entrant arrhythmia.

Phase 3 block

This type of block occurs when the cardiac rate is accelerated or after a short diastolic interval, often related to premature atrial beats. An impulse falling during a prolonged refractory period will be blocked or conducted with delay.

A later impulse which falls when the fascicle has completed its recovery will be conducted normally. This is the interpretation generally accepted for the phase 3 IVCD (Figure 16).

A problem presently under discussion involves the features of the action potential of the cells showing phase 3 block [12, 41, 42]. It has emerged that such cells present a more or less accentuated depolarization for a reduction of the maximum transmembrane potential and consequently a more or less reduced membrane responsiveness. However, such an alteration is never very accentuated, otherwise a permanent BBB would be observed.

In some studies [5, 43] the depolarization of the injured fibers coexisted with a reduction of the phase 3 action potential. However, in more recent experimental studies [12, 44, 45] a constant prolongation of the action potential has been observed even though its entity was slight.

According to other authors [12, 42, 46, 47] a tachycardia-dependent block does not necessarily mean that impulse falls on phase 3 of the preceding action potential. In fact, under certain conditions, such as acute ischemia, the refractory period has been shown to outlast the completion of the repolarization (so-called post

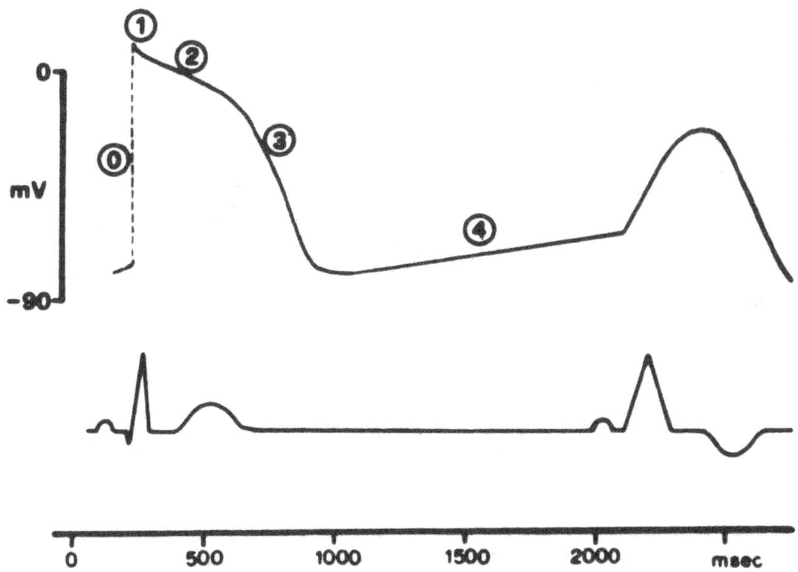

Figure 16. Schematic representation of the electrophysiological mechanisms underlying phase 3 bundle branch block. (For details see text)

repolarization refractoriness). An impulse can therefore be blocked in spite of the completion of the phase 3 action potential. If these observations are exact phase 3 block would therefore be more time-dependent than voltage-dependent since the refractoriness outlasts the action potential duration. The precise electrophysiologic mechanisms of this intermittent block cannot be determined in clinical setting where transmembrane potential records are not obtained. The terms phase 3 and phase 4 block used in clinical contest may thus be considered oversimplified and sometimes misleading. The report of Task Force I of the American College of Cardiology [48] has also cautioned against the application of several terms derived from cellular electrophysiology.

However, the term phase 3 block, used side by side with phase 4 block, is a simple way of individualizing and at the same time interrelating these two varieties of rate-dependent blocks. In general, phase 3 BBB refers to an abnormal conduction in which the refractoriness is prolonged.

Phase 4 block

This type of block occurs when the heart rate slows or after a long diastolic interval. In recent years and following the experimental observations of Singer et al. [6], bradycardia-dependent disorders were increasingly ascribed to enhanced diastolic depolarization [7, 10] (Figure 17). Singer et al. [6] reported that, when diastolic depolarization developed in Purkinje fibers, an impulse arriving late in

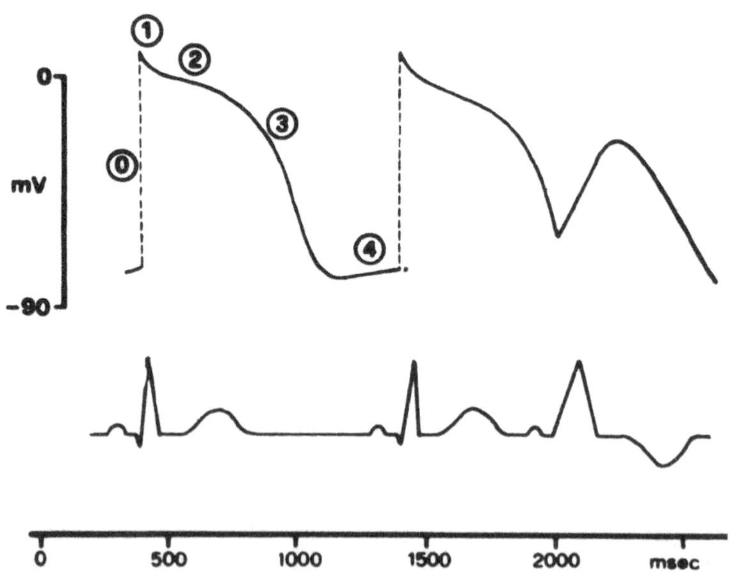

Figure 17. Schematic representation of the electrophysiological mechanisms underlying phase 4 bundle branch block. (For details see text)

these fibers during electrical diastole (phase 4) would find the transmembrane potential significantly more reduced than an impulse arriving immediately after the completion of repolarization. Since the rate and amplitude of phase 0 depolarization (the two major determinants of conductivity) would be decreased in action potential arising from such reduced (less negative) membrane potential levels [5, 36], impulse transmission was either delayed or blocked under these conditions. It is then apparent that the steeper the slope of diastolic depolarization, the greater the loss of membrane potential as well as the resultant impairment of conduction, after a given duration of electrical diastole. On the other hand, as long as the rate of phase 4 depolarization remains constant, the decrease in membrane potential would proceed with time. Thus, abnormal conduction caused by automaticity tends to appear after a longer electrical diastole, a characteristic in sharp contrast to the conduction block resulting from refractoriness, or phase 3 block.

Other clinical [11], and experimental [12] studies failed to demonstrate a temporal relationship between enhanced slope of diastolic depolarization and phase 4 intraventricular block. In fact the observation that very long diastolic intervals are sometimes necessary to show phase 4 block strongly implies that a normal or slowly rising rather enhanced slope of phase 4 depolarization is probably operative. This finding, together with the frequent failure to observe pacemaker escape in spite of long diastolic intervals, suggests that the shift of threshold potential toward zero rather than enhanced diastolic depolarization may be the most important factor in the display of phase 4 block [11, 12, 15].

Indeed, the concept of voltage-dependent conduction, i.e. of a conduction related to the voltage of the action potential at a given moment, is not sufficient to explain all cases of phase 4 block [15]. As previously mentioned, it has been recently emphasized that a tachycardia-dependent block can be explained by a time-dependent rather than a voltage-dependent mechanism. It is extremely likely, even if not yet documented, that a time-dependent mechanism may play an important part also in phase 4 block [15].

It has been shown experimentally that the cells in which a phase 4 block appear present only a slight reduction of the maximum transmembrane responsiveness. If such a reduction, in fact, were very marked, a persistent BBB would appear. Phase 4 block was always obtained after linear and very circumscribed lesions of the conducting fascicle. Conversely a more widespread lesion generally precluded the production of a phase 4 block and favored a phase 3 block [49].

Slight hypopolarization is also compatible with normal conduction [50, 51]; this finding is essential in explaining the occurrence of normal conduction in the more anticipated beats.

The concomitant occurrence of phase 3 and phase 4 block in the same fascicle can be explained by characteristic changes in the electrophysiological properties of different groups of Purkinje fibers. The presence of two groups of cells arranged in series and responding differently to changes in the cardiac cycle length appears to be the most likely interpretation as to why the conduction across the fascicle is impaired both by increasing or decreasing the heart rate [11].

Various other *alternative hypotheses* have been proposed in the past to explain the IVCD occurring after long diastolic pauses: supernormality and Wedensky phenomenon, which will be discussed later, effect of vagal impulses, momentary changes in coronary perfusion, presence of bypass fibers of Mahaim.

Since in many cases the intraventricular aberrancy develops in response to vagally mediate slowing of the sinus rate, bradycardia-dependent block was attributed to the effect of vagal impulses on conduction in the HPS [52-54]. The electrophysiological effects of parasympathetic innervation on the ventricle have not as yet been fully clarified. In vitro studies on Purkinje fibers have demonstrated that acetylcholine decreases automaticity by depressing the slope of diastolic depolarization [55, 56]. It is apparent that vagal stimulation or acetylcholine administered intravenously in intact animals can slow the discharge rate of ventricular automatic foci [56]. Very recently Martins et al. [57] observed that an increased vagal tone obtained through stimulation of the canine cervical vagi prolonged the effective refractory period similarly in endocardium and epicardium.

On the basis of the available data it seems however that vagal stimulation does not have any effect on conduction velocity in normal HPS [56, 58, 59]. On the other hand, it cannot be excluded with certainty that acetylcholine depresses the conduction velocity in ischemic proximal HPS [60] and some clinical cases would seem to support these hypotheses [52, 54, 61]. One must therefore consider the possibility that in a few cases, a phase 4 intraventricular block induced by carotid sinus massage may have a vagal genesis.

The effect of momentary change in coronary perfusion is controversial. Acute reduction of the blood supply to the proximal HPS related to prolonged diastolic pauses was thought to act through local metabolic and physiochemical changes, altering the transmembrane ionic gradient [62]. Though a possible role of acute reduction of the mean blood pressure cannot be completely ruled out, it has been shown [11, 13] that the change from normal intraventricular conduction to phase 4 BBB can occur with minimal critical slowing of the heart unaccompanied by any appreciable change in the blood pressure.

Anomalous ventricular excitation due to impulse spread along paraspecific fibers of Mahaim with prolonged refractory period has also been suggested to explain bradycardia-dependent aberrancy [63]. This mechanism must be taken into consideration when an evident initial slurring of QRS complex appears and the PR interval shortens. An electrophysiological study may clarify any doubts, showing a shortening of HV interval before the aberrant ventricular beats.

Ventricular escape beats during phase 4 block

Rosenbaum et al. [49, 64] observed in experimental studies that changes in the degree of bundle branch injury and of phase 4 block were accompanied by correlative changes in the frequency and coupling interval of escape beats from the injured fascicles, indicating the existence of a close relationship between degree of injury, phase 4 BBB and ventricular escapes within the affected fascicles.

However, in other experimental [12, 65] and clinical [11] observations a temporal relationship was not demonstrated between enhanced spontaneous diastolic depolarization and phase 4 BBB. El-Sherif et al. [12] showed that bradycardia-dependent BBB was present at the stage when diastolic depolarization and automaticity were actually depressed. When enhanced automaticity began to be observed, it was usually possible to demonstrate that phase 4 BBB did not occur at rates significantly slower than the escape rate. Similar dissociation between phase 4 BBB and ventricular escapes has also been illustrated in some clinical cases where marked variations in the critical rate for bradycardia-dependent BBB were found in repeated observations in the presence of ventricular rhythm of an almost constant rate [11].

At present it is unclear why escape ventricular beats occur in some experimental studies and not in others. Rosenbaum and El-Sherif offer an electrophysiological interpretation for the appearance or lack of appearance of these beats but an explanation of the different results obtained during experimental investigations is not given. Rosenbaum et al. [64, 66] postulate that in cases in whom ventricular escapes do not appear, concealed or abortive escapes may occur in the injured region. This hypothesis does not, however, clarify such a question. The discrepancy might lie in the varying degree of injury experimentally induced in the HPS during the various studies.

It must also be underlined that in the standard electrocardiogram it is not possible to define whether escape rhythms arise from the site of the maximal conduction disturbance in the bundle branch system. In connection with this, it has been demonstrated that in the presence of phase 4 BBB, escape rhythms arising from the AV node, His bundle, proximal portion of the diseased bundle branch or from the controlateral bundle branch system may have the same QRS configuration in conventional leads [12]. Also, during electrophysiological investigation it is not possible to define the exact ventricular area in which the ventricular escapes arise.

In a clinical setting it is not therefore possible to define any relationship between phase 4 BBB and enhanced automaticity.

OVERLAPPING

There are several factors responsible for an overlapping between normal or almost normal conduction zone and block zone.

Ashman phenomenon. The duration of the refractory period of the conducting tissues is directly proportional to the preceding cycle length as reflected by the preceding RR interval [67].

A long preceding RR interval will result in a relatively long ensuing refractory period, whereas a short preceding RR interval will result in a relatively short ensuing refractory period. In other words, the refractory period shortens with tachycardia and lengthens with bradycardia.

Intermittent intraventricular aberrancy is thus favored by a long preceding RR interval (Figure 18). This is particularly evident in cases of atrial extrasystoles with identical coupling intervals. Although atrial extrasystoles may have the same degree of prematurity, one of the extrasystoles may be conducted with aberration if preceded by a long RR interval, whereas the other may be normally conducted if preceded by a short RR interval. The same phenomenon is seen in cases of supraventricular tachycardia where, not uncommonly, it is only the second beat of the paroxysm that is conducted with aberrancy.

Concealed transeptal retrograde conduction. A concealed transeptal retrograde conduction arriving from the controlateral bundle into the impaired bundle induces a delayed activation of the latter and therefore a delayed bundle branch recovery time. The consequence is that beats following RR intervals of the same duration may demonstrate aberrancy or normal intraventricular conduction, depending on whether there has been concealed transeptal retrograde conduction or not. This mechanism must be suspected whenever a phase 3 BBB pattern appears in supraventricular premature beats and persists in subsequent cycles with the same or more prolonged duration as those preceding the premature beats, conducted without aberrancy (Figure 19). The delay by which the bundle branch showing orthograde block is activated retrogradely is about 50 msec [68, 70].

In the presence of a concealed transeptal retrograde conduction, the 'linking phenomenon' described by Rosenbaum et al. [10] may be explained. By accelerating the heart rate, the critical RR interval at which phase 3 BBB appears is shorter than that at which conduction is returned to normal when heart rate is decelerated. In fact once the BBB appears it may persist during longer cycles due to concealed transeptal retrograde conduction. Linking phenomenon is easily shown during an electrophysiological study, by accelerating and decelerating the electrical stimulation rate. It may also be observed as a spontaneous manifestation in the standard electrocardiogram (Figure 20).

It has been demonstrated experimentally that retrograde conduction in the

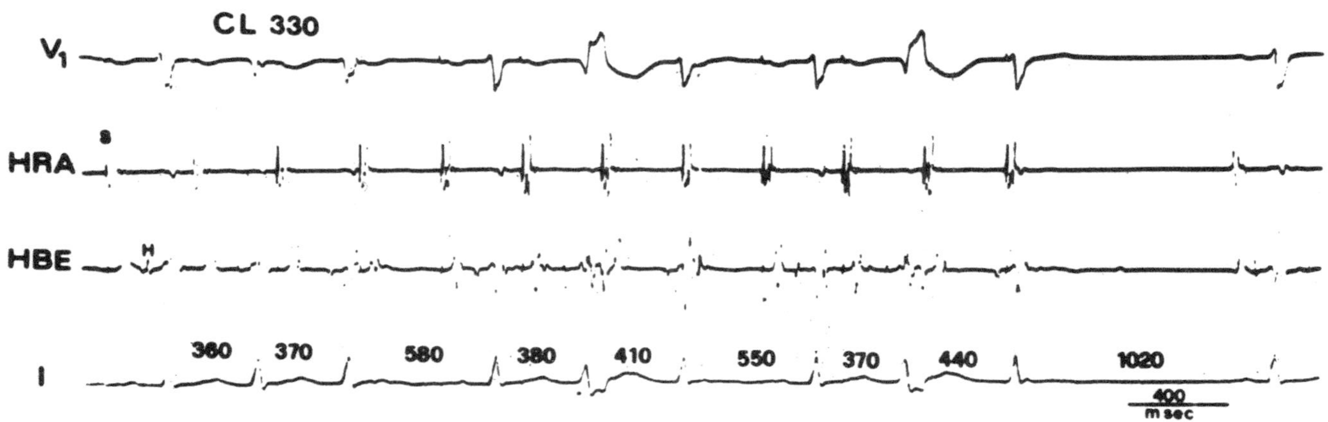

Figure 18. Ashman phenomenon. Wenckebach AV block during atrial pacing at cycle length of 330 msec. Right bundle branch block appears following RR intervals of 380 and 370 msec, when the preceding RR intervals are prolonged (580 and 550 msec, respectively). RR intervals of the same duration preceded by short RR intervals, do not show right bundle branch block

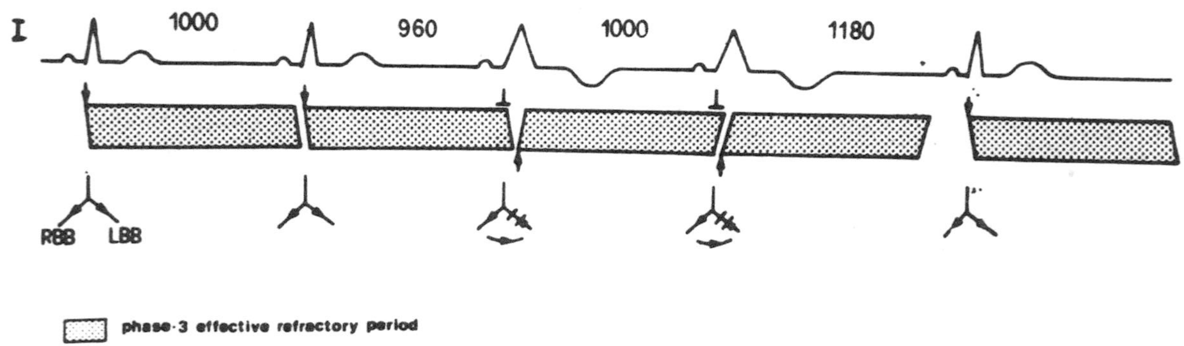

Figure 19. Diagram expressing concealed transeptal retrograde conduction, which induces overlapping during phase 3 left bundle branch block (LBBB). Intraventricular conduction is normal if the RR interval measures 1000 msec (first cycle), whereas LBBB appears when such an interval shortens to 960 msec (second cycle). The effective refractory period of the left bundle branch (LBB) lies between 960 and 1000 msec. LBB is depolarized about 50 msec later by a concealed transeptal retrograde impulse arriving from the right bundle branch. Successive cycle measures 1000 msec, but, unlike the first cycle, ends with a beat showing LBBB pattern. Owing to delay with which LBB is depolarized in the preceding beat, effective LBB cycle is not the same as RR cycle (1000 msec), but about 50 msec less (950 msec). Such a cycle lasts less than LBB effective refractory period and consequently LBBB appears. It follows that in the presence of phase 3 intraventricular block, cycles of equal duration may be ended by beats with both normal and aberrant intraventricular conduction. (Modified from Tavazzi et al. [13])

injured area tends to be preserved also during orthograde phase 4 block [20, 49]. Thus, by the same mechanism, concealed transeptal retrograde conduction may induce overlapping in the presence of phase 4 BBB.

Change of the action potential induced by variations of heart rate. These changes may be expressed by: a) variation of the action potential duration with subsequent overlapping between conduction zone and phase 3 block zone. In this regard, whereas the duration of the action potential in the normal HPS shortens with

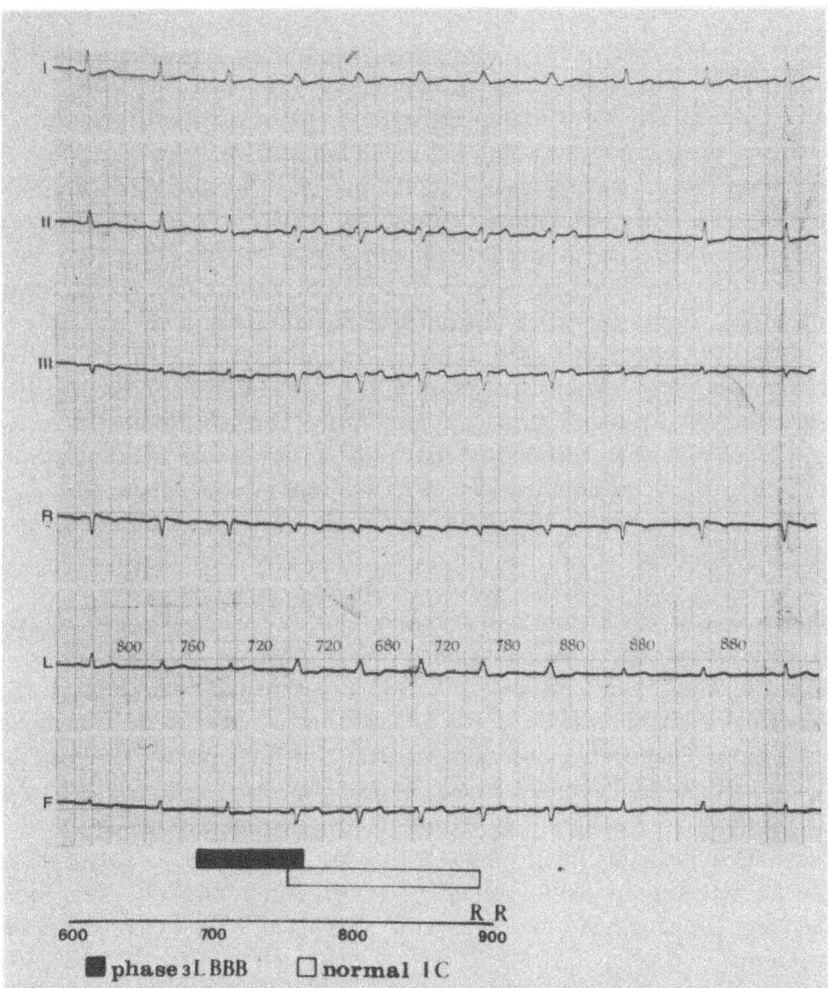

Figure 20. Linking phenomenon. Phase 3 left bundle branch block. When RR interval decreases to 720 msec, left bundle branch block pattern appears. Subsequently RR interval increases and following a cycle of 780 msec, left bundle branch block is still present. (For details see text)

increasing heart rate [5, 71, 72], in the injured HPS the action potential duration is often prolonged [72]; b) changes of the slope of the diastolic depolarization or of the maximum diastolic potential with subsequent overlapping between conduction zone and phase 4 block zone. These electrophysiological changes induced by variation of the heart rate have been demonstrated experimentally [5, 6].

Concealed premature or escape beats, which induce new conduction and block zones. These beats are not generally suspected since they are not evident in the electrocardiographic recordings [10].

Supernormal conduction is said to occur when impulse conduction is better than expected. The phenomenon has generally been observed in the setting of conduction delay and block in the HPS and represents a temporary improvement in the prevailing abnormal state of conduction [73]. It has recently been demonstrated that supernormal conduction may represent a physiological manifestation and may be induced even in the working ventricular myocardium [74, 75]. Periods of supernormal excitability were first described for nerves in 1912 by Adrian et al. [76]. Using intracellular depolarizing current, Weidmann [77] then demonstrated a period of supernormal excitability in sheep Purkinje fibers. This author showed a short period of fall or a dip (negative afterpotentials) in membrane electrical resistance corresponding to the region just preceding phase 4, or the electrical diastole. During this period the threshold potential recovered more completely than membrane potential in that excessive quantities of potassium ions may escape from the interior of the Purkinje fibers, leading to an unusual or supernormally high transmembrane potential and consequently to enhanced excitability.

The membrane potential therefore has to undergo a smaller degree of additional depolarization to reach threshold potential and thus excitation can be brought about by a weaker depolarizing current.

Recently, Spear and Moore [73, 78] experimentally demonstrated that supernormal excitability is the cause of supernormal conduction and that there exists a close temporal relationship between the two phenomena. In fact in Purkinje fibers both phenomena coincide during the cardiac cycle and respond in the same way to variations in extracellular potassium concentrations. This relationship is probably due to the fact that during the supernormal excitability period the activation potential resulting from excitation displays a very high rate of increase, a phenomenon known to be associated with increased velocity of conduction.

Experiments in which the voltage time course of the action potentials was modified by changing the pacing rate and rhythm, have shown that characteristics of the period of the supernormal excitability remained relatively unchanged in the presence of large changes in action potential duration; i.e. supernormal excitability was membrane-dependent rather than action potential configuration-dependent [79].

Since the duration of the supernormal excitability period is independent of the total duration of the action potential, reductions in action potential duration will result in the supernormal period comprising a greater percentage of the total duration of the action potential.

Other authors [80] did not find a correlation between supernormal excitability period and supernormal conduction period; they think that the conduction in supernormal phase is due to electrotonic currents which climb over the damaged area of a fascicle and depolarize the distal cells during their phase of supernormal excitability.

The duration of supernormal period may oscillate between 50 and 250 msec [81, 82].

In the standard electrocardiogram a supernormal conduction in the HPS can be suspected when, in the presence of phase 3 block, earlier premature supraventricular impulses are conducted without, or with less, aberrancy. The phenomenon may however only be apparent. In fact, whereas relatively late premature atrial impulses show BBB pattern, earlier premature supraventricular impulses can encounter sufficient AV node delay or proximal HPS delay to allow recovery of the bundle branch refractoriness. The first case has been termed type I Gap, and the second type II Gap [83].

During an electrophysiological study utilizing programmed premature atrial stimulation, a more precise evaluation can be made [72, 80, 83-90]. In type I Gap the H_1H_2 interval at which BBB disappears is longer than that at which BBB occurs. In type II Gap, the H_1H_2 interval at which normal intraventricular conduction resumes is shorter than that at which BBB appears but the H_2V_2 interval is more prolonged. The prolongation of such an interval may induce a V_1V_2 interval longer than that at which BBB appears, thus permitting the recovery of the injured bundle branch. In other cases, in which the H_2V_2 interval is prolonged but V_1V_2 is shorter than that at which BBB appears, there exists the possibility of delay in the controlateral bundle branch, inducing a synchronous ventricular activation with disappearance of the BBB pattern. When, during earlier premature atrial impulses a BBB disappears, H_1H_2 interval shortens and H_2V_2 interval remains constant, a supernormal conduction, defined also as type III gap [84], may be diagnosed (Figure 21).

Some authors [85, 91-93] have hypothesized alternative mechanisms in order to explain supernormal conduction:

i) Differential refractoriness of AV node tissues which may affect different longitudinal AV conduction pathways, or different or sequential AV junctional layers [92, 93]. Variations in the conduction in the AV node are actually recognizable during an electrophysiological study because of variations in the H_1H_2 interval. In our opinion, however, a dissociated conduction in the His

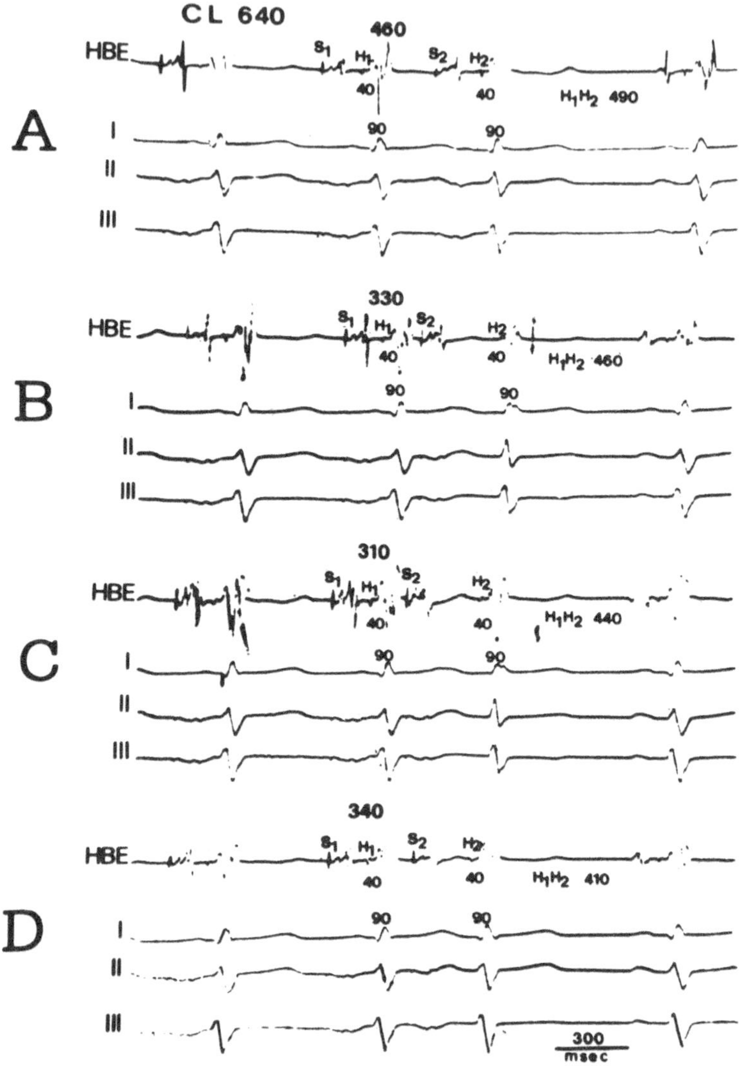

Figure 21. Supernormal conduction in the anterior fascicle. The cycle length of the basic drive is 640 msec. A_1H_1 and H_1V_1 intervals measure 80 and 40 msec, respectively. An anterior fascicular block pattern is present. In panel A, H_1H_2 interval measures 490 msec. The premature beat shows anterior fascicular block pattern (QRS: 90 msec). At shorter intervals (Panels B and C) H_2V_2 does not change and anterior fascicular block pattern disappears. The duration of the QRS complex remains at 90 msec. In Panel D, H_1H_2 interval further decreases to 410 msec. H_2V_2 interval does not change. Anterior fascicular block pattern reappears

bundle, demonstrated in experimental [94-96] and clinical [96-97] studies, and which may simulate a true supernormal conduction, is theoretically possible.

ii) Fluctuating vagal discharge related to hemodynamic changes, secondary to variations of the heart cycle, may be involved [91]. On the basis of the above mentioned data one cannot exclude that in the ischemic HPS the vagal system may in some cases condition the velocity of conduction.

However, Massumi et al. [98] have demonstrated that atropine does not abolish the supernormal conduction.

'*Pealing back*'. With this term Moe et al. [91] emphasize a pseudo-supernormal conduction related to ectopic beats which induce earlier depolarization and subsequent earlier recovery of the site of block.

Wedensky phenomena were originally described in nervous tissue and subsequently in isolated Purkinje fibers [99, 100]. These phenomena express a temporary enhancement of depressed excitability and/or conductivity and include the Wedensky facilitation and Wedensky effect.

Wedensky facilitation (Figure 22A): if the threshold potential is too high (shifted toward zero), a normal anterograde stimulus (1) arriving at the block zone will not be conducted. If a retrograde stimulus (M) arrives beyond the block it lowers temporarily the threshold potential; another anterograde stimulus of the same intensity as the first one (2a) can therefore be conducted. Later stimuli (2b) will then be blocked since the threshold potential returns to the initial values.

According to Schamroth et al. [101] a premature ventricular beat plays the same role as the stimulus M: thus one may explain the disappearance of a BBB in the supraventricular beat subsequent to a ventricular extrasystoles (Figure 23). Wedensky effect (Figure 22B): if the threshold potential is increased (shifted toward zero), an anterograde subthreshold stimulus (1) does not elicit a response. If anterograde strong above-threshold stimulus (M) is applied, it will elicit a response and will lower temporarily the threshold potential. Another anterograde stimulus (2a) of the same intensity as stimulus 1 may therefore elicit a response. Later stimuli (2b) will not elicit response in that the threshold potential returns to initial values.

The maintenance of the normal QRS complex in the second and the later sinus impulses after the ventricular extrasystoles (Figure 23) is most probably due to the Wedensky effect. Each normally conducted sinus impulse is equivalent to stimulus M and temporarily lowers the threshold potential of the depressed area with the bundle branch [101].

Thus, after a premature ventricular beat, normal conduction is probably initiated by the Wedensky facilitation and maintained by the Wedensky effect. The genesis of the decrease of the threshold potential in the Wedensky phenomena is not clear. Most likely, electronic currents play an important role [82].

'*Fatigue*' *phenomenon*. Impairment of conduction through the HPS following rapid driving has been defined as 'Fatigue' phenomenon [102, 103]. In most cases it is manifested as 2° or 3° AV block distal to His bundle, more rarely as BBB in patients with phase 3 BBB [103].

The duration and degree of 'Fatigue' in the HPS are within limits directly related to rate and duration of pacing [103]. This phenomenon may be observed following both atrial and ventricular pacing. The limited available data suggest that in a given patient, ventricular pacing results in a more prolonged 'Fatigue' effect as compared to atrial pacing at comparable levels.

Probably, fatigue phenomenon is related to transient exhaustion of the conduction capabilities in the diseased HPS [103], due to delayed regeneration of the sodium carrier in a defined area of a bundle branch [72].

Theoretically it is possible that 'Fatigue' phenomenon, or more precisely an

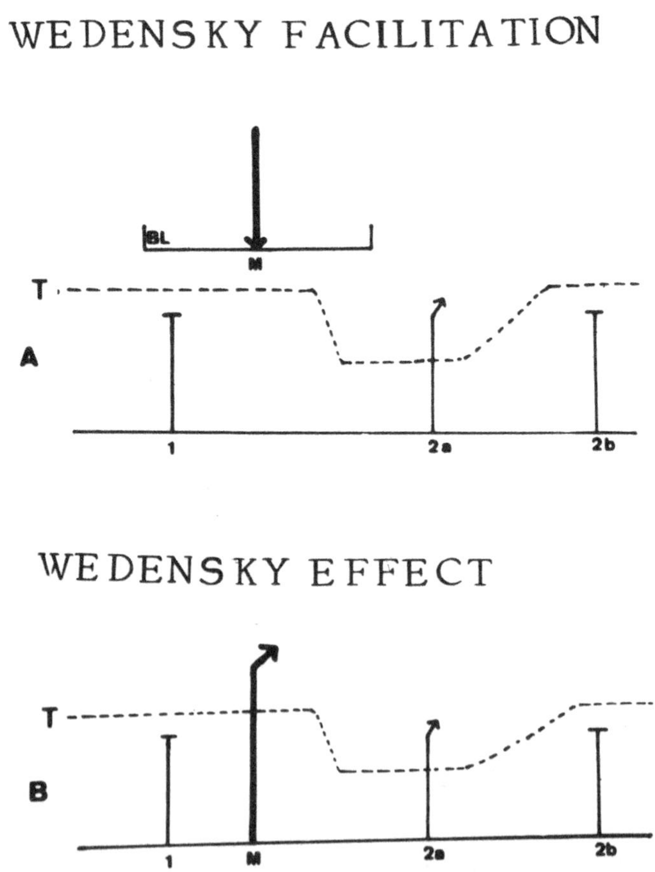

Figure 22. Diagrams of Wedensky facilitation (A) and Wedensky effect (B). BL: blocked area. T: threshold potential. (For details see text.) (Modified from Schamroth [101])

exhaustion of the conduction capabilities, may also involve the concealed transeptal retrograde conduction. In Figure 24 a record with phase 3 RBBB is reported. During atrial pacing at cycle length of 300 msec, RBBB appears and suddenly disappears without changes of HV and RR intervals. A possible interpretation of such behavior is an exhaustion of this concealed transeptal retrograde conduction which allows a normal orthograde conduction through the right bundle branch.

2:1intraventricular block

2:1 intraventricular block (or intraventricular block alternans) can occur: 1) in phase 3, 2) in phase 4, and 3) in supernormal phase. A change in rate can therefore determine the beginning or ending of alternating BBB.

Phase 3 alternans. This type of BBB alternans appears related to a refractory period prolongation of the bundle branch. It can occur in the absence of concealed transeptal retrograde conduction (Figure 25), otherwise the block would be persistent. This occurs if the effective refractory period of the bundle branch is longer than the sum of its cycle and the transeptal conduction time, but is shorter than the sum of two bundle cycles [26]. In practice a bidirectional block must be present.

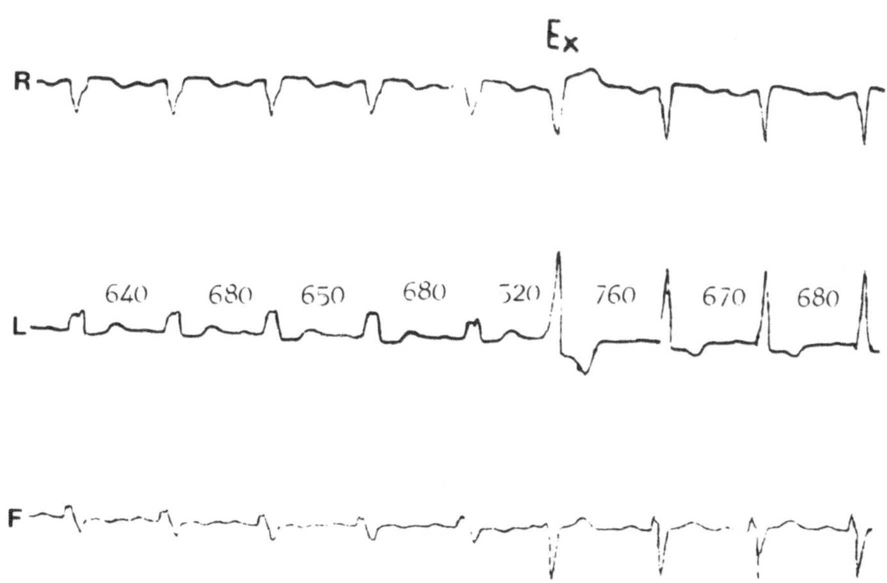

Figure 23. Wedensky facilitation and Wedensky effect. In the conducted beat following premature ventricular beat (Ex), left bundle branch block pattern disappears (Wedensky facilitation). Also, the subsequent beats show normal QRS complex (Wedensky effect). (For details see text)

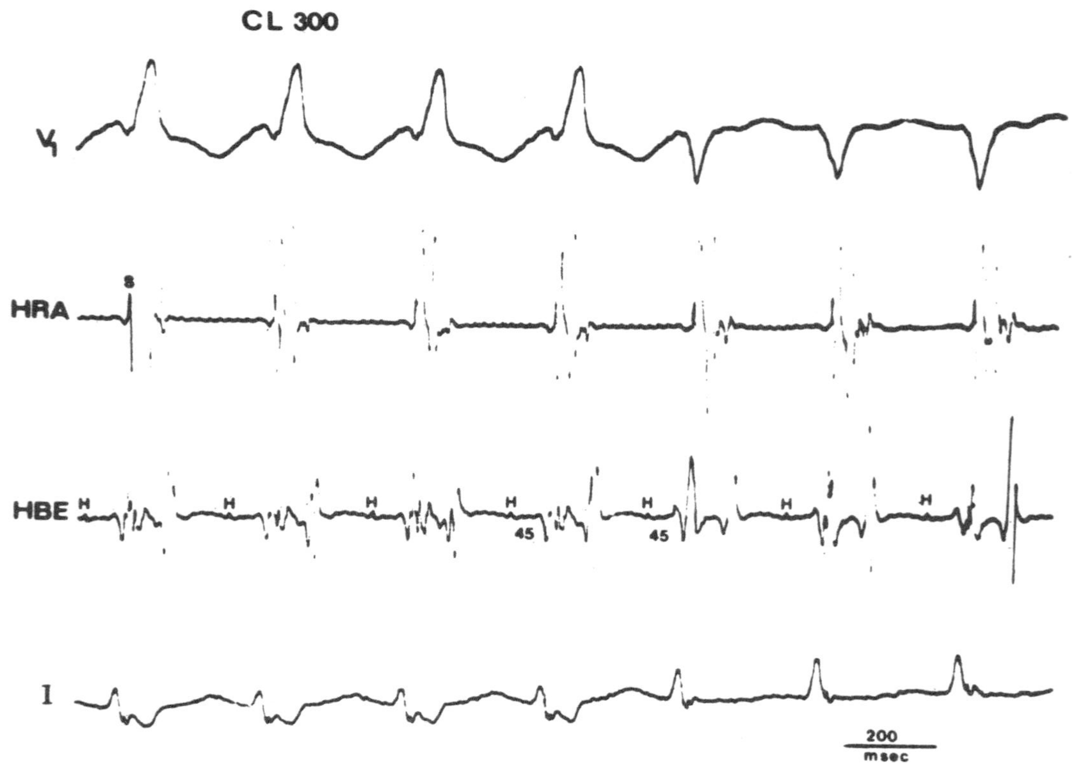

Figure 24. Phase 3 right bundle branch block. During atrial pacing at cycle length of 300 msec right bundle branch block appears and suddenly disappears without change in HV and RR intervals. A possible interpretation of such behavior is an exhaustion of the concealed transeptal retrograde conduction. (For details see text)

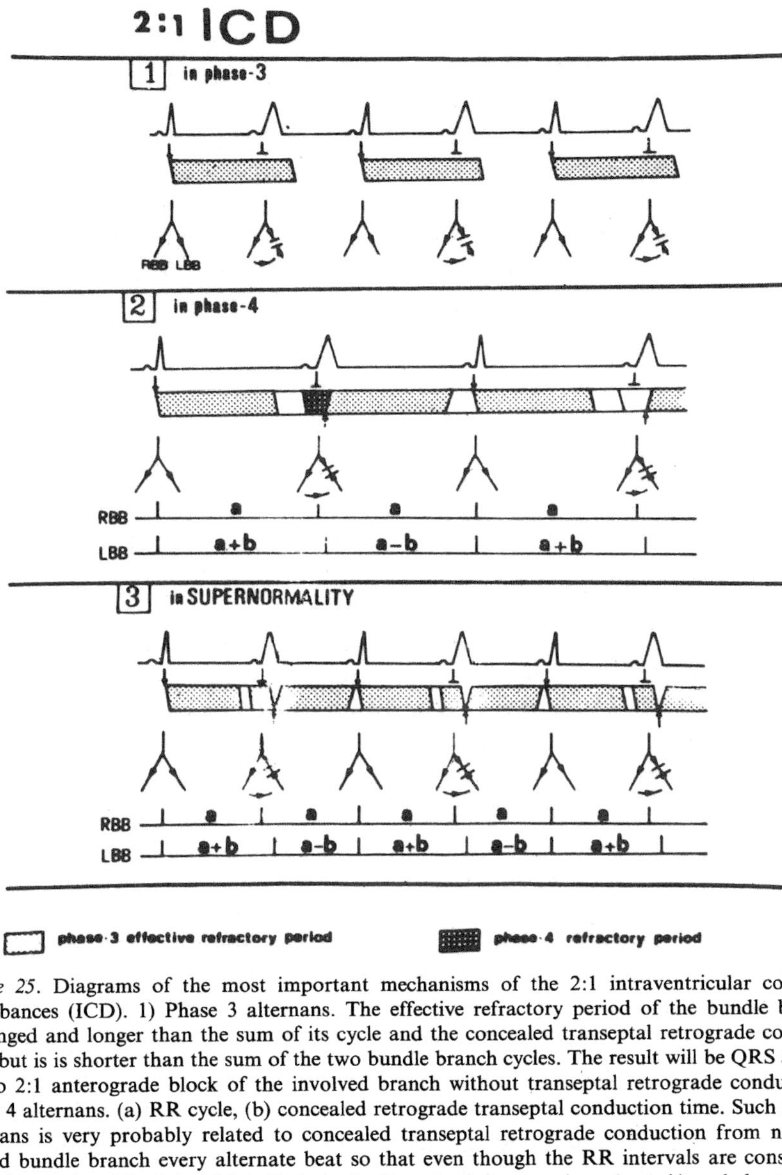

Figure 25. Diagrams of the most important mechanisms of the 2:1 intraventricular conduction disturbances (ICD). 1) Phase 3 alternans. The effective refractory period of the bundle branch is prolonged and longer than the sum of its cycle and the concealed transeptal retrograde conduction time, but is is shorter than the sum of the two bundle branch cycles. The result will be QRS alternans due to 2:1 anterograde block of the involved branch without transeptal retrograde conduction. 2) Phase 4 alternans. (a) RR cycle, (b) concealed retrograde transeptal conduction time. Such a type of alternans is very probably related to concealed transeptal retrograde conduction from normal to injured bundle branch every alternate beat so that even though the RR intervals are constant, the activation cycle of the injured bundle branch alternates between a long (a + b) and short (a − b) duration. Beats ending a short bundle branch cycle conduct normally whereas beats ending a long bundle branch cycle show bundle branch block. 3) Bundle branch block alternans in supernormal phase in subjects with phase 3 bundle branch block. Such a type of alternans occurs – as in bradycardia-dependent alternans – if in the beats with bundle branch block, a concealed retrograde conduction is present. Therefore, the activation cycle of the injured bundle branch alternates between a long (a + b) and a short (a − b) interval, even though the RR intervals are constant. In the beat following the one with bundle branch block pattern the conduction occurs in supernormal phase. In the subsequent beat, due to prolonged activation cycle of the bundle branch, the conduction occurs during the block zone following the supernormal phase. (Modified from Tavazzi et al. [13])

If the rate slows during tachycardia-dependent alternans the effective refractory period of the involved fascicle may remain longer than its cycle length but may become shorter than the sum of the latter and the transeptal conduction time. As a result a unidirectional block will be present; the bundle branch will remain unexcitable for anterograde propagation, but may become available for concealed transeptal retrograde activation which will maintain refractoriness of the bundle branch and cause 1:1 BBB [26, 69, 104]. Such unidirectional retrograde bundle branch activation in consecutive beats with slowing of the rate is postulated as the mechanism in the first part of Figure 11B. In the genesis of RBBB alternans (Figure 11A), in our opinion, a conduction in supernormal phase cannot be excluded.

Phase 4 alternans is very probably related to concealed transeptal retrograde conduction from the normal to the injured bundle branch every alterate beat, so that even though the RR intervals are constant, the activation cycle of the injured bundle branch alternates between a long and short duration (Figure 25). Beats ending a short bundle branch cycle conduct normally and beats ending a longer bundle branch cycle show BBB which is thus bradycardia-dependent. It must be assumed that the site of phase 4 BBB in every aberrant beat can be depolarized by concealed transeptal retrograde activation, even after it has become refractory to anterograde stimulation, perhaps because of a difference in the geometry of the proximal and distal ends of the bundle branch. The unidirectional nature of phase 4 block has also been demonstrated experimentally [49]; in fact it has been shown that after phase 4 anterograde block, retrograde conduction through the area of block was still possible.

Cohen et al. [26] suggest a different mechanism, i.e. that BBB during phase 4 alternans can also be bidirectional. At some point after the beginning of the aberrant beat there may be spontaneous complete depolarization of automatic cells in or near the area of block [41]. If this depolarization occurs without anterograde or retrograde propagation, it will be concealed. It is also possible that attempted transeptal retrograde conduction does not actually penetrate the area of block but that the depolarization of the large number of ventricular fibers electrotonically causes depolarization to threshold and firing of the cells in the area of the block. The interval between this spontaneous or electrotonically induced depolarization and the next beat is relatively short so that the subsequent ventricular complex does not display phase 4 block. Therefore the alternating bundle branch cycle lengths postulated in bradycardia-dependent alternans may be produced by concealed spontaneous (phase 4) or electrotonically induced diastolic depolarization of the cells of the blocked area, or by concealed depolarization into an area of unidirectional block.

BBB alternans in supernormal phase. This type of BBB postulated by Tavazzi et al. [13, 80] appears in relation to the presence of supernormal phase in the injured fascile in subjects with tachycardia-dependent BBB. A 2:1 IVCD related to supernormal phase occurs if in the beats with BBB a concealed transeptal retrograde conduction from the normal to the injured fascile is present. Thus, as in phase 4 alternans, the activation cycle of the injured bundle branch alternates between a long and short duration, even though the RR intervals are constant [13] (Figure 25). In the beat following that with BBB pattern the conduction occurs in supernormal phase with subsequent normalization of the QRS complex. In the subsequent beat, owing to the more prolonged activation cycle of the bundle branch, the conduction occurs during the block zone which follows the supernormal phase with subsequent BBB pattern. The differential diagnosis of the BBB alternans in supernormal phase must be set with the pseudo-bradycardia-dependent alternans. If at various cardiac rates, spontaneous or electroinduced, a BBB is constantly present and then disappears due to a further increase of the heart rate, as in the case of Figure 12, a BBB alternans in supernormal phase is extremely likely. An element in favor of such a type of alternans is the appearance of a true supernormal conduction zone during programmed premature atrial stimulation in subjects with tachycardia-dependent BBB. In the case of Figure 12 a supernormality zone during programmed premature atrial stimulation was not demonstrated, probably owing to the AV node prolonged refractoriness. However the electrophysiological mechanism cannot always be defined with certainty.

Pharmacological Tests

Pharmacological studies in patients with intermittent BBB [13, 29, 64, 105, 106] represent an ideal ground for the study of the electrophysiological effect of the antiarrhythmic drugs on the pathologic HPS, but unfortunately literature offers few contributions and only a few drugs have been studied.

In clinical studies [13, 29, 64, 105] it has been shown that *isoproterenol:* a) shifts significantly to the left or abolishes phase 3 BBB range; b) shifts significantly to the left phase 4 BBB range which can therefore occur during the range occupied by normal conduction in the control study; c) as a result of the first two effects, the normal conduction range shifts to the left, but its duration increases or decreases on which-ever of the two predominate; d) the coupling interval of the ventricular escapes from the injured fascicle become shorter or may appear if they are not present in the control study. These data suggest that in patients with intermittent BBB, isoproterenol shortens refractoriness in the injured fascicle and at the same time enhances automaticity, thereby moving the phase 4 BBB and the ventricular escape beats to the left. The shortening of refractoriness may be indirectely related to the restoration of membrane potential towards normal values, caused by catecholamines in injured Purkinje fibers [5, 6, 66].

Both in clinical and experimental studies [13, 29, 64] *lidocaine* causes the following effects: a) phase 3 BBB range in a few cases lengthens, in others it does not change; b) phase 4 BBB range, in some cases shifts to the left and in others it does not change; c) as a result of the two effects the duration of the normal conduction range decreases or more rarely remains unchanged. Generally when the normal conduction range is narrow, conduction in the affected fascicle is blocked entirely, whereas when the normal conduction range is wider the effects are variable; d) the ventricular escapes show a longer coupling or more commonly are totally suppressed. The effects of the lidocaine on the intermittent BBB are therefore rather complex and vary from case to case. Since this drug depresses spontaneous diastolic depolarization one should expect a shift of the phase 4 BBB range to the right with widening of the normal conduction range, because lidocaine may also shorten membrane potential duration and refractoriness [107-109]. However, in some studies the opposite occurred and the normal conduction range was decreased or abolished. A possible way of accounting for this result in which automaticity and conduction are simultaneously depressed is by postulating that lidocaine causes a significant depression of membrane responsiveness [108, 110]. Since it has shown that at therapeutic doses lidocaine has little effect on membrane responsiveness or that it may even improve it in normal Purkinje fibers [108, 109], these results suggest that the opposite effect may occur in abnormal or critically injured fibers. This suggestion is supported by the fact that it is particularly true when the normal conduction range is narrow (indicating a greater degree of injury) that lidocaine has the effect of depressing conduction further; whereas when the normal conduction range is wider (indicating less injury) the depressing effect upon conduction is less significant or absent.

In clinical studies [13, 106] *ajmaline* caused lengthening of both phase 3 and phase 4 BBB range. In several cases this drug totally suppressed the normal conduction range. The occurrence of ventricular escape beats from the injured fascicles was delayed or suppressed. These results suggest that ajmaline in injured bundle branch system induces a great prolongation of refractoriness and a significant depression of membrane responsiveness.

Amiodarone was investigated in a patient with phase 3 RBBB [29]. The drug induced depression of the conduction in the right bundle branch, expressed by prolongation of the phase 3 block range and by appearance of phase 4 RBBB with extremely narrow normal conduction range.

CLINICAL SIGNIFICANCE

Very few clinical studies concerning patients with intermittent BBB are available [13, 52, 111-116].

There are no precise data on the incidence of such blocks. Boyadjian et al. [117] encountered 15 cases (0.15 %) out of 15,000 electrocardiographic tracings and Pick

[118] 67 cases (0.13%) out of 50,000 tracings.

Phase 3 BBB was observed both in acute diseases such as myocardial infarction and myocarditis and in chronic heart diseases, whereas phase 4 BBB was almost always observed in patients with acute myocardial infarction [13].

In most studies, intermittent BBB was associated with heart disease of various type.

Coumeau et al. [52] evaluated 60 patients with intermittent LBBB; 42 suffered from hypertensive or coronary heart disease (CHD). All but one of the 14 patients reported by Bauer [111] were affected by CHD. Fish et al. [112] found heart disease, mainly CHD, in 31 out of 35 cases with intermittent BBB. In these studies the diagnosis was based on clinical-electrocardiographic criteria.

In this regard recent studies [13, 113-116] have described characteristic T-wave inversion, during normal intraventricular conduction, particularly in V_1-V_4 leads, in patients with intermittent LBBB.

Instead, during LBBB upright T waves were present in leads I, aVL, V_5 and V_6, i.e. a homophasic LBBB. These T wave abnormalities are frequent: they appeared in 58% of 12 patients described by Bauer [111], in 74% of 35 patients described by Rosenbaum et al. [119], in 43% of 30 patients reported by Luy et al. [113], in 72% of 46 patients described by Engle et al. [78], in 82% of 23 patients reported by Denes et al. [114] and in 52% of 275 patients described by Abben et al. [116]. Tavazzi et al. [13] observed that when normal conduction range was wide, the repolarization abnormalities in V_1-V_4 leads were slight, whereas when normal conduction range was narrow, the repolarization abnormalities were marked. Precordial T wave inversion during normal conduction, when associated with intermittent LBBB, has previously been attributed to ischemia [111, 113, 119], but in more recent studies [13, 114-116] patients with these ECG characteristics underwent coronary angiography and in most cases no significant obstructive lesions emerged.

It was suggested that these T-wave changes reflect an abnormality of repolarization related to previous occurrence of LBBB pattern [114, 115]. These alterations closely resemble the T-wave inversions seen after cessation of right ventricular pacing [120-122]. How the heart translates an abnormality of depolarization (LBBB) into a subsequent abnormality of repolarization is not at present clear. In the light of these data the role of CHD in the genesis of intermittent LBBB must be reevaluated since the ECG picture of anteroseptal ischemia cannot be used as sufficient evidence that CHD is the cause of intermittent LBBB.

Rare causes of intermittent BBB are: rheumatic heart diseases [52], acute infections fevers, especially diphtheria [52], thyrotoxicosis [123], siphilitic heart disease [52], and anemia [52]. Intermittent RBBB may complicate acute right ventricular stress due to pulmonary embolism [124], right heart catheterization [13, 125, 126] and various open cardiac surgical procedures [127].

A number of drugs, especially those with a depressant effect on cardiac conduction, have been responsible for the appearance of intermittent BBB. The best known of these are quinidine [128] and procainamide [129].

Intermittent BBB is generally regarded as the forerunner of a permanent conduction defect. In some cases it evolves rapidly towards the established BBB, in other cases it remains intermittent for many years [52, 130]. However at present we do not know the incidence with which intermittent BBB evolves towards the established BBB.

Generally the programmed premature atrial stimulation in normal subjects induces functional RBBB pattern as right bundle branch has a refractory period longer than that of left bundle branch. In a few subjects, programmed premature atrial stimulation induces an LBBB pattern with an effective refractory period of the left bundle branch less than 400 msec [83]. At present it is not clear if these findings express a physiologic manifestation or an initial involvement of the left bundle branch.

REFERENCES

1. Moe GK, Mendez C: Functional block in the intraventricular conduction system. Circulation 43: 949, 1971
2. Schuilenburg RM, Durrer D: Rate-dependency of functional block in the human His bundle and bundle branch-Purkinje system. Circulation 48: 526, 1973
3. Alboni P, Malacarne C, Pradella A, Masoni A: 2:1 and phase 4 peri-infarction block. Europ J Cardiol 10: 205, 1979
4. Alboni P: Il blocco periferico settale sinistro. Ipotesi fisiopatologica o nuovo elemento diagnostico? G Ital Cardiol 10: 365, 1980
5. Hoffman BF, Cranefield PF: Electrophysiology of the heart. New York: McGraw-Hill, 1960
6. Singer DH, Lazzara R, Hoffman BF: Interrelationships between automaticity and conduction in Purkinje fibers. Circ Res 21: 537, 1967
7. Massumi RA: Bradycardia-dependent bundle branch block: a critique and proposed criteria. Circulation 38: 1066, 1968
8. Singer DH, Ten Eick RE: Aberrancy: electrophysiologic aspects. Am J Cardiol 28: 381, 1971
9. Barold SS, Schamroth L: Tachycardia-dependent left bundle branch block associated with bradycardia-dependent variable left bundle branch block. A case report. Circulation 38: 216, 1973
10. Rosenbaum MB, Elizari MV, Lazzari JO, Halpern MS, Nau GJ, Levi RJ: The mechanism of intermittent bundle branch block: relationship to prolonged recovery, hypopolarization and spontaneous diastolic depolarization. Chest 63: 666, 1973
11. El-Sherif N: Tachycardia- and bradycardia-dependent bundle branch block after acute myocardial ischaemia. Br Heart J 36: 291, 1974
12. El-Sherif N, Scherlag BJ, Lazzara R, Samet P: Pathophysiology of tachycardia- and bradycardia-dependent block in the canine proximal His-Purkinje system after acute myocardial ischemia. Am J Cardiol 33: 529, 1974
13. Tavazzi L, Salerno JA, Bobba P: Meccanismo e implicazioni cliniche degli emiblocchi

e dei blocchi di branca intermittenti. Boll Soc Ital Cardiol XXXV Italian Meeting of Cardiology, 1974 p 235
14. Masoni A, Tomasi AM, Alboni P: Terapia paradossa dei blocchi in fase 3. VI National Meeting ANMCO, Verona, 1975, p 325
15. El-Sherif N, Scherlag BJ, Lazzara R: Bradycardia-dependent conduction disorders. J Electrocardiol 9: 1, 1976
16. Motte G, Fabiato A, Gorgon R, Abbaou C, Slama R: Les blocs de branche paradoussaux. Arch Mal Coeur 63, 573, 1970
17. Elizari MV, Lazzari JO, Rosenbaum MB: Phase 3 and phase 4 intermittent left anterior hemiblock. Chest 62: 673, 1972
18. Kretz A, Da Ruos O, Leguizamon P, Alumbo RJ: Delay and block of cardiac impulse caused by enhanced phase 4 depolarization in the His-Purkinje system. Br Heart J 37: 136, 1975
19. Salerno JA, Tavazzi L, Angoli L, Mussini A, Tronconi L: Phase 3 and phase 4 intermittent intraventricular conduction disturbances. VI European Meeting of Cardiology (Abstr.), Madrid, 1972
20. Elizari MV, Lazzari JO, Rosenbaum MB: Phase 3 and phase 4 intermittent left bundle branch block occurring spontaneously in a dog. Europ J Cardiol 1: 95, 1973
21. Tavazzi L, Salerno J: Disturbi della conduzione intraventricolare in fase 3 e in fase 4 coesistenti. G Ital Cardiol 3: 530, 1973
22. Motte G, Desoutter P, Fournial C, Welti JJ: Bloc en phase 3 et en phase 4 de la branche gauche du faisceau de His et conduction uniquement en phase supernormale dans la branche droite. Arch Mal Coeur 70: 789, 1977
23. Watanabe Y, Nishimura M: Terminology and electrophysiologic concepts in cardiac arrhythmias. V. Phase 3 block and phase 4 block. Part 1. Pace 2: 335, 1979
24. Watanabe Y, Nishimura M: Terminology and electrophysiologic concepts in cardiac arrhythmias. VI. Phase 3 block and phase 4 block. Part. 2. Pace 2: 624, 1979
25. Lie KI, Wellens HJ, Schuilenburg RM, Durrer D: Mechanism and significance of widened QRS complexes during complete atrioventricular block in acute inferior myocardial infarction. Am J Cardiol 33: 833, 1974
26. Cohen HC, D'Cruz I, Arbel ER, Langerdorf R, Pick A: Tachycardia- and bradycardia-dependent bundle branch block alternans. Clinical observations. Circulation 55: 242, 1977
27. El-Sherif N: Tachycardia-dependent versus bradycardia-dependent intermittent bundle branch block. Br Heart J 34: 167, 1972
28. Rosenbaum MB: The significance of phase 4 depolarization for clinical electrocardiography. Europ J Cardiol 3: 253, 1975
29. Girotti AL, Halpern MS, Elizari MV, Rosenbaum MB: Electrophysiologic and pharmacologic studies in a patient with acute myocardial infarction complicated by intraventricular and atrioventricular block. Europ J Cardiol 3: 281, 1975
30. Cohen HC, D'Cruz IA, Pick A: Effects of stable and changing rates and premature ventricular beats on transient tachycardia-, pseudobradycardia- and bradycardia-dependent bundle branch block alternans. J Electrocardiol 12: 151, 1979
31. Hodgkin AL, Keynes RO: Movement of cations during recovery in nerve. J Physiol 128: 61, 1955
32. Hodgkin AL, Keynes RD: The potassium permeability of a giant nerve fiber. J Physiol 128: 61, 1955
33. Draper MH, Weidman S: Cardiac resting and action potentials recorded with an intracellular electrode. J Physiol 115: 74, 1951
34. Reuter H: Divalent cations as charge carriers in excitable membranes. In: Progress in

biophysics and molecular biology, Butler JAV, Noble D. New York: Pergamon, 1973, p 3
35. McAllister RE, Noble O: The time and voltage dependence of the slow outward current in cardiac Purkinje fibers. J Physiol 186: 632, 1966
36. Weidman S: Resting and action potentials of cardiac muscle. Ann NY Acad Sci 65: 665. 1957
37. Noble O, Tsien RW: The kinetics and rectifier properties of the slow potassium current in cardiac Purkinje fibers. J Physiol 195: 185, 1968
38. Rosen MR: Electrophysiology of the cardiac specialized conduction system. In: His bundle electrocardiography and clinical electrophysiology, Narula OS. Philadelphia: FA Davis, 1975, p 19
39. Dominguez G, Fozzard HA: Influence of extracellular K^+concentration on cable properties and excitability of sheep cardiac Purkinje fibers. Circ Res 26: 565, 1970
40. Brooks CMcC, Hoffman BF, Suckling EE, Orias O: Excitability of the heart. New York: Grune & Stratton, 1955
41. Elizari MV, Nau GJ, Levi RJ, Lazzari JO, Halpern MS, Rosenbaum MB: Experimental production of rate dependent bundle branch block in the canine heart. Circ Res 34: 730, 1974
42. Lazzara R, El-Sherif N, Scherlag BJ: Disorders of cellular electrophysiology produced by ischemia of the canine His bundle. Circ Res 36: 444, 1975
43. Trautwein W, Gottstein V, Dudel J: Der Aktionsstrom der Myokardfaser in Sauerstoffmangel. Pflüger Arch 260: 40, 1954
44. Friedman PL, Stewart JR, Fenoglio JJ: Survival of subendocardial Purkinje fibers after extensive myocardial infarction in dogs. In vivo and in vitro correlations. Circ Res 33: 597, 1973
45. Lazzara R, El-Sherif N, Scherlag BJ: Electrophysiological properties of canine Purkinje cells in one-day-old myocardial infarction. Circ Res 33: 722, 1973
46. Fabiato A, Corabgeuf E: Facteurs cellulaires de désynchronisation électrique ventriculaire: étude sur le coeur isolé de lapin dans des conditions de perfusion normale et de dépolarisation partielle. J Physiol (Paris) 61: 277, 1969
47. Cranefield PF, Klein HO, Hoffman BF: Conduction of cardiac impulse: I. Delay, block and one way block in depressed Purkinje fibers. Circ Res 28: 199, 1971
48. Surawicz B, Uhley N, Borun R, Laks M, Crevassel, Rosen K, Nelson W, Mandel W, Lawrence P, Jackson L, Flowers N, Clifton J, Greenfield J Jr, Robles de Medina E: Task Force I: Standardization of terminology and interpretation. Am J Cardiol 41: 130, 1978
49. Elizari MV, Novakosky A, Quintero RA, Levi RJ, Lazzar JO, Rosenbaum MB: The experimental evidence for the role of phase 3 and phase 4 block in the genesis of AV conduction disturbances. In: The conduction system of the heart. Structure, function and clinical implications, Wellens HJJ, Lie KI, Janse MJ. Leiden: Stenfert Kroese, 1976, p 360
50. Van Dam RT, Hoore EN, Hoffman BF: Initiation and conduction of impulses in partially depolarized fibers. Am J Physiol 204: 1133, 1963
51. Mendez C, Erli JD, Moe GK: Indirect action of epinephrine on intraventricular conduction time. Circ Res 14: 318, 1964
52. Comeau WJ, Hamilton JGM, White PD: Paroxysmal bundle branch block associated with heart disease: a review and an analysis of the literature, with thirteen new cases and notes upon the influence of the vagus. Am Heart J 15: 276, 1938
53. Dressler W: Transient bundle branch block occurring during slowing of the heart beat and following gagging. Am Heart J 58: 760, 1969

54. Tavazzi L, Salerno JA, Chimienti M, Ray M, Bobba P: Mecanismos electrofisiologicos de los bloqueos A-V paroxisticos. In: Diagnostico y tratamiento de las arritmias cardiacas, Bayes A, Cosin J. Barcelona: Doyoma, 1978, p 343
55. Bailey JC, Greenspan K, Elizari MV, Anderson G, Fisch C: Effects of acetylcholine on automaticity and conduction in the proximal portion of the His-Purkinje specialized conduction system. Circ Res 30: 210, 1972
56. Danilo P, Rosen MR, Hordof AJ: Effects of acetylcholine on the ventricular specialized conduction system of neonatal and adult dogs. Circ Res 43: 777, 1978
57. Martins JB, Zipes DP: Effects of sympathetic and vagal nerves on recovery properties of the endocardium and epicardium of the canine left ventricle. Circ Res 46: 100, 1980
58. Hoffman BF: Neural influences on cardiac electrical activity and rhythm. In: Neural regulation of the heart, Randall WC. New York: Oxford University Press, 1977, p 289
59. Gadsby DC, Wit AL, Cranefield PF: The effects of acetylcholine on the electrical activity of canine cardiac Purkinje fibers. Circ Res 43: 29, 1978
60. Rosen MR, Hoffman BF: Vagus and ventricles. Circ Res 42: 1, 1978
61. Jonas EA, Kosowsky BD, Ramaswamy K: Complete His-Purkinje block produced by carotid sinus massage. Report of a case. Circulation 50: 192, 1974
62. Vessel H, Lowen G: Bundle branch block on cardiac slowing at a critical slow heart rate. Am Heart J 66: 329, 1963
63. Pick A: Aberrant ventricular conduction of escaped beats. Preferential and accessory pathways in the A-V junction. Circulation 13: 702. 1956
64. Rosenbaum MB, Elizari MV, Chiale P, Levi RJ, Nau GJ, Halpern MS, Lazzari JO, Novakovsky A: Relationships between increased automaticity and depressed conduction in the main intraventricular conducting fascicles of the human and canine heart. Circulation 49: 818, 1974
65. Tajima R, Nakamura Y, Murata K: Rate related block in the canine His-Purkinje system after ligation of the anterior septal artery. Observations by His bundle electrocardiography. Jap Circulation J 43: 403, 1979
66. Rosenbaum MB, Lazzari JO, Elizari MV: The role of phase 3 and phase 4 block in clinical electrocardiography. In: The conduction system of the heart. Structure, function and clinical implications, Wellens HJJ, Lie KI, Janse MJ. Leiden: Stenfert Kroese, 1976, p 126
67. Goudaux JL, Ashman R: Auricular fibrillation with aberration simulating ventricular paroxysmal tachycardia. Am Heart J 34: 366, 1947
68. Katz AM, Pick A: The transeptal conduction time in the human heart. An evaluation of fusion beats in ventricular parasystole. Circulation 27: 1961, 1963
69. Moe GK, Mendez C, Han J: Aberrant A-V impulse propagation in the dog heart: a study of functional bundle branch block. Circ Res 16: 261, 1965
70. Castellanos A Jr, Agha AS, Befeler B, Castillo CA, Berkovitz BV: A study of arrival of excitation at selected ventricular sites during human bundle branch block using close bipolar catheter electrodes. Chest 63: 208, 1973
71. Denes P, Wu D, Dhingra R, Pietras RJ, Rosen KM: The effects of cycle length on cardiac refractory periods in man. Circulation 49: 32, 1974
72. Neuss H, Thormann J, Schleppep M: Electrophysiological findings in frequency-dependent left bundle branch block. Br Heart J 36: 888, 1974
73. Spear JF, Moore EN: Supernormal excitability and conduction. In: The conduction system of the heart. Structure, function and clinical implications, Wellens KJJ, Lie KI, Janse MI. Leiden: Stenfert Kroese, 1976, p 111
74. Cabasson J, Morena H, Guimond, G, Deceuninck P, Gagne J, Cinca J, Rocca J, Sassine A, Masse C, Puech P: La phase supernormale de conduction cardiaque. Etude

expérimentale chez le chien. Arch Mal Coeur 71: 691, 1978
75. Puech P, Guimond C, Nadeau R, Morena H, Molinal, Matina D: Supernormal conduction in the intact heart. In Cardiac arrhythmias. Electrophysiology, diagnosis and management, Narula OS. Baltimore: Williams & Wilkins, 1979, p 40
76. Adrian ED, Lukas K: On the summation of propagated disturbances in nerve and muscle. J Physiol 44: 68, 1912
77. Weidmann S: Effects of calcium ions and local anesthetics on electrical properties of Purkinje fibers. J Physiol 129: 568, 1955
78. Spear JF, Moore EN: Effect of potassium on supernormal conduction in the bundle branch Purkinje system of the dog. Am J Cardiol 40: 923, 1977
79. Spear JF, Moore EN: The effect of changes in rate and rhythm on supernormal excitability in the isolated Purkinje system of the dog. A possible role in re-entrant arrhythmias. Circulation 50: 1144, 1974
80. Tavazzi L, Salerno JA, Bobba P: Intraventricular conduction in supernormal phase in intermittent bundle branch block. Circulation (Abstr.) 52(II): 248, 1975
81. Pellegrino L, Casari A, De Filippi R, Salerno JA: L'uso della xilocaina nelle aritmie cardiache associate a disturbi di conduzione. Boll Soc It Cardiol 15: 665, 1970
82. Garashi M, Ayabe T: Quantitative study of the supernormal phase of ventricular excitability in man. Am J Cardiol 36: 292, 1975
83. Gallagher JJ, Damato AN, Varghese P, Caracta A, Josephson ME, Lau SH: Alternative mechanisms of apparent supernormal atrioventricular conduction. Am J Cardiol 31: 362, 1973
84. Agha AS, Castellanos, A Jr, Wells D, Ross M, Befler B, Myerburg RJ: Type I, type II and type III Gaps in bundle branch conduction. Circulation 76: 325, 1973
85. Gallagher JJ, Damato AN, Caracta AR, Varghese PJ, Josephson ME, Lav SH: Gap in A-V conduction in man: types I and II. Am Heart J 85: 78, 1973
86. Cannom DS, Goodman DJ, Harrison DC: Electrophysiological studies in patients with rate related intermittent left bundle branch block. Br Heart J 36: 653, 1974
87. Denes P, Wu D, Dhingra RC, Amat-y-Leon F, Wyndham C, Rosen KM: Electrophysiological observations in patients with rate dependent bundle branch block. Circulation 51: 244, 1975
88. Barnay C, Medwedowsky JL, Nicolaï P, Delaahe M, Blache E: Phénomène de Gap et conduction supernormal au cours du bloc de branche gauche intermittent. Arch Mal Coeur 69: 681, 1976
89. Damato AN, Akhtar M, Ruskin J, Caracta A, Lav SH: Gap phenomena: anterograde and retrograde. In: The conduction system of the heart. Structure, function and clinical implications, Wellens KJJ, Lie KI, Janse MJ. Leiden: Stenfert Kroese, 1976, p 504
90. Abate G, Zaca'F, Polimeni RM, Alberici S, Lenzi S: I Gaps anterogradi. G Ital Cardiol 8: 374, 1978
91. Moe GK, Childers RW, Meredith J: An appraisal of 'supernormal' A-V conduction. Circulation 38: 5, 1968
92. Moore EN, Spear JF: Experimental studies on the facilitation of A-V conduction by ectopic beats in dogs and rabbits. Circ Res 29: 29, 1971
93. Schamroth L: Supernormal phase in hemiblock conduction. Br Heart J 38: 207, 1976
94. Sciacca A, Sangiorgi M: Trombe de la conduction intraventriculaire droite due à la lésion du tronc commun du faisceau de His. Acta Cardiol 12: 486, 1957
95. Fabregas R, Tse W, Han J: Conduction disturbances of the bundle branches produced by lesions in the nonbranching portion of His bundle. Am Heart J 92: 356, 1976
96. El-Sherif N, Amat-y-Leon F, Schonfield C, Scherlag B, Rosen K, Lazzara R, Wynd-

ham C: Normalization of bundle branch block patterns by distal His bundle pacing. Clinical and experimental dissociation in the pathologic His bundle. Circulation 57: 473, 1978
97. Narula OS: Longitudinal dissociation in the His bundle. Bundle branch block due to asynchronous conduction within the His bundle in man. Circulation 56: 996, 1977
98. Massumi RA, Amsterdam EA, Mason DT: Phenomenon of supernormality in the human heart. Circulation 46: 264, 1972
99. Goldenberg M, Rothberger CJ: Untersuchungen an der spezifischen Muskulatur des Hundenherzens. Z Ges Exp Med 90: 508, 1933
100. Cranefield PF, Hoffman BF: Conduction of the cardiac impulse. II. Summation and inhibition. Circ Res 28: 220, 1971
101. Schamroth L, Friedberg HD: Wedensky facilitation and the Wedensky effect during high grade A-V block in the human heart. Am J Cardiol 23: 893, 1969
102. Runge M, Narula OS: 'Fatigue' phenomenon in the His-Purkinje system (HPS). Circulation 48 (suppl IV): 102, 1973
103. Narula OS, Runge M: Accommodation of A-V nodal conduction and fatigue phenomenon in the His-Purkinje system. In: The conduction system of the heart. Structure, function and clinical implications, Wellens HJJ, Lie KJ, Janse MJ. Leiden: Stenfert Kroese, 1976, p 529
104. Edmand RE, Greenspan K, Fisch C: Effect of cycle length alternation upon the configuration of the canine ventricular action potential. Circ Res 19: 602, 1966
105. Salerno JA, Tavazzi L: Correlazioni tra automaticità e conduzione. Considerazioni su un caso di blocco di branca sinistro in fase 3 e in fase 4. G Ital Cardiol 6: 509, 1976
106. Chiale PA, Przybylsky J, Lazzari JO, Elizari MV, Rosenbaum MB: Comparative effects of Ajmaline on intermittent bundle branch block and the Wolff-Parkinson-White syndrome. Am J Cardiol 39: 651, 1977
107. Davies LD; Temte JV: Electrophysiological action of lidocaine on canine ventricular muscle and Purkinje fibers. Circ Res 24: 639, 1969
108. Bigger JT jr, Mandel WJ: Effect of lidocaine on conduction in canine Purkinje fibers and at the ventricular muscle-Purkinje fiber junction. J Pharmacol Exp Ther 172: 239, 1970
109. Biggert JT jr, Mandel WJ: Effect of lidocaine on the electrophysiological properties of ventricular muscle and Purkinje fibers. J Clin Invest 49: 63, 1970
110. Rosen MR, Hoffman BF: Mechanisms of action of antiarrhythmic drugs. Circ Res 32: 1, 1973
111. Bauer GE: Transient bundle branch block. Circulation 29: 730, 1064.
112. Fisch C, Zipes DP, McHenry PL: Rate dependent aberrancy. Circulation 48: 714, 1973
113. Luy G, Bahl O, Massie E: Intermittent left bundle branch block. A study of the effects of left bundle branch block on the electrocardiographic patterns of myocardial infarction and ischemia. Am Heart J 85: 332, 1973
114. Denes P, Pick A, Miller RH, Pietras RJ, Rosen KM: A characteristic precordial repolarization abnormality in patients with intermittent left bundle branch block. Ann Intern Med 89: 55, 1978
115. Engle TR, Shah R, De Podesta LA, Frankl WS, Krause RL: T-wave abnormalities of intermittent left bundle branch block. Ann Intern Med. 89: 204, 1978
116. Abben R, Rosen KM, Denes P: Intermittent left bundle branch block: anatomic as reflected in the electrocardiogram during normal conduction. Circulation 59: 1040, 1979
117. Boyadjian N, Van Dooren F: Raccourcissement des complexes QRS dans les blocks

intraventriculaires suite aux modifications du rythme. Acta Cardiol 6: 254, 1951

118. Pick A: Aberrant ventricular conduction. The Heart Bulletin 8: 49, 1959
119. Rosenbaum MB, Elizari MU, Lazzari JO: The hemiblocks. Oldsmar: Tampa Tracings, 1970
120. Chatterjee K, Harris AM, Davies JG, Leatham A: Electrocardiographic changes subsequent to artificial ventricular depolarization. Br Heart J 31: 770, 1969
121. Gola E, Arosio G, Riva S, Rusconi C: Alterazioni della ripolarizzazione ventricolare correlate con l'elettrostimolazione endocavitaria destra. G Ital Cardiol 2: 257, 1972
122. Antonioli GE, Alboni P, Baggioni GF, Fischer DM: Sulle alterazioni della ripolarizzazione nell'elettrocardiogramma spontaneo susseguente a stimolazione endocavitaria permanente. Cardiol Prat 25: 275, 1974
123. Di Giglio VA: Reversible bundle branch block in a case of toxis goitre. Am Heart J 15: 116, 1938
124. Bauer GE: Pulmonary embolism and pulmonary infarction. Med J Australia 1: 286, 1959
125. Simonson E: Transient right bundle branch block produced by heart catheterization in man. Am Heart J 41: 217, 1951
126. Penaloza D, Gamboa R, Sime F: Experimental right bundle branch block in the normal human heart. Am J Cardiol 8: 767, 1961
127. Bristow JD, Kassebaum DG, Starr A, Griswold HE: Observations on the occurrence of right bundle branch block following repair of ventricular septal defect. Circulation 22: 896, 1960
128. Barker PS, Johnston FD, Wilson FN: The effect of quinidine upon sinus tachycardia including the production of transient bundle branch block. Am Heart J 25: 760, 1943
129. Wallace AG, Laszo J: Mechanisms influencing conduction in a case of intermittent bundle branch block. Am Heart J 61: 548, 1961
130. Shern MA, Rytand DA: Intermittent bundle branch block. Observations with special reference to the critical heart rate. Arch Intern Med 91: 448, 1953

11. PROGNOSTIC VALUE OF HV INTERVAL IN PATIENTS WITH INTRAVENTRICULAR CONDUCTION DISTURBANCES

Several studies have emphasized the association of various intraventricular conduction disturbances (IVCD) with the development of complete heart block (CHB) located below the AV node [1-7].

The incidence of progression to CHB in patients with right bundle branch block (RBBB) associated with anterior fascicular block (AFB) is the one which has been studied most. In these patients, based on electrocardiographic analysis and follow-up observations, an incidence of CHB ranging from 6% to 21% has been reported by various investigators [2, 5, 7-10].

The patients with RBBB and posterior fascicular block (PFB) appear at higher risk of progression (21-75%) [7, 9].

However, most of these studies concerning development of CHB, in addition to being retrospective, do not specify the duration of the follow-up period. Studies with a known duration of follow-up suggest that the longer the follow-up the higher the incidence of CHB, i.e. 9% over 6.3 months [8], 13.6% over 19 months [9] and 21% over 58 months [10].

In 1973 Kulbertus concluded that the risk of developing CHB per year of follow-up was 6% after the initial manifestation of RBBB and AFB [10]. However, the same author in a subsequent paper [11] reported an incidence of CHB of less than 1%. The latter series was comprised of individuals detected by mobile screening units.

In a prospective study on the general population (mean follow-up: 10 years) there was no progression to CHB observed in the nine patients with RBBB and AFB (mean age: 58.1 years) [12].

Thus it is obvious that the risk of CHB is related to several factors and selection of patient material, i.e. hospitalized or asymptomatic out-patient cases selected from the street.

The incidence of CHB in patients with monofascicular block has been scantily investigated. Rotman et al. [13] reporting on 229 Air Force personnel, found 125 with left bundle branch block (LBBB) (mean age: 40 years) and 104 with RBBB (mean age: 36 years). Only two of those patients progressed to CHB over a mean follow-up period of 10.8 years, with an incidence of 1%. The young age of the patients must, however, be stressed.

Bath et al. [14], who followed 455 patients over 65 years of age with various

IVCD, found no progression. However, the average follow-up period was only 2 years.

Clinically it is important to detect patients with IVCD at high risk of developing CHB so that the possibility of sudden death may be prevented by a prophylactic pacemaker implantation.

Surface ECG is of limited value for this purpose as a lengthening of PR interval does not necessarily indicate a delayed conduction through the His-Purkinje system (HPS) [15-19].

It was observed that patients with a prolonged mean HV interval had a longer mean PR interval; however, in individual patients it is impossible to deduce the duration of the HV interval from the PR interval [20]. By studying in great detail the meaning of first degree AV block in patients with BBB, Levites et al. [18] drew the following conclusions:
1) in the presence of first degree AV block a significant number of these patients have a normal HV interval; 2) more than 50% of patients with a pattern of left or right bundle branch block (BBB) and right axis deviation have a prolonged HV interval regardless of the PR interval, and the correlation of PR and HV prolongation is not statistically significant; 3) in patients with a pattern of RBBB and AFB, the presence of PR prolongation suggests abnormality of the HV interval, although 30% of the patients with this finding have a normal HV interval and this interval cannot be predicted in individual patients; 4) His bundle electrocardiography is essential to determine accurately the presence of disease in the remaining fascicle or bundle branch in individual patients, whether the PR interval is normal or prolonged.

In patients with IVCD, CHB is most often localized in the HPS, so integrity of conduction in the remaining functional fibers of the HPS is critical for the final out-come and progression to CHB [21, 22]; in this regard HV interval registration is of particular usefulness.

CHRONIC INTRAVENTRICULAR CONDUCTION DISTURBANCES

The relation between HV interval and the risk of developing CHB is still a debatable issue. The subject has been investigated in a limited number of prospective studies [19, 20, 22-31]. Most groups of investigators have observed that HV prolongation in patients with chronic BBB is associated with a high risk of progression to CHB and sudden death [19, 23, 25, 26, 28, 30, 31]. Two other groups indicate a lack of such correlation [20, 22, 24, 27, 29].

Narula [30] has recently reported his updated prospective data in 95 patients with RBBB and LAD who had been followed for up to ten years (1968-78). The patients ranged in age from 49 to 91 years (mean: 72) and were divided into five groups. Group A: 26 patients, with a normal HV time ($\leq$ 45 msec) and without a documented AV block, were followed without a permanent pacemaker despite the presence of symptoms of syncope or dizziness in half of them. Group B: 16 patient received permanent pacemakers for intermittent 2° type II or 3° AV block; all had a prolonged HV time. Group C: 13 patients with symptoms of syncope or dizziness, without a documented AV block but with a prolonged HV time, received a permanent pacemaker. Asymptomatic patients [40] without AV block but a prolonged HV time were followed without a pacemaker. The latter were divided into subgroup D: 17 with HV time 46 to 55 msec, and subgroup E: 23 patients with HV time > 55 msec. The mean follow-up periods for Groups A to E were 5.4, 4.5, 4.1, 4.1 and 2.3 years, respectively. During the follow-up period, 50 of the 95 patients had died. Progression to CHB was noted in two of 26 group A, nine of the 13 group C who were alive, one of 17 group D and three of 23 group E patients. There were no sudden deaths in groups A, B and C, in contrast to two and four in groups D and E, respectively. The mortality rate per year of follow-up in groups A to E was 6.5%, 10%, 14%, 12% and 33% respectively. These data show a definite correlation between a prolonged HV time and sudden death or development of CHB.

Another group of 121 patients was followed up to 18 months by Scheinman et al. [19]. They observed a significantly greater incidence of 2° and 3° degree AV block (21%) and severe heart failure (38%) in the 42 patients with HV interval > 70 msec compared to 79 patients with HV interval < 70 msec (13% and 16%, respectively). Similarly, the incidence of sudden death differed significantly (17 vs 1%). On the other hand, the incidence of the frequency of syncope or dizziness was similar in both the groups. These authors concluded that asymptomatic and symptomatic patients with HV time > 70 msec appear to be at an increased risk of CHB.

Thirty-eight patients with RBBB and AFB (mean age: 74 years) were prospectively observed for a mean follow-up period of 28.5 months by Gupta et al. [25]. The HV interval was 55 msec or less in 17 patients (Group A), between 56 and 75 msec in 13 (Group B) and more than 75 msec in 8 (Group C). Ten patients (26%) died during the follow-up period. Of these, three were in Group A (mortality rate 8% per year), three in Group B (10% per year) and four in group C (21% per year). None of the deaths in Group A and B were sudden, while one possible sudden death occurred in Group C. Mode of death in one patient each from Group B and C remained unknown. Heart block was not seen in any patient from Group A and B, while two patients from Group C progressed to complete heart block during the follow-up period. It was concluded that patients with bifascicular block and prolonged HV tend to show a higher mortality when compared to those with normal HV intervals, and a definite risk of heart block exists in patients with HV intervals of more than 75 msec.

Altschuler et al. [28], prospectively analyzed symptomatic patients (mean age: 69.5 years) without documented heart block. To reduce the number of variables, patients were included only when 1) prior ECG monitoring and medical-neurologic evaluation failed to document heart block; 2) His bundle studies were normal or showed only HV prolongation; and 3) there was no history of a recent myocardial infarction. Of 35 patients with prolonged HV interval ($\geq$ 60 msec), 18 received permanent pacers, while 17 remained unpaced. Eighteen unpaced patients constituted the normal HV interval group. All groups had similar types of heart disease, NYHA classification, general medical condition, age and sex. All patients with normal HV intervals remained stable (no deaths or progression to heart block) for a mean follow-up period of 22 months. Among 18 patients with prolonged HV who received pacers, there were three deaths, none sudden, during a mean follow-up period of 23 months; four patients developed heart block unaccompanied by symptoms. Among 17 patients with prolonged HV intervals who were not paced, eight died (three suddenly) and three progressed to heart block with symptoms, leaving only six stable after six months follow-up. It was concluded that HV interval is of predictive value for progression to CHB.

Dini et al. [26], based on their follow-up observations (mean 26 months) in 66 patients with chronic BBB, indicated the prognostic value of HV interval. Of their 22 patients with a prolonged HV time ($>$ 55 msec) and without a pacemaker, three progressed to CHB and four died suddenly. No development of CHB or sudden deaths were noted in those patients with a normal HV time.

Similarly, in a recent Italian multicenter project [31], carried out in an attempt to clarify the prognostic value of HV interval duration after Ajmaline administration, we observed a very high risk of CHB in patients with chronic BBB and basic HV interval of 80 msec or more.

Contrary to the above reports, two other groups of investigators found no significant correlation between the duration of the HV interval and the risk of CHB [20, 22, 24, 27, 29]. Rosen's group reported on their observations in 119 patients with RBBB and AFB (mean follow-up: 1.5 years) [22] and also in 21 patients with RBBB and PFB (mean follow-up: 1.8 years) [20]. Patients with prolonged HV time ($>$ 55 msec) showed a more marked myocardial involvement; however the incidence of CHB was extremely low. None of the cases with RBBB and AFB with a prolonged HV interval progressed to AV block in the HPS, and two cases with a normal HV time manifested AV block (one distal, the other site unknown) [22]. In their series with RBBB and PFB, only one out of 21 patients (5 %) progressed to AV block in the HPS [20]. The incidence of sudden death in both of these series was very low (eight out of 119 and one out of 21, respectively) [20, 22].

In a subsequent paper [29], this group of investigators reported their updated prospective data in 452 patients with RBBB and AFB (mean follow-up: 88.8 months). Their patients ranged in age from 18 to 93 years (mean 62). 168 patients showed prolonged HV interval ($>$ 55 msec). AV block (2° or 3°) developed in 29 patients, nine with apparent cause (acute myocardial infarction, hyperkalemia, antiarrhythmic therapy) and spontaneously in 20. Cumulative annual incidence of all heart blocks for 5 years was respectively 4%, 5.9%, 8.7%, 10.1% and 11.3% and for spontaneous block was 2%, 3.2%, 5.2%, 6.7% and 7.1%. Sites of spontaneous block were probably or definitely AV nodal in 10, intra-His in one and infra-His in nine. Sudden death occurred in 14% of cases. The authors thus confirm the previous conclusions, that owing to low incidence of sudden death and of documented spontaneous development of 2° or 3° AV block, the duration of HV interval is of little predictive value.

McAnulthy et al. [27] prospectively observed 257 patients with chronic BBB (mean follow-up 2.1 years). Thirteen of their 257 patients progressed to AV block (six with HV interval $>$ 55 msec, five with HV $<$ 55 msec and two without HV measurements). Fifteen of the 50 deaths could possibly have resulted from CHB (five unknown, seven sudden and three bradycardia). Their data suggest a possible 6% mortality rate due to CHB. These authors report conclusions similar to those of Rosen's group.

Though it is difficult to explain the contradictory results, the following considerations may partly explain the differing results [30, 32]:

- Selection of patients and differences in patient population, i.e. hospitalized, symptomatic or asymptomatic out-patients selected during mass screening of general population. That may explain the different results obtained by the same author in two separate studies [10, 11].
- It is often impossible to know the duration of a BBB pattern prior to inclusion into the study. This variable may influence the outcome of a prospective study.
- The duration of follow-up period varies markedly in the various studies and the results are difficult to compare.
- The mean age of patients is highly different. Studies in a comparatively younger group of patients may show a disease process at an earlier stage than that observed in older patients. The mean ages in the series reported by Gupta et al. [25], Narula [23] and Scheinman et al. [19] were 74, 72 and 67 years, respectively. However, in all the reports indicating a lack of predictive value, the mean age of patients ranged from 61 to 63 years [20, 22, 29]. Recently, Dhingra et al. [33] investigated the effect of age on both severity of conduction defect and life history. The patients were subdivided into a younger group, aged 18 to 59 years, and an older group, aged 60. No differences in the incidence of sudden death in the two groups were observed. Progression to CHB was slightly higher in the older group, but the differences were not statistically significant. However it is possible that if the patients had been subdivided in more numerous age groups, statistically significant differences may have been found.
- Another important consideration is the relative incidence of associated diseases, i.e. hypertension, coronary artery disease (CAD), cardiomyopathy, rheumatic or congenital heart disease. In the series reported by Rosen's laboratory, the incidence of hypertension and cardiomyopathy was high (41% to 48%) and

that of CAD was low (27 %) [20, 22]. However, in the reports by Narula [30] and Scheiman et al. [19], the incidence of CAD was higher (43 % to 57 %) and that of hypertension was low. A very high percentage (18 %) of patients reported by McAnulty et al. [27] had valvular or congenital heart disease. The prognosis of BBB may reflect the clinical circumstances in which the conduction disease occurs. Recently, Dhingra et al. [34] observed a lower incidence of sudden death and progression to CHB in patients with primary conduction disease compared to those with organic heart disease. McAnulty et al. [27] reported the same conclusions, whereas Scanlon et al. [9] referred opposing data.

- The relative number of patients with syncope or dizziness vs those who are asymptomatic is another variable. However, according to our experience such symptoms appear with different frequency in the various population groups, in the various social strata and they are more frequent in women who are generally more emotional and in certain social groups scarcely acculturated. Syncopes and dizziness therefore represent highly aspecific symptoms. Perhaps for these reasons literature offers contrasting data on the relationship between syncope and HV interval prolongation. Dini et al. [26] observed higher incidence of syncope in patients with prolonged HV interval, whereas this was not evidenced by Scheinman et al. [19] or by Dhingra et al. [35].
- In some studies a single ECG pattern has been analyzed, whereas in others various IVCD have been combined into a single group [19, 26, 27, 28]. The underlying etiology and the site of lesion may differ in relation to an ECG pattern. Therefore, for the purpose of a prospective analysis, a mixing of various types of ECG pattern into a single group may further modify the results.
- Left axis deviation and right axis deviation coexisting with RBBB are not pathognomonic of a conduction defect in the fascicles of the left bundle branch. Therefore, patients with RBBB and left or right axis deviation may result from other etiologies (see Chapters 4 and 5). Consequently, those patients do not represent a homogeneous group as bifascicular block may not be present in all cases.
- Technical aspects of His bundle recording are very important to the prognostic value of the HV interval. The identification of the H potential, and the assurance that it is constituted by the depolarization of the most proximal portion of the His bundle, is at times difficult [23]. The different results in prospective studies may be related to the methods used by each investigator to validate the H potential. In some cases with a normal HV interval, the occurrence of CHB at short intervals has been reported [22, 26, 36]. In such cases the possibility that split His potentials may have been missed cannot be ignored.
- HV intervals have been measured in a variable fashion. Some investigators measured HV interval from the first rapid component or the peak of the His bundle potential; this is fraught with potential pitfalls as the proximal His bundle lesions may be missed due to slow, low amplitude potentials resulting

from a marked decrease in conduction velocity [23].

- Several histological and experimental studies have shown that an ECG pattern of BBB or fascicular block may result from an intra-His bundle lesion in the presence of normal bundle branches [37-39]. This is due to longitudinal partitioning of the His bundle into narrow cords which are insulated from each other by collagen and with relatively little cross connections between the compartments [38]. These findings have been recently confirmed by electrophysiology studies in man [40, 41]. Stimulation of the His bundle at various sites, i.e. proximal or distal to the intra-His lesion, clinically permitted the anatomic localization of the lesion responsible for an ECG pattern [40, 41]. The prognosis of patients with RBBB and LAD may vary with the site of lesion. It may be speculated that an intra-His lesion may be more critical and at greater risk of progressing to AV block than a peripheral lesion in the bundle branches. Therefore, it would be logical to evaluate each factor prospectively and separately.
- For prognostic purposes, the demonstration of CHB is a valid marker. However, for this purpose sudden death as a criterion may be potentially misleading as it may result from extracardiac etiologies. Sudden death, even when cardiogenic, may have resulted from a ventricular arrhythmia [42]. However, the demonstration of ventricular tachycardia or fibrillation as a terminal event does not necessarily exclude CHB as the primary and initiating mechanism with terminal deterioration into a ventricular arrhythmia. Furthermore, sudden death has been defined differently by various investigators, i.e. within 1 hour [19], 3 hours [20, 22], or 24 hours [27] after the onset of symptoms.

By analyzing all the above factors, the reported data suggest that a substantially prolonged HV interval in elderly patients has a predictive value of progression to CHB, provided His potentials are properly validated and the measurements are made from the earliest onset of the His potential. These conclusions are also indirectly supported by other studies [43].

It has been suggested that the use of Ajmaline may be of prognostic value in conjunction with HV measurements, due to its marked negative dromotropic effect on the HPS [36, 44-47]. It was argued that in patients with chronic BBB, this drug may permit an evaluation of the remaining functional HPS. The opinions on the utility of the Ajmaline test are however varied. Whereas some authors [22, 27, 48] do not attribute a prognostic value to any lengthening of HV interval, others [26, 45, 49, 50] hold that the risk of development of CHB, is proportional to the lengthening of the HV interval after Ajmaline administration. The duration of the HV interval after drug administration, beyond which there would be a high risk of CHB, varies in several studies to between 90 and 120 msec. In an Italian Multicenter Project we prospectively studied 85 patients (mean age: 63.7 years) with chronic BBB for a mean follow-up period of 48 months [31]. Patients with sinus node and AV node dysfunctions were not included. Six patients showed RBBB, 31 LBBB and 48 RBBB associated with AFB. After Ajmaline administration (1 mg/kg e.v.) infra-His 2° or 3° AV block (Figure 1) appeared in 11 patients; in eight of these the AV block appeared subsequently during the follow-up period. This suggests that a 2° or 3° block after Ajmaline administration is highly predictive of spontaneous progression. Of the eight patients, five presented an HV interval ≥ 70 msec, and three were asymptomatic. A marked lengthening of HV interval, even beyond 150 msec, did not demonstrate any predictive value.

Another test which aims at better identification of patients at high risk of CHB is incremental atrial pacing. This provides provocative stress of the conduction system, allowing demonstration of conduction disease not apparent during sinus rhythm. The usual response to incremental atrial pacing is the development of AV nodal Wenckebach periodicity (block proximal to H defection). Block distal to H (BDH) induced by atrial pacing is a rare manifestation – it was observed in 4% of the patients with bifascicular block [51] – and therefore it does not show sufficient sensitivity [50, 52-54]. Recently, 21 patients with bifascicular block and BDH

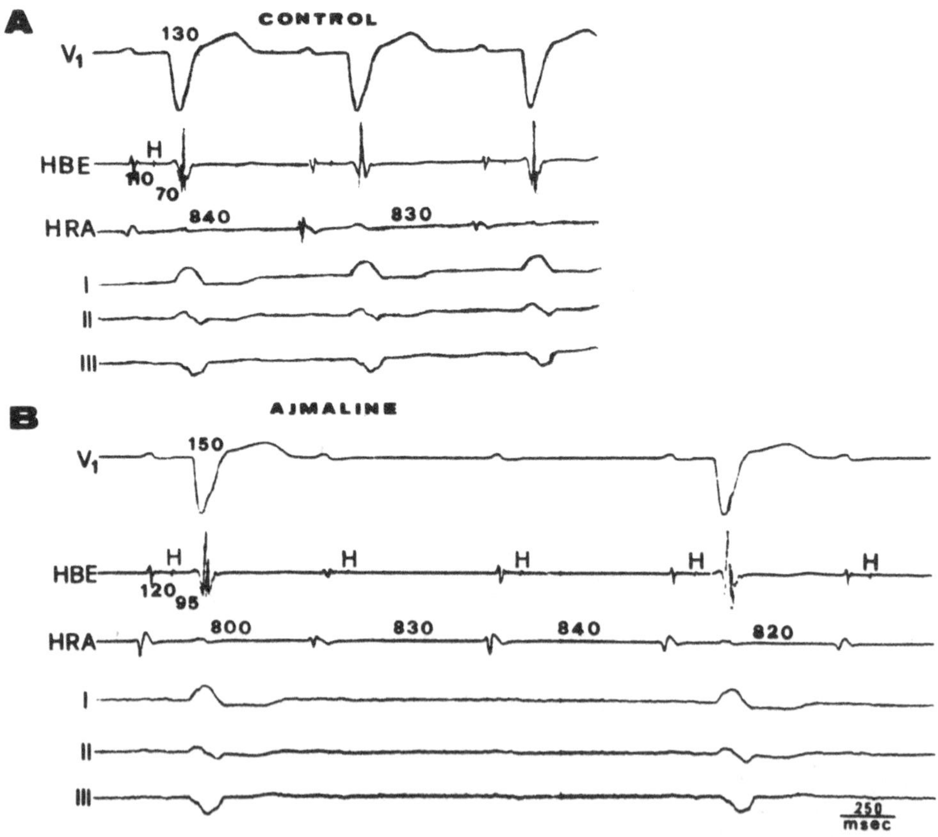

Figure 1. Patient with left bundle branch block and prolonged HV interval (70 msec). After Ajmaline administration (1 mg/kg i.v.), a 3:1, 4:1 AV block distal to His bundle appears. (For details see text)

induced by atrial pacing were followed prospectively [51]. In six, BDH was noted during pacing-induced AV nodal Wenckebach periods (at paced rates of 150-190 beats/min), with BDH in the short HH cycles after the AV nodal blocked P (long cycle). None of the six patients developed AV block during a mean follow-up of 5.3 years. This datum suggests that this type of BDH represents a functional manifestation, most probably related to the Ashman phenomenon (see Chapter 10).

In the remaining 15 patients, pacing-induced BDH was noted during intact AV nodal conduction (paced rate of 80-200 beats/min) (Figure 2). During a mean

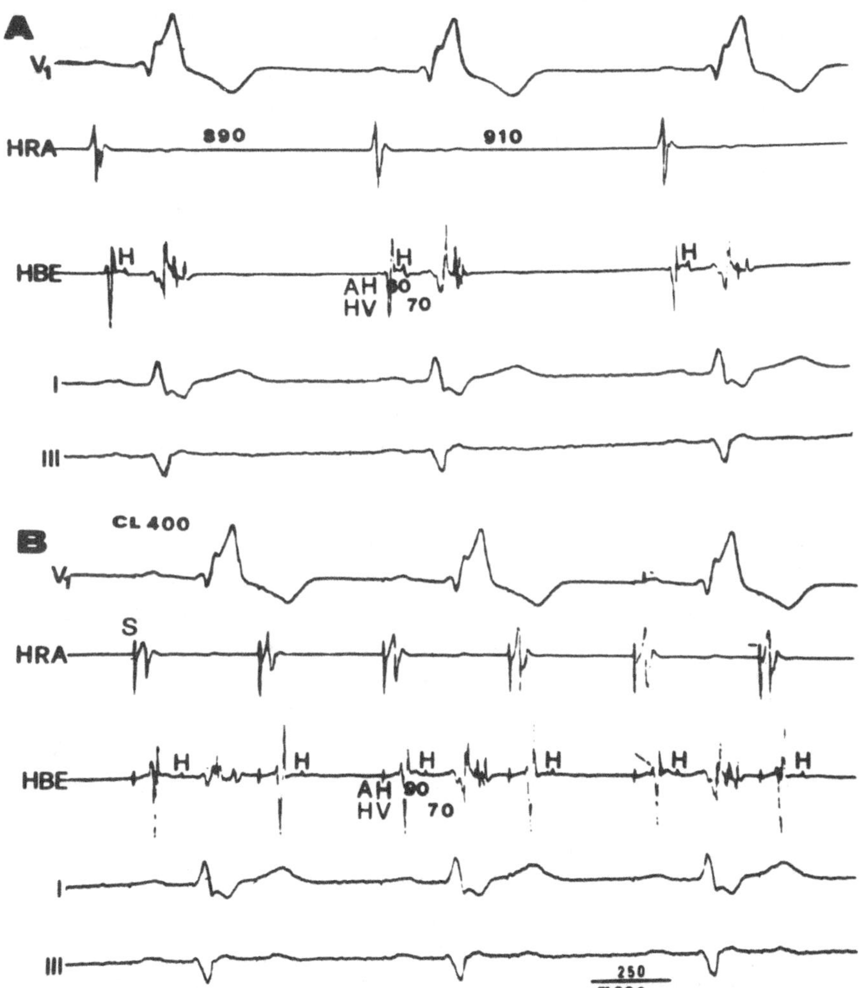

Figure 2. Patient with bifascicular block (right bundle branch block and anterior fascicular block) with prolonged HV interval (70 msec). During continuous atrial pacing (cycle length: 400 msec) a 2:1 AV block distal to His bundle with intact AV node conduction appears. (For details see text)

follow-up of 3.4 years, seven of these patients developed AV block, one had treadmill-provoked AV block and two died suddenly.

This datum suggests that pacing-induced BDH with intact AV nodal conduction expresses a marked involvement of the HPS.

These results thus prove that BDH induced by atrial pacing is an infrequent finding in patients with bifascicular block and can be functional as well as pathologic response. A BDH with intact AV nodal conduction is highly predictive of future development of CDH and sudden death.

Some authors [55-66] also believe that a ventricular pacing is useful to document a conduction disease in the HPS, not apparent during sinus rhythm. The appearance of 2° or 3° degree AV block distal to His bundle when ventricular pacing is stopped, seems to express a marked involvement of the HPS. Such behavior has in fact been observed in patients with CAD and chronic BBB showing spontaneous transient AV block. So far it is still unknown whether such pacing induced block is related to hemodynamic factors or to 'fatigue' of the diseased HPS [55]. Prospective studies are necessary in order to evaluate the prognostic value of this test.

ACUTE MYOCARDIAL INFARCTION

There are few reports concerning the implications of His bundle electrocardiograms in the setting of acute myocardial infarction (AMI) [57-65]. These recordings provide useful information about intracardiac conduction in patients with AMI.

First of all these studies have confirmed preceding hypotheses based on anatomical data in which it was postulated that conduction disturbances are usually located in the AV node following inferior infarction and in the His-Purkinje system following antero-septal infarction. Several reports with His bundle recordings in man have established this relationship between the site of block and the site of infarction [57, 58, 61, 65-67]. Of the 25 patients with inferior wall myocardial infarction reported by Lie et al. [65], the AV block was localized within the AV node in 24, and was distal to His bundle in only one patient. By contrast, in cases with an anteroseptal infarction the block was always distal to His bundle. A few rare cases of intra-His block secondary to acute inferior infarction have been reported [68, 69].

As in chronic BBB, the studies dealing with His bundle recording have confirmed that the length of PR interval is only of limited value in predicting both prolonged HV interval and development of CHB. In fact seven out of 15 patients reperted by Lie et al. [60] with bifascicular block and prolonged HV interval ($>$ 55 msec) had a normal PR interval and four of these seven progressed into complete AV block.

The discrepancy between the PR and the HV intervals is often caused by the presence of a short AH interval, probably because of an increased sympathetic tone which usually accompanies large infarcts [65].

Regarding the relationship between the duration of HV interval and the progression to CHB, Lie et al. [60, 65] reported that 11 out of 15 patients with bifascicular block and prolonged HV interval progressed into complete AV block as compared to one out of 10 patients with bifascular block and normal HV interval. This suggests that the His bundle recording in AMI is of value in identifying a group of patients with BBB and 1:1 AV conduction who are at immediate risk of CHB. This is in contrast to patients with chronic BBB since the development of chronic conduction disturbances occurs over a much longer period.

Regarding the relationship between duration of the HV interval and early mortality, there are contrasting data. The presence of a prolonged HV interval in patients with BBB, who were not in severe heart failure, was found to be associated with a significantly higher mortality. In fact 13 out of 18 patients with prolonged HV interval died compared to nine out of 19 with normal HV [60]. The same results were reported by Lichstein et al. [62]: 15 out of 23 patients with an initially abnormal HV time died, whereas only one died in the group of five with a normal HV interval. Since most of these deaths were caused by repetitive and fatal ventricular fibrillation or by the appearance of severe heart failure, the poor prognosis is probably due to extensive necrosis, involving all fascicles of the intraventricular conducting system. By contrast, Harper et al. [61] in their large review of 72 patients complicated by AV block or BBB, found that there was no difference in early mortality in patients showing BBB with normal or prolonged HV interval. Gould et al. [64] also observed that the presence or absence of a prolonged HV time did not affect hospital mortality in patients with BBB; in both groups of patients pump failure was the main cause of death.

During the acute phase of the myocardial infarction, examination of serial His bundle electrocardiograms showed variations of the HV interval [61, 62]. In six out of eight patients with an initially abnormal HV interval reported by Lichstein et al. [62], four showed a 10 to 15 msec decrease in HV time, while two showed no significant change. In two patients with an initially normal HV interval, no significant changes were observed. In the three patients with BBB reported by Harper et al. [61], in whom His bundle electrocardiogram was repeated, the variation in the HV interval between the first and the second study was within 10 msec.

The reduction in the HV time may express edema and inflammatory cell infiltration [70] and/or increased extracellular potassium released by necrotic myocardial cells during the first days of the AMI [71]. The daily variations in HV interval duration represent, however, a limit in the definition of both the clinical and prognostic value of such interval whose duration depends on the moment in which it is registered.

In conclusion, His bundle electrocardiograms provide additional information about intracardiac conduction in patients with AMI and wide QRS complexes with or without AV block. This information appears to be useful in identifying patients with BBB and intact AV conduction who are at immediate risk of developing CHB. In order to draw any definitive conclusions, repeated registrations in a large number of patients are necessary.

REFERENCES

1. Grant RP: Left axis deviation: an electrocardiographic-pathologic correlation study. Circulation 14: 233, 1956
2. Lenegre J: Contribution à l'étude des blocs de branche. Paris: Baillière, 1958
3. Unger PN, Lesser ME, Kugei VH, Lev M: The concept of masquerading bundle branch block. An electrocardiographic pathologic correlation. Circulation 17: 397, 1958
4. Pryor R, Blonunt SG: The clinical significance of true left axis deviation. Left intraventricular blocks. Am Heart J 72: 931, 1966
5. Lasser RP, Haft JI, Friedberg CK: Relationship of right bundle branch block and marked left axis deviation (with left parietal or peri-infarction block) to complete heart block and syncope. Circulation 37: 429, 1968
6. Kulbertus H, Collignon P: Association of right bundle branch block with left superior or inferior intraventricular block. Its relation to complete heart block and Adams-Stokes syndrome. Br Heart J 31: 435, 1969
7. Rosenbaum MB, Elizari MV, Lazzari JO: The hemiblocks. Oldsmar: Tampa Tracings, 1970
8. Wat TB Jr, Pruiti RD: Character, cause and consequence of combined left axis deviation and right bundle branch block in human electrocardiograms. Am Heart J 77: 460, 1969
9. Scanlon PJ, Pryor R, Blount SG: Right bundle branch block association with left superior or inferior intra-ventricular block. Clinical setting, prognosis and relation to complete heart block. Circulation 42: 1123, 1970
10. Kulbertus HE: The magnitude of risk of developing complete heart block in patients with LAD, RBBB. Am Heart J 86: 278, 1973
11. Kulbertus HE, De Leval-Rutten F, Dubois M, Petit JM: Epidémiologie et histoire naturelle du bloc de branche bilatéral partiel. In: Troubles du rythme et électrostimulation. Symposium international. Toulouse: Fournie, 1977 p 91
12. Siegman-Igra Y, Yahini JH, Goldbourt U, Neufeld HN: Intraventricular conduction disturbances: a review of prevalence, etiology, and progression for ten years within a stable population of Israeli adult males. Am Heart J 96: 669, 1978
13. Rotman M, Triebwasser JH: A clinical and follow-up study of right and left bundle branch block. Circulation 51: 477, 1975
14. Bhat PK, Watanabe K, Rao DB, Luisada A: Conduction defects in the aging heart. J Am Geriatr Soc 22: 517, 1974
15. Narula OS, Cohen LS, Samet P, Lister JW, Scherlag BJ, Hildner FJ: Localization of AV conduction defect in man by recording of the His bundle electrocardiogram. Am J Cardiol 25: 228, 1970
16. Narula OS, Samet P: Right bundle branch block with normal, left or right axis deviation: analysis by His bundle recordings. Am J Med 51: 432, 1971
17. Touboul, P, Ibrahim M: Atrioventricular conduction defects in patients presenting with syncope and normal PR interval. Br Heart J 34: 1005, 1972
18. Levites R, Haft JI: Significance of first degree heart block (prolonged PR interval) in

bifascicular block. Am J Cardiol 34: 259, 1974
19. Scheinman MM, Peters RW, Modin G, Brennan M, Lies C, Young J: Prognostic value of infranodal conduction time in patients with chronic bundle branch block. Circulation 56: 240, 1977
20. Dhingra RC, Denes P, Wu D, Chuquimia R, Amat-y-Leon F, Wyndham C, Rosen KM: Chronic right bundle branch block and left posterior hemiblock. Clinical electrophysiologic and prognostic observations. Am J Cardiol 36: 867, 1975
21. Narula OS, Scherlag BJ, Javier RP, Hildner FJ, Samet P: Analysis of the AV conduction defect in complete heart block, utilizing His bundle electrograms. Circulation 41: 437, 1970
22. Denes P, Dhingra RC, Wu D, Chuquimia R, Amat-y-Leon F, Wyndham CR, Rosen KM: HV interval in patients with bifascicular block (right bundle branch block and left anterior hemiblock). Clinical, electrocardiographic and electrophysiologic correlations. Am J Cardiol 35: 23, 1975
23. Nurula OS, Gann D, Samet P: Prognostic value of H-V intervals. In: His bundle electrocardiography and clinical electrophysiology, Narula OS. Philadelphia: FA Davis, 1975, p 437
24. Dhingra RC, Denes P, Wu D, Wyndham CR, Amat-y-Leon F, Towne WD, Rosen KM: Prospective observations in patients with chronic bundle branch block and marked H-V prolongation. Circulation 53: 600, 1976
25. Gupta PK, Lichstein E, Chadda KD: Follow-up studies in patients with right bundle branch block and left anterior hemiblock: significance of H-V interval. J Electrocardiol 10: 221, 1977
26. Dini P, Santini M, Di Mascolo R, Boschetti C, Ialongo D, Rocchi M, Masini V: Significato prognostico dell'intervallo H-V in 66 pazienti con blocco di branca cronico. G Ital Cardiol 8: 392, 1978
27. McAnulty JH, Rahimtoola SH, Murphy ES, Kauffmann S, Ritzmann LW, Kanarek, P, De Mots H: A prospective study of sudden death in 'high risk' bundle branch block. N Engl J Med 299: 209, 1978
28. Altschuler H, Fisher JD, Furman S: Significance of isolated H-V interval prolongation in symptomatic patients without a documented heart block. Am Heart J 97: 19, 1979
29. Dhingra RC, Wyndham C, Amat-y-Leon F, Denes P, Wu D, Sridhar S, Bustin AG, Rosen KM: Incidence and site of atrioventricular block in patients with chronic bifascicular block. Circulation 59: 238, 1979
30. Narula OS: Intraventricular conduction defects: current concepts and clinical significance. In: Cardiac arrhythmias: electrophysiology, diagnosis and management, Narula OS. Baltimore: Williams & Wilkins, 1979, p 114
31. Dini P, Ialongo D, Alboni P, Malacarne C, Lotto A, Finzi A, Pagnoni F, Baldi N, Morgera T, Gronda M, Rognoni G, Occhetta E, D'Aurello M: Blocchi di branca cronici: valore prognostico, sensibilità, specificità ed accuratezza predittiva dei parametri elettrofisiologici endocavitari. (In preparation)
32. Narula OS, Alboni P: Prognostic value of H-V interval in patients with chronic right bundle branch block and left axis deviation. G Ital Cardiol 9: 111, 1979
33. Dhingra RC, Wyndham C, Deedwania PC, Bauerfeind R, Swiryn S, Best D, Rosen KM: Effect of age on atrioventricular conduction in patients with chronic bifascicular block. Am J Cardiol 45: 749, 1980
34. Dhingra RC, Wyndham C, Bauernfeind R, Denes P, Wu D, Swiryn S, Rosen KM: Significance of chronic bifascicular block without apparent heart disease. Circulation 60: 33, 1979
35. Dhingra RC, Denes P, Wu D, Chuquimia R, Amat-y-Leon F, Wyndham C, Rosen

KM: Syncope in patients with chronic bifascicular block: significance, causative mechanisms, and clinical implications. Ann Intern Med 81: 302, 1974
36. Motte G, Fournial C, Bodereau P, Kevorkian M, Welti JJ: Intérêt prognostique de l'intervalle HV spontané et après Ajmaline chez les patients ayant un bloc de branche. Symposium international. Toulouse: Fourne, 1977, p 99
37. Sciacca A, Sangiorgi M: Trouble de la conduction intraventriculaire droite due à la lésion du tronc commun du faisceau de His. Acta Cardiol 12: 486, 1957
38. James TN, Sherf L: Fine structure of the His bundle. Circulation 44: 9, 1971
39. Fabregas R, Tse W, Han J: Conduction disturbances of the bundle branches produced by lesions in the nonbranching portion of His bundle. Am Heart J 92: 356, 1976
40. Narula OS: Longitudinal dissociation in the His bundle: bundle branch block due to asynchronous conduction within the His bundle in man. Circulation 56: 996, 1977
41. El-Sherif M, Amat-y-Leon F, Schonfield C, Scherlag B, Rosen K, Lazzara R, Wyndham C: Normalization of bundle branch block pattern by distal His bundle pacing. Clinical and experimental dissociation in the pathologic His bundle. Circulation 57: 473, 1978
42. Watanabe Y, Pamin Tuan JC, Dreifus LS: Role of intraventricular conduction disturbances in ventricular premature systoles. Am J Cardiol 32: 188, 1973
43. Vera Z, Mason DT, Fletcher RD, Awan NA, Massumi RA: Prolonged His-Q interval in chronic bifascicular block. Relation to impending complete heart block. Circulation 46: 53, 1976
44 Camerini F, Baldi N, Gori P, Martinoli E: L'ajmalina nello studio prognostico dei blocchi bifascicolari. E' possibile valutare il rischio di evoluzione verso il blocco totale? G Ital Cardiol 3: 380, 1973
45. Guërot C, Coste A, Valere P, Tricot R: L'épreuve à l'ajmaline dans le diagnostic du block auriculo-ventriculaire paroxystique. Arch Mal Coeur 66: 1241, 1973
46. Meilhac B, Le Pailleur C, Heulin A, Vacheron A, Guise L, Di Matteo J: Intérêt de la stimulation auriculaire et des épreuves pharmaco-dynamiques dans le diagnostic des syncopes et l'élettrocardiogrammc normal. Arch Mal Coeur 67: 775, 1974
47. Alboni P, Malacarne C, Pedroni P: Effetti elettrofisiologici dell'ajmalina sul sistema di conduzione nell'uomo. G Ital Cardiol 8: 752, 1978
48. Foster JR, Damato AN, Batsford WP: Prognostic value of His bundle recording in right bundle branch block and left anterior hemiblock: one to five year follow-up. Circulation (Abstr.) Suppl II: 183, 1975
49. Gupta PK, Lichstein E, Chadda KD: Intraventricular conduction time (H-V interval) during anterograde conduction in patients with heart block. Am J Cardiol 32: 27, 1973
50. Rossi P, Gronda M, Rognoni G: Assessment of latent atrioventricular block. Troubles du rythme et électrostimulation. Symposium international. Toulouse: Fourné, 1977, p 125
51. Dhingra RC, Wyndham C, Bauerfeind R, Swiryn S, Dewania PC, Smith T, Denes P, Rosen KM: Significance of block distal to the His bundle induced by atrial pacing in patients with chronic bifascicular block. Circulation 60: 1455, 1979
52. Berkowitz WD, Lau SH, Patton RD, Rosen KM, Damato AN: The use of his bundle recording in the analysis of unilateral and bilateral bundle branch block. Am Heart J 81: 340, 1971
53. Dodinot GH, Hua G, Mentre B, Faivre G: Stimulation auticulaire et explorations hissiennes dans les indications de l'entraînement électro-systolique au long cours. Arch Mal Coeur 66: 257, 1973
54. Rosen KM, Rahimtoola SH, Chuquimia R, Loeb HS, Gunnar R: Electrophysiological significance of first degree atrioventricular block with intraventricular conduction disturbances. Circulation 43: 491, 1973

55 Narula OS, Runge M: Accommodation of A-V nodal conduction and fatigue phenomenon in the His-Purkinje system. In: The conduction system of the heart. Structure, function and clinical implications. Wellens HJJ, Lie KI, Janse MJ:. Leiden: Stenfert Kroese, 1976, p 529
56. Fisher JD, Kulbertus HE, Narula OS: The prognostic value of the HV interval. Pace 1: 132, 1978
57. Rosen KM, Loeb HS, Chuquimia R, Sinno MZ, Rahimtoola SH, Gunnar RM: Site of heart block in acute myocardial infarction. Circulation 42: 925, 1970
58. Hunt D, Lie JT, Vohra I, Sloman G: Histopathology of heart block complicating acute myocardial infarction. Correlation with the His bundle electrogram. Circulation 48: 1252, 1973
59. Lichstein E, Gupta PK, Chadda KD, Liu HM, Sayeed M: Findings of prognostic value in patients with incomplete bilateral bundle branch block complicating acute myocardial infarction. Am J Cardiol 32: 913, 1973
60. Lie KI, Wellens HJ, Schuilenburg RM, Becker AE, Durrer D: Factors influencing prognosis of bundle branch block complicating acute antero-septal infarction. The value of His bundle recordings. Circulation 50: 935, 1974
61. Harper R, Hunt D, Vohra J, Peter T, Sloman G: His bundle electrogram in patients with acute myocardial infarction complicated by atrioventricular or interventricular conduction disturbances. Br Heart J 37: 705, 1975
62. Lichstein E, Gupta PK, Chadda KD: Long-term survival of patients with incomplete bundle branch block complicating acute myocardial infarction. Br Heart J 83: 924, 1975
63. Lotto A, Greco EM, Graziina, Salvade P, Finzi A: La registrazione dell'elettrocardiogramma hissiano nei disturbi della conduzione atrio-ventricolare nell'infarto miocardico acuto. G Ital Cardiol 5: 932, 1975
64. Gould L, Reddy C, Kim SG, Oh KC: His bundle electrogram in patients with acute myocardial infarction. Pace 2: 428, 1979
65. Lie KI, Durrer D: Conduction disturbances in acute myocardial infarction. In: Cardiac arrhythmias. Electrophysiology, diagnosis and management, Narula OS. Baltimore: Williams & Wilkins, 1979, p 140
66. Arcebal AG, Machado H, Lemberg I, Castillo CA, Castellanos A Jr: His bundle electrograms in type II (Mobitz) block occuring during acute myocardial infarction. Circulation (abstr.) 45, 46 (Suppl. 11): 125, 1970
67. Narula OS, Javier RP: Sequelae of A-V block in acute myocardial infarction. Circulation (abstr.) 45, 46 (Suppl. 11): 197, 1970
68. Rizzon P, Di Biase M: Intrahis bundle block in acute myocardial infarction. Report of two cases. J Elettrocardiol 10: 197, 1977
69. O'Callaghan AC, Jorda CF, Aguillar LR, Vila FM, Garcia RC, Marco MR: Bloqueo auriculo-ventricular intra-His en el infarto de miocardio agudo. Rev Esp Cardiol 32: 199, 1979
70. Becker AE, Anderson B, Lie KI: Bundle branch block and anteroseptal infarction. Clinicopathologic correlations. Br Heart J 40: 773, 1978
71. Hackel DB, Wagner G, Ratlif NB, Cies A, Estes EH Jr: Anatomic studies of the cardiac conduction system in acute myocardial infarction. Am Heart J 83: 77, 1972

12. NONINVASIVE RECORDING OF HIS-PURKINJE ACTIVITY

Diagnosis and evaluation of disorders in atrio-ventricular (AV) conduction are the most important purposes of His bundle electrocardiogram (HBE). The recording of His bundle (HB) potentials usually requires cardiac catheterization.

In 1973, working independently and using similar but not identical techniques of signal averaging, Berbari et al. [1] and Flowers et al. [2] in animal studies, and Lazzara et al. [3] in humans showed that His-Purkinje activity (HPA) could be recorded from the body surface. Such activity has been defined by Berbari et al. [1] G complex. Subsequent studies have confirmed the feasibility of external recording of HPA [4-13]. These methods require computer elaboration of the bioelectrical signal. In accordance with standard volume conductor theory [14] the potentials generated by the HP system should propagate to the body surface. However, these potentials are too small (less than 10 μV)) to be measured with the amplification conventionally applied to electrocardiography. A direct solution would be the use of greater amplification of the ECG signal. This approach will not be satisfactory if the signal of interest and noise are of the same order of magnitude. If there is no improvement of the signal-to-noise (S/N) ratio, the signals would remain unrecognized (Figure 1).

A similar problem of small signal detection occurs in the neurological sciences where the signal source is the brain.

For many years workers in that field have employed signal averaging as a method of improving the signal-to-noise ratio of periodic signals [15-17].

Signal averaging has been used to extract the fetal electrocardiogram [18] where the mother's ECG is considered to be noise. This method has also been utilized to enhance the fidelity of recording of the P wave [19-21].

Signal averaging can be used with periodic signal to improve the S/N ratio. Essentially, a signal averager stores information during a designated interval and sums the information of successive intervals.

In this way random components of the stored information, such as noise, will average to zero, while the desired signal will accumulate. Divisions of this sum by the number of cycles will yield an ensemble average. There are certain criteria that must be met before the average can be considered to be a valid representation of the original signal.

The contaminating noise must be random; i.e. the magnitude of the noise must have a Gaussian distribution. Also the signal of interest must be periodic or must be associated with an event such as a trigger pulse which will activate the averaging equipment. For the recording of HPA these suppositions exist. In fact, the noise originates mainly from two sources:

1) physiological noise such as muscle tremor, and
2) electronic noise from the measuring equipment.

Physiological noise in general is random with respect to the cardiac cycle. Such noise may be due in part to contraction of the intercostal muscles during respiration. Since the respiratory cycle and the cardiac cycle are not synchronous, any electrical activity associated with breathing will appear as random and therefore average to zero. Also the noise inherent in all electronic measuring equipment is random in nature.

The improvement of S/N ratio is primarily dependent upon the number (n) of cycles to be summed and is equal to $\sqrt{n}$ (i.e.: $\sqrt{128} = \times 13$.

As is evident in Figure 2, the improvement in the S/N ratio is related to the number of repetitions and occurs with the progressive disappearance of the noise, which allows us to define with greater accuracy the potentials of the HP system (G complex).

One sees clearly the necessity to sum at least 128 cycles. With further increase in the cycles an improvement in recording is not generally obtained.

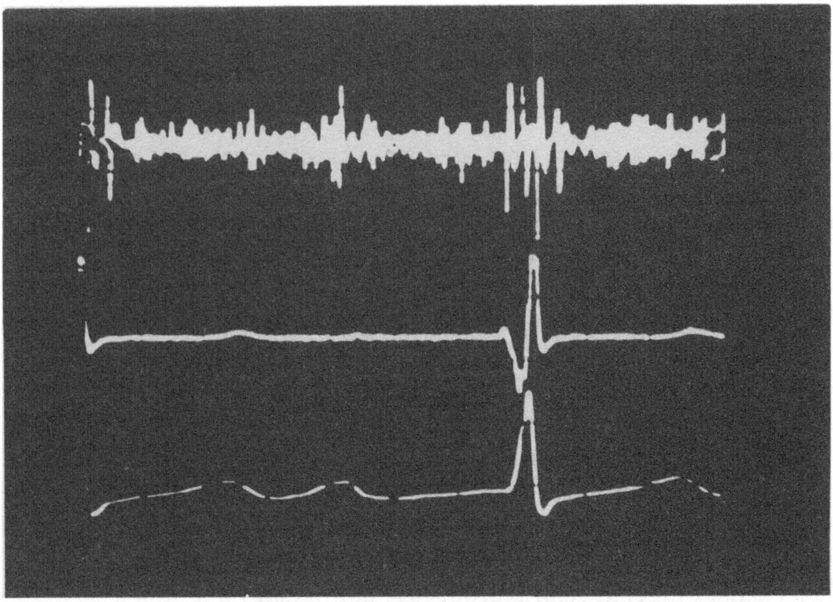

Figure 1. Top strip represents external Hiss-Purkinje activity recording with an amplification of ×97,500; middle strip represents chest bipolar lead used for the trigger (×20,000) and the bottom strip lead II. One should notice the remarkable quantity of noise introduced by the use of a high gain, which masks Hissian deflections and thus makes it necessary to use techniques which reduce the noise

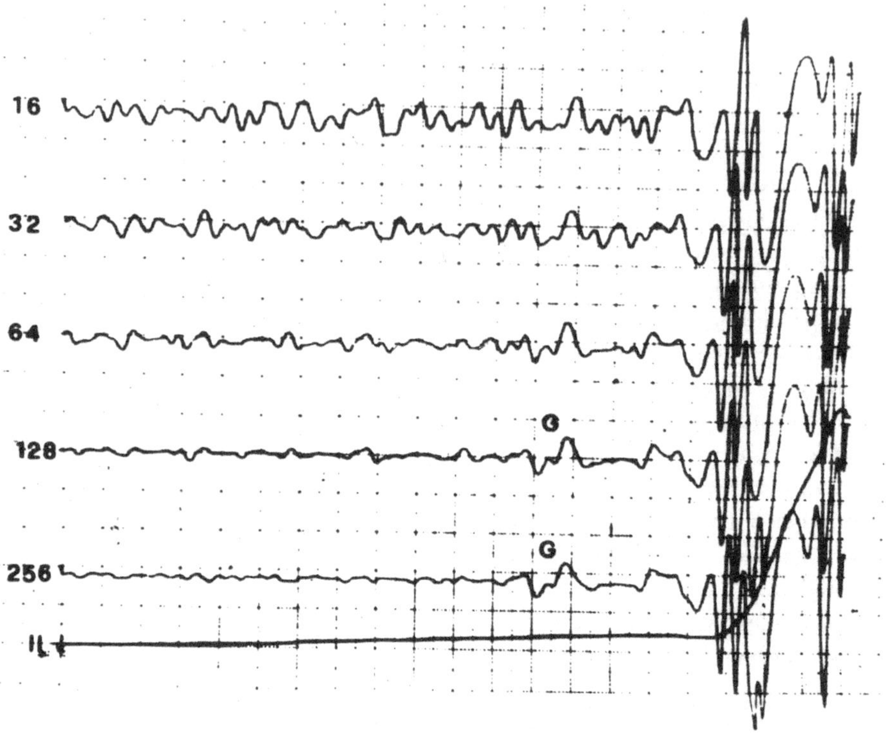

Figure 2. Number of cycles averaged in order to obtain a reproducible G complex. 128 cycles are necessary for a valid average

In order to select a precise time window of cardiac cycle, a synchronization of the RR interval for stable triggering is necessary.

In several studies [1, 2, 22] this has been done by means of an atrial spike; in this way, however, the method remains invasive because of the need for introduction of an intraatrial electrode.

Stopczyk et al. [23] modified the method by utilizing transesophageal pacing in human studies.

Subsequently, Hishimoto et al. [6] reported a successful synchronization by utilizing the amplified P waves from the esophageal lead. Furness et al. [5] utilized QRS synchronization in human studies by playing the magnetic tape recording of the precordial electrocardiogram in reverse.

We [8, 9] and others [10-12] demonstrated in humans that triggering with the QRS complex, utilizing a specially designed QRS detector and digital computer, yielded results with consistent reproducicle morphology and timing.

The patients were put in a small acoustic and electrically shielded room. A bipolar lead was attached across the patient's chest. We have mostly utilized a diagonal lead between the apex and right precordial area.

For the trigger, the extremity bipolar lead with more monophasic potential was chosen. The signal of this lead, amplified and filtered, drives a QRS detector, generating a trigger pulse when the QRS exceeds a prefixed threshold.

In a storage oscilloscope (Tektronix 5103/N/D/13) the temporal stability of the trigger is adjusted and continuously checked in order to rejet the recordings over the limit of $\pm$ 1 msec.

Once the trigger is stabilized, the averaging process is programmed in order to select a window (usually 200 msec) which occurs up to 150 msec prior and 50 msec after the trigger signal. In other words, the bioelectric signal is continuously sampled and stored in a transient memory; every trigger pulse, and therefore everything which precedes by 150 msec and which follows it by 50 msec is transferred to the storage memory.

In Figure 3 the process is schematically represented. A block diagram of the instrumentation is shown in Figure 4.

The two signals, i.e. the chest bipolar lead for His-Purkinje activity and the bipolar lead for the QRS detector, were recorded through differential preamplifier (gain: $\times$ 700) and final preamplifiers (variable gain: step $\times$ 15).

The chest bipolar lead is filtered from 60 to 300 Hz (24 db/octave). Trigger derivation is band-pass filtered from 10 to 5000 Hz (6 db/octave).

To these two leads we added a conventional electrocardiograph from which the three extremity bipolar leads I, II and III are taken.

Analysis is performed with a four channel analyzer (Data Laboratories DL 4000) connected to a microcomputer (Data Laboratories DL 450).

The analogic and alphanumeric output are displaced on an XY scope and on an XY plotter.

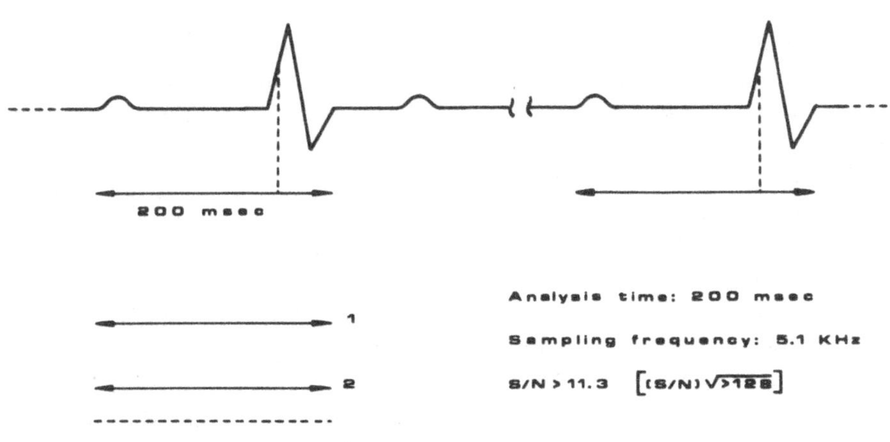

Figure 3. Scheme of the averaging process. In the top strip a scheme of two cardiac cycles is reported. The broken line expresses the point at which the trigger is produced. In the lower part of the figure the temporal relationship and the S N of the procedure are reported. (See text)

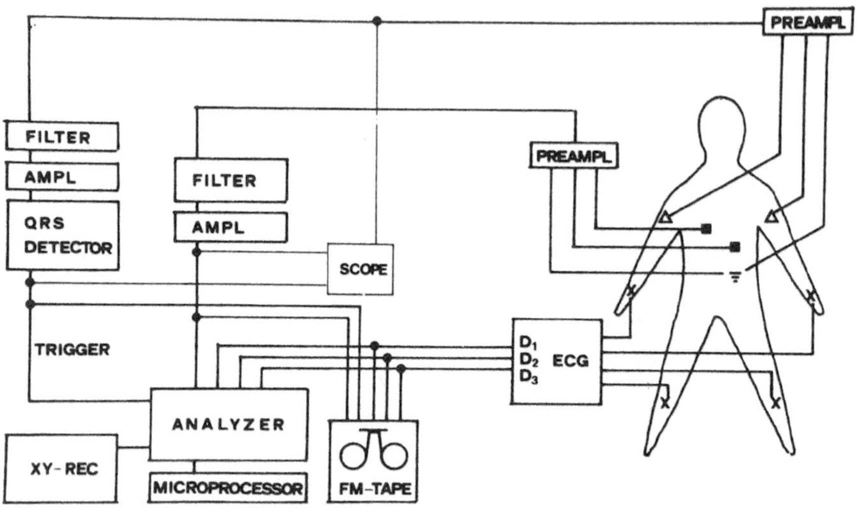

Figure 4. Block diagram of instrumentation for external recording of His bundle activity. For details see text. (From Alboni et al., with permission of G Ital Cardiol [8]))

The sampling rate is 5 kHz for 1024 samples for each channel and the sweep numbers are fixed from 128 to 512.

In this way, in the four channels of the averager, the chest bipolar lead for HPA and the three extremity bipolar leads are analyzed with the same temporal relationship.

We have modified the preceding method by utilizing all three extremity leads or the ones in which the beginning of the QRS complex appeared earlier in order to assess with greater accuracy the beginning of the ventricular activation.

A particular problem concerns the filters. Their use has two aims: to reduce the noise by narrowing as far as possible the band-pass of the amplifier and to isolate the G complex of the P wave, mainly in the cases with short PR interval, in which the P wave and HPA are overlapped.

The choice of the cut-off frequencies was made on a patient with long PR interval (250 msec) from whom it was possible not only to obtain the spectrum of the Hissian potentials and test various band-pass, but also to verify phase-lags and alterations of the HP potentials. The most critical and important part seemed to be the high pass section: highest frequency is 60 Hz (24 db/octave); beyond this frequency marked alterations in the HP potential morphology are induced.

In Figure 5 a case is reported in which in the middle recording with band-pass 30-300 Hz, the P wave overlaps with the G wave. It is therefore necessary to increase the high-pass cut off frequency to 50 Hz (top recording, band-pass 50-600 Hz) so as to isolate the G complex. The low-pass section intervenes mainly on the noise itself and does not greatly influence the morphology of the potentials; it may assume a certain importance in inducing phase-lags only when very narrow band-pass are used, related therefore to the high-pass cut off frequency. An example is reported in the third recording of Figure 5, where with a band-pass of 60-300 Hz there is a slight phase-lag of the G wave compared to the first recording.

Reproducibility of recorded signals was a prerequisite for acceptance of the cardiac origin of the signal. Figure 6 reports the tracing obtained during cruent electrophysiological study (HV interval: 50 msec) and Figure 7 the noninvasive recording of HPA in the same patient.

Atrial wave and HPA are more or less continuous and it is difficult to evaluate the beginning of the His bundle deflections. Such a beginning may however be assessed with recordings (Figure 8) which confirm the value of the GV interval, suspected in the previous recording (Figure 7). Moreover the G complex shows a similar configuration in the three averages performed.

In subjects with long PR interval it is generally easier to assess the beginning of the G complex since atrial activity ends prior to the onset of HPA and the G complex is preceded by an isoelectric interval (Figures 9 and 10).

In order to overcome the difficulty of cases whose atrial and His-Purkinje activity tend to overlap, besides acting on the filters, we at first utilized atrial pacing (Figures 11 and 12) and then Verapamil administration (Figures 13 and 14) which induces a selective prolongation of the AV node conduction, thus separating the G complex from the atrial wave. With Verapamil administration, which also induces slowing of the cardiac rate, it is possible to discriminate whether deflections interposed between the atrial wave and QRS complex are related to HBA or to atrial

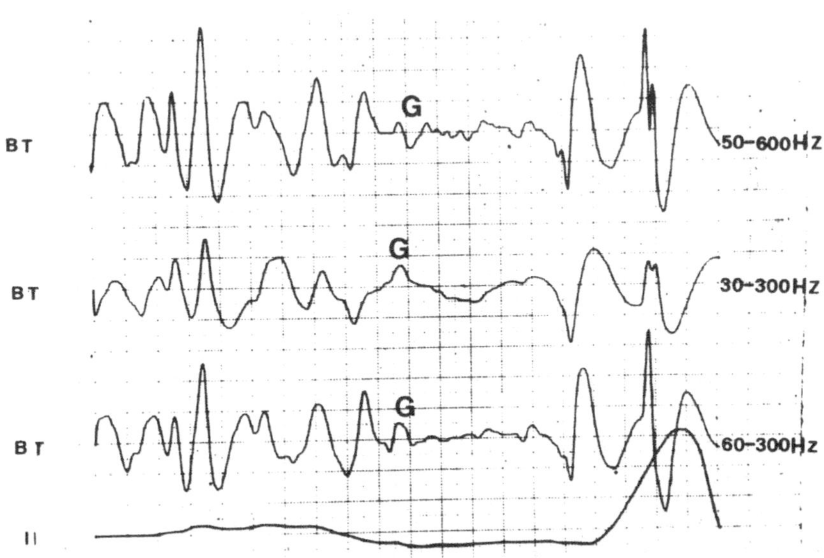

Figure 5. Effect of the filters on the His-Purkinje system waveforms. There is a slight phase shift of the waveforms in the PR segment produced by the changes of the band pass filtering

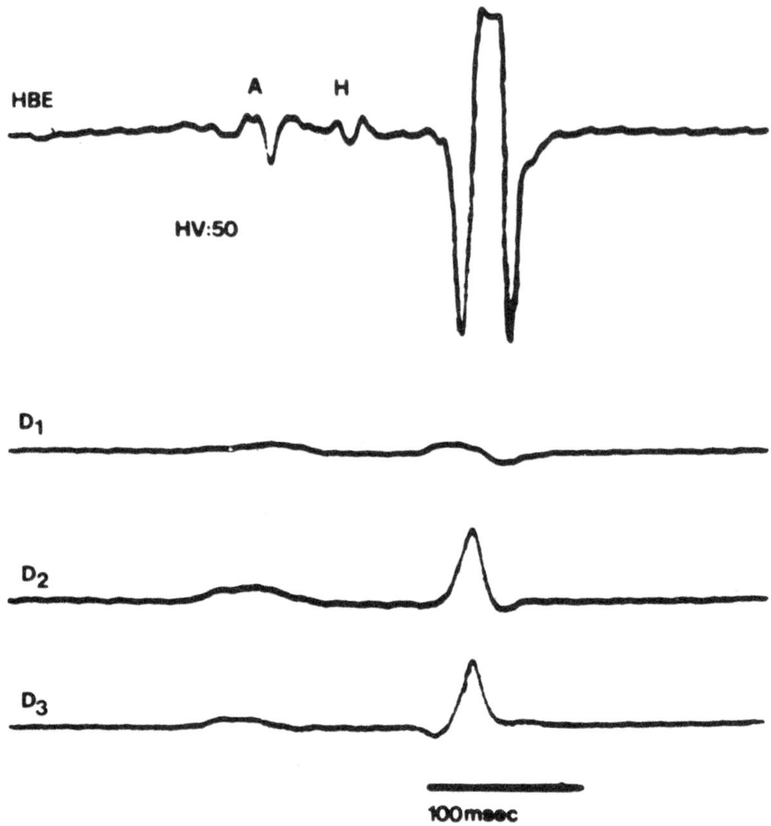

Figure 6. Intracardiac His bundle recording: HV interval measures 50 msec. HBE: His bundle electrocardiogram. D_1: lead I, D_2: lead II, D_3: lead III (From Alboni et al., with permission of G Ital Cardiol [8])

repolarization. In fact, by varying cardiac rate, the temporal relationship between atrial repolarization and QRS complex varies. If this relationship remains constant it is possible to say that high deflections are not related to atrial repolarization.

After preparing a few patients with this method, we performed a noninvasive recording of HPA, after or at the same time as the electrophysiological investigation, in 12 subjects with sinusal rhythm and 1: 1 AV conduction and in two with atrial fibrillation.

In the 12 patients with sinusal rhythm, PR interval was prolonged in five cases, in two a left bundle branch block was present, in two a right bundle branch block and in one an anterior fascicular block.

The G complex appeared in 11 patients, but only in eight was the GV interval evaluable with any precision since in the remaining cases the initial points were doubtful, varying in the diverse recordings performed (Figure 15).

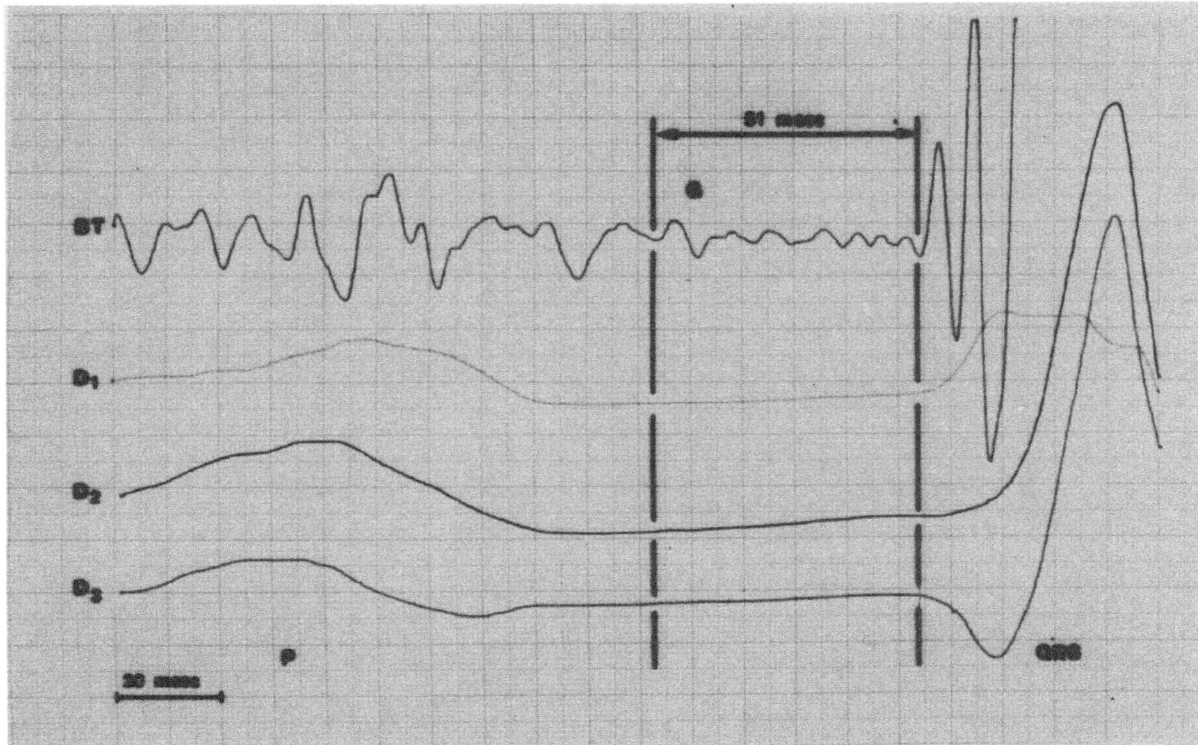

Figure 7. Noninvasive recording of His bundle activity. Same case as previous figure. The starting point of the His bundle potentials (G) is not certain as atrial and His-Purkinje waveforms remain more or less continuous. One may only presume that the GV interval measures 51 msec. BT: chest bipolar lead. (From Alboni et al., with permission of G Ital Cardiol [8])

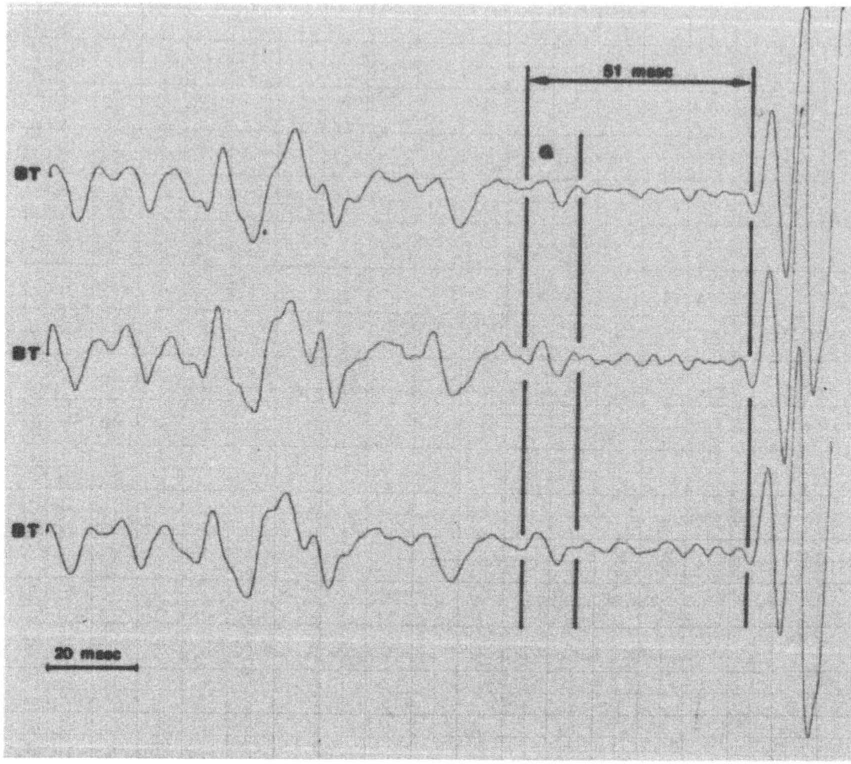

Figure 8. Same case as the previous figure. The recording was repeated three times and a good temporal relationship of the G complex is evident. (From Alboni et al., with permission of G Ital Cardiol [8])

A good correlation appeared between the HV and GV intervals. The mean value of the HV interval was 43 msec and that of the GV interval was 44.6 msec. The greatest difference observed was 5 msec.

In the two patients with atrial fibrillation, G complex was evident but it was difficult to evaluate the initial point.

COMMENT

With the averaging technique it appears possible to record the His-Purkinje activity. In fact it is unlikely that the G complex represents residual noise after averaging. The amplitude of the deflections of the G complex is much greater than the amplitude of the residual noise during the quiescent period. Moreover, of great importance is the fact that in most cases the configuration of the G complex is reproducible on repeated averages, whereas residual noise is variable.

The HV time defines activation of the HP system prior to ventricular activation. Owing to the good correlation between HV and GV intervals, it appears very

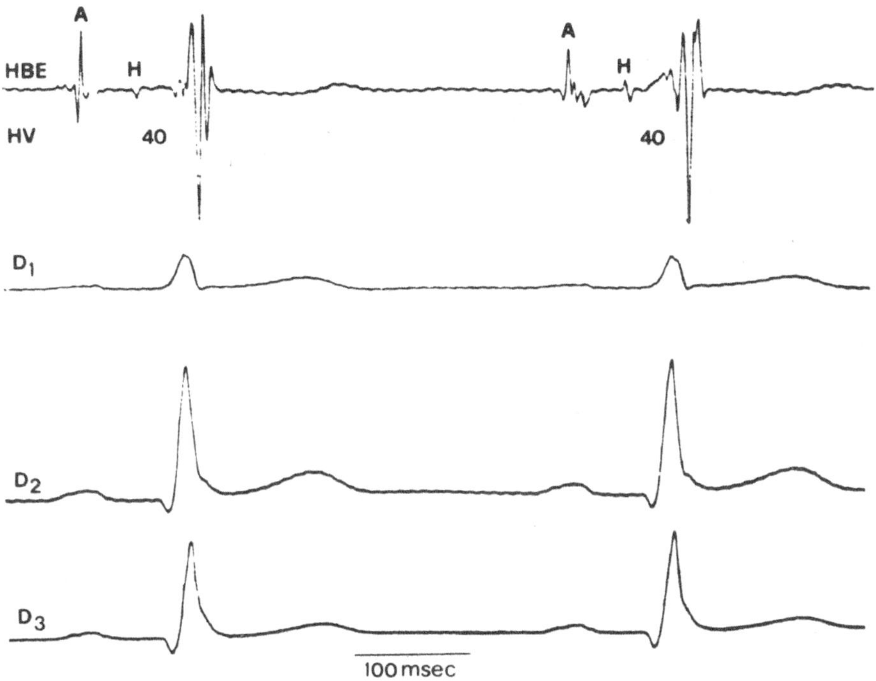

Figure 9. Intracardiac His bundle recording. HV interval measures 40 msec

likely that the first deflections of the G complex represent potentials originating from proximal His bundle. For a better definition of such a correlation further studies are however necessary since both the catheter technique and signal averaging techniques introduce certain errors in the measurements.

Specifically, the choice of measurement points, i.e. the onsets of His-Purkinje and ventricular activity, are partially subjective. Once the measurement points are chosen, regardless of their correctness, resolution is limited with both techniques.

Stable triggering is an essential prerequisite for the average technique. In the study by Furness et al. [5], it was noted that activity corresponding to the HP system was recorded in only 30% of the patients studied. The authors point out that more stable QRS detection and greater reduction of interferences would aid these recordings. These authors, in fact, used only an amplitude scheme of QRS detection for triggering; recording on magnetic tape also provided another source of noise.

Comparison of external averaged recordings, triggered with pacemaker spike and those triggered with QRS complex, showed similar temporal relationship of activity deflection to the following QRS, but the voltage of His deflection was slightly higher in the pacemaker-triggered recording [13]. The cause of the attenuation of this deflection with QRS triggering is not well understood. It is possible

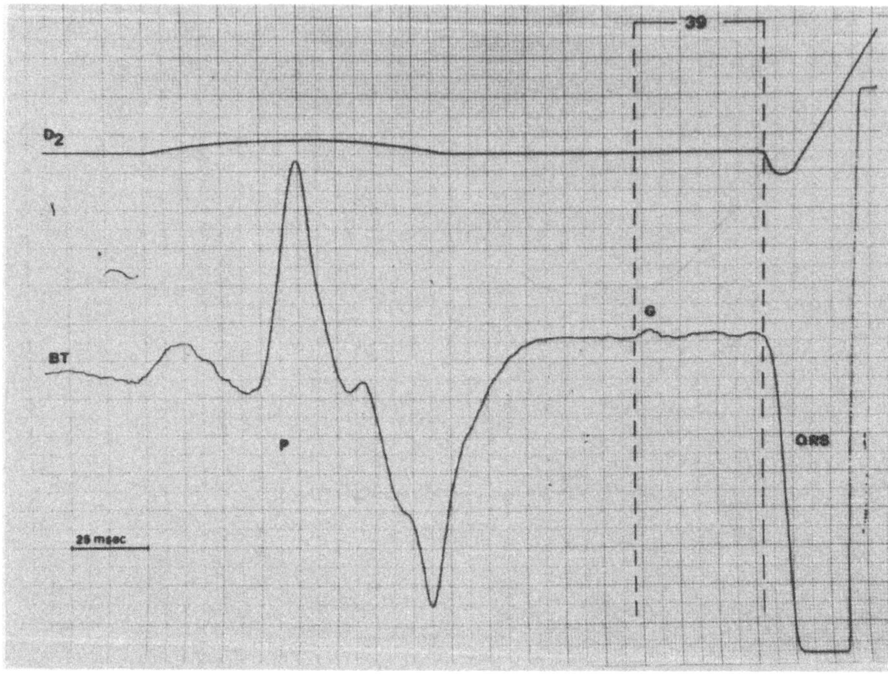

Figure 10. Noninvasive recording of His-Purkinje activity. Same case as the previous figure. The beginning of G complex is well evident in that it is preceded by an isoelectric interval. GV: 39 msec

that some degree of variability of trigger point selection on QRS existed, leading to partial cancellation of the recorded voltage during the process of averaging [13]. For practical purposes, however, the magnitude of recorded voltages appears less important than the temporal relationship, which is similar in both types of recording.

Wajszczuk et al. [13] also performed the averaged process on the direct intracardiac His bundle recording; comparison with the precordial recording showed a very similar temporal relationship, as is also evident in one of our recordings (Figure 16). Major His deflections were well seen in the averaged internal as well as external recording. The process of signal averaging performed on the direct internal recording of the His bundle did not markedly change its morphology. A discrepancy of a few milliseconds in the HP conduction time evaluated by direct intracardiac recording and by the internal averaging techniques may be attributed to trigger instability and difficulty in defining onsets of H and V signals in both techniques.

In the recordings obtained by the noninvasive method there is no definite demarcation between HP potentials and ventricular potentials – as there was in the recordings obtained by the cruent method – but some deflections of low amplitude were observed. It is not clear at present if these deflections express only residual

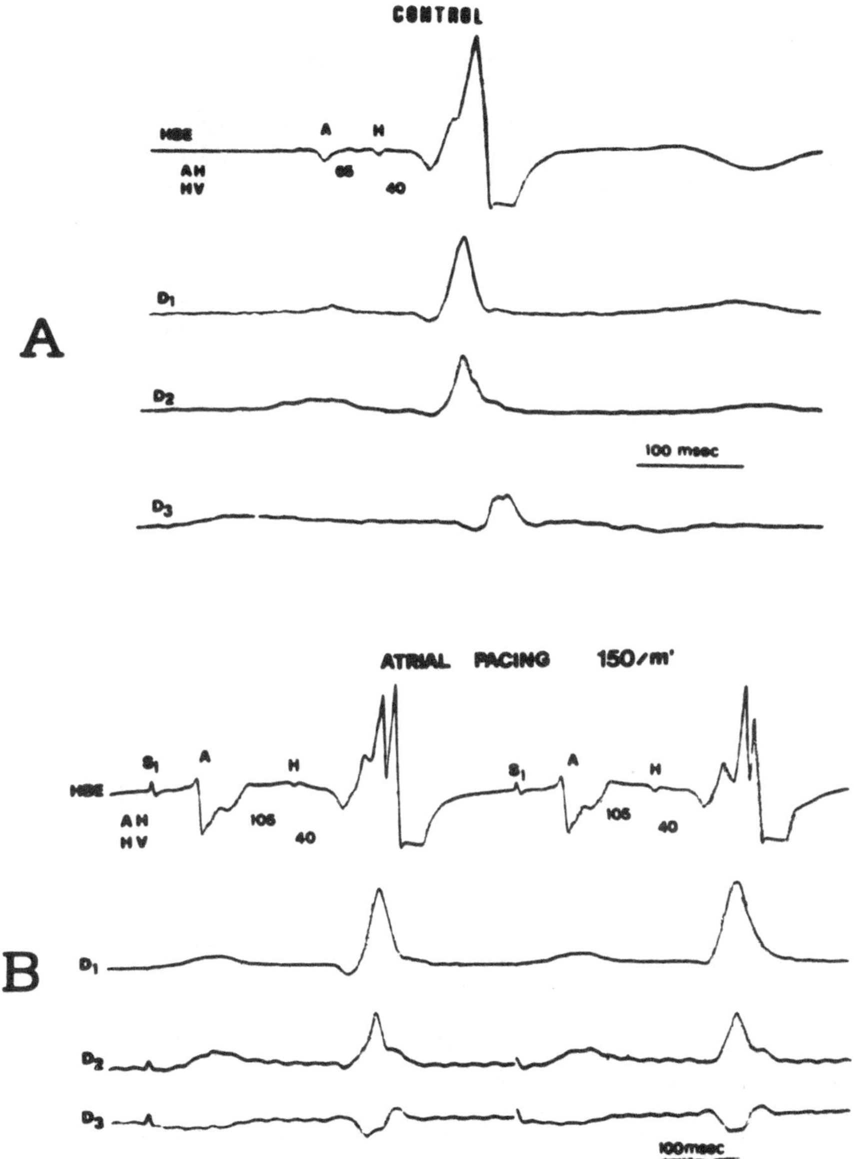

Figure 11. Intracardiac His bundle recording. A: Control study. B: Atrial pacing at cardiac rate of 150/min. HV interval does not change (40 msec) whereas AH interval increases from 65 to 105 msec

noise or also bundle branch activity.

In subjects with short or normal PR interval, overlap of atrial and HPA often prevents a clear demarcation between the two types of activity. In fact with the high gain employed, atrial activity extends much further into the PR interval than

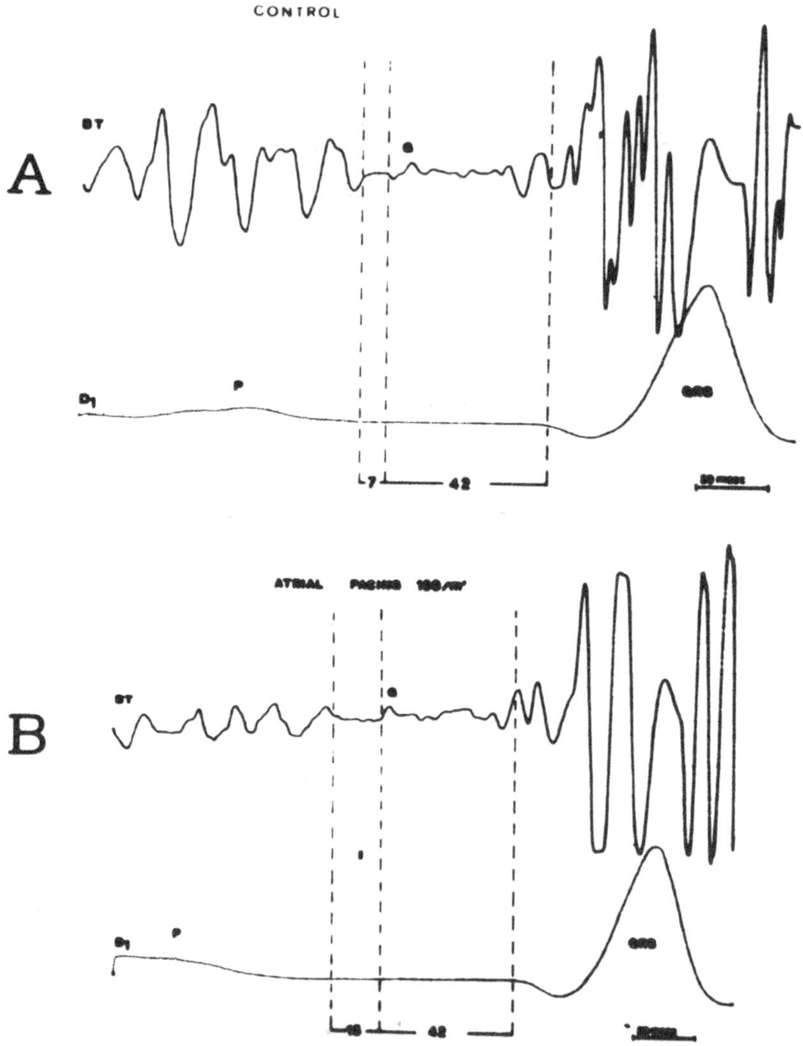

Figure 12. Noninvasive recording of His-Purkinje activity. Same case as previous figure. GV interval measures 42 msec both during control study (A) and during atrial pacing at a cardiac rate of 150/min (B). This excludes the possibility that the G complex is related to the atrial repolarization. During atrial pacing the drawing away of the G complex from the end of the P wave is evident

indicated on the standard ECG, even superimposing itself on HPA. It is also possible that some of the terminal atrial potentials might be the atrial repolarization wave. Sivertssen [24] has used signal averaging to study atrial repolarization wave from intracardiac catheter and this wave has been known to appear on the standard ECG in patients with complete heart block. This wave, being atrial in origin, would not show the same time relationship to the QRS of different cardiac

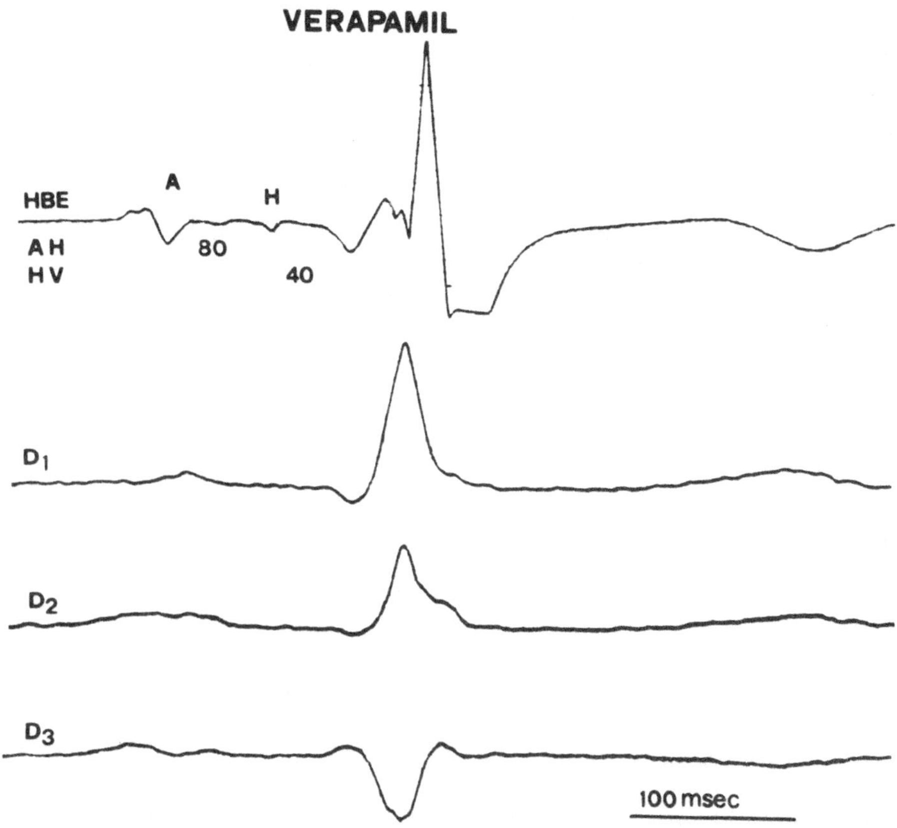

Figure 13. Intracardiac His bundle recording after Verapamil administration. Same case as the previous figure. The drug induces a prolongation of the AH interval from 65 to 80 msec, whereas HV interval does not change (40 msec)

rates. By varying the band-pass filter these problems are only minimally resolved. Of particular usefullness seems to be Verapamil administration in that by prolonging the AV node conduction, it spaces out the G complex from the atrial activity and by slowing cardiac rate it allows us to discriminate whether G complex is related to the HPA or to the atrial repolarisation.

Recently Heron et al. [25] performed HPA recordings utilizing a chest unipolar lead. These authors affirm that this new method gives better discrimination of the specific atrio-ventricular conduction pathways; in our opinion, however, in the tracings reported it does not appear possible to discriminate the HPA.

At present the noninvasive method appears to be of value in patients with acute or chronic heart disease showing: 1) long PR interval with normal or prolonged QRS complex or 2) prolonged QRS complex with normal or long PR interval. It may also be useful for subjects with junctional rhythms, as long as the P wave is completely buried in the QRS complex [22].

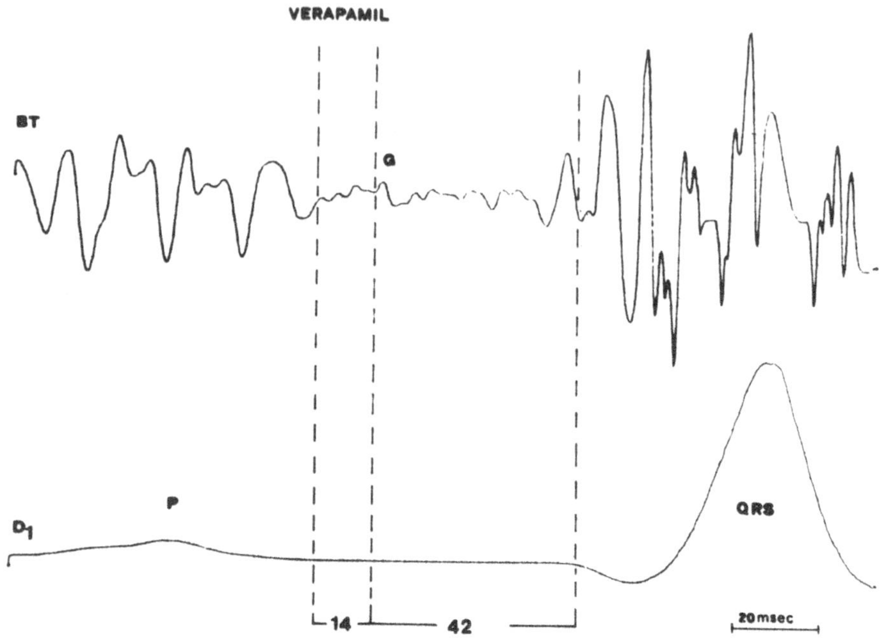

Figure 14. Noninvasive His bundle recording after Verapamil administration. Same case as the previous figure. Compared to the control tracing a drawing away of the G complex from the end of the P wave is observed, whereas GV interval does not change (42 msec). This excludes any possible relationship between the G complex and atrial repolarization

In patients with second degree AV block it is possible to record the G complex preceding the QRS complex, but it is not possible to discriminate whether the block is supra, intra or infra His. Such a differentation may be made only when the atrial pacing pulse is used as the fiducial point for the averaging window [22]; in such cases, however, the method becomes invasive.

In complete AV block, in which atrial and ventricular potentials superimpose, His bundle activity is buried in the large amplitude of atrial or ventricular potentials and cannot be extracted with the conventional techniques of signal averaging. Very recently Takeda et al. [26] resolved this problem with the appropriate compilation of ECGs by use of a simplified device, the 'automated discrimination circuit'. This circuit was designed to nullify the filtered surface ECG for a pre-set interval when triggered by an esophageal P wave or the R wave of a standard lead. The elimination intervals could be set in 10 msec increments from 10 to 1000 msec. Before deciding on which intervals were adequate for avoiding atrial and ventricular superimposition, it was essential to measure accurately the P and QRS intervals in the high-speed, magnified ECG of standard lead. In order to nullify ventricular potentials from the surface ECG, the surface signals were abolished for QT intervals plus the preceding 100 msec to assure perfect elimination of the initial

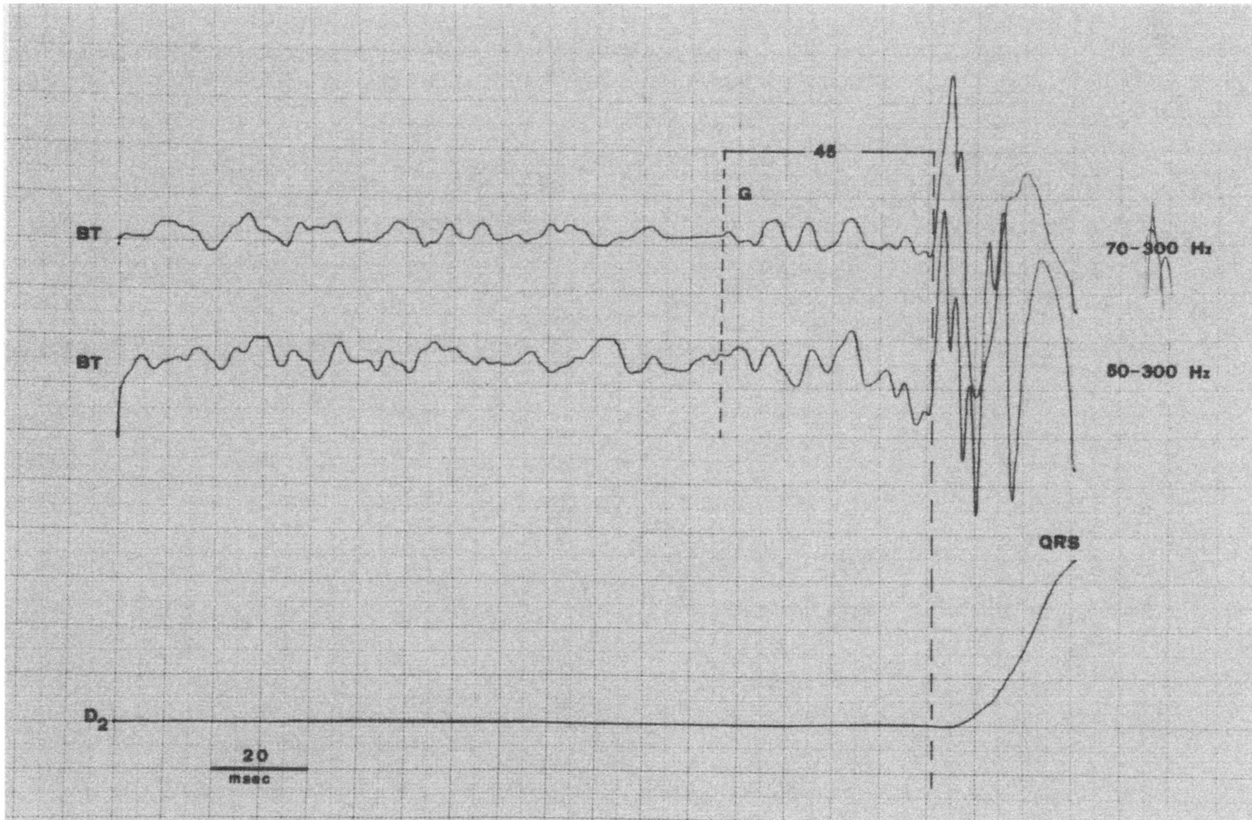

Figure 15. Noninvasive His bundle recording. In the top recording GV interval seems to measure 45 msec, whereas in the middle recording the beginning of the G complex is not well-defined. In other recordings GV interval shows marked changes and so it is not possible to evaluate it precisely

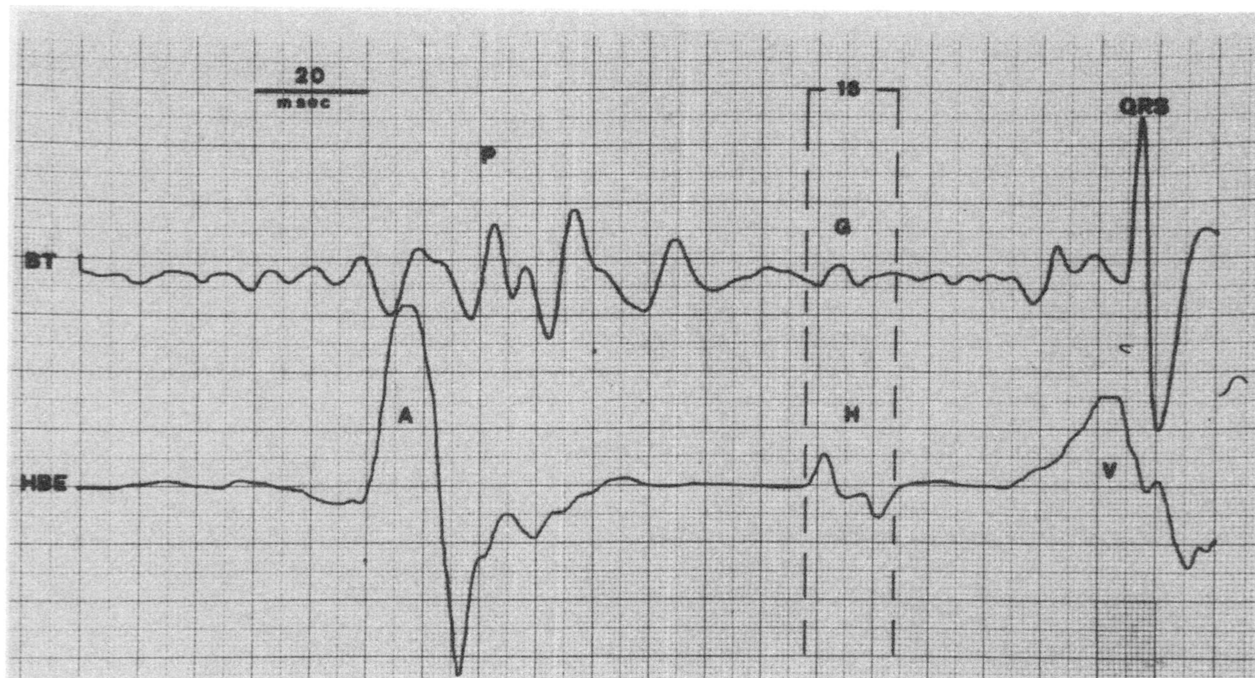

Figure 16. Effect of averaging on the direct (QRS-triggered) (bottom strip) and external (top strip) His bundle recording. The good temporal relationship between the two recordings is evident. (For details see text)

portion of the R wave contents when triggered by the ascending limb of the R waves of the standard ECG.

The postatrial segment superimposed by ventricular potentials was abolished, while the segment without ventricular superimposition remained. In order to nullify the P waves from the surface ECG, the initiation of the P waves in the esophageal ECG was delayed in comparison with those in the surface ECG because the former depicted left atrial activity and, in addition, because a short time constant shortened the duration of the P waves. Therefore it was important to start elimination at the beginning of the P waves in the surface ECG preceding the triggering point in the esophageal ECG. The preventricular segment superimposed by the P wave was abolished, while the segment without a P wave superimposition remained. After these elimination procedures, two sets of surface ECGs were available for averaging, one with P waves and ensuing intervals, the other with QRS complexes and preceding intervals. The former was passed through a signal averager that was triggered by P waves amplified from the esophageal ECG. The latter was directed to the averager triggered by the R wave of a standard lead when the recorded signals were replayed in reverse.

With this method it was possible to evaluate in a noninvasive way whether a complete AV block had a supra or infra His localization.

The noninvasive method can assume particular importance in cases with contraindications to study, such as thrombophlebitis in the leg, coagulation disorders. and serious impairment to the general state of health.

This method may be of particular usefulness in the long-term follow-up and study of the natural history of HP conduction as it may be repeated periodically.

It may also be an easy and practical way of evaluating the effects of several drugs on the HP conduction system.

In some cases, however, the G complex appears to be of low amplitude, difficult to define or even absent. Most likely in such cases the potentials generated in the intraventricular conduction system are small or their transmission to the chest surface is impaired due to the patient's chest configuration or other conditions, including emphysema or obesity.

In other cases the G complex is well-evident, but in several averages performed its beginning does not present a good temporal relationship; this is most likely due to trigger instability.

We believe that the recordings may be improved by making the trigger more stable compared to the variations in the QRS morphology related to the respiratory cycles.

REFERENCES

1. Berbari EJ, Lazzara R, Samet P, Scherlag BJ: Noninvasive technique for detection of electrical activity during the P-R segment. Circulation 48: 1005, 1973
2. Flowers NC, Horan LG: His bundle and bundle branch recordings from the body surface. Circulation 48 (Supple 48): IV-102, 1973
3. Lazzara R, Campbell R, Berbari EJ, Scherlag BJ, Myerburg RJ: Electrocardiogram of His-Purkinje system of man. Circulation 48 (Suppl IV): IV-22, 1973
4. Flowers NC, Hand RC, Orander PC, Miller CB, Walden MO, Horan LG: Surface recording of electrical activity from the region of bundle of His. Am J Cardiol 33: 384, 1974
5. Furness A, Sharrat GP, Carson P: The feasibility of detecting His-bundle activity from the body surface. Cardiovasc Res 9: 390, 1975
6. Hishimoto Y, Sawayama T: Noninvasive recording of His bundle potential in man. Simplified method. Br Heart J 37: 635, 1975
7. Berbari EJ, Lazzara R, El-Sherif N, Befeler B, Aranda JM: The His-Purkinje electrocardiogram in man. An initial assessment of its uses and limitations. Circulation 54: 219, 1976
8. Alboni P, Arslan E, Malacarne C: Registrazione esterna dell'attività elettrica del fascio di His. G Ital Cardiol 7: 532, 1977
9. Alboni P, Arslan E, Malacarne C, Masoni A: Registrazione incruenta dei potenziali elettrici del fascio di His nell'uomo. Boll Soc Ital Cardiol 22: 2044, 1977
10. Cywinski JR, McNiece JR, Ledee GJ, Ruskin J: A technique for noninvasive His-Purkinje system (HPS) recording. In: To pace or not to pace. Controversial subjects on cardiac pacing. Thalen HJ Th, Harthorne JW. The Hague: Martinus Nijhoff, 1978, p 49
11. Pernod J, Court L, Proust F, Droniou J: Enregistrement des potentiels hisiens à partir d'électrodes thoraciques de surface à l'aide d'un moyenneur. Arch Mal Coeur 71: 785, 1978
12. Vincent R, Stroud NP, Jenner R, English MJ, Woollons DJ, Chamberlain DA: Noninvasive recording of electrical activity in the PR segment in man. Br Heart J 40: 124, 1978
13. Wajszczuk WJ, Stopczyk MJ, Moskowitz MS, Zochowski RJ, Bauld T, Dabos PL, Rubenfire M: Noninvasive recording of His-Purkinje activity in man by QRS-triggered signal averaging. Circulation 58: 95, 1978
14. Plonsey R: Bioelectric phenomena. New York: McGraw-Hill, 1969
15. Brazier MAB: Evoke responses recorded from the depths of the human brain. Ann NY Acad Sci 112: 33, 1964
16. Perry NW, Childers DG: The human visual evoked. Response-method and theory. Springfield: Chares C Thomas, 1969
17. Arslan E, Teatini GP: Stimolazione ed analisi dei risultati in elettrococleografia. Pavia: CNR, 1974
18. Hon EH, Lee ST: Noise reduction in fetal electrocardiography. Am J Obstet Gynecol 87: 1086, 1963
19. Irisawa H, Seyama I: Configuration of the P wave during mild exercise. Am Heart J 71: 467, 1966
20. Brody DA, Woolsey MD, Arzbaecher RC: Application of computer techniques to the detection and analysis of spontaneous P-wave variations. Circulation 36: 359, 1967

21. Brody DA, Cox JW, McEachran AB, Giles HH, Ruesta VJ: Spatial parameters and saphe factors of the normal atrial vectorcardiogram and its scalar components. Circulation 39: 229, 1969
22. Berbari EJ, Lazzara R, El-Sherif N, Scherlag BJ: Extracardiac recordings of His-Purkinje activity during conduction disorders and junctional rhythms. Circulation 51: 802, 1975
23. Stopczyk MJ, Kopec J, Zochowsky RJ, Pieniak M: Surface recording of electrical heart activity during the PR segment in man by computer averaging technique. (Abstr.) Proc World Congr Cardiol, 1974
24. Sivertssen E: The atrial recovery wave (Pt) studied by averaging computer technique in patients with complete heart block. J Electrocardiol 5: 243, 1972
25. Heron F, Mialet G, Schuller Ch, Breton D, Perrin J, Degeorges M: Recueil et traitement des signaux d'activité électrique de voies de conduction spécifiques atrioventriculaires chez l'homme. Arch Mal Coeur 72: 48, 1979
26. Takeda H, Kitamura K, Takanashi T, Tokuoka T, Hamamoto H, Katoh T, Niki I, Hishimoto Y: Noninvasive recording of His-Purkinje activity in patients with complete atrioventricular block. Clinical application of an automated discrimination circuit. Circulation 60: 421, 1979

13. EFFECT OF ANTIARRHYTHMIC DRUGS ON INTRAVENTRICULAR CONDUCTION

Classification of antiarrhythmic drugs has always been a controversial subject. In recent years it has become increasingly so with so many new compounds appearing on the pharmacological horizon. Furthermore there is no complete understanding of either the electropharmacology of the antiarrhythmic agent or the mechanisms engendering various cardiac arrhythmias, despite the recent contributions by investigators using ultramicroelectrode and His bundle recording.

Various classifications of the antiarrhythmic drugs have been proposed [1-5] but none of these seem satisfactory. The most acceptable, at present, is the one proposed by Singh et al. [2], based chiefly on the membrane effects of the antiarrhythmic agents, which have been subdivided into several groups. An overlap in the electrophysiological effects among the groups is, of course, to be expected.

This classification excludes drugs which have a possible, but not exclusive, antiarrhythmic use and the most recent antiarrhythmic agents.

GROUP 1A

Group 1A includes quinidine, procainamide, disopyramide and ajmaline.

These antiarrhythmic agents share the dominant electrophysiologic property of blocking the fast inward sodium current during the depolarization of the cardiac membrane. This may be measured quantitatively either as a change in the maximal rate of rise of the action potential (Vmax of phase 0) or as a change in membrane responsiveness when the rate of rise is related to the level of the resting membrane potential from which the spike depolarization is initiated [2]. A reduction in the rate of rise of the action potential or in membrane responsiveness is accompanied by a decrease in conduction velocity together with an increase in the threshold of excitability. The action potential duration is not significantly affected but it often lengthens; phase 4 depolarization is instead constantly depressed. By blocking the fast inward sodium current, the class 1A antiarrhythmic agents depress intraventricular conduction.

Quinidine

Quinidine is the dextro-isomer of quinine and is employed in the management of a wide spectrum of atrial and ventricular arrhythmias. Ordinarily, quinidine is administered as quinidine sulfate, orally, intramuscularly or intravenously, but the latter route is almost never used because of the associated undesirable effects on heart and circulation.

When quinidine is administered by mouth, absorption is almost complete. After a single oral dose the plasma level attains a peak value within 1 to 2 hours. When given intramuscularly, the peak plasma level occurs at the same time as after oral administration but the value is only 70% of that attained after a comparable oral dose. The usual range of therapeutic plasma levels is between 2 and 6 μg/ml.

Quinidine is also available as long acting preparations such as quinidine polygalacturate and quinidine gluconate.

Circulating quinidine is metabolized in the liver and only about 20 to 50% is excreted unchanged in the urine. Little is known about the biologic activity of the metabolities but most are probably less active than the parent drug and most are excreted in the urine. Because quinidine depends both on hepatic metabolism and renal excretion for elimination, blood levels will depend on both hepatic and renal function.

From an electrical point of view, quinidine is the classic example of a class IA agent, since it slows intraventricular conduction, depresses spontaneous phase 4 diastolic depolarization and slightly prolongs the effective refractory period of ventricular and Purkinje fibers [6-11]. These effects have been observed not only in normal Purkinje fibers, but also in diseased ones [12].

The results of clinical studies [13, 14] are in agreement with those in vitro. The effects of quinidine on intraventricular conduction can in part be recognized electrocardiographically. The drug causes progressive prolongation of the QRS complex and sometimes of the PR interval. The prolongation of this latter interval is related to the effect of the drug on intraatrial and His-Purkinje conduction and not on AV node conduction. In fact, electrophysiological studies [15, 16] evidenced an increase in PA and HV intervals, whereas AH interval tended to be reduced. The latter effect has been attributed to the anticholinergic properties of the drug, evidenced both in animal [11, 14, 17, 18] and in man [19, 20]. Electrophysiological studies in man also evidenced a prolongation of both the effective and relative refractory periods of His-Purkinje system (HPS) after quinidine administration [16].

In clinical setting the magnitude of the effect of quinidine on intraventricular conduction does not seem to be dependent on the initial value. In the electrophysiological study by Josephson et al. [16], quinidine, administered intramuscularly, showed the same effect on HV and QRS duration in patients with bundle branch block and in those with normal intraventricular conduction.

Procainamide

Procainamide has emerged as an important antiarrhythmic drug in the treatment of ventricular arrhythmias, especially in the coronary care unit [21]. It can be administered by mouth, intramuscularly or intravenously. After an oral dose the peak plasma level and cardiac effect are usually attained within 1 to 2 hours.

The usual range of therapeutic plasma levels is between 3 and 10 μg/ml [22]. The average $t_{\frac{1}{2}}$ for elimination of procainamide is 3 to 4 hours in normal adults; for this reason the plasma level falls fairly rapidly after each dose.

Procainamide is eliminated both by hepatic metabolism and renal excretion. Between 75 and 95% of a given dose is eliminated in the urine; 30 to 60% appears as procainamide and the remainder as metabolites. Elimination of the drug in the urine is slowed down by impaired renal perfusion or by alkalinization of the urine.

On the intraventricular conduction procainamide shares all the electrophysiologic properties of quinidine since in ventricular and Purkinje fibers it decreases velocity of conduction and automaticity and prolongs the effective refractory period [14, 23-26].

In electrophysiological studies in man [27-29] it has also been demonstrated that procainamide induces a significant prolongation of conduction time and within the HPS (HV interval prolongation), an increase of the relative and effective refractory period of the HPS. Changes in QRS duration and configuration were modest, thus suggesting that the drug causes a uniform delay in HPS conduction and has little effect on ventricular muscle. In a few rare cases, however, procainamide may induce the appearance of bundle branch block pattern in patients with normal intraventricular conduction (Figure 1).

Ogunkelu et al. [30] studied effects of different doses of procainamide administered intravenously on the electrophysiological properties of the intraventricular conduction system in man. Dose-related increases in His-Purkinje conduction were observed, starting with a dose of 200 mg. After administration of 300 mg, the mean increase in HV interval was 8 msec (17%), compared to the control values; after administration of 400 or 500 mg the mean increase was 9 msec (19%). The increase in the HPS refractory period also appeared dose-related. Scheinman et al. [31] reported that in patients with bundle branch block and prolonged HV interval, large doses of procainamide (750 to 1000 mg) resulted in a mean increase in the HV interval of 11 msec (18% over control value). It would appear that the percent increase in the mean HV interval values remains approximately the same (about 18%) after large doses of procainamide in patients with intraventricular conduction troubles.

From these data it may be deduced that procainamide administered intravenously does not induce important variations in intraventricular conduction from a clinical point of view. However, at present, there do not exist data regarding investigations on the electrophysiological effects of different doses of pro-

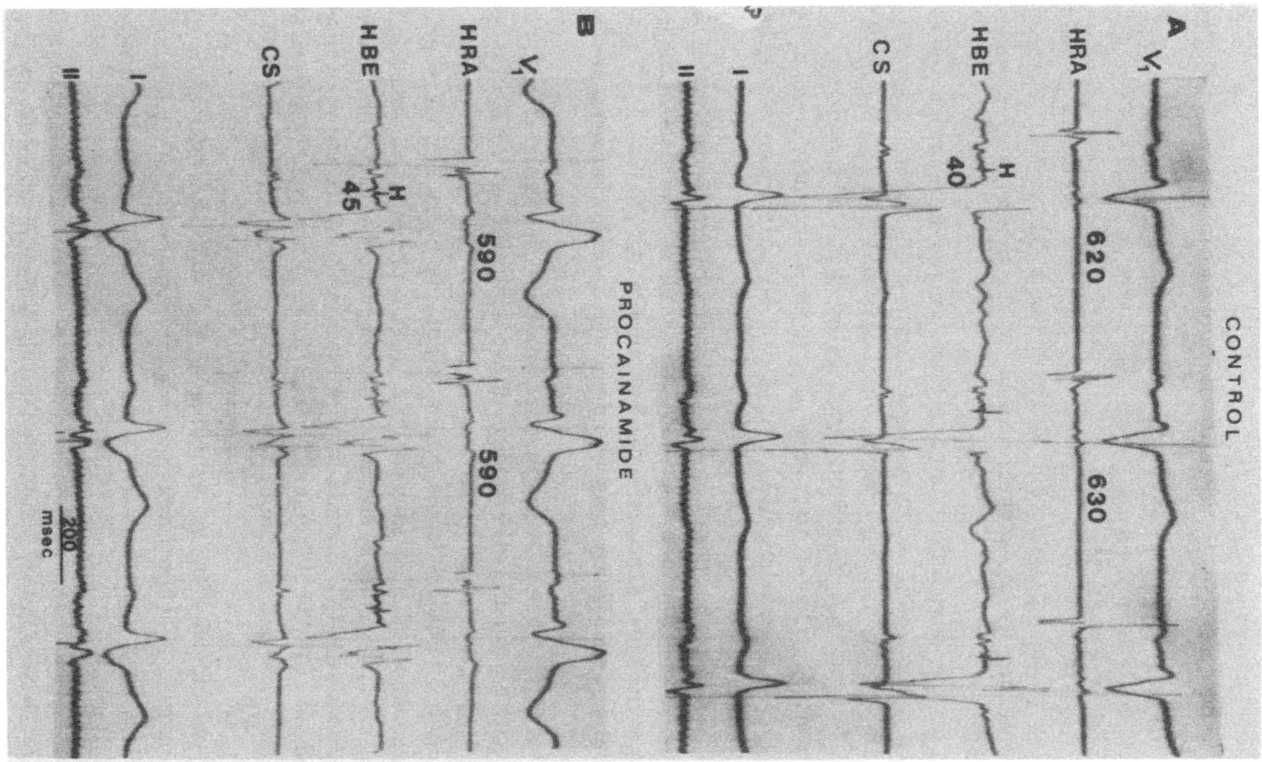

Figure 1. After procainamide administration (500 mg i.v.), slight prolongation of HV interval (40 msec vs 45 msec) and appearance of right bundle branch block can be observed. HRA: high right atrium. HBE: His bundle electrocardiogram. CS: coronary sinus

cainamide administered orally over long periods of time.

On AV node conduction, procainamide presents the same effects as quinidine, as it shows anticholinergic properties [24, 26, 32]: the AH interval, in fact, tends to be reduced, but not significantly, after a procainamide administration [27, 28, 30, 31].

Ajmaline

Ajmaline is a derivative of *Rauwolfia serpentina* [33]. In 1956, this drug was first recognized as possessing significant anti-arrhythmic effects [34]. Subsequent studies have defined its effectiveness in man for the treatment of a variety of arrhythmias [35-40].

However, clinical observations indicate brief effective duration of this drug. This has been further confirmed by pharmacological studies on excretion [41] and serum half-life [42], and by comparing the duration of action of ajmaline and other antiarrhythmic agents on fibrillation produced by electrical stimulation in the guinea-pig heart [43]. The fact that ajmaline does not accumulate in the myocardium and is rapidly excreted by the kidneys [41, 42, 44] led to a search for ajmaline derivates with more prolonged activity [44].

A new ajmaline ester has been found, 17-monochloroacetyl ajmaline (MCAA), with longer effect than ajmaline, and which appears effective in man for the treatment of supraventricular and ventricular arrhythmias [45-50].

Both ajmaline and MCAA may be administered orally, intramuscularly or intravenously.

Obayashi et al. [51] demonstrated that ajmaline has a depressant effect on conduction velocity on canine Purkinje fibers due to depression of Vmax of phase 0 and membrane respinsiveness. Moreover, ajmaline was shown to have significant depressant effect on phase 4 depolarization in Purkinje fibers. De Azevedo et al. [52] and Piwonke et al. [53] showed that MCAA presents the same electrophysiological effects. Studies in man have confirmed the results obtained in vitro.

Both ajmaline and MCAA administered intravenously induce a prolongation of HV and QRS intervals [54-59] (Figure 2). Such prolongation is more marked after ajmaline administration but is more protracted after MCAA administration [54, 60].

We observed that absolute prolongation of HV and QRS intervals is more marked in patients in whom these intervals are prolonged during the control study, while the percentage increase is almost equal in patients with normal and prolonged HV and QRS intervals [59].

At present the lack of data does not permit an accurate evaluation of the effects of ajmaline on HPS refractory periods. In the only patient in whom the evaluation was possible, we observed a prolongation in the HPS relative refractory period after ajmaline administration [59].

Ajmaline, in contrast to quinidine, also induces a prolongation in the AH inter-

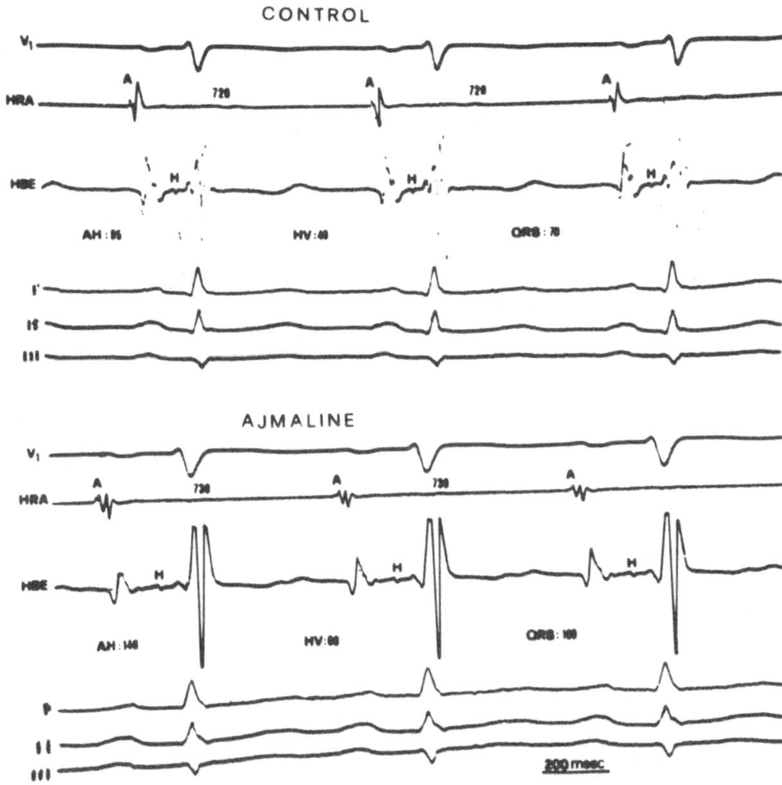

Figure 2. Ajmaline administration (1 mg/kg i.v.) induces prolongation of HV and QRS intervals (40 msec vs 60 msec and 70 msec vs 100 msec, respectively), as well as of AH interval. (From Alboni et al., with permission of G Ital Cardiol [59])

val, which is an expression of conduction slowing in the AV node [54, 58, 59]; this prolongation is less after MCAA administration [54, 56, 60].

Very recently a new derivative of ajmaline has been used, *aimaline bitartrate*, which presents electrophysiological effects of great similarity to the MCAA ones [61]. It has proved to be very efficacious in the therapy of ventricular arrhythmias [61, 62].

Disopyramide

Disopyramide phosphate, a synthetic compound, is an antiarrhythmic drug with many quinidine-like properties [63].

Clinical studies have evidenced its usefulness in the management of both supraventricular and ventricular arrhythmias [64-68]. Disopyramide phosphate, unrelated chemically to any of the antiarrhythmic agents, is available for both oral and parenteral administration. When given intravenously, disopyramide has a two-phase disappearance curve. The first, or so-called distribution phase, which reflects the equilibrium between tissue content and vascular space, has a half-life of 20 to 50 minutes. The second, or excretory phase, which reflects the disappearance of the drug from the body once tissue equilibrium has occurred, has a half-life of 2 hours [69]. The oral preparation is almost completely absorbed from the gut and rapidly eliminated in the urine and feces. After peak blood levels are reached, the biologic half-life in man is about 7 hours [69].

This drug has been shown in vitro to reduce the maximum rate of depolarization in ventricular tissues [70]. Sekiya et al. [63] also showed a prolongation of action potential duration during intracellular recording on rabbit atria, which has been confirmed in anesthetized dogs by Edwards et al. [71] recording monophasic action potentials with suction electrodes and by Levites et al. [72], who demonstrated a prolongation of effective refractory period in ischemic areas of canine heart after disopyramide administration.

In electrophysiological studies in man [73-80] these properties of the drug have been confirmed on the intraventricular conduction system. In fact, disopyramide increases HV and QRS intervals. In some studies [76, 78] this increase is statistically significant, in others it is not significant [73, 74, 75, 77]. The differences among the various results may be related to the relatively small patient size or differences in disopyramide dosings or both.

Few data are available concerning the effect of the drugs on HPS refractory periods. The relative refractory period was compared before and after disopyramide in six patients by Desai et al. [78] and in two by Josephson et al. [73]. In all cases this period increased after drug administration. The HPS effective refractory period was not determined in any patient.

Desai et al. [78] performed an electrophysiological study in 22 patients with bundle branch block before and after intravenous infusion of disopyramide (2 mg/kg). In no cases did a 2° or 3° AV block appear. The degree of prolongation of the HV interval (18 %) was similar to that (17 %) found for a roughly comparable group of patients with BBB who were studied with intravenous procainamide [31]. These data confirm the safety of intravenous disopyramide infusions in patients with bundle branch block.

This drug shows variable but not significant effects on AV node conduction: at times the AH interval may increase or decrease slightly [76, 78]. This variable effect on AV node is best explained by both its direct and vagolitic actions [18, 77, 78].

GROUP 1B

This group includes lidocaine and diphenylhydantoin. Most investigators agree that these drugs shorten the effective refractory period of Purkinje fibers without significantly changing the membrane responsiveness and conduction velocity [79-82].

The results obtained after administration of these drugs are, however, contradictory.

Lidocaine

Lidocaine is a local anesthetic which Southworth et al. [83] in 1950 demonstrated antiarrhythmic properties.

Lidocaine is primarily used to treat ventricular arrhythmias resulting from cardiac disease or digitalis toxicity; it appears less efficacious in the therapy of supraventricular arrhythmias although some authors [84] have reported satisfactory results.

Lidocaine is usually administered intravenously. Therapeutic plasma concentrations are 1-5 μg/ml [85]. Within approximately half a minute after a lidocaine injection, 70 % of the drug has left the blood and entered the highly perfused tissues and fat, while less than 1 % has been metabolized [86]. As plasma lidocaine levels fall, the diffusion gradient from tissue to blood increases and the lidocaine which initially entered the well perfused tissues diffuses back into the blood and is metabolized by the liver. The major determinants of the $t_{\frac{1}{2}}$ of lidocaine (about 3 minutes following an intravenous bolus of 50 to 100 mg) are the distribution of lidocaine in the body and hepatic metabolism, the latter being affected largely by microsomal enzymes [87].

Because of its brief duration, lidocaine must be given by continuous intravenous infusion (20-50 μg/kg/min) which must be preceded by a bolus injection, otherwise therapeutic plasma concentration is not reached. The metabolic products of the drugs are excreted in the urine; less than 10 % of administered lidocaine is excreted unmetabolized [87].

The intramuscular route of administration also appears to be efficacious in the therapy of ventricular arrhythmias [88-93].

Fehemers et al. [91] reported that following an intramuscular injection of 250 mg of lidocaine, plasma concentrations greater than 1 μg/ml were attained within 5 to 10 minutes.

In vitro studies [81, 94, 95] indicated that lidocaine has no effect on phase 0 depolarization and conduction in normal Purkinje fibers until rather high concentrations were attained. At these concentrations (11-50 μg/ml) they reported that lidocaine decreased action potential amplitude, Vmax and membrane responsiveness.

Lidocaine dramatically shortens the action potential duration of Purkinje fibers [95]. Although the decrease in action potential duration induced by the drug is accompanied by shortening of the effective refractory period, several studies indicate that the refractoriness does not decrease as much as the action potential.

Other in vitro studies [96, 97], suggest that lidocaine exorts a differential effect on healthy and diseased tissues but the results appear to be contradictory. Sasyniuk et al. [96] reported that, compared with normal Purkinje fibers, subendocardial Purkinje fibers surviving myocardial infarction demonstrated markedly decreased action potential amplitudes and a minimal rate of depolarization of phase 0 in response to lidocaine.

Prolongation of the interval from the Q wave to the electrocardiogram recorded over infarcted muscle after a lidocaine administration has been described [98]. In contrast, there was no effect in normal tissue in the dog 2 hours after myocardial infarction. El-Sherif et al. [97] demonstrated that lidocaine selectively slowed conduction in reentrant pathways of ischemic cardiac muscle, but it did not effect conduction in normal muscle. The same results have been reported by Rosen et al. [99-101] and by Wald et al. [12]. On the other hand, Bigger et al. [94] observed that lidocaine improved conduction in Purkinje fibers when the drug acted on partially depolarized fibers.

Even the effects of the drug on diseased intact heart appear to be contradictory.

Rosen et al. [102] studied the effect of lidocaine in 10 patients with arrhythmias in the presence of arteriosclerotic, primary or hypertensive heart disease and reported that at various pacing rates lidocaine had no effect on the HV interval. Kunkel et al. [103] reported no change in the His-Purkinje conduction time or QRS duration in 10 patients with right or left bundle branch block after administration of lidocaine. Bekheit et al. [104] studied conduction intervals before and after lidocaine in 10 patients, four of whom had a prolonged HV interval. They found no significant effect on the intraventricular conduction system, even in the patients with impaired conduction.

Contrasting results have been observed by Gupta et al. [105], who evaluated the effect of lidocaine in 16 patients with prolonged HV interval, six of whom had earlier shown transient 2° or 3° AV block. Lidocaine administration produced complete heart block distal to His bundle in two. A third patient, with an HV interval of 70 msec, showed 2° AV block distal to H deflection during atrial pacing after administration of lidocaine but not before. An additional patient, observed clinically to have alternating right and left bundle branch block, experienced cardiac standstill after the injection.

Similar results have been reported by Roos et al. [106] in patients with bundle branch block with or without acute myocardial infarction. These authors, moreover, did not encounter a shortening of HPS refractory periods, observed by Josephson et al. [107] in normal patients.

In an animal study, Gerstenblith et al. [108] observed that lidocaine, after ischemic damage of the intraventricular conduction system, significantly increased HV time during sinus rhythm and at all pacing rates. It also resulted in advanced His-Purkinje conduction defects including His bundle block and right bundle branch block in these animals. These authors postulated that lower pH in the infarct zone, greater extracellular potassium concentration, local metabolic products due to ischemia may be responsible for these effects of lidocaine in diseased intraventricular conduction system.

These data, even though they are contradictory, suggest that lidocaine should be used cautiously in patients with bundle branch block. However, all the studies show that this drug does not have significant effects on AV node conduction.

Diphenylhydantoin

Diphenylhydantoin (DPH), chemically analogous to barbiturates, was introduced as an antiarrhythmic agent in 1950 by Harris et al. [109]. It is effective in the management of ventricular arrhythmias and also arrhythmias resulting from digitalis toxicity [110-112].

DPH may be administered by either the intravenous or oral route. DPH plasma levels of 10-18 μg/ml are regarded as the therapeutic range [113], although some cardiac arrhythmias, particularly those resulting from digitalis toxicity, may respond to lower plasma levels.

Only 1% to 5% of the DPH in the body is excreted unchanged by the kidneys [114]. inactivation of the remaining drug results from metabolism in the liver by the mixed function oxidase system; it is then excreted in the urine [115].

As for lidocaine, cellular electrophysiological effects of DPH depend above all on the concentration of DPH and the electrophysiological condition of the fibers. When resting membrane potential, Vmax of phase 0 and action potential amplitude are normal, therapeutic concentrations of DPH do not have any effect on conduction but significantly shorten the action potential duration. The effective refractory period is also decreased, although the reduction is not as great as the reduction in action potential duration [116].

Available experimental data indicate that DPH also depresses the slope of phase 4 depolarization of Purkinje fibers [116]. The increased slope of spontaneous diastolic depolarization induced by catecholamines or digitalis is also depressed by the drug [116].

High concentrations of DPH depress Vmax of phase 0 and membrane responsiveness [116, 117].

According to some authors [116], DPH improves membrane resting potential and conduction in diseased Purkinje fibers; according to others [12] it depresses these parameters.

In the intact heart, therapeutic levels of DPH do not significantly slow conduction in the HPS (do not alter the HV interval in the His bundle electrocardiograms) nor do they slow conduction in ventricular muscle; there is no significant effect of the drug on the QRS complex [118-122]. Instead DPH shortens the relative and effective refractory period and consequently improves conduction of premature impulses in the ventricular conduction system and ventricular muscle in both canine and human hearts.

In agreement with several in vitro studies it has been reported that in the presence of bundle branch block, DPH speeds His-Purkinje conduction in the intact heart. This occurred in the canine heart after conduction had been depressed by toxic concentrations of procainamide [123].

Also in the clinical setting, Haiat et al. [124] described a case of right bundle branch block and left posterior fascicular block associated with atrial tachycardia; the intravenous administration of 250 mg of DPH restored normal intraventricular conduction. The normalization of conduction was not rate-related since the conduction disturbances were previously observed at a slower rate.

Further electrophysiological investigations are required in order to clarify the effects of DPH on diseased HPS in clinical setting.

The effects of DPH on AV node conduction are variable; however in most cases this drug shortens AH interval, most probably owing to the anticholinergic effect [120, 121].

GROUP II

Included in this group are the beta-adrenergic blocking agents, i.e. propanolol and other drugs which interfere with the uptake and release of the sympathetic nervous system transmitters.

Beta-adrenergic blocking drugs

The beta-adrenergic blocking drugs bind to the beta receptor and thereby prevent the interaction between the catecholamines and receptor which results in the physiologic response.

A number of beta-receptor blocking drugs are now becoming available for clinical use. The one most studied in a clinical setting is propanolol which seems to be efficacious in a wide spectrum of atrial and ventricular arrhythmias, particular when sympathetic influences represent the most important cause of arrhythmia. Propranolol can be administered intravenously or orally. Many doubts exist regarding the clinical meaning of the plasma levels of propranolol in that 90% to 95% of the drug in the intravascular compartment is bound to plasma proteins [125] and measured plasma levels include both the bound and unbound drug. Probably only the unbound drug can interact with the beta receptors and is pharmacologically active [126].

Almost 95% of propranolol in the body is metabolized and very little is excreted unaltered in the urine [127]. Most of the metabolism occurs in the liver but there is some evidence that propranolol may be metabolized in the lung as well [128]. The effects of propranolol on intraventricular conduction depend on several factors including 1) whether catecholamines are present and if so, which effects they are exerting on the action potential; 2) the condition of tissue, i.e. are action potentials normal or are they depressed, and 3) the presence or absence of direct effects of the drug [129].

In concentrations low enough to cause beta receptor blockade but no direct membrane effect, propranolol does not alter the normal resting membrane potential and Vmax of Purkinje and ventricular muscle fibers [130-133].

When in such fibers values for these parameters are abnormally low, catecholamines may increase them. In this case beta receptor blockade might depress conduction by removing the catecholamine effect.

Propranolol also has direct membrane effects which are exerted at very high concentrations: 10 to 100-fold higher than necessary for the beta blocking action. These effects probably result from actions of this drug to decrease Na^+ conductance [134]. The concentrations which depress the normal action potential are far higher than the antiarrhythmic blood levels in humans. However, it is possible that much lower concentrations would exert a direct effect on diseased Purkinje fibers. At present we do not know if the drug exerts a direct effect on Vmax of phase 0 and conduction of slow response action potentials which are not dependent on catecholamines. In low concentrations beta blockers do not affect repolarization and refractoriness of Purkinje or ventricular fibers when these tissues are not being superfused with catecholamines [129].

In the presence of high doses of catecholamines the effect of propranolol on action potential duration and refractoriness is complex and variable [129] and so far it has not been well defined.

Propranolol prevents the enhanced spontaneous diastolic depolarization in Purkinje fibers caused by catecholamines [129]. This drug will therefore slow the rate of spontaneous impulse initiation or abolish it in cells under the influence of catecholamines. This effect is probably one of the most important antiarrhythmic actions of beta receptor blockade. In clinical setting propranolol has not evidenced significant effects on conduction and refractoriness in the intraventricular conduction system. In man, the therapeutic doses of propranolol do not alter the HV interval in the His bundle electrocardiogram and do not affect the relative and effective refractory period of the HPS [135-137] (Figure 3).

Instead this drug slightly slows the AV node conduction [135-137]. Other beta receptor blocking agents, like Pindolol, Tolamolol, Practolol, Metaprolol, Oxprenolol, Tenormine present electrophysiological effects in man which are very similar to those of propranolol [136, 138-143].

GROUP III

This group includes drugs like Amiodarone and Bretylium, whose main elec-

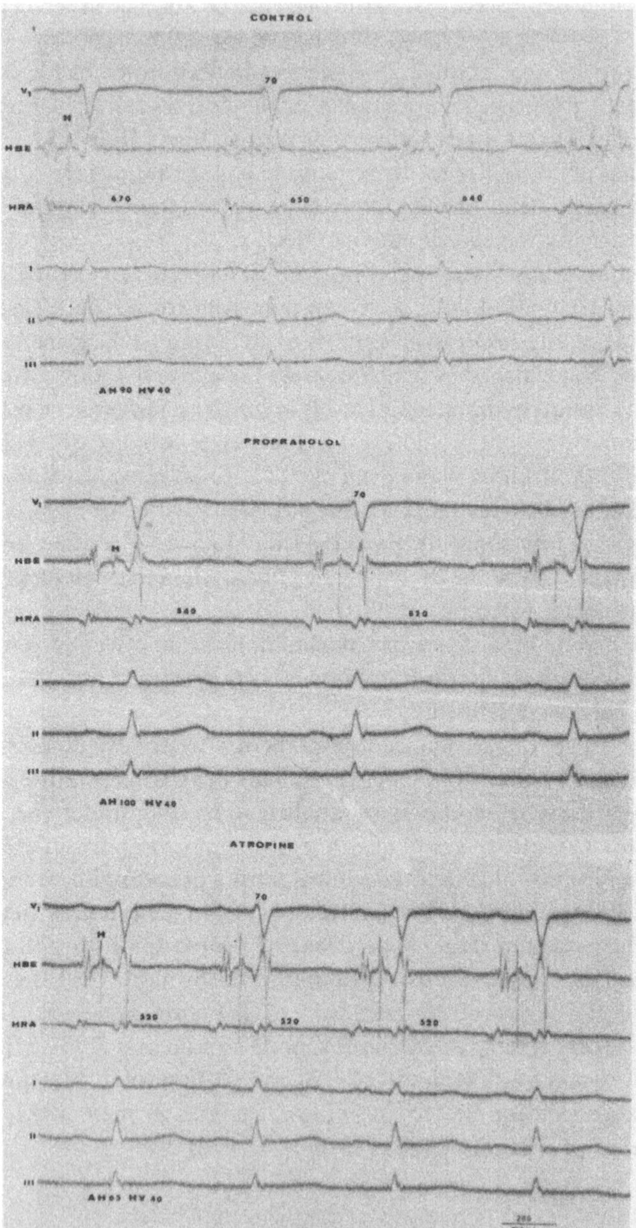

Figure 3. Propranolol (0.2 mg/kg i.v.) and atropine (0.04/mg/kg i.v.) do not change either HV or QRS duration

trophysiological effect is the prolongation of the refractory periods of the cardiac conduction system.

Amiodarone

Amiodarone, a benzofuran derivative, is a new antagonist of adrenergic excitation which does not produce competitive blockade of adrenoreceptors [144]. This drug is remarkably effective in the treatment of a wide variety of atrial and ventricular arrhythmias [145-147].

Amiodarone can be administered orally or intravenously. When administered by mouth it is reported to be absorbed slowly and fairly well, though somewhat variably (about 50%) [148]. The half-life has not been determined, though it has been estimated that the body concentration is diminished by only 16% to 34%, 30 days after administration of the drug has been stopped [148]. Such body stores may explain the persistance of amiodarone antiarrhythmic effect for as long as 30 to 45 days after drug administration has been discontinued [147].

An in vitro study by Singh et al. [149] showed that amiodarone prolongs the action potential duration of ventricular muscle and Purkinje fibers without altering resting membrane potential or automaticity.

Prolongation of ventricular refractory periods has also been demonstrated by Cabasson et al. [150] in dog, and by Ollson et [151] in man by registering monophasic action potentials with suction electrodes.

Rosenbaum et al. [147] have also observed a decrease in the maximal rate of rise of the action potential, a depression of membrane responsiveness and a slowing of conduction in the ventricular and Purkinje fibers after amiodarone administration. These authors have thus demonstrated that this drug shows electrophysiological properties similar to those of Group IA drugs.

Electrophysiological studies in man evidenced that amiodarone does not have an effect on the HPS conduction (Figure 4), or rather it induces only in a few cases a slight prolongation of HV interval, whereas it constantly prolongs the refractory periods of the HPS.

The drug constantly slows the AV nodal conduction [152-156]. So far, however, there are no data on the electrophysiological effects of amiodarone after protracted chronic therapy.

Bretylium

Bretylium tosylate was originally introduced as an antihypertensive agent until irregular absorption and side effects resulted in its withdrawal.

The demonstration that it increased the fibrillation threshold of the ventricular myocardium in dog [157] and protected against experimental digitalis-induced arrhythmias, has led to further evaluation. Clinical studies have demonstrated its usefulness in the treatment of ventricular arrhythmias [158-160].

The in vitro electrophysiological effects of bretylium have been investigated by With et al. [161] and by Bigger et al. [162]. Both groups showed that bretylium did not depress conduction and automaticity in Purkinje fibers, the only significant effect being the very striking prolongation that it produced in the repolarization phase of the action potential. The prolongation of the action potential duration with the associated increase in the effective refractory period in all probability

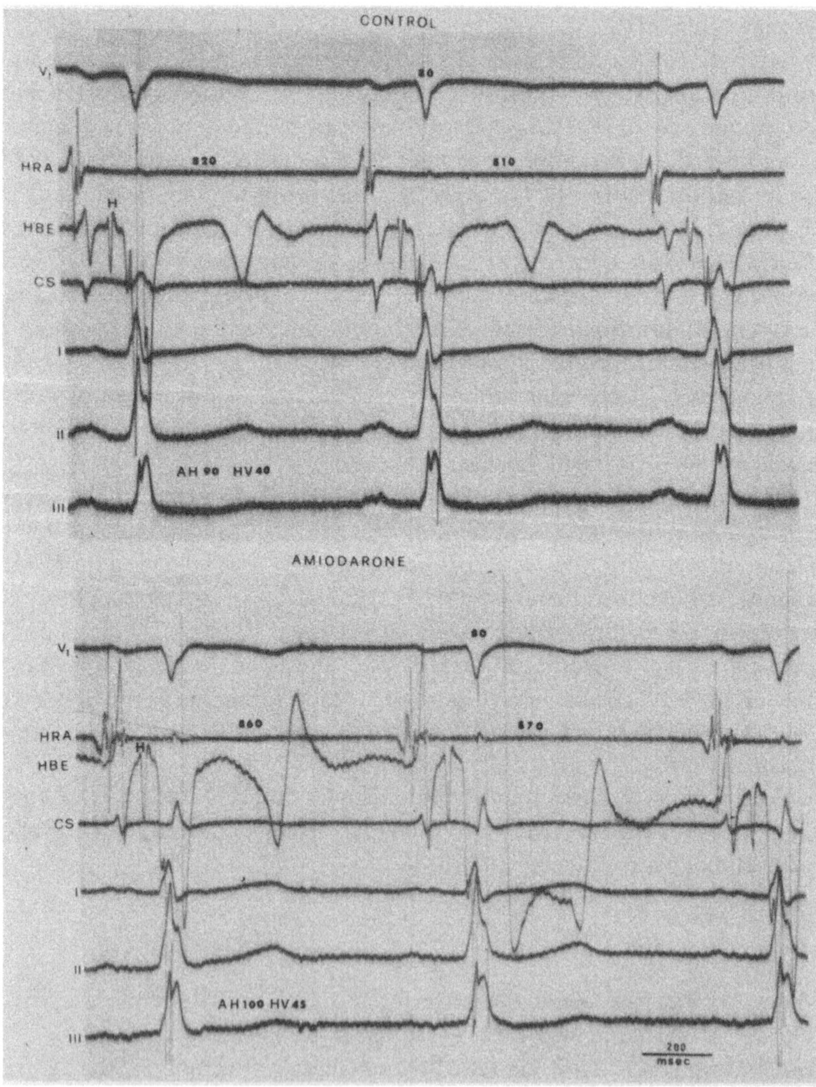

Figure 4. Amiodarone administration (200 mg i.v.) induces slight prolongation of HV interval (40 msec vs 45 msec) without any variation of QRS duration

constitutes, at least in part, the mechanism of the drug's antiarrhythmic action. Insufficient data do not permit an evaluation of electrophysiological effects of bretylium on intraventricular conduction system in man.

GROUP IV

Included in this group are the drugs which block the transmembrane influx of calcium, i.e. the slow channel, without affecting to any significant degree the transmembrane influx of sodium through the fast channel. At present verapamil is the sole example of an agent with class IV type actions which has reached clinical practice.

Verapamil

Verapamil, a papaverine derivative, was introduced as a coronary vasodilator in 1962 by Haas et al. [163].

Subsequently, intravenous administered verapamil has been repeatedly shown to be extremely effective in terminating episodes of supraventricular tachycardia in patients with and without Wolff-Parkinson-White syndrome [164-166]. The effectiveness of orally administered verapamil in treating arrhythmias has been less well documented than the efficacy of the drug given intravenously.

Little has been reported concerning the clinical pharmacology of verapamil. Following oral administration, the drug is 80% absorbed within 3 hours [167] and maximal plasma levels are attained in 2 hours. On intravenous administration. distribution to the various body compartment is rapid, only 1% of the dose being detectable in plasma 15 minutes following injection [167].

Metabolism of verapamil occurs largely in the liver [168]. The metabolic products reportedly have little biologic activity. Eighty percent of a given dose is excreted as metabolites in the bile within 10 hours of drug administration; another 20% is excreted as metabolites in urine over 48 hours [167]. The observation that verapamil markedly depresses contractility of ventricular muscle fibers without altering the transmembrane action potential suggested to Fleckenstein [169] that the drug interferes with Ca^{++} mobilization or utilization. Subsequent investigators have attempted to localize and further define the actions of verapamil. In voltage clamp experiments on cat ventricular trabeculae, verapamil caused a disappearance of the late slow inward current which may be carried by Ca^{++}, with only suppression of the initial rapid inward Na^{+} current which is responsible for the fast upstroke of the cardiac action potential [170].

The depressant effect of verapamil on the slow inward current in these voltage clamp experiments was overcome by increasing the Ca^{++} concentration gradient across the cell membrane. It was therefore concluded that one of the major actions of verapamil is to block the slow inward Ca^{++} current in cardiac fibers [170]. Subsequently, investigations have suggested that although verapamil does block the inward current carried by Ca^{++}, it also inhibits a slow current carried by Na^{+}. Hence, its primary action may be on the slow channel itself and not specifically on calcium [171].

In isolated Purkinje fibers at low to moderate concentrations, verapamil exerts little or no effect on action potential amplitude or maximal rate of rise of phase 0; moreover, the drug does not change significantly the effective refractory period of normal Purkinje fibers [172-174]. On the other hand, it does depress diastolic spontaneous depolarization which originates at normal levels of membrane potential in canine Purkinje fibers [172]. The mechanism of this inhibitory effect on normal spontaneous diastolic depolarization has not been identified.

The electrophysiological properties of verapamil on diseased Purkinje fibers appear to be more complex. Recently El-Sherif et al. [175] demonstrated that the drug improved conduction enhancing electrophysiological properties of depressed Purkinje fibers. Such improved conduction, according to these authors, is due to a direct electrophysiologic action on altered membrane response.

Verapamil would therefore have the opposite effects to those of the class IA drugs and of lidocaine on ischemic Purkinje fibers, on which such drugs impair conduction. Both mechanisms, further depression and block or improvement of conduction may induce an antiarrhythmic effect [175, 176]. According to other authors [177], however, the improvement of conduction in depressed Purkinje fibers is not necessarily related to a direct action on membrane response, but a reduction in the contractile performance or metabolic requirement, or both. The experimental models which have been used do not permit a distinction between the relative contributions of each of these factors.

In man, verapamil administered intravenously does not affect intraventricular conduction (HV and QRS intervals do not change), whereas it constantly prolongs conduction time through AV node [165, 178, 179] (Figure 5).

CARDIOACTIVE DRUGS WITH POSSIBLE ANTIARRHYTHMIC USE

Included in this group are drugs with a possible but not exclusive antiarrhythmic use like digitalis, atropine, and beta-adrenergic agents.

Digitalis

Despite the extensive investigation of the actions of digitalis there are still many questions concerning the electrophysiological mechanisms underlying therapeutic and toxic effects of digitalis. Its antiarrhythmic effect has been attributed to both a direct effect on membrane action potential and to cholinergic action mediated by

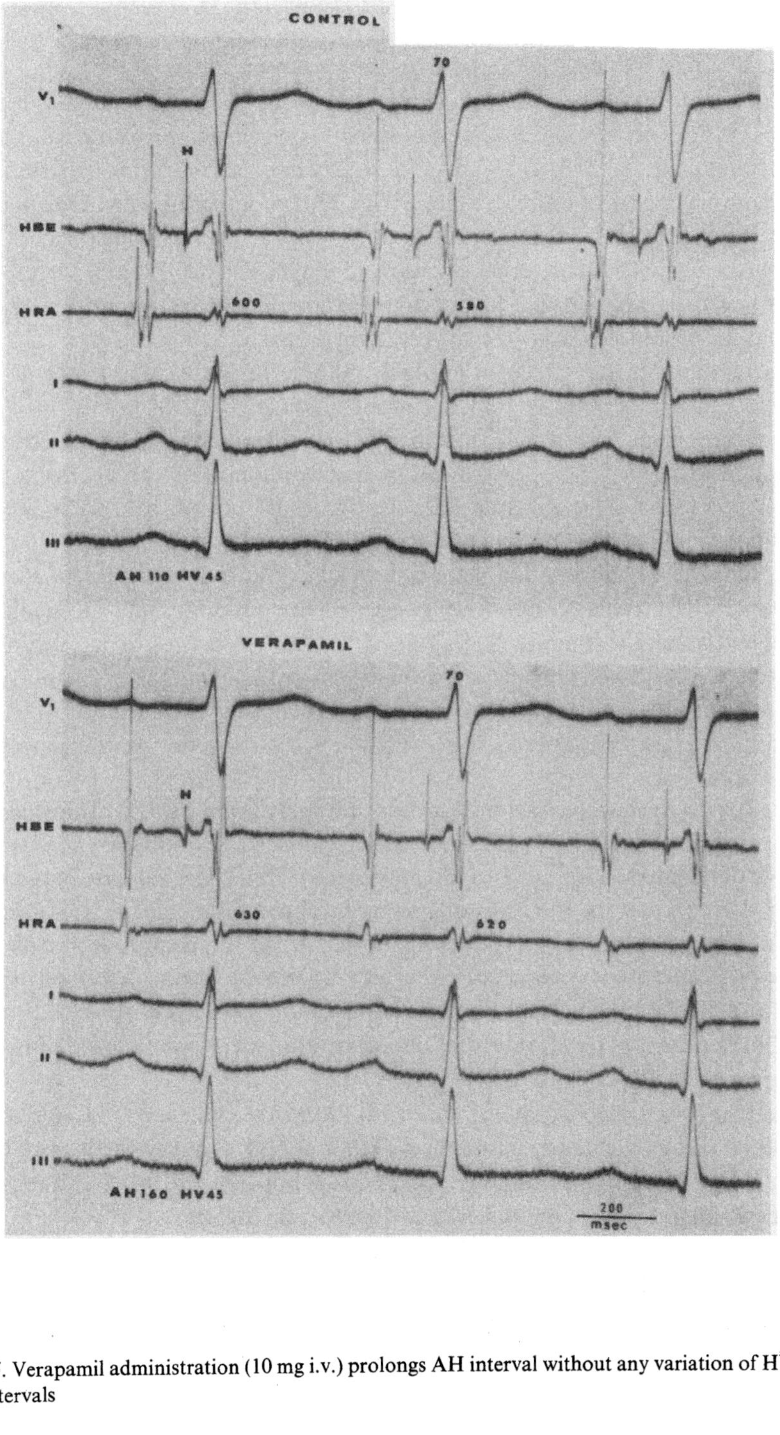

Figure 5. Verapamil administration (10 mg i.v.) prolongs AH interval without any variation of HV and QRS intervals

the vagus nerve [180]. Most of the antiarrhythmic effects of digitalis are the result of its action on sinus node and AV node.

The changes induced by digitalis on the action potential of Purkinje fibers are diverse according to various concentrations of the drug. At therapeutic concentrations it does not change conduction velocity on cells of intraventricular conduction system but induces a small, and somewhat variable, prolongation of the voltage-time course of repolarization [181]. This prolongation has been attributed to an increase in membrane resistance to potassium ion flux which occurs following perfusion with a low concentration of digitalis [180, 181]. With more prolonged perfusion periods (or higher digitalis concentrations) membrane resistance decreases and repolarization is accelerated [181].

The cholinomimetic effects of digitalis on the ventricle have not been defined so far, but it does not seem to play an important role.

With very high doses (or with prolonged perfusion periods) the toxic manifestations of digitalis appear, evidenced by marked alterations of the Purkinje fiber action potentials. They include decrease in resting membrane potential, action potential amplitude and Vmax of phase 0 [180].

Although these alterations were initially attributed to changes in membrane resistance [181], other studies have suggested that an additional mechanism may be involved; i.e. the binding of digitalis with ($Na^+ + K^+$)-ATPase and resultant interferences with active transport [180]. Such binding has the effect of depleting intracellular potassium concentration and/or increasing intracellular sodium concentration. These alterations are responsible for a reduction in the resting membrane potential.

Digitalis administered at high doses not only modifies the transmembrane action potential, but also induces alterations in the slope of phase 4 depolarization of cells of the intraventricular conduction system [180]. The increase in the slope of phase 4 may result in the attainment of threshold potential and a spontaneous rhythm, or in a transient sequence of oscillations of membrane potential and subsequent electrical quiescence. The latter event has been described for atrial [182] and ventricular specialized conduction cells [183-186] and referred to as a low amplitude potential [186], transient depolarization [184] or enhanced diastolic depolarization [183].

Electrophysiological studies in man [187-190] have evidenced that digitalis does not alter intraventricular conduction (HV and QRS intervals do not change) whereas it constantly slows AV node conduction (Figure 6). In these studies, however, digitalis was administered at therapeutic dosages.

Information concerning the effects of digitalis on the HPS refractory periods in man is limited. In a study by Przybyla et al. [189], in two patients in whom an evaluation was possible, digitalis did not change significantly the effective refractory period of the HPS. Gomes et al. [190], using the ventricular extrastimulus technique, evaluated the effects of digitalis on retrograde conduction and refractoriness of the HPS and ventricular myocardium in 17 patients. After treatment with ouabain, there was a significant decrease in the refractory periods of the ventricular muscle; in contrast, there was no significant change in retrograde His-Purkinje conduction and refractoriness. The same authors [191], in a study on the canine heart, observed that therapeutic doses of ouabain had no effect on anterograde conduction velocity within the HPS but did increase anterograde His-Purkinje refractoriness in seven out of 12 dogs. The apparent differences in the latter anterograde study in dog and the retrograde study in man may be related to 1) the use of different experimental models, because anterograde refractoriness may not

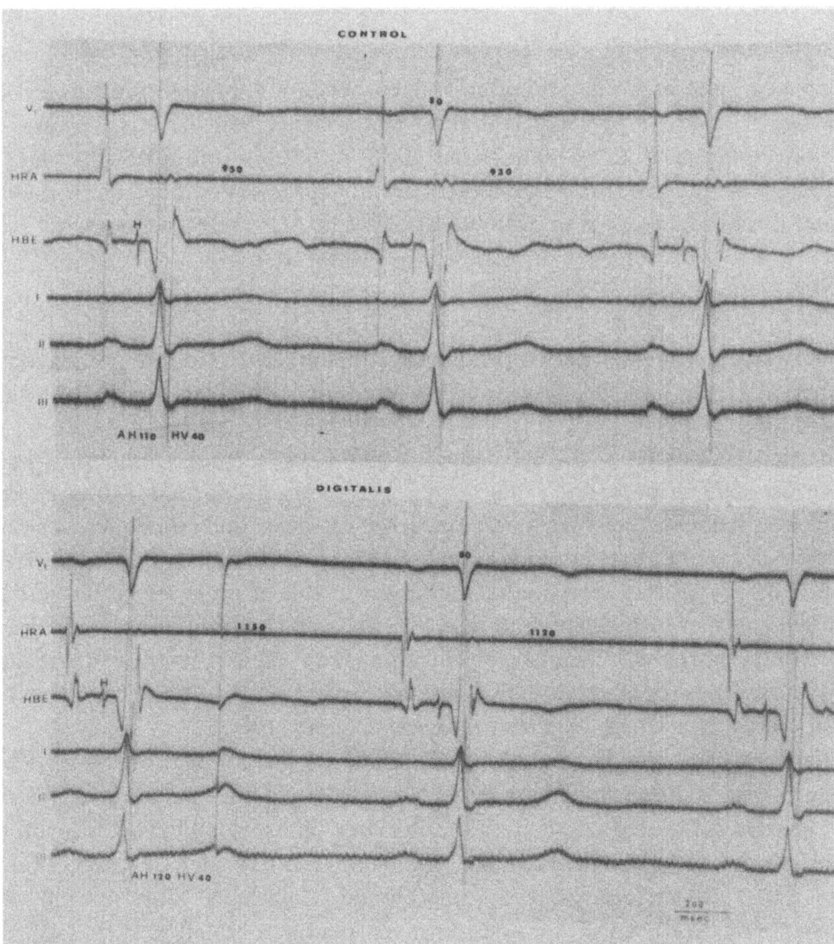

Figure 6. Digitalis administration (digitoxin, 1 mg i.v.) does not show any effect on HV and QRS intervals

correlate with retrograde HPS refractoriness; 2) to the use of different cycle lengths and 3) to species differences [190].

The few electrophysiological data available in the literature suggest that, in spite of a few discrepancies on the effect of digitalis on the HPS refractory periods, the drug does not significantly alter the intraventricular conduction in man.

There are not sufficient data available on the electrophysiological effects of the drug in patients with bundle branch block to draw definite conclusions, but some clinical studies of patients with electrocardiographic signs of digitalis toxicity have not evidenced intraventricular conduction impairment related to the drug's effect [192, 193].

Atropine

Atropine is used as an antiarrhythmic agent when a depressed function of sinus node or AV node is present. This drug has no effect on the His-Purkinje conduction; in fact, it does not induce variations in the HV and QRS intervals [194] (Figure 3). At present, once again, there are not sufficient data available on either animal or man to be able to evaluate its effect on HPS refractoriness.

Beta-adrenergic agents

Beta-adrenergic agents, i.e. isoproterenol, dopamine and dobutamine, may be used as antiarrhythmic drugs when a depressed function of sinus node or AV node is present.

In vitro studies [195-197] have shown that beta-receptor stimulation has no effect on resting potential, Vmax and overshoot of normal Purkinje fibers. Moreover, it does not change membrane responsiveness and consequently conduction velocity is not affected. Beta-adrenergic stimulation accelerates repolarization of the Purkinje fiber action potentials; however, this effect is seen after perfusion with isoproterenol which stimulates only beta-receptors [196]. In fact norepinephrine, which probably stimulates both alpha and beta receptors in the heart, slightly prolongs repolarization but this effect may be due to alpha receptor stimulation which overwhelms the beta adrenergic effect [196].

The electrophysiological effects of beta-adrenergic stimulation by catecholamines on diseased Purkinje fibers are different from the effects on normal fibers. In vitro studies of isolated ventricular and Purkinje fibers which have low membrane potentials due to mechanical trauma, anoxia or cold have demonstrated that catecholamines can restore the resting membrane potential to more normal values (hyperpolarization), thus improving intraventricular conduction [195, 198].

Electrophysiological studies in man [199-201] evidenced that beta-adrenergic agents usually have no effect on conduction in the specialized conduction system. Administration of isopreterenol [199, 200] and dobutamine [201] did not change

HV and QRS intervals (Figures 7 and 8). Only Dhingra et al. [202] and Masini et al. [203] observed in some cases a shortening of HV interval after isoproterenol and dopamine administration. In several studies it emerged that the beta-adrenergic agents shorten the relative refractory period of HPS [200-202]. In none of the

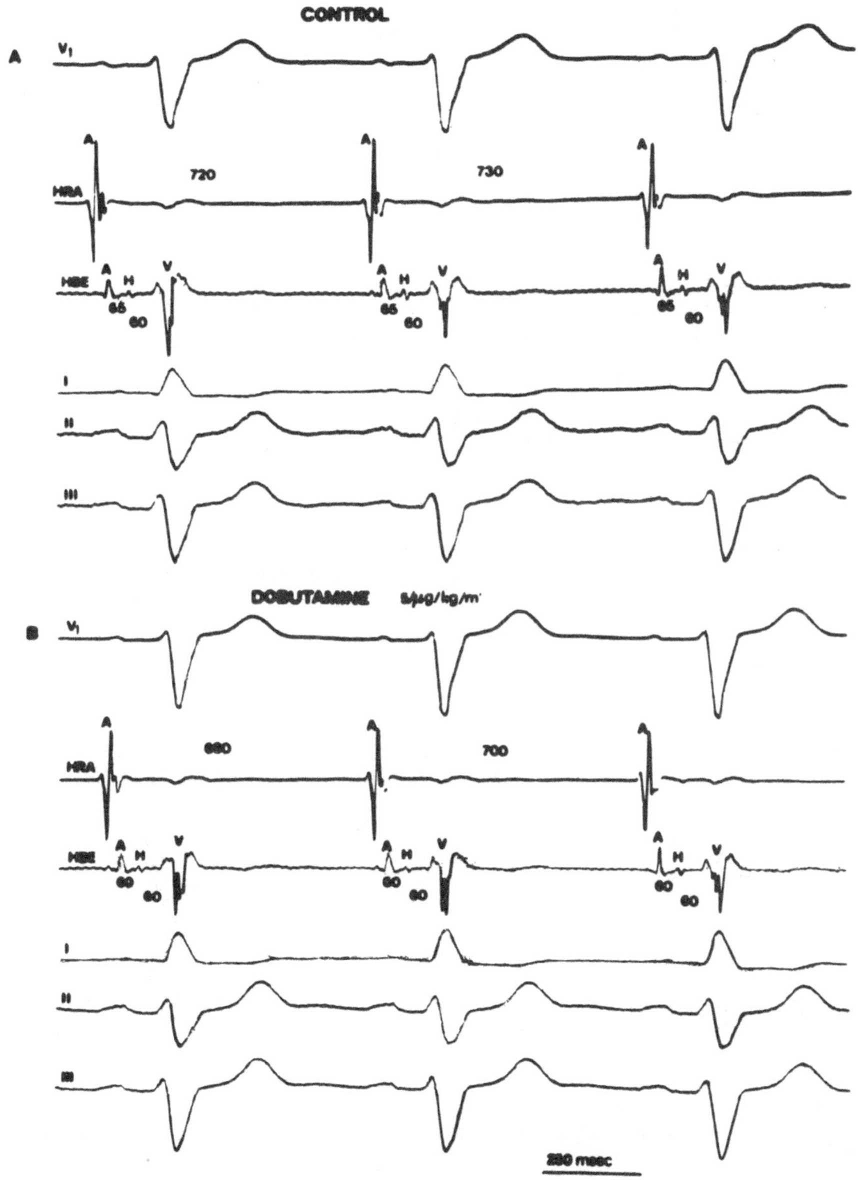

Figure 7. During infusion of 5 μg/kg/min dobutamine, HV and QRS intervals do not change

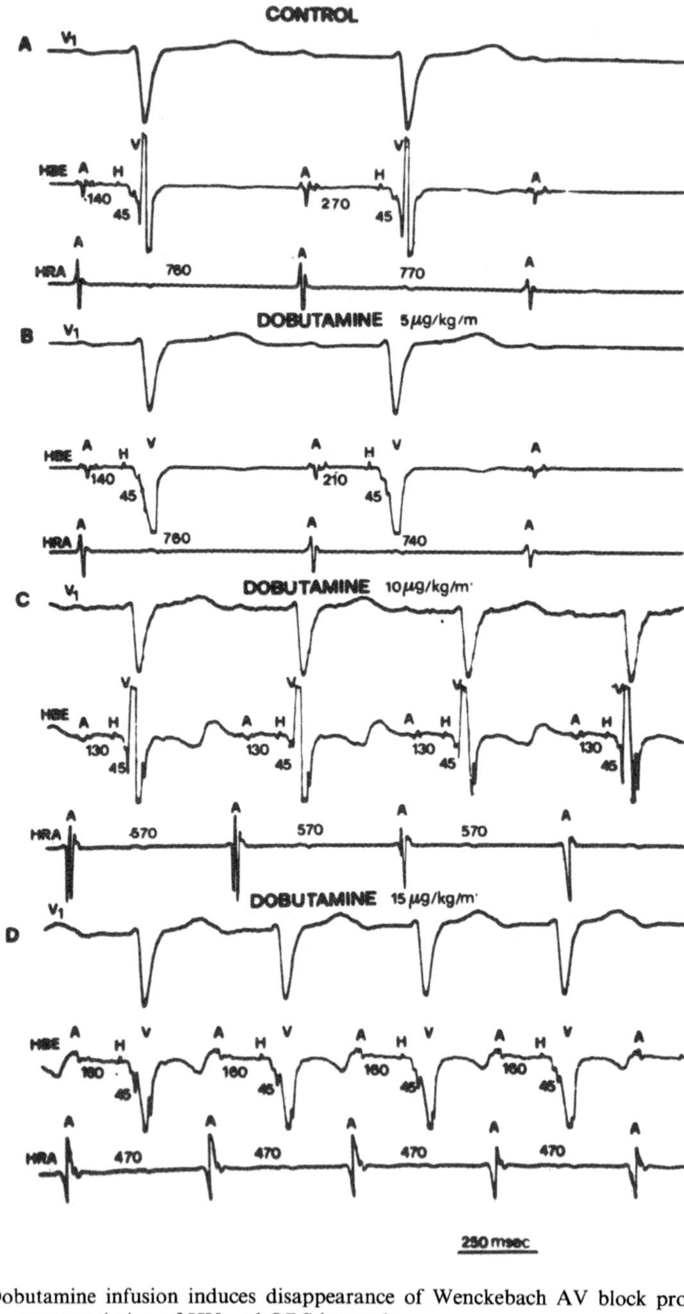

Figure 8. Dobutamine infusion induces disappearance of Wenckebach AV block proximal to His bundle without any variation of HV and QRS intervals

reported cases, however, has it been possible to assess the effect of these drugs in HPS effective refractory period.

NEW ANTIARRHYTHMIC AGENTS

Recently introduced into the clinical setting are several antiarrhythmic agents like aprindine, bunaphtine, encainide, ethmozim, mexiletine, propraphenone. and tocainide, which represent promising advances for the therapy of cardiac arrhythmias.

Aprindine

Aprindine was developed and used initially in Belgium. This drug possesses some structural similarities to procainamide, lidocaine, and propranolol in that all four agents consist of an aromatic residue, an intermediate chain, and an amino group with two ethyl groups attached [204].

Several studies established aprindine as an effective antiarrhythmic agent against a variety of supraventricular and ventricular arrhythmias occurring in patients with different types of heart disease [204-207].

Aprindine is effective when administered orally or intravenously. It is metabolized in the liver [205]; approximately 40% to 85% of a given dose is eliminated in the urine, and as much as 35% is eliminated in the feces [205, 208]. Elimination of aprindine has been explained using a two compartment model [209]. The early, rapid phase has a $t_{\frac{1}{2}}$ of 0.5 to 2.7 hours and the later, slower phase has a $t_{\frac{1}{2}}$ of 12.5 to 66 hours. Effective plasma levels of aprindine have been reported to range between 0.32 and 6.6 μg/ml [205].

Microelectrode studies of isolated cardiac preparations indicate that aprindine slows intraventricular conduction. In fact the drug decreases action potential amplitude and Vmax of phase 0 of Purkinje fibers [210, 211]. It appears to shorten action potential duration and effective refractory period of bovine and canine Purkinje fibers [210, 211]. Aprindine has been reported to decrease Purkinje fibers automaticity [210, 211].

Electrophysiological studies in man evidenced that aprindine constantly increased HV and QRS intervals [138, 212-214] (Figure 9). AV nodal conduction is also constantly slowed. At present there are no data on the electrophysiological effects of the drug on HPS refractoriness in man.

On the basis of the above-mentioned data, aprindine appears to induce electrophysiological effects which are very similar to those of group IA drugs.

Very recently, *moxaprindine*, a derivative of aprindine which possesses antiarrhythmic properties in the dog, was submitted for clinical experimentation. The first results are promising [215]. This drug induces in man the same electrophysiological effects as aprindine [216].

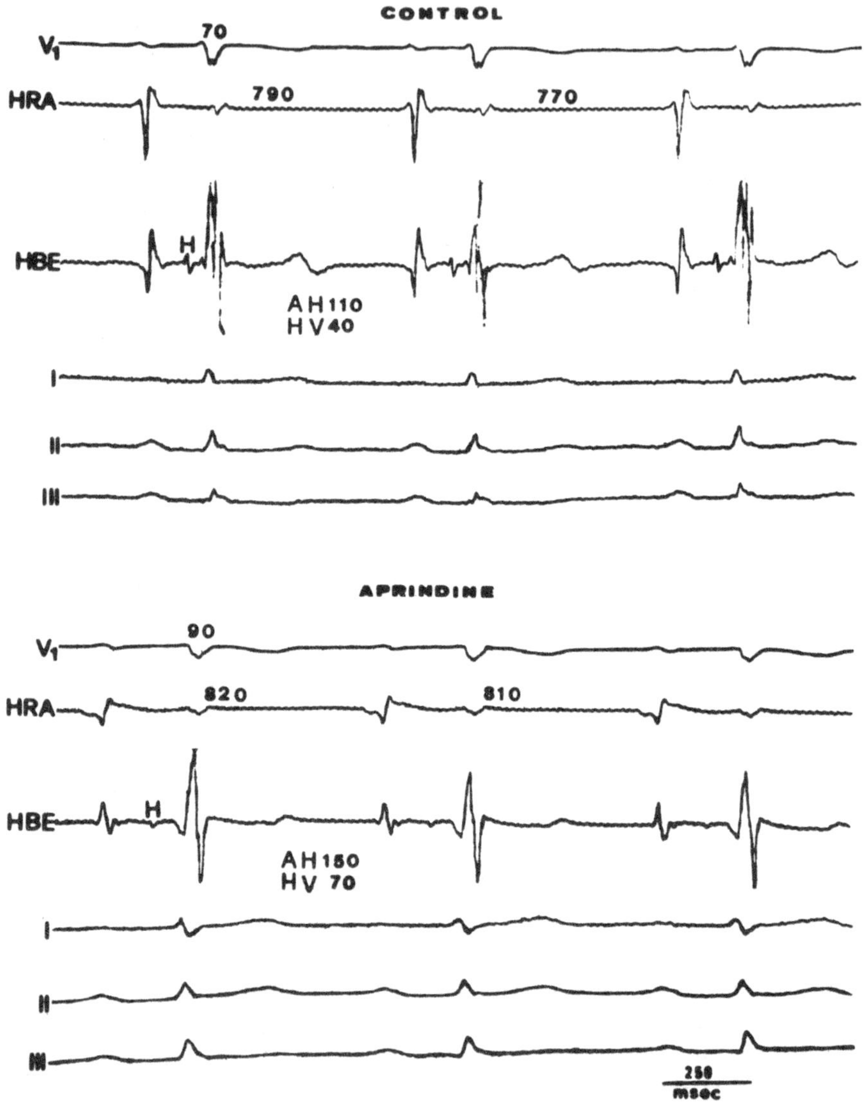

Figure 9. Aprindine administration (2 mg/kg i.v.) prolongs both HV and QRS intervals

Bunaphtine

Bunaphtine, a synthetic compound with antiarrhythmic properties, was first used in Italy. Several studies [217-220] have established bunaphthine as an effective antiarrhythmic agent especially in ventricular arrythmias.

The drug is effective when administered orally, intramuscularly or intravenously. It is metabolized in the liver and eliminated mainly in the urine [220]. Plasma concentration levels showed that bunaphtine is cleared from the blood in two different stages: $t_{\frac{1}{2}}\alpha = 9.5$ min and $t_{\frac{1}{2}}\,\beta = 84.7$ min [220]. Antiarrhythmic effect was observed in connection with the first distribution phase and it was even more evident when plasma concentrations varied between 3 and 4 μg/ml.

Microelectrode study [221] of isolated cardiac preparations showed that the drug slightly decreases action potential amplitude and Vmax of phase 0; furthermore it prolongs action potential duration and effective refractory period.

Effects of bunaphtine on right ventricular monophasic action potentials were investigated in man by Bonatti et al. [222, 223], who found that the drug, administered intravenously, increases the action potential duration, together with an effective refractory period prolongation. The decrease in action potential amplitude and Vmax were either minimal or absent.

Electrophysiological investigations in man [224, 225] showed an inconstant prolongation of HV and QRS intervals (Figure 10); the effect on AV node conduction is variable and not significant. Bunaphtine thus induces electrophysiological effects which are very similar to those of amiodarone.

Encainide

Encainide is a newly developed benzanilide derivative that has shown promising antiarrhythmic properties in various short-term animal models [226, 227]. Its chemical structure does not resemble that of any of the known antiarrhythmic drugs.

In isolated cardiac Purkinje fibers, encainide has a direct membrane depressant action, reducing action potential amplitude and Vmax of phase 0. It decreases action potential duration without significantly affecting refractoriness and also decreases automaticity [228].

Sami et al. studied its electrophysiological effects in the dog [229] and in man [230]. Encainide prolonged HV and QRS intervals, but no significant changes were noted in AV nodal conduction. In no case was it possible to evaluate relative or effective refractory periods of HPS. The results of these studies suggest that encainide resembles class IA antiarrhythmic agents.

Ethmozim

Ethmozim, a phenothiazine derivative, was developed and used initially in the USSR [231]. Early reports in this country have shown that ethmozim effectively controls ventricular arrhythmias in experimental animals and in man [231-233]; such results have been confirmed in subsequent studies carried out in the USA [234] and in the USSR [235].

Ethmozim is administered orally. Its pharmacokinetics in man have not been fully defined. The drug is well absorbed and appears not to be excreted in its native

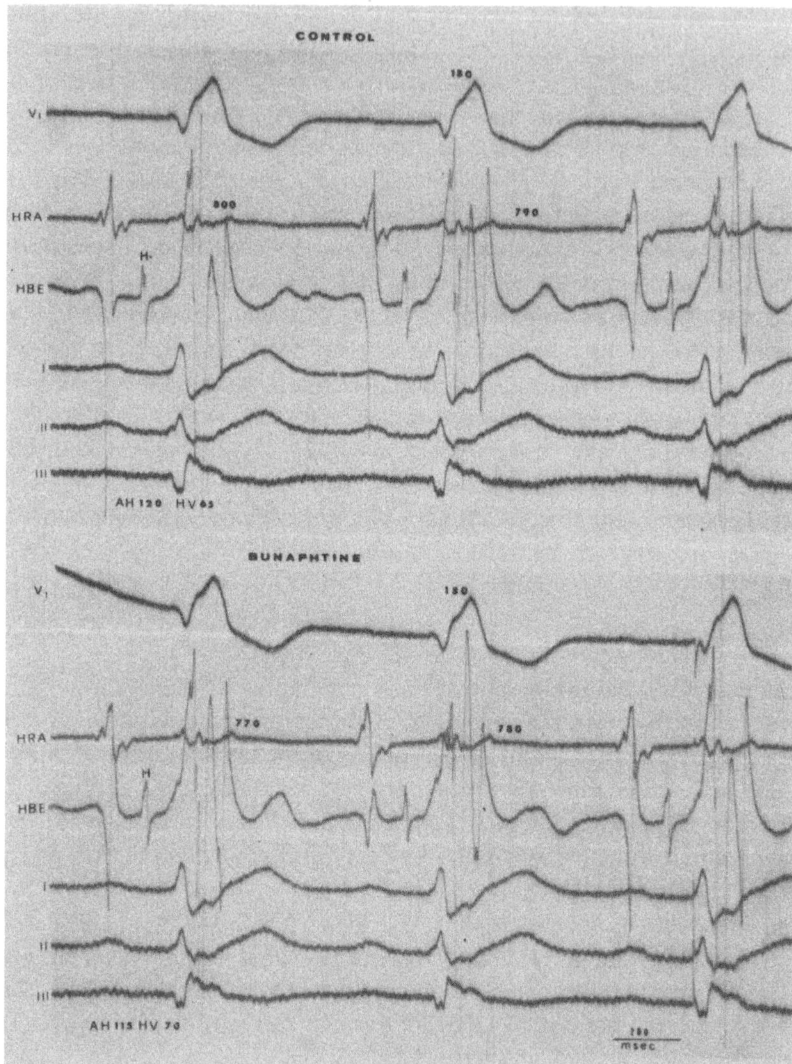

Figure 10. Bunaphtine administration (2 mg/kg i.v.) slightly prolongs HV interval, whereas QRS duration does not change

form in either feces or urine. The exact nature of its metabolites is not known and it is not clear whether they possess antiarrhythmic property themselves.

In isolated non-ischemic canine Purkinje fibers, ethmozim demonstrated electrophysiologic characteristics similar to lidocaine [236, 237]. The drug produced a dose-dependent decrease of maximum upstroke velocity of phase 0 depolarization. The action potential duration and effective refractory periods were markedly shortened. Unlike lidocaine, ethmozim did not affect the slope of phase 4 depolarization of spontaneous automatic Purkinje fibers. However, in ischemic Purkinje fibers, ethmozim did decrease the slope of phase 4 depolarization [234]. Electrophysiological studies have not yet been performed in man.

Mexiletine

Mexiletine is a new antiarrhythmic drug chemically similar to lidocaine, effective also when administered orally. It has been found to be effective in the treatment of acute and chronic ventricular arrhythmias associated with diverse cardiac disease [238-240]. Mexiletine is almost completely absorbed followed oral administration. Prescott et al. [24] found that in healthy individuals peak plasma levels are reached 2 to 4 hours after mexiletine, 3 mg/kg. However, in patients with myocardial infarction, peak plasma levels were not reached for 4 to 6 hours. Therapeutic plasma levels have been reported to range between 0.5 and 2 μg/ml [239]. The average half-life of elimination ($t_{\frac{1}{2}}$) in healthy individuals is approximately 10 hours after an oral dose, whereas in patients with myocardial infarction, $t_{\frac{1}{2}}$ ranged from 7.8 to 25.3 and from 6.7 to 18.5 hours for intravenous and oral administration, respectively [241]. Following intravenous injection, plasma mexiletine concentration decreases very rapidly. Normally, mexiletine is eliminated metabolically by the liver, with less than 10% excreted unchanged in the urine. Studies using microelectrode techniques have shown that mexiletine decreases the Vmax of phase 0 depolarization in ventricular and Purkinje fibers; moreover, it shortens action potential duration and effective refractory period [242]. Phase 4 depolarization was not significantly altered by mexiletine at concentrations which suppressed the rate of spontaneous action potential [242].

In an electrophysiological study in man [243], mexiletine (200 to 250 mg i.v.) increased slightly, but not significantly, the HV interval. The effective refractory period of HPS, determined in five patients, increased constantly. In four of these five patients, however, intraventricular conduction disturbances were known to exist prior to administration of mexiletine. In another study [244], 20 patients having coronary heart disease received mexiletine 3 mg/kg i.v. The drug had no effect on HV intervals and the relative refractory period of the HPS was significantly decreased. QRS interval was prolonged in eight out of nine patients. The electrophysiological effects of mexiletine on HPS in man thus appear different in these two studies. Further investigations are still required. The drug does not have any significant effects on the AV node conduction [243, 244].

Propaphenone

Propaphenone (2-2-(hydroxy)-3-(propylamino)-propoxy-3-phenyl propiophenonehydrochloride) has recently been introduced in the clinical setting as an antiarrhythmic agent. It appears to be effective in suppressing chronic recurrent supraventricular and ventricular tachycardias, tachyarrhythmias and ectopic beats [245-248].

Propaphenone can be administered orally or intravenously. It appears effective at plasma levels of about 1.3 μg/ml [249]. The clinical pharmacology of this drug has still not been sufficiently investigated.

Bergamann et al. [250] studied the in vitro effects of propaphenone in ventricular and Purkinje fibers of the rabbit. The drug induced a marked reduction in the maximal rate of rise of phase 0 whereas the resting membrane potential was not significantly affected. The effective refractory time was increased by a variable amount of propaphenone, the maximum increase being 10%. While the qualitative effects were similar, there were quantitative differences between the effects produced by propaphenone on the action potentials of the Purkinje and myocardial fibers. Reduction in the amplitude of the action potential for the Purkinje fibers was much more marked than for myocardial fibers. The response of Purkinje fibers regarding the maximum rate of rise in the action potential in response to propaphenone was 50% greater than that for the fibers of the working myocardium.

An electrophysiological study in man [251] evidenced that propaphenone constantly prolongs HV and QRS intervals. In no case have the HPS refractory periods been assessed. Propaphenone thus presents electrophysiological effects which are very similar to those of group IA drugs but in contrast to these it also induces a marked depression of the AV node conduction.

Tocainide

Tocainide is a new antiarrhythmic drug, chemically similar to lidocaine. Unlike lidocaine, however, tocainide is also effective when administered orally. It has been found to be effective against chronic ventricular arrhythmias associated with a variety of cardiac diseases [213, 252, 253]. Tocainide appears to be rapidly and well absorbed with peak serum levels occurring 60 to 90 minutes after drug administration.

Therapeutic plasma concentration levels range between 6 and 12 μg/ml [213]. Renal excretion of unchanged drug average 40%; 60% of the drug presumably undergoes hepatic degradation [254].

In one in vitro study by Gerstenblith et al. [255], it was reported that tocainide decreases maximal rate of rise of phase 0 and action potential duration of isolated Purkinje fibers. The effective refractory period tends to decrease. In addition, ouabain-induced automaticity of Purkinje fibers was abolished by tocainide.

Andersen et al. [250] performed an electrophysiological study in 12 patients, some of whom had intraventricular conduction disturbances; they did not observe variations in HV and QRS intervals after drug administration. In no case was it possible to assess the HPS refractoriness. The AH interval increased slightly.

Table 1 reports the effects of antiarrhythmic drug on HV and QRS intervals and HPS refractoriness.

Table 1. Effect of antiarrhythmic drugs on HV and QRS intervals and HPS refractoriness

Antiarrhythmic drugs	HV interval	QRS interval	Relative and effective refractory periods of HPS
Quinidine	↑	↑	↑
Procainamide	↑	↑	↑
Ajmaline	↑	↑	*
Disopyramide	↑	↑	↑
Lidocaine	↑ ↔	↔	↔ ↓
Diphenylhydantoin	↔	↔	↓
Propranolol	↔	↔	*
Amiodarone	↑ ↔	↑ ↔	↑
Verapamil	↔	↔	*
Digitalis	↔	↔	*
Atropine	↔	↔	*
Beta-adrenergic agents	↔	↔	↓
Aprindine	↑	↑	*
Bunaphtine	↑ ↔	↑ ↔	↑
Encainide	↑	↑	*
Mexiletine	↑ ↔	↑ ↔	↑ ↔ ↓
Propaphenone	↑	↑	*
Tocainide	↔	↔	*

↑ increase
↓ decrease
↔ unchanged
* insufficient data available

COMMENT

The antiarrhythmic agents which greatly depress intraventricular conduction are the class IA drugs: quinidine, procainamide, ajmaline, disopyramide, as well as aprindine, encainide and propaphenone. In the presence of bundle branch block, lidocaine may also impair intraventricular conduction.

It may be speculated that the slowing of conduction is one mechanism by which these drugs prevent or abolish reentrant ventricular arrhythmias, but at the same time this mechanism may be dangerous as it can induce a complete AV block distal to His bundle in patients with bundle branch or bifascicular block. Complete AV block in patients treated with these antiarrhythmic agents is particularly dangerous since such drugs decrease the slope of phase 4 depolarization and the rate of the ventricular rhythm will be very slow.

If the use of these drugs is necessary in patients with bundle branch block, a close, careful follow-up of the patients is recommended.

On the other hand it is always inadvisable to administer these drugs in conjunction in patients with bundle branch block, not only because the interaction of various antiarrhythmic agents still remains unclear, but mainly because there is more likely to be, at least in theory, a progression to complete AV block distal to His bundle due to a summation effect on intraventricular conduction.

However, for a better evaluation of the indications and contraindications of these drugs in patients with intraventricular conduction disturbances, a repetition of the electrophysiological investigations would be required after long periods of chronic oral therapy. Such studies have not yet been performed.

These antiarrhythmic agents should be used in low dosages in the presence of hepatic failure as they are all, more or less, metabolized in the liver.

The same is valid in the presence of renal failure as these drugs are eliminated mainly in the urine, with the exception of verapamil, which is mainly excreted as metabolites in the bile.

Finally it should be emphasized that hypopotassemia may completely nullify the depressive or antiarrhythmic effects of these drugs, while hyperpotassemia or concomitant administration of potassium salts may enhance the depressant effect on intraventricular conduction [257, 258].

At present, however, there are no available electrophysiological data regarding safety of antiarrhythmic agents in patients with marked electrolyte abnormalities.

REFERENCES

1. Vaughan Williams EM: The classification of antiarrhythmic drugs. In: Symposium on cardiac arrhythmias, Sandol E, Fleusted-Jensen E, Olesen Kh. Sodertalje, Sweden: AB Astra 1970, p 449
2. Singh BN, Hauswirth O: Comparative mechanism of action of antiarrhythmic drugs. Am Heart J 87: 367, 1974
3. Dreifus LS, Ogawa S: Quality of the ideal antiarrhythmic drug. Am J Cardiol 39: 466, 1977
4. Ferrari M, Maragno I, Melacini P: Una classificazione dei farmaci antiaritmici quale indicazione alla terapia clinica. In: Le nuove frontiere delle aritmie, Furlanello F, Disertori M. Lanzetta L. Padua: Piccin, 1977, p 185
5. Touboul P, Attalah G, Gressard A, Michelon G, Chatelain MY, Delahaye JP: Effets électrophysiologiques des agents antiarythmiques chez l'homme. Tentative de classification. Arch Mal Coeur 72: 72, 1979
6. Hoffman BF: The action of quinidine and procaine amide on single fibers of dog ventricle and specialized conduction system. Ann Bras Ciencias 29: 365, 1957
7. West TC, Amory DW: Single fiber recording of the effects of quinidine at the atrial and pacemaker sites in the isolated right atrium of the rabbit. J Pharmacol Exp Ther 130: 183, 1960
8. Gettes LS, Surawicz B, Shive JC: Effect of high K, low K on QRS duration and

ventricular action potential. Am J Physiol 203: 1135, 1962
9. Watanabe Y, Dreifus LS, Likoff WL: Electrophysiological antagonism and synergism of potassium and antiarrhythmic agents. Am J Cardiol 12: 702, 1963
10. Conn Hl Jr, Luchi RJ: Some cellular and metabolic considerations relating to the action of quinidine as a prototype antiarrhythmic agent. Am J Med 37: 685, 1964
11. Wallace AG, Cline RE, Sealy WC, Young WG, Troyer WG: Electrophysiological effects of quinidine. Circ Res 19: 960, 1966
12. Wald RB, Vaxman MB, Downar E: The effect of antiarrhythmic drugs on depressed conduction and unidirectional block in sheep Purkinje fibers. Circ Res 46: 612, 1980
13. Heissenbuttel RH, Bigger JT Jr: The effects of oral quinidine on intraventricular conduction in man: correlation of plasma quinidine with changes in QRS duration. Am Heart J 80: 453, 1970
14. Moe GK, Abildskov JA: Antiarrhythmic drugs. In: The pharmacologic basis of therapeutics, 4th edn, Goodman LS, Gilman A. New York: Macmillan, 1970, p 709
15. Damato AN, Lau SH: The clinical value of the electrogram of the conduction system. Progr Cardiovasc Dis 13: 119, 1970
16. Josephson ME, Seides SF, Batsford WP, Wisfogel GM, Akhtar M, Caracta AR, Lau SH, Damato AN: The electrophysiological effects of intramuscular quinidine on the atrioventricular conducting system in man. Am Heart J 87: 55, 1974
17. Watanabe Y, Dreifus L: Interactions of quinidine and potassium on atrioventricular transmission. Circ Res 20: 434, 1967
18. Mirro MJ, Watanabe AM, Bailey JC: Electrophysiological effects of disopyramide and quinidine on guinea pig atria and canine cardiac Purkinje fibers. Dependence on underlying cholinergic tone. Circ Res 46: 660, 1980
19. Sokolow M, Perloff DB: The clinical pharmacology and use of quinidine in heart disease. Progr Cardiovasc Dis 3: 316, 1961
20. Marriott HJL: Rational approach to quinidine therapy. Mod Concepts Cardiovasc Dis 31: 745, 1962
21. Kock-Weser J: Antiarrhythmic prophylaxis in ambulatory patients with coronary heart disease. Arch Intern Med 129: 763, 1972
22. Giardina EGV, Heissenbuttel RH, Bigger JT Jr: Intermittent intravenous procaine amide to treat ventricular arrhythmias. Ann Intern Med 78: 183, 1973
23. Woske H, Belford J, Fasier FN: The effect of procainamide on excitability, refractoriness and conduction in the mammalian heart. J Pharmacol Exp Ther 107: 134, 1953
24. Weidman S: Effects of calcium ions and local anesthetic on electrical properties of Purkinje fibers. J Physiol 129: 568, 1955
25. Hoffman BF: The possible mode of action of antiarrhythmic agents. In: The myocardial cell, Briller S, Coon H. Philadelphia: University of Pennsylvania Press, 1966, p 251
26. Helfant RH, Scherlag BJ, Damato AN: The electrophysiological properties of diphenylhydantoin sodium as compared to procainamide in the normal and digitalis intoxicated dog. Circulation 36: 108, 1867
27. Rosen KM, Lisi KR, Berkowitz WS: The effect of procaineamide on atrioventricular and intraventricular conduction in man. Circulation (Abstr) 39: Suppl III:III-173, 1969
28. Josephson ME, Caracta AR, Ricciutti MA, Lau SH, Damato AD: Electrophysiologic properties of procainamide in man. Am J Cardiol 33: 596, 1974
29. Reddy CP, Damato AN, Akatar M, Dhatt M, Gomes JAC, Calon AH: Effect of procainamide on reentry within the His-Purkinje system in man. Am J Cardiol 40: 957, 1977
30. Ogunkelv JB, Damato AN, Akatar M, Reddy CP, Carata AR, Lau SH: Electro-

physiologic effects of procainamide in subtherapeutic to therapeutic doses on human atrioventricular conduction system. Am J Cardiol 37: 724, 1976
31. Scheinman MM, Weiss AN, Shafton E, Benowitz N, Rowland M: Electrophysiologic effects of procaineamide in patients with intraventricular conduction delay. Circulation 49: 522, 1974
32. Wedd AM, Blair HA, Warner RS: The action of procaine amide on the heart. Am Heart J 42: 399, 1951
33. Siddiqui S, Siddiqui RH: The alkaloids of *Rauwolfia serpentina* Benth. Part I. J Ind Chem Soc 9: 539, 1932
34. Arora RB, Madan BR: Antiarrhythmics. VI. Ajmaline and serpentine in experimental cardiac arrhythmias. J Pharmacol Exp Ther 117: 62, 1956
35. Kleinsorge H: Klinische Untersuchungen über die Wirkungsweise des Rauwolfia-alkaloids Ajmaline bei Herzrhythmusstörungen insbesondere der Extrasistolie. Med Klin 54: 409, 1959
36. Puech P, Latour H, Hertault J, Grolleau R: L'ajmaline injectable dans les tachycardies paroxystiques et le syndrome WPW. Comparaison avec la procainamide. Arch Mal Coeur 57: 897, 1964
37. Bazika V, Lang TW, Pappelbaum S, Corday E: Ajmalin, a rauwolfia alkaloid for the treatment of digitoxis arrhythmias. Am J Cardiol 17: 227, 1966
38. Bianchi C, Beccari E: L'ajmalina nella terapia delle aritmie cardiache. Sperimentazione policentrica pianificata. Min Med 57: 1273, 1966
39. Farinelli A, Zanardi A, Degli Atti B, Longhini C, Alvisi A: Rilievi clinici sull'impiego dell'ajmalina in talune aritmie accessuali. Min Cardioangiol 16: 1047, 1968
40. Wellens HJJ, Durrer D: Effect of procaine amide, quinidine and ajmaline in the Wolff-Parkinson-White syndrome. Circulation 50: 114, 1974
41. Kleinsorge A. Gaida P: Quantities and rates of excretion of the *Rauwolfia* alkaloid ajmaline following different methods of administration. Arzneim Forsch 11: 1100, 1961
42. Kleinsorge H. Gaida P: Behaviour of the serum level after intravenous injection of ajmaline. Klin Wschr 40: 149, 1962
43. Petter A, Zipf K: Zur antifibrillaren Herzwirkung von Ajmaline, Brom-Ajmalin, Chinidin und Novocainamid. Arch Exp Pharmacol 243: 519, 1962
44. Capra C: Sull'attività antiaritmica di alcuni derivati dell'ajmalina. Il Farmaco 19: 865, 1964
45. Vorgatti E, Pascucci E, Mavulis A, Magnani B: Risultati clinici preliminari sull'attività antiaritmica di un derivato acetilato dell'ajmalina: la dicloroacetilajmalina. Boll Soc Ital Card 8: 494, 1963
46. Botti G, Visioli O, Barbaresi F, Lazzari GB: Primi risultati sperimentali sull'attività antiaritmica di un derivato acetilato dell'ajmalina: la dicloroacetilajmalina. Boll Soc It Card 11: 135, 1966
47. Cocour V, Enesco R, Sirbulesco R, Pompilian P: La di-monocloroacetilajmalina nel trattamento delle alterazioni del ritmo cardiaco. Min Med 61: 16, 1970
48. Coumel P, Bouvrain Y: Pharmacodynamics and clinical results in 95 cases. In: Concepts on the mechanisms and treatment of arrhythmias, Gensini GG. New York: Futura, 1974, p 97
49. Pretolani E: Clinical studies on the antiarrhythmic properties of MCAA. In: Concepts on the mechanisms and treatment of arrhythmias, Gensini GG. New York: Futura, 1974, p 125
50. Ross P, Messina G, Giampaolo P, Cernigliaro C: Rapporto tra concentrazione plasmatica ed effetto antiaritmico della di-monocloroacetilajmalina. G Ital Cardiol 4: 444, 1974

51. Obayashi K, Mandel WJ: Electrophysiological effects of ajmaline in isolated cardiac tissue. Cardiovasc Res 10: 20, 1976
52. De Azevedo IM, Dreifus LS, Watanabe Y: Electrophysiologic effects of new ester of ajmaline 17-monochloroacetyl ajmaline hydrochloride (MCAA). Europ J Cardiol 2: 321, 1975
53. Piwonka RW, Canniff PC, Healey JF: Electrophysiological effects of a new antiarrhythmic agent in cardiac tissue. In: Concepts on the mechanisms and treatment of arrhythmias, Genzini GG. New York: Futura, 1974, p 219
54. Knippel M, Cadel A, Mazzini C, Figini A, Rovelli F: Effetti dell'ajmaline e della dimonocloroacetilajmalina sulla conduzione atrioventricolare ed intraventricolare nell'uomo. G Ital Cardiol 1: 321, 1971
55. Camerini F, Baldi N, Gori P, Martinoli E: L'ajmalina nello studio prognostico dei blocchi bifascicolari. E' possibile valutare il rischio di evoluzione verso il blocco totale? G Ital Cardiol 3: 880, 1973
56. Jacovella G, Santini M, Dini P, Alliegro A, Floris B, Masini V: Effect of 17-monochloroacetylajmaline (MCAA) upon conduction and excitability of the human heart. In: Concepts on the mechanisms and treatment of arrhythmias, Gensini GG. New York: Futura, 1974, p 151
57. Meilhac B, Le Pailleur C, Heulin A, Vacheron A, Guise L, Di Matteo J: Intérêt de la stimulation auriculaire et des épreuves pharmaco-dynamiques dans le diagnostic des syncopes à électrocardiogramme normal. Arch Mal Coeur 67: 775, 1974
58. Morena H, Chaltiel G, Denis B, Rossignol B, Machecourt J, Martin Noel P: Effets dromotropes des associations médicamenteuses. Premiers resultats sur l'association deslanoside-ajmaline. Arch Mal Coeur 70: 749, 1977
59. Alboni P, Malacarne C, Pedroni P: Effetti elettrofisiologici dell'ajmalina sul sistema di conduzione nell'uomo. G Ital Cardiol 8: 752, 1978
60. Guerot CL, Valere PE, Castillo-Fenoy A, Coste A, Morice MC: Action comparée de l'ajmaline et du chloracetylajmaline sur la conduction auriculo-ventriculaire de l'homme. Coeur Med Int 14: 129, 1975
61. Seipel L, Both A, Breithardt G, Gleichman V, Loogen F: Action of antiarrhythmic drugs on His bundle electrocardiogram and sinus node function. Acta Cardiol (Suppl) 18: 251, 1974
62. Shigenobu K, Kasuya J, Ishiko J, Fukada J: The actions of N-propyl Ajmaline on experimental arrhythmias and electrophysiological properties of the heart. Chem Pharm Bull 22: 2329, 1974
63. Sekiya A, Vaughan Williams EM: A comparison of the antifibrillatory actions and effects on intracellular cardiac potentials of Pronethalol, Disopyramide and Quinidine. Br J Pharmacol 21: 473, 1963
64. Colonna D, Sorouche M, Tep T, Calisti G: Le traitement des troubles du rythme cardiaque par la disopyramide. Coeur Med Int 7: 455, 1968
65. Granier J: La disopyramide nel trattamento delle alterazioni ritmiche. Min Med 61: 3718, 1970
66. Mathur PP: Cardiovascular effects of a newer antiarrhythmic agent, disopyramide phosphate. Am Heart J 84: 764, 1972
67. Hulting J, Rosenhamer G: Antiarrhythmic and haemodynamic effects of intravenous and oral disopyramide in patients with ventricular arrhythmia. J Int Med Res (Suppl I), 4: 9, 1976
68. Mizgala HF, Huvell PR: Acute termination of cardiac arrhythmias with intravenous disopyramide. J Int Med Res (Suppl I) 4: 82, 1976
69. Ranney RE, Dean RR, Karim A, Radzialowski FM: Disopyramide phosphate: phar-

macokinetic and pharmacologic relationship of a new antiarrhythmic agent. Arch Int Pharmacodyn Ther 191: 162, 1971
70 Yen BK, Sung P, Scherlag BJ: Effects of disopyramide on electrophysiological and mechanical properties of the heart. J Pharm Sciences 62: 1924, 1973
71. Edwards IR, Martin JF, Ward JW: The effect of disopyramide on in vivo measurement of monophasic action potential in canine heart muscle. J Intern Med Res (Suppl I): 4: 26, 1976
72. Levites R, Anderson GJ: Electrophysiological effects of disopyramide phosphate during experimental myocardial ischemia. Am Heart J 98, 339, 1979
73. Josephson ME, Caracta AR, Lau S, Gallagher JJ, Damato AN: Electrophysiological evaluation of disopyramide in man. Am Heart J 86: 771, 1973
74 Befeler B, Castellanos A Jr, Wells DE, Vagueiro MC, Yen BK: Electrophysiological effects of the antiarrhythmic agent disopyramide phosphate. Am J Cardiol 35: 282, 1975
75. Spurrell RAJ, Thorburn CW, Camm J, Sowton E, Deuchar DC: Effects of disopyramide on electrophysiological properties of specialized conduction system in man and on accessory atrioventricular pathway in Wolff-Parkinson-White syndrome. Br heart J 37: 861, 1975
76. Marrott PK, Ruttley MSI, Winterbottom JT, Muit JR: A study of the acute electrophysiological and cardiovascular action of disopyramide in man. Europ J Cardiol 4: 303, 1976
77. Birkhead JS, Vaughan Williams EM: Dual effect of disopyramide on atrial and atrioventricular conduction and refractory periods. Br Heart J 39: 657, 1977
78. Desai JM, Scheinman M, Peters R, O'Young J: Electrophysiological effects of disopyramide in patients with bundle branch block. Circulation 59: 215, 1979
79. Bigger JF, Bassett AL, Hoffman BF: Electrophysiological effects of diphenylhydantoine in canine Purkinje fibers. Circ Res 22: 221, 1968
80. Bigger JT, Mandel WJ: Effects of lidocaine on the electrophysiological properties of ventricular muscle and Purkinje fibers. Circ Res 22: 221, 1968
81. Davis LD, Temte JV: Electrophysiological actions of lidocaine on canine ventricular muscle and Purkinje fibers. Circ Res 24: 639, 1969
82. Mandel WS, Bigger JT: Effect of lidocaine on sino-atrial node and atrial fibers. Am J Cardiol 25: 113, 1970
83. Southworth JL, McKusick VA, Peirce EC, Rawson FL Jr: Ventricular fibrillation precipitated by cardiac catheterization. JAMA 143: 717, 1950
84. Cotoi S, Luca C: Effetti della lidocaina nelle aritmie sopraventricolari. G Ital Cardiol 6: 433, 1976
85. Hoffman BF, Bigger JT Jr: Antiarrhythmic drugs. In: Drill's pharmacology in medicine, 4th edn Palma JR. New York: McGraw-Hill, 1971, p 824
86. Benowits N, Forsyth RP, Melmon KL, Rowland M: Lidocaine disposition kinetics in monkey and man. I. Prediction by a perfusion model. Clin Pharmacol Ther 16: 87, 1974
87. Sung CY, Truant AP: The physiological disposition of lidocaine and its comparison in some respects with procaine. J Pharmacol Exp Ther 112: 432, 1954
88. Scott DB, Jerson PJ, Vellani CW, Julian DG: Plasma lignocaine levels after intravenous and intramuscular injection. Lancet 1: 41, 1970
89. Alboni P: La lidocaina intramuscolare nel trattamento delle aritmie. G Ital Cardiol 1: 581, 1971
90. Bellet S, Roman L, Kostis JB, Fleischmann D: Intramuscular lidocaine in the therapy of ventricular arrhythmias. Am J Cardiol 27: 291, 1971

91. Fehmers MCO, Dunning AJ: Intramuscularly and orally administered lidocaine in the treatment of ventricular arrhythmias in acute myocardial infarction. Am J Cardiol 29: 514, 1972
92. Sarnoff SJ: Plasma levels of lidocaine after intramuscular administration. Am J Cardiol 29: 520, 1972
93. Rossi P, Lombardi M, Lotto A, Puddu V: La lidocaina per via intramuscolare nella prevenzione delle complicazioni e della mortalità nell'infarto miocardico acuto. Studio a doppio cieco di 246 casi. G Ital Cardiol 6: 220, 1976
94. Bigger JT Jr, Mandel WJ: Effect of lidocaine on canine Purkinje fibers and at the ventricular muscle-Purkinje fiber junction. J Pharmacol Exp Ther 172: 239, 1970
95. Bigger JT Jr, Mandel WJ: Effect of lidocaine on transmembrane potentials of ventricular muscle and Purkinje fibers. J Clin Invest 49: 63, 1970
96. Sasyniuk BI, Kus T: Comparison of the effects of lidocaine on electrophysiological properties of normal Purkinje fibers and those surviving acute myocardial infarction. Fed Proc (Abstr) 33: 476, 1974
97. El-Sherif N, Scherlag BJ, Lazzara R: Re-entrant ventricular arrhythmias in the late myocardial infarction period. IV. Mechanism of action of lidocaine. Circulation 56: 395, 1977
98. Kupersmith J, Antam EM, Hoffman BF: In vivo electrophysiological effects of lidocaine in canine acute myocardial infarction. Circ Res 36: 84, 1975
99. Rosen MR, Merker C, Pippenger CE: Effects of clinically relevant plasma lidocaine concentrations on electrophysiologic properties of canine Purkinje fibers. Circulation 48 (Suppl) IV: 209, 1973
100. Rosen MR, Hoffman BF, Wit AL: Electrophysiology and pharmacology of cardiac arrhythmias. V. Cardiac antiarrhythmic effects of lidocaine. Am Heart J 89: 526, 1975
101. Rosen MR, Merker C, Pippenger CE: The effects of lidocaine on the canine ECG and electrophysiologic properties of Purkinje fibers. Am Heart J 91: 191, 1976
102. Rosen KM, Lau SH, Weiss MB, Damato AN: The effect of lidocaine on atrioventricular and intraventricular conduction in man. Am J Cardiol 25: 1, 1970
103. Kunkel F, Rowland M, Scheinman MM: The electrophysiological effects of lidocaine in patients with intraventricular conduction defects. Circulation 49: 894, 1974
104. Bekheit S, Murtagh JG, Fletcher E: Effect of lignocaine on conducting system of human heart. Br Heart J 35: 305, 1973
105. Gupta PK, Lichstein E, Chadda KD: Lidocaine-induced heart block in patients with bundle branch block. Am J Cardiol 39: 550, 1974
106. Roos JC, Dunning A: Effects of lidocaine on impulse formation and conduction defects in man. Am Heart J 89: 686, 1975
107. Josephson ME, Caracta AR, Gallagher JJ, Damato AN: Effects of lidocaine on refractory periods in man. Am Heart J 84: 1778, 1972
108. Gerstenblith G, Scherlag BJ, Hope RR, Lazzara R: Effect of lidocaine on conduction in the ischemic His-Purkinje system in dog. Am J Cardiol 42: 587, 1978
109. Harris AS, Kodernot RH: Effects of diphenylhydantoin sodium (Dilantin) sodium and phenobarbital sodium upon ectopic ventricular tachycardia in acute myocardial infarction. Am J Physiol 163: 505, 1950
110. Leonard WA: The use of diphenylhydantoin (Dilantin) sodium in the treatment of ventricular tachycardia. Arch Inter Med 101: 714, 1958
111. Mercer EN, Osborn JA: The current status of diphenylhydantoin in heart disease. Ann Inter Med 67: 1084, 1967
112. Eddy JD, Singh SP: Treatment of cardiac arrhythmias with phenytoin. Br Heart J 4: 270, 1969

113. Bigger JT Jr, Schmidt DH, Kutt H: Relationship between the plasma level of diphenylhydantoin sodium and its cardiac antiarrhythmic effects. Circulation 38: 363, 1968
114. Kutt H: Biochemical and genetic factors regulating Dilantin metabolism in man. Ann NY Acad Sci 179: 704, 1971
115. Maynert EW: The metabolic fate of diphenylhydantoin in the dog, rat and man. J Pharmacol Exp Ther 130: 275, 1960
116. Bigger JT Jr, Bassett AL, Hoffman BF: Electrophysiological effects of diphenylhydantoin on canine Purkinje fibers. Circ Res 22: 221, 1968
117. Bassett AL, Bigger JT Jr, Hoffman BF: Prospective action of diphenylhydantoin on canine Purkinje fibers during hypoxia. J Pharmacol Exp Ther 173: 336, 1970
118. Helfant RH, Scherlag BJ, Damato AN: The electrophysiological properties of diphenylhydantoin sodium as compared to procaine amide in the normal and digitalis intoxicated heart. Circulation 36: 108, 1967
119. Rosati RA, Alexander JA, Schall SF, Wallace AG: Influence of diphenylhydantoin on electrophysiological properties of the canine heart. Circ Res 21: 757, 1967
120. Damato AN, Berkowitz WD, Patton RD, Lau SH: The effect of diphenylhydantoin on atrioventricular and intraventricular conduction in man. Am Heart J 79: 51, 1970
121. Caracta AR, Damato AN, Josephson ME, Riccuittu MA, Gallagher JJ, Lau SH: Electrophysiologic properties of diphenylhydantoin. Circulation 47: 1234, 1973
122. Bissett JK, De Soyza NDB, Kane JJ, Murphy ML: Improved intraventricular conduction of premature beats after diohenylhydantoin. Am J Cardiol 33: 493, 1974
123. Helfant RH, Scherlag BJ, Damato AN: Use of diphenylhydantoin sodium to dissociate the effects of procainamide on automaticity and conductions in the normal and arrhythmic heart. Am J Cardiol 20: 280, 1967
124. Haiat R, Chapelle M, Benaim R: Effect of diphenylhydantoin on intraventricular conduction disturbance: report of a case. J Electrocardiol 5: 197, 1972
125. Evans GH, Shand DG: Disposition of propranolol. IV. Independent variation in steady state circulating drug concentration and half-life as a result of plasma drug binding in man. Clin Pharmacol Ther 14: 494, 1973
126. Nies AS, Whand DG: Clinical pharmacology of propranolol. Circulation 52: 6, 1975
127. Shand DG, Nuckolls EM, Oates JA: Plasma propranolol levels in adults, with observations in four children. Clin Pharmacol Ther 11: 112, 1970
128. Walle T, Gaffney TE: Propranolol metabolism in man and dog: mass spectrometric identification of six new metabolites. J Pharmacol Exp Ther 182: 83, 1972
129. With AL, Hoffman BE, Rosen MR: Electrophysiology and pharmacology of cardiac arrhythmias. IX. Cardiac electrophysiologic effects of beta adrenergic receptor stimulation and blockade. Part C. Am Heart J 90: 795, 1975
130. Davis LD, Temte JV: Effects of propranolol on the transmembrane potentials of ventricular muscle and Purkinje fibers in the dog. Circ Res 23: 661, 1968
131. Coltart DJ, Meldrum SJ: The effect of racemic propranolol, dextropropranolol and racemic practolol on the human and canine cardiac transmembrane action potential. Arch Int Pharmacodyn 192: 188, 1971
132. Strauss HC, Bigger JT Jr, Hoffman BF: electrophysiological and beta-receptor blocking effects of MJ 1999 om dog and rabbit cardiac tissue. Circ Res 26: 661, 1970
133. Kumakura S, Somani P: The effects of LB-46, a β-adrenoceptor blocking drug on isolated normal and ouabain intoxicated Purkinje fibers of the dog. Europ J Pharmacol 25: 335, 1974
134. Wu CH, Narashashi T: Mechanism of action of propranolol on squid axon membranes. J Pharmacol Exp Ther 184: 155, 1973
135. Berkowitz WD, Wit AL, Lau SH, Steiner C, Damato AH: Effects of propranolol on

cardiac conduction. Circulation 40: 855, 1969
136. Smithen CS, Balcon R, Sowton E: Use of His potentials to assess changes in atrioventricular conduction produced by a series of beta-adrenergic blocking agents. Br Heart J 33: 955, 1971
137. Seides SF, Josephson ME, Batsford WP, Weisfogel GM, Lau SH, Damato AN: The electrophysiology of propanolol in man. Am Heart J 88: 733, 1974
138. Seipel L, Both A, Breithardt G, Gleichmann U, Loogen F: Action of antiarrhythmic drugs on His bundle electrogram and sinus node function. Acta Cardiol, Suppl XVIII, 251, 1974
139. Dini P, Santini M, Di Mascolo R, Milazzotto F, Jacovella G: Effetti elettrofisiologici del pindololo in pazienti con disturbi della eccito-conduzione. VI Congr. Naz ANMCO Rome: Pozzi, 1975, p 322
140. Alboni P, Malacarne C, Tomasi AM, Masoni A: Effetti del tolamololo sulla eccito-conduzione nell'uomo. G Ital Cardiol 7: 862, 1977
141. Di Biase M, Guglielmi R, Scarcia A, Chiddo A, Rizzon P: Electrophysiologic properties of intravenous oxprenolol in man. J Electrocardiol 10: 267, 1977
142. Rizzon P, Di Biase M, Chiddo A, Mastrangelo D, Sorgente L: Electrophysiologic properties of intravenous metoprolol in man. Br Heart J 40: 650, 1978
143. Di Biase M, Favale S, Rizzon P: Electrophysiologic properties of intravenous tenormine in man. Europ J Cardiol 9: 333, 1979
144. Charlier R: Cardiac actions in the dog of a new antagonist of adrenergic excitation which does not produce competitive blockade of adrenoreceptors. Br J Pharmacol 39: 668, 1970
145. Coumel P, Bouvrain Y: Etude clinique des effets pharmacodynamiques et antiarythmiques de l'amiodarone. J Agrèges 6: 69, 1973
146. Fauchier JP, Brochier M, Raynaud R: Etude clinique des effets anti-arythmiques ventriculaires de l'amiodarone (orale et injectable). Ann Cardiol Angeiol 22: 427, 1973
147. Rosenbaum MB, Chiale PA, Halpern MS, Nau GJ, Przybylski J, Levi RJ, Lazzari JO, Elizari MV: Clinical efficacy of Amiodarone as an antiarrhythmic agent. Am J Cardiol 38: 934, 1976
148. Broekhuysen J, Laurel R, Sion R: Etude comparée du transit et du métabolisme de l'amiodarone chez diverses espèces animales et chez l'homme. Arch Inter Pharmacodyn Thér 177: 340, 1969
149. Singh BN, Vaughan Williams EM: The effect of amiodarone, a new anti-anginal drug, on cardiac muscle. Br J Pharmacol 39: 657, 1970
150. Cabasson J, Puech P, Melle JM, Guimond G, Bachy C, Sassine A: Analyse des effets électrophysiologiques de l'amiodarone par l'enregistrement simultane des potentiels d'action monophasiques et du faisceau de His. Arch Mal Coeur 69: 691, 1976
151. Olsson SB, Brorson L, Varnauskas E: Class 3 antiarrhythmic action in man. Observations from monoplasic action potential recordings and amiodarone treatment. Br Heart J 35: 1255, 1973
152. Curry PVC: Fundamentals of arrhythmias: modern methods of investigation. In: Cardiac arrythmias. The modern electrophysiological approach, Krikler D, Goodwin JF. London: WB Saunders, 1975, p. 39
153. Disertori M, Molinis G, Vergara G, Bettini R, Furlanello F: Effetti dell'amiodarone sulla conduzione atrio-ventricolare e ventricolo-atriale nella sindrome di Wolff-Parkinson-White. G. Ital Cardiol 6: 792, 1976
154. Touboul H, Huerta F, Porte J, Delahaye JP: Bases électrophysiologiques de l'action antiarythmique de l'amiodarone chez l'homme. Arch Mal Coeur 69: 845, 1976

155. Wellens HJJ, Lie KI, Bar FW, Wesdorp JC, Dohmen HJ, Duren Dr, Durrer D: Effect of amiodarone in the Woll-Parkinson-White syndrome. Am J Cardiol 38: 189, 1976
156. Waleffe A, Bruninx P, Kulbertus HE: Effects of amiodarone studied by programmed electrical stimulation of the heart in patients with paroxysmal re-entrant supraventriular tachycardia. J Electrocardiol 11: 253, 1978
157. Bacaner M: Bretylium tosylate for suppression of induced ventricular fibrillation. Am J Cardiol 17: 528, 1966
158. Terry G, Vellani CW, Higgins MR, Doig A: Bretylium toxylate in treatment of refractory ventricular arrhythmias complicating myocardial infarction. Br Heart J 32: 21, 1070
159. Dhurandhar RW, Teasdale SJ, Mahon WA: Bretylium tosylate in the management of refractory ventricular fibrillation. Can Med Ass J 105: 161, 1971
160. Berstein JG, Koch-Weser J: Effectiveness of bretylium tosylate against refractory ventricular arrhythmias. Circulation 45: 1024, 1972
161. Wit AL, Steiner C, Damato AM: Electrophysiological effects of bretylium tosylate on single fibers of the canine specialized conduction system and ventricle. J Pharmacol Exp Ther 173: 344, 1970
162. Bigger JT, Jaffe CC: The effect of bretylium tosylate on the electrophysiological properties of ventricular muscle and Purkinje fibers. Am J Cardiol 27: 82, 1971
163. Haas, H, Hartfelder G: α-Isopropyl-α-[N-methyl-N-homoveratril)-δ-aminopropyl]-3,4-dimethoxyphenyl-acetonitril, eine Substanz mit Coronargefässerweiternden Eigenschaften. Arzneimittel Forsch 12: 549, 1962
164. Schamroth L, Krikler DM, Garrett C: Immediate effects of intravenous verapamil in cardiac arrhythmias. Br Med J 1: 660, 1972
165. Krikler D: Verapamil in cardiology. Europ J Cardiol 2: 10, 1974
166. Spurrell RAJ, Krikler M, Sowton E: Concealed bypass of the A-V node in patients with paroxismal supraventricular tachycardia revealed by intracardiac electrical stimulation and intravenous verapamil. Am J Cardiol 33: 590, 1974
167. Rosen MR, Wit AL, Hoffman BF: Electrophysiology and pharmacology of cardiac arrhythmias. VI. Cardiac effects of Verapamil. Am Heart J 89: 665, 1975
168. Belz GG, Bender F: Therapie der Herzrhythmusstörungen mit Verapamil. Stuttgart: Gustav Fischer, 1974
169. Fleckenstein A: Specific inhibitors and promotors of calcium action in the excitation-contraction coupling of heart muscle and their role in the prevention or production of myocardial lesions. In: Calcium and the heart, Harris P, Opie LH. New York: Academic Press, 1971, p 135
170. Kohlhardt M, Baver B, Krause H, Fleckenstein A: New selective inhibitors of the transmembrane Ca conductivity in mammalian myocardial fibers. Experientia 15: 288, 1972
171. Shigenobu K, Schneider JA, Sperelakis N: Verapamil blockade of slow Na^+ and Ca^{++} responses in myocardial cells. J Pharmacol Exp Ther 190: 280, 1974
172. Rosen MR, Ilvento JP, Gelband H, Merker C: Effects of verapamil on electrophysiologic properties of canine cardiac Purkinje fibers. J Pharmacol Exp Ther 189: 414, 1974
173. Zipes DP, Besch HR, Watanabe AM: Role of the slow current in cardiac electrophysiology. Circulation 51: 761, 1975
174. Dershm GH, Han J: Effects of Verapamil on action potentials of Purkinje fibers. J Electrocardiol 13: 67, 1980
175. El-Sherif N, Lazzara R: Reentrant ventricular arrhythmias in the late myocardial infarction period. 7. Effect of Verapamil and D-600 and the role of the slow channel. Circulation 60: 605, 1979

176. Fazzini PF, Marchi F, Pucci P: Azione antiaritmica del Verapamil nell'infarto miocardico acuto. Considerazioni sul possibile meccanismo d'azione. G Ital Cardiol 7: 940, 1977
177. Elharrar V, Gaum WE, Zipes DP: Effect of drugs on conduction delay and incidence of ventricular arrhythmias induced by acute coronary occlusion in dogs. Am J Cardiol 39: 544, 1977
178. Husaini MH, Kvasnicka J, Rysen L, Holmberg S: Action of Verapamil in sinus node, atrioventricular, and intraventricular conduction. Br Heart J 35: 734, 1973
179. Rizzon P. Di Biase M, Calabrese P, Brindicci G, Chiddo A: Electrophysiologic evaluation of intravenous Verapamil in man. Europ J Cardiol 6: 179, 1977
180. Hoffman BF: Effects of digitalis on electrical activity of cardiac membranes. In: Basic and clinical pharmacology of digitalis, Marks BH, Weissler AM. Springfield: Charles C. Thomas, 1972, p 118
181. Kassebaum DC: Electrophysiological effects of strophantin on the heart. J Pharmacol Exp Ther 140: 329, 1963
182. Hashimoto K, Moe GK: Transient depolarizations induced by acetylstrophanthidin in specialized tissue of dog atrium and ventricle. Circ Res 32: 618, 1973
183. Davies LD: Effect of changes in cycle length on diastolic depolarization produced by ouabain in canine Purkinje fibers. Circ Res 32: 206, 1973
184. Ferrier GR, Saunders JH, Mendez C: A cellular mechanism for the generation of ventricular arrhythmias by acetylstrophanthidin. Circ Res 32: 600, 1973
185. Hogan PM, Wittenberg SM, Klocke FJ: Relationship of stimulation frequency to automaticity in the canine Purkinje fiber during ouabain administration. Circ Res 32: 377, 1973
186. Rosen MR, Gelband H, Merker C, Hoffman BF: Mechanisms of digitalis toxicity: effects of ouabain on phase 4 of canine Purkinje fiber transmembrane potentials. Circulation 47: 681, 1973
187. Damato AN, Lau SH: Clinical value of the electrocardiogram of the conducting system. Progr Cardiovasc Dis 13: 119, 1970
188. Puech P, Grolleau R: L'enregistrement endocavitaire des potentiels du tissu de conduction. Rev Prat 22: 1207, 1972
189. Przybyla AC: Effects of digoxine on atrio-ventricular conduction pattern in man. Am J Cardiol 33: 344, 1974
190. Gomes JA, Dhatt MS, Akhtar M, Carambas CR, Rubenson DS, Damato AN: Effects of digitalis on ventricular myocardial and His-Purkinje refractoriness and reentry in man. Am J Cardiol 42: 931, 1978
191. Gomes JA, Damato AN, Bobb G, Lau S: The effect of digitalis on refractoriness of the intact canine His-Pukinje system. Circulation 58: 284, 1978
192. Gaultier M. Fournier E, Efthymiou ML, Freaville JP, Jouannot P, Dentan M: Intoxications digitaliques aiguës (70 observations). Bull Soc Med Hop 119: 247, 1968
193. Ollagnier J: Digitaliques et conduction cardiaque coeur. Med Int 17: 537, 1978
194. Akhtar M, Damato AN, Caracta AR, Batsford WP, Josephson ME, Lau SH: Electrophysiologic effects of atropine on atrioventricular conduction studied by His bundle electrogram. Am J Cardiol 33: 333, 1974
195. Hoffman BF, Singer DH: Appraisal of the effects of catecholamines on cardiac electrical activity. In: New adrenergic blocking drugs: their pharmacological, biochemical and clinical actions, Moran N. Ann NY Acad Sci 139: 914, 1967
196. Giotti A, Ledda F, Mannaioni PF: Effects of noradrenaline and isoprenaline in combination with α and β-receptor blocking substances on the action potential of cardiac Purkinje fibers. J Physiol 229: 99, 1973

197. Wit AL, Hoffman BF, Rosen RR: Electrophysiology and pharmacology of cardiac arrhythmias. IX. Cardiac electrophysiologic effects of beta adrenergic receptor stimulation and blockade. Part A. Am Heart J 90: 521, 1975
198. Trautwein W, Schmidt RZ: Zur Membranwirkung des Adrenalin an der Herzmuskelfaser. Pflügers Arch 271: 715, 1960
199. Cannom DS, Rider A, Stinson EB, Harrison DC: Electrophysiologic studies in the denervated transplanted heart. II. Response to norepinephrine, isoproterenol and propranolol. Am J Cardiol 36: 859, 1975
200. Vargas G, Akhtar M, Damato AN: Electrophysiologic effects of isoproterenol on cardiac conduction system in man. Am Heart J 90: 25, 1975
201. Masoni A, Alboni P, Malacarne C, Codeca' L: Effects of Dobutamine on electrophysiological properties of the specialized conduction system in man. J Electrocardiol 12: 361, 1979
202. Dhingra RC, Winslow E, Pouget J, Rahimtoola S, Rosen KM: The effect of isoproterenol on atrioventricular and intraventricular conduction. Am Heart J 90: 25, 1975
203. Masini G, Gherardi C, Dianda R, Cuccu E: Effetti della dopamina sulla conduzione atrio-ventricolare ed intraventricolare. G Ital Cardiol 3: 545, 1973
204. Kesteloot H, Van Mieghem W, De Geest H: Aprindine (AC 1802). A new antiarrhythmic drug. Acta Cardiol 28: 145, 1973
205. Fasola AF, Carmichael R: The pharmacology and clinical evaluation of aprindine, a new antiarrhythmic agent. Acta Cardiol (Suppl) 18: 317, 1974
206. Fasola AF, Noble RJ, Zipes DP: Treatment of recurrent ventricular tachycardia and fibrillation with aprindine. Am J Cardiol 39: 903, 1977
207. Pouleur H, Chaudron JM, Reyns P: Effects of disopyramide and aprindine on arrhythmias after acute myocardial infarction. Europ J Cardiol 5: 397, 1977
208. Murphy PJ: Metabolic pathways of aprindine. Acta Cardiol (Suppl) 18: 131, 1976
209. Delcroix C, Martin L, Van Durme JP, Kesteloot H, Hagemeijer F, Mbuyamba P, Deblecker M: Model for exchange kinetics of aprindine in man after single and multiple doses. Acta Cardiol (Suppl) 18: 177, 1974
210. Verdonck F, Vereecke J, Vleugels A: Electrophysiological effects of aprindine on isolated heart preparations. Europ J Pharm 26: 338, 1974
211. Steinberg MI, Greenspan K: Intracellular electrophysiological alterations in canine cardiac conducting tissue induced by aprindine and lignocaine. Cardiovasc Res 10: 236, 1976
212. Greene HL, Reid PR, Schaeffer AH: Prolongation of cardiac conduction times by intravenous aprindine in man. Am J Cardiol 42: 1002, 1978
213. Zipes DP, Troup PJ: New antiarrhythmic agents. Amiodarone, Aprindine, Disopyramide, Ethmozim, Mexiletine, Tocainide, Verapamil. Am J Cardiol 41: 1005, 1978
214. Vergara G, Disertori M, Molinis G, Inama G, Antonini L, Del Favero A, Stefenelli C, Furlanello F: Studio degli effetti elettrofisiologici dell'aprindine nell'uomo con particolare riferimento alla sindrome da preeccitazione ventricolare. G Ital Cardiol 9: 597, 1979
215. Kesteloot H, Van de Werf F, Marchandise B, Sluyts R: Influence of moxaprindine treatment on ventricular arrhythmias occurring during maximal exercise stress testing. Acta Cardiol 34: 301, 1979
216. Waleffe A, Mary-Rabine L, Kulbertus HE: Study of moxaprindine with programmed electrical stimulation of the heart in patients with reentrant tachyarrhythmias. Am J Cardiol 45: 640, 1980
217. Beani L: Profilo farmacologico di un nuovo antiaritmico: la bunaftide. Boll Soc It

Card 17: 1279, 1972
218. Lotto A, Lomanto B, Bossi M: Prime esperienze nell'impiego clinico di un nuovo antiaritmico: la bunaftide. Cardiol Prat 23: 123, 1972
219. Masini G, Cuccu E, Zanetti L: Sull'impiego della bunaftide nel trattamento ambulatoriale di alcuni disturbi del ritmo cardiaco. Boll Soc It Card 17: 1173, 1972
220. Rossi P, Carcano G, Rognoni G, Cernigliaro C, Calcaterra G: Correlazione fra concentrazioni plasmatiche ed effetto antiaritmico della bunaftide. G Ital Cardiol 6: 1048, 1976
221. Ferroni A, Monticelli G: Electrophysiological aspects of the action of bunaphtine on single cardiac muscle fibres. Pharmacol Res 5: 151, 1973
222. Bonatti V, Finardi A, Cabasson J, Botti G: L'effetto della bunaftide sui potenziali di azione monofasici del miocardio atriale e ventricolare destro nell'uomo. Nota preliminare. G Ital Cardiol 6: 440, 1976
223. Bonatti V, Finardi A, Cabasson J, Botti G: Studio sul meccanismo d'azione della bunaftide mediante registrazione dei potenziali d'azione monofasici del miocardio nell'uomo. Nota conclusiva. G Ital Cardiol 6: 1378, 1976
224. Scibilla G, Bonatti V, Pavarani A, Tagliavini S, Botti G: Effetto sul fascio di His di una nuova sostanza antiaritmica, la bunaftide. Cardiol Prat 24: 79, 1973
225. Grazi S, Romano S, Bonazzi O, Pozzoni L, Cavoretto D, Gardumi L, Sardella F: Effetti di un nuovo antiaritmico, la bunaftide, sulla conduzione intraatriale, atrioventricolare ed intraventricolare dello stimolo. Cardiol Prat 25: 213, 1974
226. Byrne JE, Gomoll AW: Antiarrhythmic activity of MJ 9067. Fed Proc (Abstr) 32: 812, 1973
227. Byrne JE, Gomoll AW: Antiarrhythmic properties of MJ 9067 in acute animal models. J Pharmacol Exp Ther 200: 147, 1977
228. Gibson JK, Somani PF, Bassett A: Effect of MJ 9067 on transmembrane potentials of canine cardiac Purkinje fibers (Abstr). Pharmacology 18: 169, 1976
229. Sami M, Mason JW, Oh G, Harrison DC: Canine electrophysiology of Encainide, a new antiarrhythmic drug. Am J Cardiol 43: 1149, 1979
230. Sami M, Mason JW, Peters F, Harrison DC: Clinical electrophysiologic effects of Encainide, a newly developed antiarrhythmic agent. Am J Cardiol 44: 526, 1979
231. Kaverina NV, Senova DP, Vikhlyayev YI, Ul'yanova OV: Antiarrhythmic properties of ethmozine. Farmako Toksikol 33: 693, 1970
232. Votchal BY, Lozinskiy LG: Efficacy of a new antiarrhythmic drug, ethmozim. Klin Med (Mosk) 10: 16, 1971
233. Senova ZP, L'Vov MV: Mechanism of the antiarrhythmic effect of ethmozim. Farmakol Toksikol 36: 703, 1973
234. Morganroth J, Pealman AS, Dunkam WB, Horowitz LN, Josephson ME, Michelson EL: Ethmozim: a new antiarrhythmic agent developed in the USSR. Efficacy and tolerance. Am Heart J 98: 621, 1979
235. Podrid PJ, Lyakishev A, Lown B, Mazur N: Ethmozim, a new antiarrhythmic drug for suppression of ventricular premature complexes. Circulation 61: 450, 1980
236. Danilo P, Langman WB, Rosen MR, Hoffman BF: Effects of phenothiazine analog, EN 131, on ventricular arrhythmias in the dog. Europ J Pharmacol 45: 127, 1977
237. Ruffy R, Rozenshtraukh L, Elharrar V, Zipes DP: Cardiac electrophysiologic properties of ethmozim. Clin Res (Abstr) 25: 557, 1977
238. Campbell NPS, Kelly JG, Shanks RG, Chaturvedi NC, Strong JE, Partridge JF: Mexiletine (Ko 1173) in the management of ventricular arrhythmias. Lancet 2: 404, 1973
239. Talbot RG, Nimmo J, Julian DG, Clark RA, Nielson JMM, Prescott LF: Treatment

of ventricular arrhythmias with mexiletine (Ko 1173). Lancet 2: 399, 1973
240. Heger JJ, Nattel S, Rinkenberger RL, Zipes DP: Mexiletine therapy in 15 patients with drug-resistant ventricular tachycardia. Am J Cardiol 45: 627, 1980
241. Prescott LF, Clements JD, Pottage A: Absorption, distribution and elimination of mexiletine. Postgrad Med J (Suppl) 53: 50, 1977
242. Weld FM, Bigger JT, Swistel D, Bordiuk J, Lau YH: Electrophysiological effects of mexiletine (Kö 1173) on ovine cardiac Purkinje fibers. (In preparation)
243. Roos JC, Paalman ACA, Dunning AJ: Electrophysiological effects of mexiletine in man. Br Heart J 38: 1261, 1976
244. McComish M, Kitson D, Robinson CC, Jewitt DE: Clinical electrophysiological effects of mexiletine. Postgrad Med J 53 (Suppl I): 85, 1977
245. Beck OA, Kramer KD, Wolff R, Muller A, Hochrein H: Propafenon, ein neues Antiarrhythmikum zur Therapie tachycarder und extrasystolischer Herzrhythmusstörungen. Med Klin 70, 95: 1975
246. Ador E, Heeger I: Propafenon, ein neues Antiarrhythmikum. Dtsch Med Wschr 101: 1318, 1976
247. Kock R: Zur Propafenon-wirkung bei ventrikularer Arrhythmie. In: Fortschritte in der Pharmakotherapie von Herzrhythmusstörungen I, Hochrein H, Hapke HJ, Beck OA. Internationales Propafenon-Symposium. Stuttgart: Gustav Fischer, 1977, p 84
248. Fazzini PF, Marchi F, Santoro GM, Pucci P, Zambaldi G: Profilo di un nuovo antiaritmico: il proprafenone. Contributo casistico in terapia clinica. (In preparation)
249. Keller K, Meyer-Estorf G, Beck OA, Hochrein H: Correlation between serum concentration and pharmacological effect of atrioventricular conduction time of the antiarrhythmic drug. Europ J Pharmacol 13: 17, 1978
250. Bergamann M, Bolte HD: Elektrophysiologische Untersuchungen mit Propafenon in myokardialen Einzelfasern. In: Fortschritte in der Pharmakotherapie von Herzrhythmusstörungen I, Hochrein H, Hapke HJ, Beck OA. Internationales Propafenon-Symposium. Suttgart: Gustav Fischer, 1977, p 84
251. Seipel L, Both A, Breithardt G, Loogen F: Die Wirkung neuer Antiarrhythmika (Aprindin, Propafenon, Ci 661) auf die intrakardiale Anregungsleitung und die Sinusknotenautomatik beim Menschen. (Personal communication)
252. McDevitt DG, Nies AS, Wilkinson GR, Smith RF, Woosley RL, Oates JA: Antiarrhythmic effects of a lidocaine congener, tocainide, 2-amino-2, 6-propionoxylidide in man. Clin Pharmacol Ther 19: 396, 1976
253. Lewinter MM, Englel RE, Karliner JS: Tocainide therapy for treatment of ventricular arrhythmias: assessment with ambulatory electrocardiographic monitoring and treadmill exercice. Am J Cardiol 45: 1045, 1980
254. Harrison DC, Meffin PJ, Winkle RA: Clinical pharmacokinetics of antiarrhythmic drugs. Prof Cardiovasc Dis 20: 217, 1977
255. Gerstenblith G, Spear JF, Moore EN: Electrophysiological effects of a new antiarrhythmic drug. Clin Res 21: 419, 1973
256. Anderson JL, Mason JW, Winkle RA, Meffin PJ, Fowles RE, Peters F, Harrison DC: Clinical electrophysiologic effects of tocainide. Circulation 57: 685, 1978
257. Pamintuan JC, Dreifus LS, Watanabe Y: Comparative mechanism of antiarrhythmic agents. Am J Cardiol 26: 512, 1960
258. Watanabe Y, Dreifuss LS, Likoff W: Electrophysiologic antagonism and synergism of potassium and antiarrhythmic agents. Am J Cardiol 12: 702, 1963

14. PACEMAKER THERAPY IN PATIENTS WITH INTRA-VENTRICULAR CONDUCTION DISTURBANCES

The scope and clinical application of cardiac pacing have rapidly evolved and expanded since its inception nearly two decades ago.

The many conduction disturbances currently amenable to pacemaker therapy include those which are well established and others for which the role of pacing is less certain and controversial; among these latter there are various forms of intraventricular conduction disturbances (IVCD).

The therapeutic problems are different if IVCD are observed in patients with chronic or acute heart disease.

INDICATION FOR PACING IN PATIENTS WITH CHRONIC INTRAVENTRICULAR CONDUCTION DISTURBANCES

Complete AV block distal to His bundle

Complete AV block distal to His bundle represents the most commonly encountered type of acquired complete AV block. It is characterized by an idioventricular escape rhythm without a preceding H potential with a rate frequently less than 40 beats/min.

In most cases this form of AV block is secondary to coronary artery disease or to idiopathic intraventricular conduction disease.

Cerebral symptoms, including Morgagni-Adams-Stock attacks, are frequently present. Congestive heart failure and other manifestations of pump failure secondary to a slow and unstable ventricular rate may occur.

Implantation of a permanent cardiac pacing is indicated in all patients with complete AV block distal to His bundle whether symptoms exist or not, due to high risk of ventricular asystole.

2° AV distal to His bundle

When a 2° AV block is localized in the His-Purkinjie system (HPS), in most cases it manifests itself as advanced degree AV block (2:1, 3:1, etc.) or as Mobitz type II.

This latter form of block is characterized by a constant PR interval and sudden failure of AV conduction of an atrial impulse. More commonly, Mobitz type II is recognized by a fixed bundle branch or bifascicular block during conduction and intermittent loss of ventricular conduction when AV block occurs in the remaining functioning fascicle. When AV block is distal to the His bundle, the atrial electrocardiogram is followed by a His bundle potential.

One very rarely observes Mobitz type I AV block in the HPS [1-3].

All patients with 2° AV block distal to His bundle require permanent cardiac pacing because of the increased proclivity toward complete heart block (CHB) and its serious consequences.

Symptomatic chronic bundle branch block

When patients with chronic bundle branch block (BBB) or bifascicular block complain of syncope or dizziness and an intermittent 2° or 3° AV block is documented, all the authors recommended a permanent pacemaker implantation as such a finding very often progresses to persistent CHB.

When the AV block is not documented, it is essential to exclude other causes responsible for syncope or dizziness, such as neurologic diseases, gastrointestinal bleeding, hypertrophic cardiomyopathy, aortic stenosis, paroxysmal tachyarrhythmias, sinus node dysfunction, orthostatic hypotension and vagally induced syncope.

Continuous ECG monitoring is warranted if pertinent diagnostic information is not ascertained from the clinical and laboratory examination.

If during ECG monitoring, syncope and dizzines do not appear, a His bundle study becomes necessary in order to assess the HPS conduction time, i.e. HV interval. In fact, surface ECG is of limited value for this purpose as a lengthening of PR interval does not necessarily indicate a delayed conduction through the HPS [4-7].

If in symptomatic patients with chronic BBB the HV interval is prolonged, most of the authors [7-14] recommend permanent pacemaker implantation, despite the absence of a documented AV block.

The results of several studies suggest this procedure.

Narula [12] has reported that in all symptomatic patients, without a documented AV block but with a prolonged HV interval, who received a pacemaker and were alive at the end of the follow-up period, a CHB was subsequently documented. Scheinman et al. [7] reported six cases with prolonged HV interval and negative Holter recordings, who within 22 days developed 2° or 3° AV block. Altschuler et al. [11] followed 35 symptomatic patients with HV interval prolongation without documented heart block. Eighteen of these patients received a permanent ventricular pacemaker (paced group), while the other 17 remained unpaced (unpaced group). Among the paced group there were three deaths, none sudden, during a mean follow-up of 23 months; four patients developed asymptomatic CHB. Among the unpaced group, eight patients died (three suddenly) and three progressed to CHB with symptoms, leaving only six stable after a 6 month follow-up.

McAnulty et al. [15], however, do not recommend permanent ventricular pacing in these patients if there is no documentation of 2° or 3° degree AV block. However their conclusions should be reassessed, considering the fact that two of their 13 patients who developed CHB died in hospital while awaiting a permanent pacemaker implantation.

Symptomatic patients with normal HV interval, in the absence of a documented AV block, are not candidates for a pacemaker implantation [13, 16]. According to our experience, and that of others [17], the appearance of CHB in patients with normal HV interval is an extremely rare occurrence.

However, if the symptoms continue to recur without explanation, continuous Holter monitoring for several days is warranted.

Asymptomatic patients with chronic bundle branch block

The indication for prophylactic pacemaker insertion in asymptomatic patients with chronic BBB and prolonged HV interval is highly controversial.

Pacemaker insertion is not recommended by Dhingra et al. [18-20] or by McAhulty et al. [15] under these circumstances as they do not believe that HV interval duration has a predictive value of developing CHB. Others, however, recommend a prophylactic pacemaker implantation in selected asymptomatic elderly patients with a markedly prolonged HV interval (> 70 msec.) and bifascicular block of greater than three years duration and/or when associated with 1° AV block [10, 21-23].

In the study by Scheinman et al. [7] the incidence of sudden death in patients with chronic BBB associated with an HV interval of 70 msec or more was 17 % and progression to 2° or 3° AV block was 21 %. By contrast, in this prospective study, sudden death and development of 2° or 3° AV block remained less than 3 % when HV interval was less than 70 msec. However these authors recommend a close follow-up, without pacemaker implantation.

We insert permanent ventricular pacing in those asymptomatic patients with chronic BBB and prolonged HV interval who show 2° or 3° AV block after Ajmaline administration, or block distal to His bundle with intact AV nodal conduction during incremental atrial pacing. Such pharmacological and pacing-induced blocks, although they appear very rarely in the asymptomatic patients, are highly predictive of future development of CHB and sudden death (see Chapter II).

However, at present prophylactic pacemaker insertion in asymptomatic patients with chronic BBB and prolonged HV interval remains a controversial issue.

Prophylactic preoperative pacing

The stress of anesthetic induction and surgery might predispose patients with chronic BBB, particulary those with bifascicular block, to CHB.

Thus the problem of whether to insert a prophylactic preoperative temporary pacing in such patients arises.

The literature offers little on this topic; moreover, most studies performed are retrospective [24-27].

The medical records of 30 patients who underwent 36 surgical procedures were analyzed by Berg et al. [24]. Twenty-sic of these patients had right bundle branch block (RBBB) associated with anterior fascicular block (AFB), the remaining four having left bundle branch block (LBBB) and 1° AV block. Twenty-five (83%) patients had evidence of underlying cardiac disease and two patients gave prior history of syncope and dizziness. No 2° or 3° AV block after surgical procedure was documented in any patient.

We studied 94 patients with RBBB and AFB submitted to various types of surgery. The appearance of 2° or 3° degree block was not observed in any of these cases [25].

An analysis of 38 patients with bifascicular block who underwent surgical or endoscopic procedures was carried out by Wenkataram et al. [26]. Seven patients had additional 1° or 2° AV block. The authors report that two of these seven developed bradyarrhythmias requizing treatment. They concluded that in patients with bifascicular block and 1° or 2° AV block pacemaker insertion may be warranted. However, the form of bradyarrhythmia observed in this subset of patients is not specified.

Thirthy-eight patients undergoing 74 surgical and other procedures were studied by Pirzada et al. [27] to determine the need for prophylactic temporary pacing in bifascicular block. The preoperative cardiac rhythms were atrial fibrillation in two patients, stable junctional rhythm in one patient, 2:1 AV block of Mobitz type II in one patient and sinus rhythm with 1:1 AV conduction in the remaining patients. Six patients had prolonged PR interval and two had one or more syncopal episodes.

Only the patient with Mobitz II AV block was observed to go into transient CHB at the time of recovery from anesthesia and required ventricular pacing to maintain normal blood pressure.

In the few prospective studies performed the same results were reported [28, 29]. Kunstadt et al. [28] studied 24 patients with bifascicular block who underwent 38 operations, 13 of which were performed after insertion of a prophylactic pacemaker. Constant intra operative ECG monitoring did not disclose any episode of 2° or 3° AV block.

Another 44 patients with RBBB and AFB who underwent a total of 52 operations were followed by Pastore et al. [29]. One patient gave a history of syncope.

All patients had continuous ECG monitoring throughout anesthesia induction, operation and surgical recovery. The preoperative cardiac rhythms were atrial fibrillation in two patients, atrial tachycardia with block in one patient, atrial flutter in one patient and sinus rhythm in the remaining patients.

Temporary pacemakers were inserted preoperatively in six patients, mostly because of PR prolongation in the preoperative electrocardiogram. There was only one episode of transient CHB out of the 52 operative procedures.

The few available data would suggest that non-cardiac surgical procedures do not represent an important risk factor in patients with bifascicular block. Therefore the stress of surgery and the drugs in use for anesthesia do not seem to depress significantly the intraventricular conduction.

In this connection, Santini et al. [30] performed His bundle electrocardiogram in 11 patients with syncope and IVCD (five LBBB, two RBBB, four bifascicular block) before and after administration of Pentothal 0.20 g i.v., succinylcholine 1 mg/kg i.v. and breathing of Fluothan 1 % or Ethrane.

Only succinylcholine showed a negative dromotropic effect on the HPS; in two patients a transient CHB distal to His bundle appeared and in the other nine HV interval duration increased by 5 %.

On the basis of the above-mentioned data we believe that prophylactic preoperative pacing in asymptomatic patients with bifascicular block is not necessary. However, administration of succinylcholine is not advisable in such patients.

In the other hand there are too few cases reported of patients with bifascicular block and syncopes who have undergone surgical procedures to be able to draw any conclusions. We believe that these patients must first undergo all clinical and electrophysiological examinations before an operation in order to assess the genesis of the syncopes and any eventual need for permanent pacemaker implantation. If such examinations are not possible because the operation is urgent, we recommend, as a precaution, the insertion of prophylactic temporary pacing to determine afterwards the need for permanent pacing.

In patients with chronic BBB who must undergo open heart surgery, the problem of whether to insert a temporary pacemaker or not does not exist as the present trend is to perform prophylactic cardiac pacing in all patients, independent of the presence of automaticity or conduction troubles, due to the frequent appearance of these complications during and after cardiosurgery procedure [31, 32].

INDICATION FOR PACING IN PATIENTS WITH INTRAVENTRICULAR CONDUCTION DISTURBANCES IN ACUTE MYOCARDIAL INFARCTION

Much controversy still exists as to the indication for cardiac pacing during acute myocardial infarction (AMI) complicated by IVCD. These controversies are primarily due to different data reported by various authors on the incidence of early and late death and early and late progression to CHB.

Temporary pacing

The insertion of a temporary pacemaker during AMI may have a prophylactic objective in patients with 1:1 AV conduction and therapeutic objective in patients with 2° or 3° AV block.

Regarding the indications of prophylactic temporary pacing there are not sufficient data to draw any definite conclusions.

During AMI, hospital mortality is higher in patients with IVCD (24-55 %) compared to those without interventricular block (12-22 %) and appears above all to be related to the high incidence of several heart failure due to extensive myocardial damage (33-42).

Also, the risk of developing CHB is increased when BBB complicates AMI [35, 37, 43-57].

In patients with BBB in whom a CHB has appeared, the hospital mortality is very high (70-90 %) [48, 50, 53, 58-62]; it is generally accepted that the poor prognosis in those patients is mainly due to marked extension of the infarction rather than to conduction trouble itself.

A problem which is yet unresolved is whether the insertion of a propylactic pacemaker reduces hospital mortality in patients with BBB.

In the study by Fenig et al. [50], of 11 patients showing CHB who were prophylactically paced, four died (36 %) compared with 11 out of 15 patients (73 %) in whom the pacemaker was inserted after the occurrence of CHB. Waters et al. [54] described 15 patients with BBB showing CHB: hospital mortality was 40 % in the five who already had prophylactic pacemakers and 50 % in the ten in whom the pacemaker was inserted after the development of CHB. Nimetz et al. [56] reported very similar results in their 15 patients; five were prophylactically paced, of whom two (40 %) died, while the remaining ten received this treatment after the onset of CHB and of whom six (60 %) died. The procedure was considered life-saving in two cases. Godman et al. [48] reported 13 deaths in 15 patients (86 %) showing CHB who were prophylactically paced and 21 deaths in 26 patients (81 %) who received a pacemaker after CHB developed. Stephens et al. [63] compared a retrospective series of 25 patients who were not paced, with a prospective group of 12 patients with bifascicular block who were paced; although three patients in the first group died from sudden CHB, the difference in mortality between the two series was not significant.

Although these reports make it impossible to reach a reliable conclusion about the place of prophylactic pacing in reducing hospital mortality, it would appear that in some cases this procedure may be life-saving. It is therefore necessary to identify those parameters which indicate a very high risk of CHB in patients who are not inevitably destined to die from pump failure.

Infarct location does not appear to influence the risk of CHB in patients with AMI and IVCD. High degree AV block was as common with inferior or posterior infarctions (20 %) as with anterior infarctions (25 %) [57].

Also, PR interval prolongation does not appear to increase significantly the risk of developing CHB [57, 61]. It was observed that the presence of 1° AV block was associated with a 25% incidence of progression to high degree AV block compared to 19% incidence in patients with normal PR interval. Furthermore, over one third of the patients who developed CHB did so suddenly without 1° or 2° AV block [57].

The type of intraventricular block appears to be the most important factor in identifying the patients at high risk of developing CHB.

The highest incidence of progression was observed in patients with RBBB and posterior fascicular block (PFB). Such incidence varied between 25% and 65% [34, 48, 53, 57, 63, 64].

The incidence of high degree AV block appears high also in patients with RBBB and AFB, varying between 10% and 40% [34, 40, 46, 48, 53, 57, 63-65].

In patients with isolated RBBB and in those with LBBB there is less tendency toward progression; in the former a high degree AV block was observed in 14-32% of the cases, in the latter in 10-20% [34, 40, 51, 57, 65].

Some authors [56, 57, 61], analyzing separately the patients with preexistent and those with acquired BBB, observed that only the latter were at high risk of progression. However, in 40-83% of reported cases BBB was already present at admission [61] and a previous ECG had not recorded or was not available for comparison; consequently it is not possible to define in such cases whether the BBB is preexistent or acquired.

HV interval seems to correlate well with the risk of progression (see Chapter II). Further studies are, however, required in order to draw any definite conclusions. Moreover, His bundle electrocardiography is a more complicated procedure than the relatively simple introduction of an electrode wire connected to a pacemaker and, at least so far, does not seem to play a practical role in the management of these patients. External His bundle recording, if perfected, may prove to be a useful tool in the future.

According to Lie et al. [61], a prophylactic pacemaker is not necessary in patients with BBB of delayed onset (later than 24 hours) or of short duration (less than 6 hours) since in these patients a low incidence of progression has been observed. The cases reported are however too few in order to draw any conclusions.

On the basis of the above-mentioned data we believe that insertion of a temporary prophylactic pacemaker is warranted in all patients with bifascicular block and in those with new or indeterminate onset RBBB or LBBB (Table 1).

We do not consider these indications as final, but only as a precautionary measure until the risk factors of developing CHB have been clarified.

In spite of the fact that in these patients a prophylactic pacemaker does not seem to affect significantly the immediate prognosis, we believe it is warranted for the following reasons:

- In some individual cases without severe heart failure, prophylactic pacing may be life-saving [35, 36, 38, 47, 50, 56, 57, 66-68].
- The presence of a prophylactic pacemaker makes the onset of CHB a hemodynamically smooth and clinically undetectable event in several patients, obviating the necessity for electrode catheter insertion under emergency conditions.
- The temporary pacemaker is useful in suppressing ventricular arrhythmias – frequent in patients with AMI complicated by IVCD [68] – by overdrive and also allows safer use of lidocaine in patients with BBB. The danger that this drug may precipitate CHB is small but it may do so in patients with bifascicular block [69, 70]. It is not certain when the temporary pacemaker should be removed. According to Lie et al. [61] it should be left 'in situ' about five days as the development of CHB usually occurs within this period.

Table 1. Indications for pacing in acute myocardial infarction complicated by intraventricular conduction disturbances

Prophylactic temporary pacing
- Right bundle branch block associated with anterior fascicular block
- Right bundle branch block associated with posterior fascicular block
- New or indeterminate onset right bundle branch block
- New or indeterminate onset left bundle branch block

Therapeutic temporary pacing
- 2° or 3° atrioventricular block

Permanent pacing
- Survivors with transient 2° or 3° atrioventricular block

Permanent pacing

Regarding late mortality in patients with myocardial infarction, there are few and contrasting data. Furthermore the results reported by several authors are difficult to compare because of the different number of patients, the different in hospital mortality rate and duration of follow-up periods.

From the few studies in which the overall late mortality of patients with IVCD has been compared to that of patients without intraventricular block, it appears higher in the former [40, 42, 57, 62] (see Chapter 9).

The incidence of sudden death is also moderately higher in patients with BBB, but it is similar to that of patients with chronic BBB without myocardial infarction [34, 71].

In these patients the mechanism of sudden death remains speculative. Several data suggest that ventricular fibrillation is the major cause [72-76]. Unfortunately we are still in the dark as to the part that an abrupt development of CHB plays in the genesis of sudden death and we do not know whether insertion of a permanent demand pacemaker reduces the sudden late mortality rate in these patients.

However, an extraordinarily high incidence of late sudden death was noted in patients with AMI and BBB, who have developed transient high degree AV block and who were subsequently discharged from the hospital with normal AV conduction [35, 36, 44, 47, 57, 77]. In these cases a dramatic reduction in sudden death has been reported after the institution of permanent demand pacing [35, 36, 57, 77].

Atkins et al. [35], combining their cases with those of Scanlon et al. [47] and Godman et al. [44], noted that of the 21 patients with RBBB associated with AFB who had transient CHB during AMI, eight out of eight with permanent pacemakers were alive at an unspecified postdischarge period, whereas 11 of the 13 without permanent pacemakers had died suddenly. Similar findings have been reported by Waugh et al. [36] who observed ten unpaced patients for one year, five of whom died suddenly and two of whom developed syncope, while seven patients were permanently paced with no sudden deaths or syncope during a one year follow-up period. In the study by Ritter et al. [77], all five patients who did not have permanent pacing died suddenly with a mean survival of 2-4 months after hospital discharge; 12 patients received permanent pacemakers and had a significantly improved prognosis with a mean survival time of 18 months; six patients were still alive at an average follow-up time of 20 months.

In an American Multicenter Project [57] it was reported that 26 patients not continuously paced had a markedly higher incidence of sudden death or recurrent high degree AV block compared to 20 patients continuously paced (65% vs 10%) during the first year of follow-up.

Nimetz et al. [56] and Ginks et al. [78] did not observe a decreased incidence of late sudden death in the paced patients compared to the unpaced ones. However the analysis of seven series [35, 36, 47, 54, 56, 77, 78], into which the patients reported by Nimetz and Ginks were inserted, revealed a late mortality rate of 51% in the non-paced group and 12% in the paced group [62].

These findings therefore show that the institution of a demand permanent pacemaker in patients with AMI, BBB and transient CHB increases longevity by preventing sudden death.

The mechanism of sudden death remains speculative in these cases, since pacemaker therapy appeared to be partially protective against sudden death in this subset of patients and since several episodes of recurrent high degree AV block were observed in the non-paced patients [57, 62]. Therefore, abrupt CHB, and not ventricular fibrillation, may play a prominent role in the genesis of sudden death in these patients.

An uninterrupted use of temporary and permanent pacemakers in patients who survive high degree AV block during AMI complicated by BBB would, therefore, seem advisable (Table 1).

It has singled out another group of patients with BBB, who did not have high degree AV block or significant cardiac failure during myocardial infarction, but who were nevertheless at high risk of sudden death during the year after the infarction. This group consisted of patients with documented previous myocardial infarction and acute anterior or indeterminately located infarcts. The incidence of late sudden death (within one year) was 35% compared to 7% in similar patients without BBB [57]. Unfortunately in these patients a control group is not available to allow assessment of the possible protective effect of long-term pacing.

REFERENCES

1. Narula OS, Samet P: Wenckebach and Mobitz type II A-V block due to lesions within the His bundle and bundle branches. Circulation 41: 957, 1970
2. Puech P, Grolleau R, Latour H, Dufoix R, Cabasson J, Robin J: L'enregistrement de l'activité électrique du faisceau de His dans les blocks A-V spontanés. Arch Mal Coeur 63: 784, 1970
3. Narula OS: Current concepts of atrioventricular block. In: His bundle electrocardiography and clinical electrophysiology, Narula OS. Philadelphia: FA Davis, 1975, p 139
4. Narula OS, Scherlag BJ, Javier RP, Hildner FJ, Samet P: Analysis of the A-V conduction defect in complete heart block, utilizing His bundle electrograms. Circulation 41: 437, 1970
5. Touboul P, Ibrahim M: Atrioventricular conduction defects in patients presenting with syncope and normal PR interval. Br Heart J 34: 1005, 1972
6. Levites R, Haft J: Significance of first degree heart block (prolonged PR interval) in bifascicular block. Am J Cardiol 34: 259, 1974
7. Scheinman MM, Peters RW, Modin G, Brennan M, Lies C, Young J: Prognostic value of infranodal conduction time in patients with chronic bundle branch block. Circulation, 56: 240, 1977
8. Gupta PK, Lichstein E, Chadda KD; Follow-up studies in patients with right bundle branch block and left anterior hemiblock: significance of H-V interval. J Electrocardiol 10: 221, 1977
9. Wu D, Rosen KM: Clinical judgement is not sufficient for the management of conduction defects (indications for diagnostic electrophysiologic studies). Cardiovasc Clinic 8: 203, 1977
10. Dini P, Santini M, Di Mascolo R, Boschetti C, Ialongo D, Rocchi M, Masini V: Significato prognostico dell'intervallo HV in 66 pazienti con blocco di branca cronico. G Ital Cardiol, 8: 392, 1978
11. Altschuler H, Fisher JD, Furman S: Significance of isolated HV interval prolongation in symptomatic patients without a documented heart block. Am Heart J, 97: 19, 1979
12. Narula OS: Intraventricular conduction defects: current concepts and clinical significance. In: Cardiac arrhythmias. Electrophysiology, diagnosis and management, Narula OS. Baltimore: Williams & Wilkins, 1979, p 114
13. Narula OS, Alboni P: Prognostic value of H-V interval in patients with chronic right bundle branch block and left axis deviation. G Ital Cardiol 9: 111, 1979
14. Dini P, Ialongo D, Alboni P, Malacarne C, Lotto A, Finzi A, Pagnoni F, Baldi N, Morgera T, Gronda M, Rognoni G, Occhetta E, D'Aurelio M: Blocchi di branca cronici: valore prognostico, sensibilità, specificità ed accuratezza predittiva dei parametri elettrofisiologici endocavitari. (In preparation)
15. McAnulty JH, Rahimtoola SH, Murphy ES, Kauffmann S, Ritzmann LW, Kanarek P, De Mots H: A prospective study of sudden death in 'high risk' bundle branch block. N

Engl J Med 299: 209, 1978
16. Narula OS, Gann D, Samet P: Prognostic value of HV interval. In: His bundle electrocardiography and clinical electrophysiology, Narula OS. Philadelphia: FA Davis, 1975, p 437
17. Fischer JD, Kulbertus HE, Narula OS: The prognostic value of the H-V interval. Pace 1: 132, 1978
18. Dhingra RC, Denes P, Wu D, Chuquimia R, Amat-y-Leon F, Wyndham C, Rosen KM: Chronic right bundle branch block and left posterior hemiblock. Clinical electrophysiologic and prognostic observations. Am J Cardiol 36: 867, 1975
19. Dhingra RC, Denes P, Wu D, Wyndham CR, Amat-y-Leon F, Towne WD, Rosen KM: Prospective observations in patients with chronic bundle branch block and marked H-V prolongation. Circulation 53: 600, 1976
20. Dhingra RC, Wyndham C, Amat-y-Leon F, Denes P, Wu D, Sridhar S, Bustin AG, Rosen KM: Incidence and site of atrioventricular block in patients with chronic bifascicular block. Circulation 59: 238, 1979
21. Vera Z, Mason DT, Fletcher RD, Awan NA, Massumi RA: Prolonged His-Q interval in chronic bifascicular block. Circulation 46: 53, 1976
22. Haft JI: Clinical indications for the His bundle electrogram. Cardiovasc Med 2: 449, 1977
23. Heft JI: The H-V interval and patients with bifascicular block. J Electrocardiol 10: 1, 1977
24. Berg R, Kotler MN: The significance of bilateral bundle branch block in the preoperative patient. A retrospective electrocardiographic and clinical study in 30 patients. Chest 59: 62, 1971
25. Alboni P, Fischer DM, D'Agostino F: Il rischio operatorio in portatori di blocchi mono e bifasciculari. Min Med 64: 2294, 1973
26. Venkataraman K, Madias JE, Nood WB: Indications for prophylactic preoperative pacemakers in patients with right bundle branch block and left anterior hemiblock. Chest 68: 501, 1975
27. Pirzada FA, Venkataraman JE, Madias JE, Hood WB Jr: Prophylactic preoperative pacing. In: To pace or not to pace. Controversial subjects on cardiac pacing, Thalen HJ Th, Harthorne JW. The Hague: Martinus Nijhoff, 1978, p 82
28. Kunstadt D, Punja M, Cagin N, Fernandes P, Levitt B, Yuceo-Glu YZ: Bifascicular block: a clinical and electrophysiologic study. Am Heart J 86: 173, 1973
29. Pastore JO, Yurchak PM, Janis KM, Murphy JD, Zir LM: The risk of advanced heart block in surgical patients with right bundle branch block and left axis deviation. Circulation 57: 677, 1978
30. Santini M, Carrara P, Benhar M, Lazzari G, Rocchi M, Dini P, Di Mascolo R, Alliegro A, Messina G, Masini V: L'anestesia generale nei disturbi della conduzione intraventriculare. G Ital Cardiol 7: 917, 1977
31. Rabagd G, Fraile J, De Vega NG, Moreno T: Cardiac pacing in open heart surgery. In: To pace or not pace. Controversial subjects on cardiac pacing, Thalen HJTh, Harthorne JW. The Hague: Martinus Nijhoff, 1978, p 91
32. Byrd CL: Pacemaker therapy in cardiac surgery. In: Cardiac pacing. A concise guide to clinical practice, Variale P, Naclerio EA. Philadelphia: Lea & Febiger, 1979, p 185
33. Col JJ, Weinberg SL: Incidence and mortality of intraventricular conduction defects in acute myocardial infarction Am J Cardiol 29: 344, 1972
34. Scheinman M, Brenman B: Clinical and anatomic implications of intraventricular conduction block in acute myocardial infarction. Circulation 46: 753, 1972
35. Atkins JM, Leshen SJ, Blomqvist G, Mullins CB: Ventricular conduction blocks and

sudden death in acute myocardial infarction: potential indications for pacing. N Engl J Mede 288: 281, 1973
36. Waugh RA, Wagner GS, Haney TL, Rosati RA, Morris JJ: Immediate and remote prognostic significance of fascicular block during acute myocardial infarction. Circulation 48: 765, 1973
37. Rizzon P, Di Biase M, Baissus C: Intraventricular conduction defects in acute myocardial infarction. Br Heart J 36: 660, 1974
38. De Vita C, De Ponti C, Pioselli D, Bossi M: I disturbi di conduzione intraventricolare in corso di infarto miocardico acuto. Prognosi immediata e a distanza. G Ital Cardiol 5: 513, 1975
39. Medrano GA: Bloques bifasciculares y de ramas del haz de His en el infarto del miocardio. Arch Inst Cardiol Mex 47: 750, 1977
40. Blanc JJ, Boschat J, Granatelli D, Morin JF, Germa D, Penther PH: Bloc de branche complet et infarctus du myocarde. Histoire naturelle. Etude comparative. Arch Mal Coeur 71: 43, 1978
41. Hindman MC, Wagner GS, Jaro M, Atkins JM, Scheinman MM, DeSanctis RW, Hutter AH, Yeatman L, Rubenfire M, Pujura C, Rubin M, Morris JJ: The clinical significance of bundle branch block complicating myocardial infarction. 1. Clinical characteristics, hospital mortality, and one year follow-up. Circulation 58: 679, 1978
42. Michalopoulos A, Athanasopoulos C, Lekakis J: The fate of patients with intraventricular conduction disturbances complicating acute myocardial infarction. Acta Cardiol 34: 189, 1979
43. Hunt D, Sloman G: Bundle branch block in acute myocardial infarction. Br Med J 1: 85, 1969
44. Godman MJ, Lassers BW, Julian DG: Complete bundle branch block complicating acute myocardial infarction. N Engl J Med 282: 237, 1970
45. Norris RM, Croxsen MS: Bundle branch block in acute myocardial infarction. Am Heart J 79: 728, 1970
46. Roos JC, Dunning AJ: Right bundle branch block and left axis deviation in acute myocardial infarction. Br Heart J 32: 847, 1970
47. Scanlon PJ, Pryor R, Blount SG: Right bundle branch block associated with left superior or inferior intraventricular block associated with acute myocardial. Circulation 42: 1135, 1970
48. Godman MJ, Alpert BA, Julian DG: Bilateral bundle-branch block complicating acute myocardial infarction. Lancet 2: 345, 1971
49. Lim CH, Toh CCS, Low LP: Atrioventricular and associated intraventricular conduction disturbances in acute myocardial infarction. Br Heart J 33: 947, 1971
50. Fenig S, Lichstein E: Incomplete bilateral bundle branch block and A-V block complicating acute anterior wall myocardial infarction. Am Heart J 84: 38, 1972
51. Scheidt S, Killip T: Bundle branch block complicating acute myocardial infarction. JAMA 222: 919, 1972
52. Lichstein E, Gupta PK, Chadda KD, Liu HM, Sayeed M: Findings of prognostic value in patients with incomplete bilateral bundle branch block complicating acute myocardial infarction. Am J Cardiol 32: 913, 1973
53. Lie KI, Wellens JJ, Schuelenburg RM, Becker AE, Durrer E: Factors influencing prognosis of bundle branch block complicating acute anteroseptal infarction: the value of His bundle recordings. Circulation 50: 935, 1974
54. Waters DD, Mizgala HF: Long-term prognosis of patients with incomplete bilateral bundle branch block complicating acute myocardial infarction: role of cardiac pacing. Am J Cardiol 34: 1, 1974

55. Gann D, Balachandran PK, El-Sherif N, Samet P: Prognostic significance of chronic versus acute branch block in acute myocardial infarction. Chest 67: 298, 1975
56. Nimetz AA, Shubrooks SJ, Hutter AM, DeSanctis RW: The significance of bundle branch block during acute myocardial infarction. Am Heart J 90: 439, 1975
57. Hindam MC, Wagne GS, Jaro M, Atkins J, Scheinman A, DeSanctis E, Hutter AH, Yeatman L, Rubenfire M, Pujura C, Rubin M, Morris J: The clinical significance of bundle branch block complicating acute myocardial infarction. 2. Indications for temporary and permanent pace-maker insertion. Circulation 58: 689, 1978
58. Friedberg CK, Cohen H, Donoso E: Advanced heart block as a complication of acute myocardial infarction. Role of pacemaker therapy. Progr Cardiovasc Dis 10: 466, 1968
59. Norris RM: Heart block in posterior and anterior myocardial infarction. Br Heart J 31: 352, 1969
60. Voridis E, Plessas S, Mallios K, Cokkinos D: Blocs complets droits et bifasciculaires au cours de la phase aiguë de l'infarctus du myocarde. Arch Mal Coeur 66: 1193, 1973
61. Lie KI, Durrer D: Conduction disturbances in acute myocardial infarction. In: Cardiac arrhythmias. Electrophysiology, diagnosis and management, Narula OS. Baltimore: Williams & Wilkins, 1979, p 140
62. Constans R, Marco J, Berthoumieu H, Alibelli MJ, Dardenne P: Devenir des infarctus du myocarde compliqués en phase aiguë de troubles de la conduction. Arch Mal Coeur 72: 957, 1979
63. Stephens MR, Fadayomi MO, Davies GJ, Muir JR: The clinical features and significance of bifascicular block complicating acute myocardial infarction. Europ J Cardiol. 3: 289, 1975
65. Marriot HJL, Hogan RN: Hemiblock in acute myocardial infarction. Chest 58: 342, 1970
65. Basualdo CAE, Haraphonge M, Rossel RE: Intraventricular blocks in acute myocardial infarction. Chest 67: 75, 1975
66. Norris RM, Mercer CJ, Croxon MS: Conduction disturbances due to anteroseptal myocardial infarction and their treatment by endocardial pacing. Am Heart J 84: 560, 1972
67. Levy S, Castellanos A Jr, Arcebal A, Lemberg L: Le bloc de branche droit avec hémibloc gauche à la phase aiguë de l'infarctus du myocarde. Pronostic et rôle de l'entraînement électrosystolique. Arch Mal Coeur 68: 497, 1975
68. Lichstein E, Letafati A, Gupta PM, Chadda KD: Continuous holter monitoring of patients with bifascicular block complicating anterior wall myocardial infarction. Am J Cardiol 40: 860, 1977
69. Lichstein E, Chadda KD, Gupta PK: Atrioventricular block with lidocaine therapy. Am J Cardiol 31: 277, 1973
70. Gupta PK, Lichstein E, Chadda KD: Lidocaine-induced heart block in patients with bundle branch block. Am J Cardiol 33: 487, 1974
71. Dhingra RC, Denes P, Wu D, Chuquinia R, Amat-y-Leon F, Wyndham C, Rosen KM: Syncope in patients with chronic bifascicular block: significance, causative mechanisms, and clinical implications. Ann Inter Med 81: 302, 1974
72. Wilson C, Pantridge JF: ST segment displacement and early hospital discharge in acute myocardial infarction. Lancet 2: 1284, 1973
73. Vismara LA, Amsterdam EA, Mason DT: Relation of ventricular arrhythmias in the late hospital phase of acute myocardial infarction to sudden death after hospital discharge. Am J Med 59: 6, 1975
74. Calvert A, Lown B, Gorlin R: Ventricular premature beats and anatomically defined coronary heart disease. Am J Cardiol 39: 627, 1977

75. Schulze RA, Humphries JO, Griffith LSS, Ducci H, Achuff S, Baird MG, Mellits ED, Pitta B: Left ventricular and coronary angiographic anatomy: relationship to ventricular irritability in the late hospital phase of acute myocardial infarction. Circulation 55: 839, 1977
76. Califf RM, Burke JM, Behar VS, Margolis Jr, Wagner GS: Relationships among ventricular arrhythmias, coronary artery disease and angiographic and electrocardiographic indicators of myocardial fibrosis. Circulation 57: 725, 1978
77. Ritter WS, Atkins JM, Blomqvist CG, Mullins DB: Permanent pacing in patients with transient trifascicular block during acute myocardial infarction. Am J Cardiol 38: 205, 1976
78. Ginks WR, Sutton R, Oh W, Leatham A: Long-term prognosis after acute anterior infarction with atrioventricular block. Br Heart J 39: 186, 1977

SUBJECT INDEX

GPSR Compliance

The European Union's (EU) General Product Safety Regulation (GPSR) is a set of rules that requires consumer products to be safe and our obligations to ensure this.

If you have any concerns about our products, you can contact us on ProductSafety@springernature.com

In case Publisher is established outside the EU, the EU authorized representative is:

Springer Nature Customer Service Center GmbH
Europaplatz 3
69115 Heidelberg, Germany

Batch number: 10607220

Printed by Printforce, the Netherlands